OXFORD MEDICAL PUBLICATIONS

Cancer in children: clinical management

Cancer in children: clinical management

FIFTH EDITION

Edited by

P.A. Voûte

Emeritus Professor of Paediatric Oncology, Emma Kinder Ziekenhuis, Academic Medical Centre, University of Amsterdam, The Netherlands

A. Barrett

Professor of Oncology, University of East Anglia, School of Medicine, Health Policy and Practice, Norwich, UK

Michael C.G. Stevens

Professor of Paediatric Oncology, University of Bristol, UK

Hubert N. Caron

Professor of Paediatric Oncology, Emma Kinder Ziekenhuis, Academic Medical Centre, University of Amsterdam, The Netherlands

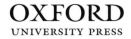

OXFORD

UNIVERSITY PRESS

*This book has been printed digitally and produced in a standard specification
in order to ensure its continuing availability*

OXFORD
UNIVERSITY PRESS

Great Clarendon Street, Oxford OX2 6DP

Oxford University Press is a department of the University of Oxford.
It furthers the University's objective of excellence in research, scholarship,
and education by publishing worldwide in

Oxford New York

Auckland   Cape Town Dar es Salaam Hong Kong Karachi
Kuala Lumpur Madrid Melbourne Mexico City   Nairobi
New Delhi Shanghai Taipei Toronto
With offices in
Argentina Austria Brazil Chile Czech Republic France Greece
Guatemala Hungary Italy Japan South Korea Poland Portugal
Singapore Switzerland Thailand Turkey Ukraine Vietnam

Oxford is a registered trade mark of Oxford University Press
in the UK and in certain other countries

Published in the United States
by Oxford University Press Inc., New York

© Oxford University Press 2005

ISBN   978-0-19-852932-3

Printed and bound in Great Britain by CPI Antony Rowe, Chippenham and Eastbourne

Foreword

From the first tentative steps in the 1950s and 1960s of treating children with cancer not just with surgery, but firstly with radiotherapy and then progressively more intensive chemotherapy, the outlook for most children who develop leukaemia and cancer has dramatically improved. Now about three-quarters of patients are living long term, and for some tumours results are even better in countries with adequate resources. Sadly, for about 80 per cent of the world's children the diagnosis and management of childhood cancer remains far from optimal and in most cases non-existent. Quite early on it was recognized in resource-rich countries that for these rare conditions all the specialists involved needed to work together in a collaborative fashion to deliver optimal care. Increasingly, international collaboration enabled us to optimize therapy more rapidly. Such collaboration proved to be extremely beneficial for the individual patient. *Cancer in Children*, now in its 5th edition, perfectly reflects that collaborative approach, with authors from around the world writing on joint assessments of how to investigate and then treat the common cancers. Each year many of the authors have taught on an annual educational programme at the International Society of Paediatric Oncology meeting. These workshop educational sessions have further enhanced the sharing of knowledge and expertise. State-of-the-art descriptions of what it is basic and essential for management and the up-to-date revision of such guidelines in the light of new evidence are a fundamental feature of this text. As President of the International Society of Paediatric Oncology, I welcome this new edition and I hope that its readers will find it as informative and useful as I have.

Professor Tim Eden
President, International Society of Paediatric Oncology
August 2005

Preface

The editions of this book, of which this is the fifth, have spanned the years from 1975, through 1986, 1992, and 1998 to 2005. In these 30 years, the different editors have seen great changes in the treatment of children with cancer. This difference in treatment from 1975 to 2005 stems from intensive international cooperation in clinical work. Clinical trials have taught us that cure of many children is possible. As many children are cured, we begin to see what the side effects of treatment are. Recognition of these effects of treatment has brought changes in treatment approaches, resulting in the same, and sometimes even better, cure rates with less treatment.

Since the unravelling of the human genome, advances in molecular biology and then the understanding of proteomics, are changing completely future treatment approaches.

We have tried to bring these issues to the attention of our readers and we hope that this book will serve as a useful bridge between basic science and the clinical treatment of children with cancer.

We should like to thank contributors to this edition and all others who have helped with the preparation of this book, and especially Sara Chare for her assistance.

A. Barrett
H.N. Caron
M.C.G. Stevens
P.A. Voûte

Contributors List

Mr Charles A. Stiller,
Senior Research Fellow,
Childhood Cancer Research Group,
University of Oxford,
Oxford, UK

G.J Draper

Dr Oskar A. Haas,
Professor of Clinical Chemistry & Laboratory
Medicine, CCRI,
St Anna's Children's Hospital, Vienna

Professor Rogier Versteeg,
Professor in Genetics and Pediatric Oncology,
Academic Medical Center,
Amsterdam

Professor Gilles Vassal,
Professor of Oncology,
Paediatrician and Pharmacologist,
Institut Gustave Roussy,
France

Dr Arnauld Verschuur,
Pediatric Haematologist/Oncologist,
Emma Children's Hospital AMC,
Amsterdam, The Netherlands

Dr Elizabeth Fox

Dr Peter C. Adamson,
Division Chief,
Clinical Pharmacology and Therapeutics,
Children's Hospital of Philadelphia, USA

Dr Andreas Schuck,
Consultant Radiation Oncologist,
University Hospital Muenster,
Muenster, Germany

Professor Hélène Martelli,
Professor of Medicine,
Hôpital de Bicêtre, France

Dr Marianne D. van de Wetering,
Paediatric Oncologist,
Emma Children's Hospital,
Amsterdam, The Netherlands

Dr Bob F. Last,
Clinical Psychologist,
Academic Medical Center,
Amsterdam, The Netherlands

Dr Martha A. Grootenhuis,
Research Psychologist,
Academic Medical Center,
Amsterdam, The Netherlands

Helen Irving,
Senior Staff Specialist,
Royal Children's Hospital,
Brisbane, Australia

Dr Meriel E.M. Jenney,
Consultant Paediatric Oncologist,
Llandough Hospital,
Cardiff, UK

Dr Kjeld Schmiegelow,
Consultant Paediatric Haematology/
Oncology,
University Hospital,
Rigshospitalet, Denmark

Dr Goran Gustafsson,
Associate Professor,
Childhood Cancer Research Unit,
Karolinska Unit,
Stockholm, Sweden

Dr Brenda Gibson,
Consultant Paediatric Haematologist,
Royal Hospital for Sick Children,
Glasgow, Scotland

Dr Geoff Shenton,
Specialist Registrar in Haematology,
Royal Hospital for Sick Children,
Glasgow, Scotland

Dr Catherine Patte,
Service de pediatrie,
Institut Gustave Roussy, France

Dr Odile Oberlin,
Paediatric Oncologist,
Institut Gustave Roussy, France

Prof. Dr. Helmut Gadner,
Professor of Paediatrics,
University of Vienna,
Vienna, Austria

Dr Nicole Grois,
St Anna Children's Hospital,
Vienna, Austria

Prof. Dr. Richard Pötter,
Professor of Medicine,
University of Vienna, Austria

Prof. Dr. Thomas Czech,
Assistant Professor,
University of Vienna Medical School,
Vienna, Austria

Prof. Dr. Karin Dieckmann,
Radiotherapist,
University of Vienna,
Vienna, Austria

Prof. Dr. I. Slavc,
Associate Professor,
Department of Paediatrics,
University of Vienna Medical School,
Vienna, Austria

Prof. Dr. D. Wimberger-Prayer,
University Hospital,
Vienna, Austria

Prof. Dr. H. Budka,
Professor of Neuropathology,
Institute Director,
Institute of Neurology,
University of Vienna, Austria

Dr Gianni Bisogno,
Consultant Pediatric Oncologist,
Hospital of Padova,
Padova, Italy

Dr Christophe Bergeron,
Résponsable du Département d'oncologie
pédiatrie,
Centre Léon Bérard,
Lyon, France

Dr Stefan S. Bielack,
Department of Pediatric Haematology and
Oncology,
University of Muenster, Germany

Dr Mark L. Bernstein,
Clinical Professor of Pediatrics,
University of Montreal,
Montreal,
Quebec, Canada

Dr Michael Paulussen,
Paediatric Oncologist,
University Children's Hospital,
Muenster, Germany

Prof. Dr. Heinrich Kovar,
Associate Professor of Molecular Biology,
Children's Cancer Research Institute,
Vienna, Austria

Prof. Dr. Heribert Jürgens,
Professor of Paediatric Haematology and
Oncology,
Universitaetskinderklinik, Germany

Dr Beatriz de Camargo,
Head of the Paediatric Department,
Hospital do Cancer,
Saô Paolo, Brazil

Dr Kathryn Pritchard-Jones,
Senior Lecturer in Paediatric Oncology,
Institute of Cancer Research,
Surrey, UK

Prof. Dr. Hubert N. Caron,
Editor

Professor A.D.J. Pearson,
Professor of Paediatric Oncology,
Sir James Spence Institute,
Newcastle-upon-Tyne, UK

Prof. Dr. Ulrich Göbel,
Professor of Paediatrics,
Heinrich-Heine University,
Düsseldorf, Germany

Dr Gabriele Calaminus,
Consultant Paediatric Oncologist,
University Children's Hospital,
Düsseldorf, Germany

Dr Dominik T. Schneider,
Paediatrician,
Heinrich-Heine University,
Düsseldorf, Germany

Professor Hitoshi Ikeda,
Professor of Pediatric Surgery,
Dokkyo University School of Medicine,
Koshigaya, Japan

Dr Tadashi Matsunaga,
Lecturer of Paediatric Surgery,
Chiba University,
Chiba, Japan

Prof. Dr. Yoshiaki Tsuchida,
Director,
Gunma Children's Medical Center,
Gunma, Japan

Dr Guillermo L. Chantada,
Assistant Physician,
Hospital J.P. Garrahan,
Buenos Aires, Argentina

Dr Enrique Schvartzman,
Consultant of Haemato-oncology Unit,
Hospital de Pediatria,
Buenos Aires, Argentina

Dr David A. Walker,
Reader in Paediatric Oncology,
Nottingham, UK

Contents

Chapter 1

The epidemiology of cancer in children

C. A. Stiller and G. J. Draper

Introduction

Although childhood cancer is rare, accounting for less than 1 per cent of all cancer in industrialized countries, it is of great scientific interest for a number of reasons. Several types of cancer are virtually unique to childhood, whereas the carcinomas most frequently seen in adults, those of lung, female breast, stomach, large bowel, and prostate, are extremely rare among children. Some of the most striking progress in cancer treatment has been made in paediatric oncology. Investigation of childhood tumours has led to major advances in the understanding of the genetic aetiology of cancer. In this chapter we consider the classification of childhood cancer, the principles of cancer registration, incidence and survival rates, and aetiology.

Classification

The great majority of malignant neoplasms occurring in adults are carcinomas, and so the *International Classification of Diseases*, by which cancers other than leukaemias, lymphomas, mesothelioma, Kaposi sarcoma and cutaneous melanomas are classified purely by site of origin, is reasonably satisfactory for the presentation of their incidence rates. In contrast, childhood cancers exhibit great histologic diversity and often arise in embryonal precursor cells. Some types of tumour can arise in many different primary sites. Therefore it is more appropriate for childhood cancers to be classified according to histology and site. The current standard classification is the *International Classification of Childhood Cancer*,[1] with groups defined by the codes for morphology in addition to topography in the second edition of the *International Classification of Diseases for Oncology* (ICD-O). A new version, based on codes in the third edition of ICD-O, is in preparation. The classification contains 12 main diagnostic groups, most of which are divided into subgroups. The main groups are as follows: I leukaemia; II lymphomas and reticuloendothelial neoplasms; III central nervous system and miscellaneous intracranial and intraspinal neoplasms; IV sympathetic nervous system tumours; V retinoblastoma; VI renal tumours; VII hepatic tumours; VIII malignant bone tumours; IX soft tissue sarcomas; X germ cell, trophoblastic, and other gonadal neoplasms; XI carcinomas and other malignant epithelial neoplasms; XII other and unspecified malignant neoplasms. Most of these groups are limited to malignant neoplasms, but there are two exceptions. Benign and unspecified intracranial and intraspinal tumours, including choroid plexus papilloma, ganglioglioma, non-malignant gliomas, craniopharyngioma, pituitary adenoma, pinealoma, meningioma, and tumours of unspecified type are included in group III because they are recorded by many cancer registries. For the same reason, non-malignant intracranial and intraspinal germ cell tumours are also included (in group X).

Childhood cancer registration

The aim of a cancer registry is to collect information on all cases of cancer occurring within a geographically defined population. Sometimes there are insufficient resources to maintain a population-based registry, but nevertheless it may be possible to collect similar data on all cases seen in one or more hospitals or pathology departments. In the absence of population-based data, these series can still yield much useful information, and several population-based cancer registries trace their origins to hospital or pathology series. The amount of data collected on each case varies enormously between registries, but the minimum consists of the patient's name (or other unique personal identifier), sex, date of diagnosis and age at diagnosis, and sufficient information on the primary site and histologic type of the neoplasm for it to be coded according to whatever system is used, preferably ICD-O. Most registries collect the patient's date of birth where known, as this is particularly useful for linking data on the same patient from different sources and for detecting duplicates. The basis of diagnosis is also usually recorded, at least to the extent of whether there was histologic verification. There can be many different sources of information, of which the most frequently used are clinical records, pathology records, death certificates, and other cancer registries. The registration data should be checked for internal consistency. Computer programs which do this for age, sex, primary site, and histologic type are included in the IARC Technical Report *International Classification of Childhood Cancer*.[1] The IARC monograph, *Cancer Registration: Principles and Methods*,[2] gives detailed information on many aspects of setting up and maintaining a cancer registry. The operating methods of many individual registries are described in *International Incidence of Childhood Cancer*, Volume II.[3] Recommendations on registry practices and guidelines on confidentiality are given in a recent publication by the European Network of Cancer Registries.[4]

Population-based general cancer registries, including patients of all ages, now cover the whole or part of about 100 countries. As childhood cancer accounts for a very small proportion of all cancer, registries which restrict their coverage to children are able to collect more detailed information on each case. There are population-based childhood cancer registries in several countries or parts of countries in Europe, the Americas and Oceania. These registries are often operated in close collaboration with paediatric oncologists; in Germany, for example, there is a common follow-up system for the childhood cancer registry and for clinical trials. In many countries where there is no national population-based cancer registration, including the USA, Japan, and Spain, registers of patients are maintained by national organizations of paediatric oncologists or by clinical trial groups.

Incidence

Incidence in Great Britain

Table 1.1 gives numbers of cases and incidence rates for the 12 main groups and principal subgroups of the International Classification of Childhood Cancer in Great Britain during the period 1987–1996. The pattern of incidence is typical of that found among the mainly White populations of industrialized countries in Europe, North America, and Oceania, although some of the rates are towards the lower end of the usual range for these populations. The total age-standardized annual incidence was 134 per million children, giving a cumulative risk of 1 in 514 of developing cancer during the first 15 years of life. About a third of all childhood cancers are leukaemias, predominantly acute lymphoblastic leukaemia (ALL). Brain and spinal tumours are the second most common diagnostic group, accounting for about a quarter of registrations, with astrocytomas being the most frequent histologic type. Lymphomas account for 9–10 per cent, and non-Hodgkin lymphoma (NHL) has a somewhat higher incidence than Hodgkin disease. Neuroblastoma and Wilms tumour, the two most frequent embryonal tumours of childhood, each account for 6–7 per cent of registrations, as do soft tissue sarcomas, while retinoblastoma accounts for 3 per cent. Nearly all the remaining cases are bone sarcomas, germ cell tumours, and epithelial tumours. Of this last group, malignant melanoma, skin carcinoma, and thyroid carcinoma are the most frequent, but none of them accounts for more than 1.5 per cent of all childhood cancer.

Within childhood, the total incidence of cancer is highest (180 per million) in the first 5 years of life, compared with about 100 per million for the age group 5–14 years. The age–incidence distribution varies considerably between diagnostic groups. There is a marked peak in the incidence of ALL at age 2–3 years. Early age peaks are also found for all the distinctive embryonal tumours. The highest incidence of neuroblastoma, retinoblastoma, and hepato-blastoma is in the first year of life, but the peak for Wilms tumour occurs slightly later. In contrast, Hodgkin disease and bone sarcomas are virtually never seen before the age of 2 years, and their incidence increases steeply throughout childhood and adolescence. Among boys, the incidence of testicular germ cell tumours is highest in early childhood, and the start of the sharp increase in incidence during adolescence and early adulthood is barely noticeable before the age of 15; among girls, ovarian germ cell tumours are rare until the postpubertal increase, which begins at an earlier age than among boys.

International variations

There is considerable systematic variation in the many types of childhood cancer between different regions of the world and between ethnic groups in the same country.[3,5]

Leukaemia

In the USA, there is a substantially lower incidence of ALL in the Black population and the early childhood peak is very much attenuated. In contrast, there is little evidence of ethnic variation in the incidence of childhood leukaemia in the UK; in particular the pattern of occurrence of ALL among both Black children and children of South Asian ethnic origin is very similar to that among White children, with a marked peak in early childhood. In many developing countries of Asia and Latin America the early childhood peak is also less marked and the total incidence is again lower. A similar pattern has been found in the former socialist countries of central and eastern Europe, although there are indications that a more marked early childhood peak is evolving.[6] There is little international variation in the incidence of acute non-lymphoblastic leukaemia (ANLL).

Lymphomas

Childhood Hodgkin disease has a relatively high incidence, particularly among younger children, in developing countries of Latin America and the Middle East. Lymphomas, both Hodgkin disease and NHL, are more common among South Asian children in the UK than among White children, and the excess of Hodgkin disease is again greatest among younger children. The highest incidence of Burkitt lymphoma, sometimes as large as 80 per million, is found in a broad geographic band of tropical Africa where malaria is endemic, and the incidence is also high in Papua New Guinea; in both of these regions, Burkitt lymphoma is the most common childhood cancer. Elsewhere it is harder to identify patterns of incidence for Burkitt lymphoma since many cases have been registered simply as NHL. The incidence of all

Table 1.1. Childhood cancer in Great Britain, 1987–1996: numbers of registrations; age-specific, age-standardized (World Standard Population), and cumulative incidence rates, and sex ratio

Diagnostic group	Total registrations	Annual rates per million by age group			Age-standardized rate per million	Cumulative rate per million	Sex ratio (M/F)
		0–4 years	5–9 years	10–14 years			
All cancers	13904	180.2	103.2	105.9	133.8	1947	1.2
I Leukaemia	4413	67.1	31.9	23.8	43.1	614	1.3
Acute lymphoblastic	3580	56.2	26.9	16.3	35.2	497	1.3
Acute non-lymphocytic	674	8.8	4.2	6.0	6.5	95	1.1
Chronic myeloid	87	1.3	0.4	0.7	0.8	12	1.8
Other specified	13	0.1	0.1	0.2	0.1	2	0.6
Unspecified	59	0.8	0.3	0.6	0.6	8	1.3
II Lymphomas	1298	6.2	12.5	18.4	11.8	185	2.3
Hodgkin disease	508	0.9	4.3	9.5	4.5	73	2.1
NHL including Burkitt lymphoma	756	5.0	7.8	8.6	7.0	107	2.3
Miscellaneous reticuloendothelial	10	0.1	0.1	0.1	0.1	1	9.0
Unspecified	24	0.2	0.3	0.3	0.2	3	3.0
III Brain and spinal tumours	3309	33.2	33.4	26.4	31.3	465	1.1
Ependymoma and choroid plexus	328	5.2	2.1	1.8	3.2	46	1.3
Astrocytoma	1383	13.3	13.9	11.7	13.0	195	1.0
Primitive neuroectodermal	665	7.5	7.1	4.0	6.4	93	1.5
Other gliomas	410	3.0	5.2	3.4	3.8	58	1.0
Other specified	337	2.3	3.5	3.8	3.1	48	1.2
Unspecified	186	2.0	1.5	1.8	1.8	26	1.0
IV Sympathetic nervous system tumours	938	21.6	3.4	0.7	9.6	128	1.2
Neuroblastoma	925	21.4	3.3	0.6	9.5	127	1.2
Other	13	0.2	0.1	0.1	0.1	2	0.4
V Retinoblastoma	439	11.3	0.6	0.0	4.6	60	1.0
VI Renal tumours	793	16.6	4.0	1.1	8.1	109	1.0
Wilms tumour etc	771	16.6	3.9	0.6	7.9	106	1.0
Renal carcinoma	20	0.0	0.1	0.5	0.2	3	1.5
Other	2	0.1	–	–	0.0	0	–
VII Hepatic tumours	128	2.5	0.5	0.5	1.3	18	2.0
Hepatoblastoma	101	2.4	0.2	0.2	1.0	14	2.1
Hepatic carcinoma	27	0.1	0.3	0.3	0.2	4	2.0

Table 1.1. (continued) Childhood cancer in Great Britain, 1987–1996: numbers of registrations; age-specific, age-standardized (World Standard Population), and cumulative incidence rates, and sex ratio

Diagnostic group	Total registrations	Annual rates per million by age group			Age-standardized rate per million	Cumulative rate per million	Sex ratio (M/F)
		0–4 years	5–9 years	10–14 years			
VIII Bone tumours	568	0.8	4.0	11.6	5.0	82	1.0
Osteosarcoma	304	0.2	2.3	6.4	2.7	44	1.0
Chondrosarcoma	13	0.0	0.1	0.3	0.1	2	2.3
Ewing sarcoma	227	0.5	1.6	4.5	2.0	32	1.1
Other specified	13	0.0	0.0	0.3	0.1	2	0.6
Unspecified	11	0.1	0.1	0.1	0.1	2	0.6
IX Soft tissue sarcomas	1012	12.5	7.6	8.3	9.7	142	1.2
Rhabdomyosarcoma	574	8.6	4.6	2.7	5.6	80	1.4
Fibrosarcoma etc.	118	0.9	0.8	1.6	1.1	17	1.1
Kaposi sarcoma	3	–	0.1	–	0.0	0	0.5
Other specified	252	2.3	1.7	3.2	2.4	36	1.1
Unspecified	65	0.7	0.4	0.8	0.6	9	1.3
X Germ cell and gonadal tumours	455	5.9	1.9	5.0	4.4	64	0.8
CNS germ cell	133	0.9	1.0	1.9	1.2	19	1.5
Other non-gonadal germ cell	113	2.8	0.1	0.2	1.2	15	0.3
Gonadal germ cell	190	2.2	0.7	2.4	1.8	27	1.1
Gonadal carcinoma	16	–	0.1	0.4	0.1	2	0.1
Other gonadal	3	0.1	0.0	–	0.0	0	0.5
XI Epithelial tumours	458	1.2	2.8	9.3	4.1	66	0.8
Adrenocortical carcinoma	15	0.2	0.1	0.1	0.1	2	0.2
Thyroid carcinoma	55	0.1	0.3	1.3	0.5	8	0.4
Nasopharynx carcinoma	25	–	0.1	0.6	0.2	4	2.1
Melanoma	157	0.6	1.2	2.7	1.4	23	0.7
Skin carcinoma	74	0.2	0.5	1.5	0.7	11	1.1
Other carcinoma	132	0.2	0.6	3.1	1.2	19	0.9
XII Other and unspecified malignant neoplasms	93	1.2	0.6	0.8	0.9	13	0.6
Other specified	15	0.2	0.1	0.1	0.1	2	0.5
Other unspecified	78	1.0	0.5	0.7	0.7	11	0.7

NHL, non-Hodgkin lymphoma; CNS, central nervous system.
Source: National Registry of Childhood Tumours.

NHL, including Burkitt lymphoma, is relatively high in Mediterranean countries and the Middle East and in some Latin American countries.

Brain and spinal tumours

In the USA, the incidence of brain and spinal tumours is lower among Black than among White children, while in Britain, children of South Asian, and perhaps especially Indian, ethnic origin also have a lower incidence. In developing countries the recorded incidence of brain and spinal tumours is often low, sometimes as little as 5 per million. It is unclear to what extent this reflects under-ascertainment, particularly in areas without neurological services, rather than a reduced underlying risk.

Neuroblastoma

The recorded incidence of neuroblastoma in several countries is much higher than in the UK, particularly in the first year of life, possibly because of increased detection of otherwise silent tumours during routine health checks. In Japan, and parts of some other countries, mass biochemical screening for neuroblastoma has led to particularly high incidence rates in infancy. In the USA, neuroblastoma has a lower incidence among Black than among White infants, but the rates are similar for the two ethnic groups at the age of 1 year and above. Recorded incidence in developing countries is often very low, but in some African registries it is similar to that among Black children in the USA. Thus it seems likely that there is little variation in underlying risk, and that recorded incidence reflects the proportions of tumours that are diagnosed and registered.

Retinoblastoma

Retinoblastoma occurs in two distinct forms, heritable and non-heritable. Heritable retinoblastoma includes all cases of bilateral retinoblastoma and a few children with unilateral tumours, and the incidence is relatively constant throughout the world. Non-heritable retinoblastoma is always unilateral and there are large variations in incidence, with substantially higher rates in many developing countries, particularly in sub-Saharan Africa.

Wilms tumour

Variations in the incidence of Wilms tumour depend largely on ethnic group rather than geographic area. Black children in the USA, the UK, and Africa have a higher incidence than White children, although their age distributions are similar. Children of East Asian ethnic origin in the USA and Asia have a lower incidence than White children, and the deficit is more marked after the first year of life.

Liver tumours

Hepatoblastoma has apparently constant incidence throughout the world. The incidence of hepatic carcinoma in children is highest in regions of the world where the disease is also common among adults, namely East and Southeast Asia, Melanesia, and sub-Saharan Africa. Nearly all childhood cases in these high-risk regions occur in chronic carriers of hepatitis B.

Sarcomas

Of the two principal types of childhood bone sarcoma, osteosarcoma appears to have a similar incidence in most populations, although it may be lower in Asia. In contrast, there are striking variations in the incidence of Ewing's sarcoma. This tumour has very low incidence in East and Southeast Asia, and among Black populations in Africa, the USA, and the UK.

Rhabdomyosarcoma is the most common soft tissue sarcoma of childhood in most populations. In much of South and East Asia, and also among Asian children in the UK, its incidence is rather less than among White children. Kaposi sarcoma is extremely rare in children in most regions of the world, but in East and Central Africa, where it is endemic among adults, the incidence among children was about 2 per million in about 1970. Since then, there have been very large increases, and rates of over 50 per million were recorded in the 1990s. The great majority of the increase is clearly related to the AIDS epidemic, which has been particularly severe in the region.

Other cancers

Germ cell tumours are somewhat more common in East Asia than in other regions of the world.

By far the highest incidence of childhood thyroid carcinoma, around 80 per million, has been recorded in areas of Belarus contaminated by radiation from the Chernobyl nuclear reactor explosion. Some extra cases may have been detected particularly early by intensive screening, and it is well known that thyroid cancer in other populations can be undetected for many years after onset. However, although the true size of the excess risk is hard to determine, its existence is not in doubt, both because the rates were 50 times greater than those seen elsewhere and because of the aggressive histologic type in many cases. Further evidence for an effect of short-lived radioactive fallout is provided by the return of incidence to normal levels among children conceived since the accident.

The highest incidence of nasopharyngeal carcinoma among children is in North Africa, a region of intermediate risk for adults, where it can account for up to 10 per cent of all childhood cancers. In East Asian countries, where incidence is highest among adults, children have only a moderately elevated incidence, up to 0.8 per million, while in the USA the incidence among Black children is about 1 per million, nine times that among Whites in the same country.

There is an exceptionally high incidence of skin carcinoma, both squamous cell and basal cell, among children in Tunisia, where the great majority of cases are associated with xeroderma pigmentosum. Malignant melanoma has a very high incidence in Australia and New Zealand, where it is also a very common cancer among adults, resulting from high levels of sun exposure.

Trends in incidence

The most striking increases in incidence of any childhood cancers, those relating to Kaposi sarcoma in East and Central Africa and to thyroid carcinoma in areas close to Chernobyl, have been described above. Otherwise, any changes have been much more modest. (Of course, the very large increases in recorded incidence of neuroblastoma in Japan and some other areas with population screening represent increased detection rather than a change in underlying risk.) The best documented trend concerns ALL, the most common childhood cancer in all developed countries. The early childhood peak started to emerge in mortality data in England and Wales in the 1920s, and it was certainly well established among White children in the USA by the early 1940s. A further modest rise, particularly in early childhood, took place in some Western countries until the late 1970s. Meanwhile, increasing incidence in early childhood among the Black population in the USA led to the emergence of a moderate peak in the age–incidence curve for this ethnic group. Small increases have also been observed in some Western populations for a number of other childhood cancers, notably brain tumours, neuroblastoma, and soft tissue sarcomas. However, it is not yet clear how much of these increases is attributable to changes in diagnostic practice rather than in underlying risk.

Clusters

A cluster of cases of a disease can be defined as the occurrence of a substantially larger number of cases than expected in a small geographically defined population, usually during a short period of time. There have been many reports of clusters of childhood leukaemia and other cancers. Among the most well known are those in the vicinity of some nuclear installations, although it is now generally accepted that they are unlikely to result from radiation exposure. Reported clusters need to be investigated carefully, the first stage being to check that the details of diagnosis, dates, and location are correct and the incidence rate is indeed high. Cluster investigations may yield clues to the aetiology of the particular cases or of the disease in general, although they are usually disappointing in this respect. It is also important to address the concerns of the local population, often with respect to the role of possible environmental pollution. In order to systematize the investigation of clusters, guidelines have been published in several countries, including the UK.[7]

Survival rates

In contrast with the very small improvements in prognosis that have occurred for many of the common adult cancers, the past 40 years have seen dramatic increases in the survival rates for most types of childhood cancer. Table 1.2 shows the 5-year survival rates for children in the UK diagnosed in successive quinquennia between 1962 and 1996 separately for the principal diagnostic groups. During this period, survival improved substantially for virtually all diagnostic groups, although the main advances for different types of cancer have occurred at different times. In the 1960s, there were particularly marked improvements in the prognosis for children with Hodgkin disease and Wilms tumour. The 1970s saw large improvements for a

Table 1.2. Actuarial 5-year survival rates (per cent) for children diagnosed with the principal diagnostic groups in the UK in the period 1962–1996

	1962–1966	1967–1971	1972–1976	1977–1981	1982–1986	1987–1991	1992–1996
ALL	4	17	44	56	70	75	81
ANLL	2	2	7	17	30	47	54
Hodgkin disease	39	68	81	89	89	93	94
NHL (including Burkitt lymphoma)	17	21	26	45	67	76	78
CNS	37	37	43	48	54	57	68
Neuroblastoma	18	17	19	31	43	41	53
Retinoblastoma	88	86	86	88	90	95	96
Wilms tumour	29	43	62	76	80	82	80
Osteosarcoma	17	18	22	25	47	51	57
Ewing sarcoma	25	23	40	34	45	68	61
Rhabdomyosarcoma	25	23	33	44	58	59	66
Gonadal germ cell	55	52	56	74	90	94	96
All cancers	24	29	42	51	62	67	73

Source: National Registry of Childhood Tumours.

wide range of diagnoses, most notably ALL and NHL. In the 1980s, survival rates increased for children with ANLL, bone sarcomas, and germ cell tumours. By 1992–1996, 5-year survival exceeded 50 per cent for all the diagnostic groups shown. Analyses of data from the EUROCARE collaboration have shown substantial variation across Europe in survival rates for many childhood cancers.[8] Survival tended to be highest in the Nordic countries and lowest in Eastern Europe. Unlike some adult cancers, survival from childhood cancer in Western Europe is similar to that in the USA.[9]

The spectacular increases in survival rates described here are undoubtedly largely due to advances in treatment and supportive care. However, at the same time as these developments in therapy, there was also a substantial movement towards concentration of treatment at relatively few specialist centers, at some of which very large numbers of children are treated. Also, whereas at one time there were national clinical trials only for acute leukaemia and a handful of other diagnostic groups, in many countries there are now national or international trials and studies open for entry of children with all but the rarest types of cancer, and the proportions of eligible children that are entered in these trials have also increased. For several diagnostic groups, survival rates have been found to be higher among children who were treated at specialist centres or who were entered in clinical trials regardless of the treatment arm.[10,11]

Follow-up

As survival rates have improved for nearly all childhood cancers, the number of long-term survivors has greatly increased and these survivors already include a substantial number of adults. Several large studies of survivors from childhood cancer are now in progress, addressing such topics as the criteria for cure, quality of life, risk of second primary neoplasms, fertility, and the health of the survivors' offspring. Late effects and long-term follow-up are discussed from a clinical point of view in Chapter 11. Here, we summarize the epidemiologic data. Although late relapses can occur, the great majority of 5-year survivors can be regarded as cured; only one-tenth of them die of recurrent tumour or a treatment-related cause during the ensuing 10 years.[12–14] The risk of developing a second primary neoplasm within 25 years of diagnosis of childhood cancer is about 4 per cent, four to six times the risk in the general population.[15,16] However, the risks vary considerably between different types of childhood cancer, being especially high among survivors of heritable retinoblastoma. It should also be stressed that these risk estimates, at least for longer intervals following diagnosis, are based on survivors who were treated before the era of intensive chemotherapy, although of course many received radiotherapy. Also, little is yet known about the risks to survivors beyond the age of about 40, when the population incidence of several common cancers begins to rise markedly.

Some forms of treatment for cancer cause infertility, but many survivors go on to have children of their own. Most children of survivors are still very young. It is particularly important to follow up the offspring of survivors of cancer in childhood for two reasons. Some childhood cancers are known to have a predominantly genetic aetiology and the risk of transmission to future generations needs to be assessed. The question of whether treatment-related germ cell mutagenesis causes cancer, congenital malformations, or other genetic disease in the offspring of survivors also needs to be studied, and the risks, if any, estimated. Estimates of the risks to offspring of survivors are discussed in the section on genetic epidemiology below.

Aetiology of childhood cancer

Little is known about the causes of childhood cancer. International comparisons of the type described above, together with case–control and cohort studies, have suggested a variety of possible aetiologic factors, but these have seldom been convincing or replicated in further studies. On the other hand, studies of the genetics of childhood cancer have been much more rewarding, both in their practical application to problems of childhood cancer and in terms of basic science. The literature on aetiology up to 1997 was reviewed in detail by Little[17] and more recent studies are covered by Stiller;[18] these sources should be consulted for further references.

Environmental factors

Possible environmental causes of childhood cancer have been investigated in a large number of studies. The factors that have attracted most attention are radiation, both ionizing and non-ionizing, and the role of infections in the child, the mother, and the community. The other factors studied include parental characteristics, environmental exposures of both child and parents, particularly *in utero* exposures, and occupational exposures of both parents. Concern about possible environmental causes of genetic damage has led to studies of preconception exposures of the parents.

Ionizing radiation

Probably the first, and still the largest, case–control study of childhood cancer was that carried out by Dr Alice Stewart and her colleagues. An early report from this study claimed that antenatal radiography, used mainly in the third trimester of pregnancy for obstetric reasons, significantly increased the probability of the subsequent child developing cancer. Although this result was initially greeted with considerable scepticism, it is now widely accepted as correct; the most useful presentation of the results is that by Bithell and Stewart.[19] For children born between about 1945 and 1965 there was a 40–50 per cent increase in the risk of childhood cancer if the mother was subjected to abdominal radiography about two or three times during pregnancy. It should be emphasized that antenatal radiography probably caused at most about 5 per cent of childhood cancers, even when it was more widely used and doses were higher than they are now. Both the number of pregnant women subjected to radiography and the doses of radiation have greatly decreased since the time of Stewart's work; indeed, radiography has largely been replaced by ultrasound. There is no evidence that ultrasound causes childhood cancer.

Other childhood exposures to radiation, for example that used in treating tinea capitis in early childhood or, particularly, the large doses given during radiotherapy, are also carcinogenic. The possibility that some childhood cancers are caused by natural radiation (gamma, radon) has been suggested. Case–control studies have shown no significant association with radon exposure. On the usual assumption of a linear dose–response relationship for the carcinogenic effects of radiation, one would expect some cases to be caused by background gamma radiation. However, in the only case–control study based on individual household measurements, there was no indication of increased risk of childhood cancer with increasing dose levels.[20]

The report that caused the most public concern and scientific interest in this area was probably that by Gardner et al.,[21] which suggested that paternal preconception exposure to ionizing radiation could lead to childhood leukaemia. Because of the relatively small doses involved (from employment in the nuclear industry) doubts were raised about the validity of this finding, although the study appeared to be epidemiologically sound. Subsequent reports, in particular two large overlapping studies of UK radiation workers including those employed Sellafield and elsewhere,[22,23] were reviewed by the Committee on Medical Aspects of Radiation in the Environment.[24] This Committee suggested that there was unlikely to be any simple causal relationship.

Non-ionizing radiation

Ultraviolet radiation from sunlight is known to cause melanoma and other skin cancers. Concern has been expressed for more than 20 years over possible carcinogenic effects of electromagnetic fields arising from electric power transmission and use, from both power lines and domestic exposure. However, despite a very large research effort, the question of whether such exposures do have carcinogenic effects is unresolved. Analysis of pooled data from case–control studies has shown no evidence of raised risk of childhood leukaemia with exposure to power frequency fields at the level experienced by more than 95 per cent of children in Western countries.[25] A doubling of risk has been found at the very highest exposure levels but the explanation is unknown, although it may be partly due to selection bias; only a tiny fraction of childhood leukaemia cases could be attributable to electromagnetic fields.

Parental occupation and socio-economic status

Any association observed between childhood disease and parental occupations may reflect either specific exposures or lifestyle factors associated with particular occupations. Furthermore, a parent may well be in the same occupation before the conception of the child, during pregnancy, and subsequently; thus it may be difficult to determine whether any observed association is attributable to exposure occurring before conception, *in utero*, or postnatally.

Many papers analysing occupation in general or specific occupations, using a variety of study designs, have been published. It is inevitable that in a large series of studies, some of which include analysis of many different occupations, a number of statistically significant results will be reported. In such circumstances it is necessary to determine whether there is consistency between different studies and whether there is any evidence of a dose–response effect, i.e. in this instance, whether the risk is higher for children of parents who have been more heavily exposed to the suspected occupational mutagen or who have worked longer in the occupation. As judged by these criteria, there is as yet no sufficient evidence that any parental occupation is causally associated with childhood cancer. However, in a review of 48 published studies some biologically plausible associations were found in more than one study and these, in particular, merit further investigation.[26]

Of course, occupational category is closely related to socio-economic status. Thus, if there is an effect of lifestyle or standards of living on childhood cancer, this could appear as an effect of an occupation which happens to be in the high-risk group as defined by socio-economic status. The possibility of such an association with socio-economic status has been investigated in both case–control studies and 'ecologic' studies, i.e. by comparing incidence rates for areas classified according to the socio-economic status of their resident populations. There is good evidence that the incidence of childhood leukaemia increases with increasing socio-economic status, but the reasons for this are unknown.

Infections

The possible role of infections, especially viruses, in the aetiology of childhood cancer has been studied in a number of ways. Viruses are known to be implicated in some human cancers. Worldwide, the most important numerically among children are Burkitt lymphoma, Hodgkin disease, and nasopharyngeal carcinoma (Epstein–Barr virus), liver carcinoma (hepatitis B), and Kaposi sarcoma (HIV and HHV8).[27] Case–control studies have included analyses of exposures to infectious illnesses of both the children themselves and their mothers while pregnant. Positive findings have been reported, but there is no conclusive evidence from these studies. Perhaps the most persuasive evidence for the involvement of an infectious agent in childhood leukaemia comes from studies of clustering and incidence rates in different geographic areas.

Kinlen,[28] in a remarkable series of studies, has shown that childhood leukaemia rates have increased in a variety of different situations in which people from several different areas come together, resulting in 'population mixing'. His explanation is that such situations are conducive to the spread of an infectious agent or agents among a previously unexposed, and therefore susceptible, group, and that childhood leukaemia may be represent an unusual response to such agents.[28] It is not suggested that leukaemia itself is an infectious disease. Under the 'delayed infection' hypothesis, children who are protected from exposure to infection in infancy have an abnormal immune response to infection subsequently, and this occasionally results in leukaemia.[29] This is supported by, among other epidemiologic findings, a deficit of common infections and social contact in infancy among children with ALL and a raised risk of ALL in first-born children.

Other possible aetiologic factors

A wide variety of other possible factors has been studied. The cell types involved in childhood cancers and the shape of the age distribution, with a peak for the typical cancers of childhood at a very early age, have led many investigators to concentrate on events occurring during pregnancy or even before conception.

Preconception factors

The fact that some childhood cancers are attributable to germ cell mutations has led many investigators to study parental exposure to possible mutagens. Such studies have included various types of exposure to ionizing radiation (including the occupational exposures mentioned above) and to chemicals. Again, no consensus has emerged.

In utero **exposures** The effects of *in utero* ionizing radiation have already been referred to. It is well known that diethylstilboestrol (DES) given to pregnant women to avert threatened miscarriage can cause vaginal adenocarcinoma in their daughters, although these occur mainly in young women rather than children. DES ceased to be used over 30 years ago and, in the absence of evidence for any transgenerational effect, no more DES-associated cases of childhood cancer are expected to arise. A number of positive findings relating to other drugs given to women during pregnancy have been published, but no firm causal associations have been established. Similarly, smoking in pregnancy has been widely studied but is not established as a risk factor for any specific childhood cancer.[30]

Postnatal exposures Ionizing radiation and infections have already been discussed. Many other environmental factors have been studied but, again, there is no consensus. The suggestion by Golding *et al.*[31] that intramuscular vitamin K, given to neonates to prevent vitamin K deficiency bleeding, doubles the risk of childhood cancer led to a series of further studies. Analysis of pooled data from six case–control studies found little evidence for a raised risk of childhood cancer with intramuscular vitamin K,[32] although interpretation was hampered by the poor quality of much of the vitamin K data. Other medications have occasionally been reported as risk factors and, of course, cytotoxic drugs given in the course of treatment for cancer are known causes of further cancers, but there is no evidence to suggest that any substantial numbers of childhood cancers are attributable to these or other drugs.

Genetic epidemiology

A detailed discussion of the genetic aspects of childhood cancer is given in Chapter 2. In the present chapter we concentrate on the estimation of risks of childhood cancer for family members of affected children and for individuals who have genetic conditions known to predispose to childhood cancer.

The most obvious example of a genetically determined cancer is retinoblastoma. About 40 per cent of cases have the heritable form of this disease. The pattern of inheritance is that of a dominant autosomal gene with about 90 per cent penetrance, but in fact the gene Rb1 is the first example of a tumour suppressor gene; about 90 per cent of individuals who inherit the mutated form of this gene from a parent subsequently suffer a mutation of the wild-type (normal) allele, leading to loss of heterozygosity and the development of retino-blastoma. These individuals are now also known to be at increased risk of a variety of other cancers.

There is an obvious genetic element in some other childhood cancers, notably Wilms tumour, but the pattern of inheritance in Wilms tumour is a great deal more complicated and the proportion of clearly hereditary cases is much smaller.

A variety of childhood cancers and some adult cancers, notable premenopausal breast cancer, are observed in the Li–Fraumeni familial cancer syndrome.[33] The risk of childhood cancer is roughly 20 times that in the general population. Germ-line mutations of the TP53 tumour suppressor gene are responsible for the high risk and distinctive pattern of cancer in many Li–Fraumeni families, but other genes have been implicated in some families apparently without TP53 mutations.

Some familial aggregations arise through the association of childhood and adult tumours with known genetic disease such as neurofibromatosis, tuberous sclerosis, Fanconi's anaemia, ataxia telangiectasia, xeroderma pigmentosum, and Bloom's syndrome, although the actual number of cases of childhood cancer in which these conditions occur is rather small.[34] There are also well-documented associations with congenital abnormalities; the strongest association with such a condition is Down syndrome, which occurs in a small percentage of cases of childhood leukaemia.

Relatives of affected children

Various authors have studied the siblings, twins, offspring, and, to a lesser extent, the parents of children with cancer.

Siblings and twins

If one child in a family has malignant disease, then, in the absence of any further information about the existence of genetic disease in that family, and excluding twins and retinoblastoma, the siblings of that child have approximately double the risk of the general population, i.e. a risk of approximately 1 in 250 compared with the average risk of about 1 in 500.[35] (NB. The estimate for the population risk is larger than that given previously.) As more has become known about the genetic element in childhood cancer, the risk estimates have increased for families where familial syndromes have been identified, while those for the remaining families have decreased. In a more recent study, the excess of cancer among siblings of children and adolescents with cancer could be entirely accounted for by familial syndromes.[36] However, in families where there is one child with cancer, a cancer syndrome may not be recognized as such until after a further sibling has been diagnosed with cancer. In providing genetic counselling in the absence of such additional information, i.e. where there is at that time no indication of a cancer syndrome in that particular family, it should be assumed that the increased risk for siblings referred to above applies. A doubling of the risks for siblings compared with the general population implies that half of the families with two affected children are in fact due to chance. (Incidentally, this implies that laboratory studies of these families will be expected to find nothing of interest at least 50 per cent of the time.) It should be emphasized that the risk is less than 1 in 250 for siblings who are a few years old when the affected child is diagnosed. The estimated risk is also lower if there are other children in the family who are not affected.

The risks are higher if there are two affected children in the family and where there is known genetic disease of a type associated with cancer. In the special case of retinoblastoma, the risk for a subsequent sibling following an apparently sporadic case of retinoblastoma, i.e. where there is no previous family history, appears to be about 2 per cent if the disease in the affected sibling is bilateral, and 1 per cent if it is unilateral.[37] This is lower than has previously been suggested, and is lower still if there are other siblings who are not affected.

The risk that the co-twin of a twin with cancer will also be affected is of particular concern, and more so if the twins are monozygous. In general, both twins and childhood cancer are too rare for any quantitative estimates of risk to be made. It seems likely that the risk for a dizygotic co-twin of an affected case will be at least as high as that for ordinary siblings, but no data are available. Nearly all the published cases of childhood cancer in twins are like-sexed pairs and are known or assumed to be monozygous. The fact that in case reports of affected twin pairs the two children almost invariably have the same diagnosis and tend to be diagnosed at the same age is an indication that such cases may be genetic in origin. One would expect there to be an increased risk for the monozygous co-twins of affected cases, but in general there are insufficient data to estimate such risks; the fact that the co-twins of the great majority of cases do not develop cancer[38] implies that the risk to co-twins is, in general, not very high. The exception to this is childhood leukaemia, where perhaps 25 per cent of co-twins of monozygotic cases also develop the disease(see also Chapter 2). However, many of these cases are due to *in utero* transfer of leukaemia cells rather than being genetically determined.

Risks to offspring and parents

The risks to offspring of childhood cancer survivors correspond well to those from the studies of siblings. In general they are low, the main exception being for retinoblastoma, although even here, as for siblings, the risks in cases of sporadic retinoblastoma appear to be lower than previously suggested: for a child of a unilateral case, and where it is not known whether the disease is of hereditary type, the estimated risk is 1 per cent.[37] After the exclusion of hereditary cancer syndromes there is no evidence of a significantly raised risk of cancer among the offspring of survivors.[39] Similarly, there is no evidence that the parents of children with cancer have an increased risk of cancer in the absence of known hereditary syndromes.[40]

References

1. **Kramárová E, Stiller CA, Ferlay J, et al.** (1996). *The International Classification of Childhood Cancer.* IARC Technical Report No. 29. Lyon: IARC.
2. **Jensen OM, Parkin DM, MacLennan R, Muir CS, Skeet RG** (eds) (1991). *Cancer Registration: Principles and Methods.* IARC Scientific Publications No.95. Lyon: IARC.
3. **Parkin DM, Kramárová E, Draper GJ, et al.** (eds) (1998). *International Incidence of Childhood Cancer,* Volume 2. IARC Scientific Publications No 144. Lyon: IARC.

4. Tyczynski JE, Démaret E, Parkin DM (eds) (2003). Tyczynski JE, Démaret E, Parkin DM, editors. *Standards and Guidelines for Cancer Registration in Europe. The ENCR recommendations. Vol 1.* IARC Technical Report No.40. Lyon: IARC.

5. Stiller CA, Parkin DM (1996). Geographic and ethnic variations in the incidence of childhood cancer. *Br Med Bull* 52, 682–703.

6. Hrusák O, Trka J, Zuna J, Poloucková A, Kalina T, Stary J (2002). Acute lymphoblastic leukemia incidence during socioeconomic transition: selective increase in children from 1 to 4 years. *Leukemia* 16, 720–5.

7. Arrundale J, Bain M, Botting B, *et al.* (1997). *Handbook and Guide to the Investigation of Clusters of Diseases.* Leeds: Leukaemia Research Fund Centre for Clinical Epidemiology, University of Leeds

8. Gatta G, Corazziari I, Magnani C, *et al.* (2003). Childhood cancer survival in Europe. *Ann Oncol,* 14 (Suppl 5), 119–27.

9. Gatta G, Capocaccia R, Coleman MP, Gloeckler Ries LA, Berrino F (2002). Childhood cancer survival in Europe and the United States. *Cancer* 95, 1767–72.

10. Stiller CA (1994). Centralised treatment, entry to trials and survival. *Br J Cancer* 70, 352–62.

11. Stiller CA, Eatock EM (1999). Patterns of care and survival for children with acute lymphoblastic leukaemia diagnosed between 1980–94. *Arch Dis Child* 81, 202–8.

12. Robertson CM, Hawkins MM, Kingston JE (1994). Late deaths and survival after childhood cancer: implications for cure. *BMJ* 309, 162–6.

13. Möller TR, Garwicz S, Barlow L, *et al.* (2001). Decreasing late mortality among five-year survivors of cancer in childhood and adolescence: a population-based study in the Nordic countries. *J Clin Oncol* 19, 3173–81.

14. Mertens AC, Yasui Y, Neglia JP, *et al.* (2001). Late mortality experience in five-year survivors of childhood and adolescent cancer: the Childhood Cancer Survivor Study. *J Clin Oncol* 19, 3163–72.

15. Hawkins MM, Stevens MCG (1996). The long term survivors. *Br Med Bull* 52, 898–923.

16. Neglia JP, Friedman DL, Yasui Y, *et al.* (2001). Second malignant neoplasms in five-year survivors of childhood cancer: childhood cancer survivor study. *J Natl Cancer Inst* 93, 618–29.

17. Little J (1999). *Epidemiology of Childhood Cancer.* IARC Scientific Publications No 149. Lyon: IARC.

18. Stiller CA. (2004). Aetiology and epidemiology. In: Pinkerton CR, Plowman PN, Pieters R (eds) *Paediatric Oncology* (3rd edn). pp 3–24 London: Arnold.

19. Bithell JF, Stewart AM (1975). Pre-natal irradiation and childhood malignancy: A review of British data from the Oxford survey. *Br J Cancer* 31, 271–87.

20. UK Childhood Cancer Study Investigators (2002). The United Kingdom Childhood Cancer Study of exposure to domestic sources of ionising radiation. 2: Gamma radiation. *Br J Cancer* 86, 1727–31.

21. Gardner MJ, Snee MP, Hall AJ, Powell CA, Downes S, Terrell JD (1990). Results of case–control study of leukaemia and lymphoma among young people near Sellafield nuclear plant in West Cumbria. *BMJ* 300, 423–9.

22. Draper GJ, Little MP, Sorahan T, *et al.* (1997). Cancer in the offspring of radiation workers: a record linkage study. *BMJ* 315, 1181–8.

23. Roman E, Doyle P, Maconochie N, Davies G, Smith PG, Beral V (1999). Cancer in children of nuclear industry employees: report on children aged under 25 years from nuclear industry family study. *BMJ* 318, 1443–50.

24. Committee on Medical Aspects of Radiation in the Environment (COMARE) (2002). *Seventh Report: Parents Occupationally Exposed to Radiation Prior to the Conception of their Children. A Review of the Evidence Concerning the Incidence of Cancer in their Children.* Chilton, Didcot, UK: NRPB

25. **Ahlbom A, Day N, Feychting M,** *et al.* (2000). A pooled analysis of magnetic fields and childhood leukaemia. *Br J Cancer* **83**, 692–8.

26. **Colt JS, Blair A** (1998). Parental occupational exposures and risk of childhood cancer. *Environ Health Perspect* **106**, 909–25.

27. **Parkin DM, Pisani P, Muñoz N, Ferlay J** (1999). The global health burden of infection associated cancers. *Cancer Surv* **33**, 5–33.

28. **Kinlen LJ** (1995). Epidemiological evidence for an infective basis in childhood leukaemia. *Br J Cancer* **71**, 1–5.

29. **Greaves M** (2002). Childhood leukaemia. *BMJ* **324**, 283–7.

30. **Boffetta P, Trédaniel J, Greco A** (2000). Risk of childhood cancer and adult lung cancer after childhood exposure to passive smoking: a meta-analysis. *Environ Health Perspect* **108**, 73–82.

31. **Golding J, Greenwood R, Birmingham K, Mott M** (1992). Childhood cancer, intramuscular vitamin K, and pethidine given during labour. *BMJ* **305**, 341–6.

32. **Roman E, Fear NT, Ansell P,** *et al.* (2002). Vitamin K and childhood cancer: analysis of individual patient data from six case–control studies. *Br J Cancer* **86**, 63–9.

33. **Varley JM** (2003). Germline *TP53* mutations and Li–Fraumeni syndrome. *Hum Mutat* **21**, 313–20.

34. **Lindor NM, Greene MH, The Mayo Familial Cancer Program** (1998). The concise handbook of family cancer syndromes. *J Natl Cancer Inst* **90**, 1039–71.

35. **Draper GJ, Heaf MM, Kinnier Wilson LM** (1977). Occurrence of childhood cancers among sibs and estimation of familial risks. *J Med Genet* **14**, 81–90.

36. **Winther JF, Sankila R, Boice JD,** *et al.* (2001). Cancer in siblings of children with cancer in the Nordic countries: a population-based cohort study. *Lancet* **358**, 711–17.

37. **Draper GJ, Sanders BM, Brownbill PA, Hawkins MM** (1992). Patterns of risk of hereditary retino-blastoma and applications to genetic counselling. *Br J Cancer* **66**, 211–19.

38. **Draper GJ, Sanders BM, Lennox EL, Brownbill PA** (1996). Patterns of childhood cancer among siblings. *Br J Cancer* **74**, 152–8.

39. **Sankila R, Olsen JH, Anderson H,** *et al.* (1998). Risk of cancer among offspring of childhood-cancer survivors. *N Engl J Med* **338**, 1339–44.

40. **Olsen JH, Boice JD, Seersholm N, Bautz A, Fraumeni JF** (1995). Cancer in the parents of children with cancer. *N Engl J Med* **333**, 1594–9.

Chapter 2

Genetics of childhood malignancies

Oskar A. Haas

> Cancer can be seen as the consequence of a chaotic process, a combination of Murphy's Law and Darwin's Law*: anything that can go wrong will, and in a competitive environment, the best adapted survive and prosper.
>
> W. Wayt Gibbs, *Scientific American* July 2003, p. 49

*. . . and, of course, also Mendel's Laws, which I take liberty to add as author of this chapter.

Setting the stage

The healthy human body is a complex linked system of cells that is composed of several dynamic equilibria whose disturbances result in disease. In this context, cancer can be viewed as a genetic disease deriving from the territorial expansion of a mutant somatic cell clone, which disrupts the organism's physiologic balance between ordered cell production, differentiation, and elimination. Consequently, the characteristic pathology of the neoplasm results from the interaction between the expanding mass and its specific somatic environment.[1] Thus mutations that collectively corrupt cellular control pathways of a single immature or undifferentiated precursor cell can be viewed as the ultimate cause of cancer. However, cancer is not a deterministic genetic disease because continuous destabilization of the genome during the self-perpetuating process of neoplastic transformation also involves characteristics, physiologic factors, and exposures that not only induce but also influence the probability of mutation. Thus the ensuing concept of a multistep evolution of cancer implies that spurts of mutations propagate tumour development via a Darwinian process of natural selection whose essential components are cell proliferation, genetic diversification, environmental pressure, competition, and adaptation.[2] The important point here, which is commonly overlooked, is that the internal and external environments influence and modify the behaviour of genes as much as genes themselves determine their intracellular and extracellular milieu. Therefore the environment plays a significant role in the selection of mutations that are appropriately adapted for the successful survival of genetically destabilized cells.[3]

The internal and external homeostatic conditions of a developing host differ significantly from those of a fully mature one. Therefore it is not surprising that the spectrum of haematologic malignancies and solid tumours, as well as their biologic features and response to therapy, varies markedly between children and adults. The vast majority of childhood malignancies result from errors that take place during early stages of cell differentiation, tissue maturation, and organ development.[4,5] The cellular self-organization into organs during embryonic development is driven by cell–cell communication. Disturbances in this process often result in disease. Genetic destabilization of productive progenitor cells creates a large amount of heterogeneity. Particular circumstances can provide one or the other of the affected cells with increased fitness and survival advantages, which are the first steps on the path to tumour development. Additional factors that contribute to the formation of the diversity of tumours in children and adults include a different susceptibility in the stem cell population that is injured by mutations as well as the type and numbers of mutations that are necessary to induce a fully malignant phenotype. Thus the predominance of specific types of mesenchymal tumours may reflect a combination of the high cell turnover during early and mid-fetal development that makes certain precursor cell populations more vulnerable to DNA replication errors, and the limited number of mutations that are necessary for the induction of overt disease. Moreover, the number and nature of cooperating mutations required to induce a fully malignant phenotype probably also varies depending on the initiating lesions. The low frequency of adult types of epithelial neoplasms in children, on the other hand, is in agreement with the idea that their development requires several more genetic alterations and steps and consequently a much longer time to become clinically apparent.[5,6]

Rather than listing the specific cytogenetic and molecular changes that characterize individual types of childhood malignancies in this chapter, we intend to focus more on these conceptual aspects of the role and significance of genetics in childhood cancer. Several unusual views and inspiring theories that have been put forward recently provide the basis for exploring how, when, and where mutations are generated, how particular patterns of genetic abnormalities emerge, in which way they reflect particular internal and external environmental conditions, and why recurrent patterns of genomic imbalances are so specifically linked with distinct types of tumours in both children and adults. In particular, concentrating on childhood malignancies illustrates that much can be learnt from studying rare conditions.[7] The relevance of the clues stretches far beyond the particular disease entity. Thorough analyses of genetic alterations, especially those occurring in haematologic neoplasms in infants and twins, have recently provided some striking insights into the time course and the potential steps and mechanism of the transformation process.[7,8] This knowledge is essential for understanding the biology, pathology, and clinical behaviour of the ensuing tumours and eventually for devising more effective and less harmful treatment strategies. Moreover, as an added bonus, genetic studies of childhood malignancies also help to elucidate the normal physiologic developmental processes of cells, organs, and the human organism. Last but not least, they also add to understanding of the pathogenesis of adult tumour forms.

Genetic information

The information provided in this section derives mainly from the very instructive and inspiring article by Hood and Galas,[9] as well as from a compilation of several other recently published excellent review articles on this topic.[10,11]

Processing and utilization

Cells, organs, and organisms consist of heterogeneous components that are organized in distinct levels and interact within large networks. At the core of biologic complexity resides DNA, the immortal molecule of life that encodes genomic information and fuels the process of molecular self-organization. Although the DNA structure provides an immediate explanation for mutation and variation, change, species diversity, evolution, and inheritance, it does not automatically provide a mechanism for understanding how the environment interacts at the genetic level.[11]

The two main elements of genomic information operate across three time spans: evolution, development, and physiology. Genes encode the RNA and protein machinery of life, whereas the regulatory networks define how these genes are expressed in time, space, and amplitude. The regulatory networks consist of two major components: the transcription factors, and the sites in the control regions of genes to which they bind, such as promoters, enhancers, and silencers. Long-term information is stored almost exclusively in the genome and short-term information in the proteome. As becomes evident from the changing morphologic patterns during the development from a fertilized egg to an adult organism, it is not so much the genes, but rather the regulatory networks that play the crucial role in this process. Consistent with this view, individual cells utilize only the very small part of the genome that is necessary to maintain their function, development, and differentiation at a given time point, and by far the largest proportion of their genome always remains inactive. This also applies to neoplastic tissues, although it must be remembered that in this situation the genome is additionally continuously perturbed and rearranged.

The DNA-encoded information flows from a gene to the environment in a distinct fashion which is subject to a variety of regulatory feedback loops and environmental influences. At each successive layer, the information becomes more complex and information can be added or altered for any given element. This includes, for example, the flexible remodelling of the chromatin configuration, RNA splicing, and protein modification (Fig. 2.1). The further the

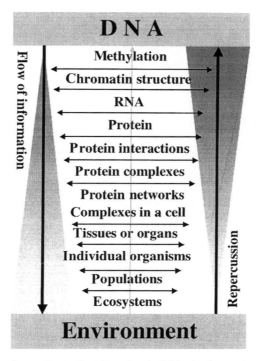

Fig. 2.1 The world according to DNA. The DNA of an individual cell encodes all the information that is necessary to form the complexity of the whole organism. Conversion of information takes place at several distinct levels and is a plastic and flexible process that is subject to many feedback loops and both intra- and extracellular environmental influences.

flow of information drifts away from the DNA, the more it is influenced and modified by the intra- and extracellular environment, and especially by other cells or chemical gradients. The elementary building blocks organize themselves into recurrent patterns and functional modules that shape the discrete cellular functions, such as gene regulatory circuits and metabolic pathways. The cellular interactions are cooperative and self-enhancing, and their autocatalytic feedback properties provide the means of altering strategies and adapting to changes in the internal and external environments. Moreover, cells and organisms also modulate the strength of the interaction with neighbouring units to increase their fitness, the maximum of which occurs at the boundary of order and chaos.

During the embryonic and fetal periods, cells increase dramatically in number, mature, and become specialized to form tissues and organs. An adult human body consists of an estimated 10^{14} cells and approximately 300 distinguishable cell types. During a human lifetime approximately 10^{17} cells are produced in total. Two hundred million cells are lost and renewed per minute, which is equivalent to a cell turnover of one body mass every 35 days. Thus this highly ordered and structured agglomeration of cells exists in an intricately labile balance. This permanent consumption and loss of cells has to be compensated by continuous cell renewal processes, whose starting points are highly specialized tissue-specific stem cells. The derived daughter cells differentiate along well-defined pathways. To counter cell production and maintain the necessary steady state, the controlled physiologic elimination of cells by apoptosis occurs in both the fetus and the adult. Intriguingly, however, and as will be explained later, apoptosis also has the catastrophic potential to promote mutation and genome instability. Therefore the fundamental idea is that a combination of deregulated proliferation and suppressed apoptosis constitutes the minimal platform upon which all neoplasms reside.[1,2]

Epigenetic inheritance and imprinting

Genetically determined differences in gene activity are usually attributed to DNA sequence variations, such as polymorphisms and mutations. However, the facts (e.g. the phenotypic traits of twins and cloned animals, with their supposedly identical DNA make-up, can still vary considerably) imply that a DNA-sequence-independent and environmental modulation of the transcribed genetic information must be at least as important as the original DNA-derived message itself. The main player in this process is the dynamic plasticity of the chromatin organization, which exerts a profound control over gene expression and other fundamental cellular processes. Such heritable, but DNA-sequence-independent, regulatory mechanisms of gene expression govern the flexible conversion of the DNA-encoded information into cell- and tissue-specific gene activity patterns. This is summarized under the umbrella term 'epigenetics'.[12]

The most important regulator is the reversible methylation of gene promoters and the inextricably linked methylation and acetylation of the associated histone proteins. Although these modifications can be altered by a variety of factors, they can also remain remarkably stable and be passed on to future generations. This kind of cellular memory ensures that fundamental decisions regarding turning individual genes or groups of genes on or off need to be made only once and that daughter cells inherit identical repressed or activated transcription states. This provides an efficient mechanism for cellular differentiation. Since such patterns of epigenetic information are also replicated, mutated, and selected in the somatic environment, they should, like the DNA sequence itself, also evolve by Darwinian mechanisms.[3]

The classic example of the phenomenon of epigenetic inheritance at the generational level is imprinting. This type of non-Mendelian inheritance of specific traits results from the parent of origin-specific transmittance and the parent of origin-specific monoallelic usage of specific genes. Since many of these genes encode fetal growth factors and their receptors, imprinting plays an important role in fetal development. Paternally expressed genes enhance fetal growth, whereas maternally expressed genes suppress it. In mammals, for example, the gene encoding insulin-like growth factor 2 (IGF-2) is only expressed from the paternal copy of the gene, whereas the H19 gene is expressed solely from the maternal allele. The uncoordinated expression of these and other genes can cause various developmental disturbances and diseases, including overgrowth and tumour-predisposition syndromes, the prototype of which is the well-known Beckwith–Wiedemann syndrome.[13]

However, epigenetic mechanisms play a much more profound role in neoplasia and are instrumental in virtually every step in its initiation and progression. Patterns of DNA methylation and chromatin structure are severely altered and include genome-wide hypomethylation as well as regional hypermethylation of specific promoters.[12]

DNA integrity, DNA repair, and cell-cycle checkpoint control

The preservation of its genomic information is of paramount importance for a cell. This task requires sophisticated surveillance and maintenance machinery, because DNA is a highly thermolabile molecule that is permanently jeopardized by a variety of internal and external noxious agents.[14] The two essential parts of this machinery are the DNA damage checkpoint system and the DNA repair enzymes.[2,11] The complex surveillance system somehow senses genome injury and arrests the cell cycle at specific checkpoints in the G_1, S, G_2, and M phases, activates DNA repair networks, or induces programmed cell death (apoptosis).

The two major categories of mechanistically distinct events of genome damage are those which affect chromosome numbers, and those which alter chromosome structure. The former most likely reflect malfunction of the mitotic chromosome segregation apparatus, whereas the latter point to irregularities in DNA repair processes. Potential contributors to chromosome mis-segregation include centrosome dysfunction, anaphase checkpoint malfunction, and cytokinesis failure.[15]

Activation of the repair system not only stimulates transcriptional programmes and the movement of the DNA repair proteins to sites of DNA damage, but also regulates the telomere length. Thus the potential sources of genomic destabilization comprise defective copying, excessive damage, ineffectual repair, and faulty segregation. The outcome of DNA damage is diverse and generally harmful. Severe damage is lethal to the cell, or at least severely deleterious to its proliferation. Insufficient repair, on the other hand, converts less severe DNA corruptions into permanent mutations, whose irreversible long-term effects contribute to ontogenesis.

In an analogous fashion, malfunction of the telomeres also adds significantly to chromosome breakage, fusion, and mis-segregation. Telomeres consist of arrays of repetitive sequences that protect the chromosome ends from degradation during cell growth and differentiation. Gradual shortening during successive cell divisions eventually results in crisis and cell death. Neoplasms circumvent this fate both by inactivating the cell death pathway and by switching on telomerase. This enzyme helps to maintain telomere length, thereby rendering the cell immortal.[16,17] Thus passage of cells through a crisis in the setting of deactivated DNA damage checkpoints provides a mutational mechanism that can generate a variety of cancer-initiating genetic alterations.[17] Although the replicative potential of tumour-forming precursor cells in infants and children is still considerably higher than that of the epithelial cells of aging adults, telomerase is nevertheless activated in a variety of childhood tumours. One explanation for this phenomenon might be that in this setting it may be necessary to maintain the proliferative potential of a tissue that has already been transformed rather than trigger tumour initiation by rescuing senescent cells, as is the case in adults. This would also explain the much more pronounced karyotype instability and complexity of chromosome rearrangements in the epithelial tumours of adults compared with those in the mesenchymal tumours and leukaemias of the young.

Allocation of an appropriate repair system is not a trivial process, as the choice depends on where and in which physiologic context DNA strand breaks occur in the genome.[2,11,14] Therefore a particular DNA repair pathway may be appropriate or normal in one situation, but inappropriate or abnormal in another. Point mutations arise from faulty repair of DNA base damage, mis-incorporated DNA bases, or spontaneous or induced deamination of methylated cytosines. Small-scale DNA damage is reversed through base excision, nucleotide excision, and mismatch repair, whereas DNA double-strand breaks (DSBs) can be repaired with high fidelity through homologous repair. Unrepaired and unprotected DSBs, including ex-posed telomere ends, are fusogenic and joined to other double-strand DNA ends. Inappropri-ate repair by the non-homologous end-joining (NHEJ) system generates structural gene and chromosome rearrangements. Repetitive inter- or intragenic simultaneous or consecutive breakage–fusion–breakage cycles may then lead to very complex structural rearrangements. The fact that break-originating processes, such as deletions, insertions, inversions, amplifica-tions, and translocations, are particularly abundant in cancer indicates that this pathway of NHEJ is frequently involved. It acts as an emergency repair of broken chromosomes, but at the cost of fidelity. This is further corroborated by the increased incidence of tumours in humans with repair deficiency syndromes and is also backed up by experimental evidence from knockout mice lacking the corresponding genes.[15]

In addition, irregularities that occur during DNA synthesis and replication can also generate substrates for recombination and give rise to gross chromosomal aberrations. Thus, in the absence of external sources of DNA damage, the increased formation of destabilizing DSBs can also be triggered by endogeneous metabolic defects or enhanced irregular DNA excision repair. The preliminary observations that exposure of preterm infants to diagnostic X-rays did not increase leukaemogenic fusion transcripts whereas epidemiologic evidence points to an asso-ciation between neonatal oxygen supplementation and leukaemia are of particular interest in this context. Thus gratuitous repair may be an important source of spontaneous mutation.

Finally, failure in DNA damage signalling is probably at least as harmful as a specific DNA repair defect. It allows mutagenic repair of DNA damage while lowering the rate of apoptotic cell death. Thus, in terms of the costs and benefits of DNA repair, stopping for repairs can be a fatal strategy in a hostile environment.[3] For instance, concurrent defects in the nucleotide excision repair and cell-cycle control systems would provide such a situation in which repairs could take place without stopping. It is a destabilizing and risky venture, but it might be the only option in a mutagenic 'war zone', as expressed so vividly by Breivik in a recent article.[3]

Genetic susceptibility and predisposition

Although the vast majority of childhood malignancies appear to occur sporadically, their early age of onset suggests that underlying inherited constitutional genetic defects might provide a strong predisposing influence.[18,19] Overall, more than 600 genetic predisposition factors have been recognized so far. They include rare high-penetrant DNA mutations and epigenetic defects as well as more common genetic polymorphisms that influence individual response to environmental exposure.[20] The classic constitutional mutations in children include sporadic chromosome anomalies as well as chromosome and gene defects that are inherited according to the Mendelian laws, i.e. autosomal dominant, autosomal recessive, and X-linked traits. More common genetic traits, such as those that influence the metabolic activation or detoxification of carcinogenic chemicals, are probably important determinants of population risk although they pose low individual risk. Intriguing mouse breeding experiments have led to the provocative speculation that offspring of parents with relatively divergent DNA sequences might be less susceptible to mitotic recombination and therefore more protected from cancer than those of less divergent parents.

Furthermore, the age-related differences that exist in susceptibility to environmental toxicants are noteworthy. Experimental and epidemiologic data indicate that, apart from predisposing genetic traits or ethnicity, the very young may have a heightened risk because of their differential exposure and physiologic immaturity.[18] For example, relative to body weight, infants and children take in appreciably more food, water, air, and any carcinogens contained therein than adults. Moreover, increased absorption and retention of toxicants, reduced detoxification and repair, and the higher rate of cell proliferation may constitute additional factors that contribute to the higher internal dose of toxicants and greater genetic damage to infants and children compared with similarly exposed adults.[18] Moreover, preliminary observations also suggest that the risk of leukaemia initiation *in utero* may be modified by dietary as well as genetic factors.[7]

Types and consequences of cytogenetic and molecular genetic alterations

Gene, chromosome, and genome mutations

Human neoplasms exhibit genome modifications that range from subtle point mutations to dramatic gains and losses of whole or parts of chromosomes.[21] Such chromosome aberrations are the visible hallmarks of gene deregulation and genome instability.[2] It is noteworthy that acquired cancer-associated mutations never occur constitutionally. Three distinct types of genome instability contribute directly or indirectly to the unbalanced expression of genes: chromosome instability, microsatellite instability, and epigenetic instability (discussed above).

The term 'chromosome instability' includes not only gains and losses of entire chromosomes, but also gains and losses of chromosome parts (deletions and duplications) and amplifications as well as structural rearrangements (translocations, inversions, and insertions).[15] Microsatellite instability, on the other hand, results from a defective mismatch repair system, which particularly affects DNA repeat sequences and causes surprisingly little chromosome instability. It is a specific hallmark of various inherited and sporadic forms of adult cancers, but is not instrumental in the pathogenesis of childhood forms of cancer.

One of the hotly debated questions at present is whether chromosomal aneuploidy or gene mutation comes first, and which type of aberration matters most.[15] A compromise suggestion is that aneuploidy may collaborate with intragenic mutations during tumorigenesis by altering the dosage of thousands of genes, thereby accelerating the accumulation of oncogenes and the loss of tumour suppressor genes. In contrast with the most common forms of carcinomas in the adult, the genome of leukaemia, lymphoma, and sarcoma is not as scrambled and often remains quite stable and within the diploid range. This distinction is important, because it implies that such specific changes result from an early single hit, whereas the more complex and clonally unstable changes reflect a more pronounced underlying defect in chromosome and genome maintenance. Even aneuploidy exhibits relatively stable chromosome complements in these malignancies, probably because it arises from a rare event in a tumour founder cell rather than from a catastrophic destabilization of the genome in senescent cells, as is generally the case in carcinomas.[15]

Aneuploidy in childhood malignancies

Three extraordinary types of aneuploidy are of particular interest: constitutional trisomy 21, hyperdiploid acute lymphoblastic leukaemia (ALL), and pseudotriploid neuroblastoma.

Constitutional trisomy 21 is a condition that predisposes to a self-limiting transient myeloid proliferative disease (TMD) as well as to progressive haematologic malignancies.[22] TMD occurs exclusively during the postnatal period, whereas true leukaemias develop later, within the first few years of life. The most common form is acute megakaryocytic leukaemia (AML-M7). TMD and AML-M7 are related clonal diseases which, except for the age of onset, are virtually indistinguishable by any currently available diagnostic measures. Although the responsible factor was suspected to reside on chromosome 21 itself, it was recently proved that mutations of the X-linked GATA1 gene are the culprit. Since these mutations occur in the fetal liver and arrest the differentiation of the megakaryopoietic lineage, they are found in both TMD and AML-M7 and are the long-sought cause of leukaemic transformation.[22]

Although the mechanism leading to the increased chromosome number in hyperdiploid ALL with 51–65 chromosomes still remains unknown, there is good evidence that a single non-disjunction event must lead to the non-random gain of the trisomic chromosomes 4, 6, 10, 14, 17, 18, 20, and X and the tetrasomic chromosome 21.[23] Once formed, the abnormal karyotype remains remarkably stable. The ensuing imbalances may either enhance the proliferation capacity of early lymphoid cells solely through a change in dosage or relative dosage of a set of genes or, in a similar process, block differentiation. This has recently been supported by gene expression studies, which have revealed that genes on chromosomes X and 21 are comparatively more expressed than others. The reason that specific gene mutations are not considered very important in this type of disease also derives from the fact that they generally lack structural rearrangements.[24]

The extraordinary biology and behaviour of neuroblastoma ranges from life-threatening progression to maturation into ganglioneuroblastoma and spontaneous regression.[25] The latter is one of the most unusual aspects of infants with stage IV-S, a disseminated disease form that may involve liver, skin, and/or bone marrow, but not cortical bones or distal lymph nodes. Genetically, these tumours are characterized by a pseudotriploid karyotype that usually consists of pure non-random numerical changes. Specifically, they also lack the typical markers for progressive and late stages, such as MYCN amplification and 1p deletions. Moreover, such favourable neuroblastomas rarely, if ever, evolve into unfavourable ones. When, how, and why pseudotriploidy arises remains as enigmatic as its role in the unusual disease process.

Cancer genes and deregulated signal transduction pathways

Cancer-associated abnormalities disturb the regulatory circuits that govern normal cell physiology and homeostasis.[2] The dominant paradigm is that four to ten mutations need to disrupt the right genes to alter five or six different regulatory systems on the path to malignancy (Table 2.1).[6] The most important gene classes that are implicated in cancer are the gatekeeper genes that control cell growth and death and the caretaker genes that maintain genome integrity.

Table 2.1. Six essential alterations in cell physiology that collectively dictate malignant growth[6]

Self sufficiency in growth signals

Insensitivity to growth-inhibitory (antigrowth) signals

Evasion of programmed cell death (apoptosis)

Limitless replicative potential

Sustained angiogenesis

Tissue invasion and metastasis

Members of either class can act as oncogenes or tumour suppressor genes. Cellular proto-oncogenes normally function as positive regulators of cell growth, whereas tumour suppressor genes serve as negative ones. Members of both classes interact and cooperate in distinct signal transduction pathways, one or the other of which is disrupted in virtually every benign and malignant human neoplasm.[2] The most prominent examples of characteristic and specific karyotype and gene rearrangements encountered in childhood malignancies are listed in Table 2.2.

Oncogenes are frequently activated by gain of function mutations or fusions with other genes. They may also become aberrantly activated through amplification, increased promoter activity, or protein stabilization. The best-known examples of gain of function mutation are probably those of the RAS genes. Reciprocal chromosome rearrangements result in the illegitimate recombination or juxtaposition of two normally separate genes.[8] The ensuing fusion genes generate either a hybrid mRNA and a chimeric protein with novel properties, such as an altered transcriptional regulation or activated kinase, or deregulate a partner gene. The former type of fusion is common in immature forms of B-cell precursor ALL, AML, and sarcomas, whereas the latter is a typical feature of mature B- and T-cell acute leukaemias and lymphomas. In the case of the formation of a chimeric fusion gene, this first or initiating event needs to be complemented with mutant or activated kinases, such as FLT3 tandem duplications or c-KIT mutations, to lead to malignant transformation.[2,11] The cytogenetic manifestations of high-level amplifications are double-minute chromatin bodies (DM) or homogeneously staining regions (HSR). Such gene amplifications cause an overexpression of the affected gene(s). The prototypic example from childhood malignancies is the MYCN amplification in neuroblastoma, which is a hallmark of advanced stages with a poor outcome.[25]

Tumour suppressor genes, on the other hand, are inactivated by physical loss (deletion), loss of function mutations, or epigenetically by promoter methylation. Whereas a mutation in one allele is enough to activate an oncogene permanently, both alleles usually have to be knocked out to inactivate a tumour suppressor gene completely.[26] Knudson's classic two-hit model[26] derived from his studies of hereditary and acquired forms of retinoblastoma and stipulates that the inherited or acquired mutation or loss of a single allele of a tumour suppressor gene should lead to a reduction of the gene dosage. In this model, the diminished expression remains below the tissue-specific thresholds that could interfere with the control of fundamental cellular processes. According to the model, tumours develop only when the function of the second allele is also lost. However, in other instances a monoallelic disruption of such a tumour suppressor gene alone may be sufficient to create a cellular phenotype that promotes tumour genesis, without the necessity of an inactivation of the second allele. Such a haplo-insufficiency of particular caretaker genes may immediately result in defective DNA repair and increased

Table 2.2. Representative examples of the most relevant chromosomes and gene rearrangements encountered in childhood haematologic neoplasms and solid tumours

Type of neoplasm	Abnormality		Genetic consequence	Remarks
	Chromosome level	Gene level		
ALL	t(12;21)(p13;q22)	TEL/AML1	Hybrid mRNA	Most common rearrangement in ALL, favourable marker
ALL	t(4;11)(q21;q23)	MLL/AF4	Hybrid mRNA	Most common rearrangement in infants, unfavourable marker
ALL	Hyperdiploidy	?	?	Non-random gains of chromosomes X, 4, 6, 10, 14, 17, 18, 21
Pre-B ALL	t(1;19)(q23;p13)	E2A/PBX1	Hybrid mRNA	Highly specific marker
ALL and CML	t(9;22)(q34;q11)	BCR/ABL	Hybrid mRNA	Unfavourable marker in ALL
B-cell ALL and lymphoma	t(8;14)(q24;q32)	MYCC/IGH	Constitutive MYCC activation	Most common of three variants
T-cell ALL and lymphoma	–	SIL/TAL-1	Constitutive TAL-1 activation	Most common gene rearrangment in T-ALL
T-cell ALL and lymphoma	t(8;14)(q24;q11)	MYCC/TCR	Constitutive MYCC activation	
T-cell ALL and lymphoma	t(1;14)(p34;q11)	TAL-1/TCR	Constitutive TAL-1 activation	Rare, but most common of several variants
ALL/AML	t(7;12)(q36;p13)	TEL/HLXB9	Hybrid mRNA*	Occurs exclusively in infants
AML-M2	t(8;21)(q22;q22)	AML1/ETO	Hybrid mRNA	Highly characteristic
AML-M3	t(15;17)(q21;q11)	PML/RARA	Hybrid mRNA	Occurs exclusively in promyelocytic leukaemia
AML-M4Eo	inv(16)(p13;q22)	CBFB/MYH11	Hybrid mRNA	Highly characteristic
AML-M5	t(9;11)(p22;q23)	MLL/AF9	Hybrid mRNA	One of the most common of 50 MLL gene fusions
AML-M7	t(1;22)(p13;q13)	OTT/MAL	Hybrid mRNA	Occurs exclusively in infant cases

Table 2.2. (continued) Representative examples of the most relevant chromosomes and gene rearrangements encountered in childhood haematologic neoplasms and solid tumours

Type of neoplasm	Abnormality		Genetic consequence	Remarks
	Chromosome level	Gene level		
AML	t(5;11)(q35;p11)	NUP98/NSD1	Hybrid mRNA	Occurs exclusively in childhood AML
AML/MDS	−7 or +8	?	?	Highly characteristic, but not specific
Ewing sarcoma	t(11;22)(q24;q21)	EWS/FLI1	Hybrid mRNA	Most common of several variants
Alveolar rhabdomyosarcoma	t(2;13)(q35;q14)	PAX3/FKHR	Hybrid mRNA	Most common of several variants
Neuroblastoma	HSR and DM	MYCN	High-level amplification	Unfavourable marker
Neuroblastoma	del(1)(p36)	?	?	Unfavourable marker
Neuroblastoma	Pseudotriploidy	?	?	Favourable marker, spontaneous remissons
Wilms tumour	del(11)(p13)	WT1	(Biallelic) inactivation	Germ line and/or somatic
Retinoblastoma	del(13)(q14)	RB1	(Biallelic) inactivation	Germ line and/or somatic

ALL, acute lymphoblastic leukaemia; AML, acute myeloblastic leukaemia; CML, chronic myeloid leukaemia; MDS, myelodysplastic syndrome
*Only occasionally.

genetic instability and thereby induce somatic mutations in other tumour suppressor genes and oncogenes in a much shorter period of time. However, tumours influenced by haplo-insufficiency usually have a later age of onset when compared with those caused by biallelic inactivation.[27]

Novel insights into the origin of reciprocal gene rearrangements

Chromosome abnormalities initiating childhood ALL might arise spontaneously and frequently as accidental by-products of the endogenous proliferative, apoptotic, or metabolic stress of haemopoiesis.[8] The production of a functional chimeric fusion gene requires not only the simultaneous presence of DSBs in two chromosomes, but also their proximity at a particular time point, perhaps in a repair complex.[8] Although DSBs can occur randomly throughout the genome, they may nevertheless cluster in particularly vulnerable regions, such as open chromatin configurations and chromosomal scaffold attachment sites. The increased incidence of secondary leukaemias with an *MLL* gene rearrangement in children who had previously been treated with topoisomerase II inhibitors instigated experiments that helped to resolve this issue. They revealed that DNA cleavage at this particular locus results from chromatin fragmentation during the initial stages of drug-induced apoptosis. These findings provided the basis for the fascinating hypothesis that such reciprocal rearrangements are commonly generated by rescuing early stage apoptotic cells by means of emergency NHEJ repair.[8] It also helped to partly explain the non-randomness of such recurrent rearrangements and the fact that they can be generated by very heterogeneous stimuli, such as increased cell turnover during physiologic B-cell development, cytostatic drugs, radiation or even viral infections. The detection of DNA-sequence patterns that are typical for NHEJ repair at the respective fusion sites render it likely that this is the predominant route for the generation of the majority of leukaemia- and sarcoma-associated chimeric fusion genes.

Translocations that involve the immunoglobulin (*IG*) and T-cell-receptor (*TCR*) loci, on the other hand, lead solely to a constitutive overexpression of the respective fusion partner without altering its gene structure; for example *MYCC* in the case of the Burkitt-lymphoma-associated t(8;14)(q24;q32). In contrast with the chimeric fusion genes, these types of gene fusions are commonly mediated by the RAG proteins and V(D)J recombinase. Under physiologic conditions, these enzymes promote somatic recombination in precursor B and T cells, which is a prerequisite for the generation of the *IG* and *TCR* repertoire.

More than 600 reciprocal chromosome rearrangements have been identified so far. They are highly specific markers for particular subentities of haematologic malignancies and solid tumours. The breakpoints of more than 285 such translocations and inversions have already been cloned and the approximately 280 genes involved have been characterized. Interestingly, only a small number of genes are frequently involved, whereas a large number are involved in a few or single rearrangements (Table 2.3).

Analysis and evaluation of genetic alterations

Particular features of neoplasms can be studied at any of the levels outlined in Figure 2.1.[2] In particular, the genome itself and several of the subsequent levels can be investigated with two different, but complementary, approaches, namely morphologically using microscopy and chemically using molecular genetic techniques.[16,21] The morphologic methods include all types and variations of light and fluorescence microscopy techniques, such as conventional cytogenetics and fluorescence *in situ* hybridization (FISH). On the other hand, all molecular

Table 2.3. The top 10 most frequently involved genes

Gene	No. of partners	Associated neoplasms
MLL	50	ALL and AML
IGH	21	B-cell lymphoma and ALL
ETV6	21	ALL and AML
NUP98	18	AML, T-ALL
BCL6	15	Lymphoma
RET	12	Papillary thyroid carcinoma
ALK	12	Lymphoma
EWSR1	11	Ewing sarcoma family
RUNX1	10	ALL and AML
E2A	5	Childhood ALL

ALL, acute lymphoblastic leukaemia; AML, acute myeloblastic leukaemia.

genetic methods aim to obtain information about the composition of a particular DNA or RNA sequence for comparison with a known reference.[9] Although the large number of methods are based on a few general principles, most of them have evolved into highly complex technologies whose application usually requires very sophisticated and expensive technical equipment. Examples of these methods are Southern blot analyses, as well as all types of polymerase chain reactions (PCRs) and DNA sequencing. Separation of the DNA- and RNA-based FISH methods from the cellular and nuclear topologic context led to the development of microarray or chip technology, which simultaneously allows the comparative analysis and evaluation of several thousand sequences.[10,28] The expectation is that technologies such as bacterial artificial chromosome (BAC) microarrays for the high-resolution detection of genetic changes and cDNA-based, oligonucleotide-based, or high-throughput proteomics approaches for the detection of gene expression will eventually facilitate the characterization of the complex network of interactions that are associated with the development of neoplasms.[2,16] However, it has been pointed out that these spectacular technologies are seductive and sometimes corrupting, and one should not commit the mortal sin of genomics and confuse throughput with output and data with knowledge.[10]

The selective forces of the internal and external environment

The two sides of mutagens and carcinogens

The external environment always exerts its influence on the DNA level in combination with genetic and acquired susceptibility.[11,18] Cancer-promoting agents not only leave their footprints on DNA, but also shape the somatic evolution of the entire genome of cancer cells.[3] Epidemiologic surveys together with clinical observations and intricate genetic analyses provide an increasing variety of illustrative examples for this idea, particularly in leukaemias of infants and young children.[8] Although it is becoming increasingly evident that genetic instability is a non-random event, the currently prevailing assumption is that mutagens and carcinogens damage the genome randomly and that the environmental risk for cancer is a direct consequence of exposure to environmental mutagens. However, this proposal has recently been challenged.[3,29] Based particularly on analyses and comparisons of *in vitro* and *in vivo* incidence and distribution rates of point mutations in various tumours and cell cultures, several researchers now consider that this originally plausible hypothesis is, to a large extent, unsupported by evidence. They believe that the contribution of environmental factors to point mutagenesis is negligible, except for very specific circumstances, such as exposure to solar radiation, chemo- and radiotherapy, or the *in vitro* exposure of cells. As an alternative, they suggest that most tumour-associated mutations result primarily from endogenous processes, such as errors during the turnover of undamaged DNA, whereas environmental conditions would be more likely to select than induce such 'oncomutations'.[3,29] One of the arguments is that the likelihood of DNA polymerase errors remains the same, irrespective of whether DNA bases are excised from damaged or undamaged DNA. Moreover, a DNA turnover rate of 1% per cell per day would require much more intensive DNA repair than the excision repair of even a million DNA damage sites.

At first glance this novel view of the role of mutagens appears counter-intuitive, but on further consideration it seems quite plausible. It fits very well with what we have discovered within the last few years about the molecular foundation of fusion genes. Regardless of the specific mechanism of their induction—be it chromosome breakage, cellular endonucleases, chemical interactions with topoisomerase II inhibitors or RAG-mediated cleavage—the final common denominator is an endogenous process, the NHEJ repair.[8]

The significance of (cancer) stem cells

Although tumour-initiating mutations may theoretically take place in any type of proliferating cell, they are only likely to have a clonal advantage in the context of a particular developmental pathway.[8] This is obviously the case when pluripotent stem cells or committed progenitor cells are the target. Therefore it comes as no surprise that cancer cells not only share the self-renewal and differentiation capabilities of normal stem cells, but also utilize the same tissue-specific and tissue-dependent signalling pathways. Since stem cells are mostly non-cycling cells, they should not be particularly susceptible to DNA damage. However, their utilization during periods of increased cell demand such as during fetal development and the maturation and activation of the immune system, as well as during regenerative rebounds, might render them significantly more vulnerable. Moreover, the self-renewal machinery is already activated in stem cells and it may be much simpler and require fewer mutations to maintain it than to reactivate it completely.[8]

Stem cells are essential for embryogenesis and for the preservation of many tissues.[30] The observation that many aspects of tumour development mimic organogenesis gone awry fuelled the idea that tumour growth and metastasis may be driven in a similar fashion by a small, but specialized, population of cancer stem cells. This hypothesis was further corroborated by the results of *in vitro* and *in vivo* clonogenic assays that were obtained with a variety of tumour tissues and cell lines. This fascinating and intellectually challenging concept has tantalizing and wide-ranging implications for cancer research as well as for cancer treatment.[30] If confirmed, it will necessitate a shift in diagnostic and therapeutic endeavours from the currently more general quantitative to a very specialized qualitative level. It will probably prove more difficult to identify and characterize the properties of these comparatively rare cancer stem cells than it was to single out the normal ones. As in normal differentiating cell lineages, cancer stem cells can most probably be distinguished from most of their more harmless descendants only by virtue of subtle functional differences, and not on the basis of their shared rearranged genetic make-up. To cure cancer it would be sufficient to simply kill these cancer stem cells rather than to eliminate the whole bulk of neoplastic cells. A successful therapy would then appear as 'spontaneous remission'. The concept of cancer stem cells also explains why even complete clinical and molecular remissions might spare cells that eventually cause a relapse. As is the case with normal stem cells in the physiologic situation, cancer stem cells could even prove to be more resistant to chemotherapeutics than their more 'mature' offspring. Despite their high sensitivity, the techniques currently employed for the detection of minimal residual disease would then prove insufficient to discriminate between these functionally heterogeneous cells. Finally, the shutting down or regression of transformed stem cells could also lead to spontaneous remissions, such as those regularly encountered in TMD and 4S-stage neuroblastoma.

The role of deterministic and stochastic information

Selective growth can arise in a cellularly autonomous fashion by mutation in the prospective cancer cell, by differences in the regulatory microenvironment, or more usually by some combination of both.[2,31] The environment provides deterministic and stochastic stimulating and inhibiting information to this process.[26] Deterministic information comprises specific predetermined signals, for example growth factors and hormones, whereas stochastic information appears primarily as random noise. However, driven by chance, it can also be converted into signals under special circumstances. One example of such a process in a physiologic situation is the genetically determined generation of antibody diversity.[26] Pre- and postnatal development, maturation, and challenge of the immune system, in particular, generate an enormous genetic diversity, and incidentally also provide the fateful repertoire of mutations that trigger the development of the various forms of childhood ALL. Screening of umbilical cord blood as well as the peripheral blood of healthy adults indicates that a variety of leukaemic fusion genes are generated much more frequently than the incidence of the respective leukaemias would suggest.[32] This implies that one or more additional genetic hits and selective steps are required for the disease to develop. In the aetiology of childhood ALL, for example, the proliferative stress associated with deficient infectious exposure in infancy and an abnormal immune response to subsequent delayed common infections should constitute pivotal factors, according to Greaves' hypothesis.[5] A well-established example of a stochastic trigger is the contribution of malaria to the development of endemic Epstein–Barr-virus-positive Burkitt lymphoma.

Childhood cancer: a disease of disturbed prenatal development
Solid tumours

As early as 1877, the German pathologist Julius Cohnheim first formulated the theory that most childhood malignancies arise when the delicate balance between growth, development, and differentiation of early fetal organogenesis is disrupted. This theory is based on the histopathologic demonstration of putative premalignant lesions at autopsy that resemble neuroblastoma and Wilms tumour (nephrogenic rests) and, more recently, on the detection of leukaemia-specific fusion genes in the umbilical cord blood and Guthrie cards of healthy neonates.[4,5,8,32] The high frequency of such events (approximately 1–5 per cent) suggests that paediatric cancers may be initiated at a high rate, but with only a low risk of penetrance to malignancy.[8,32] Depending on their particular genetic make-up, such premalignant lesions may regress, mature, or progress. Regression and maturation are features that are unique to certain childhood malignancies and virtually never encountered in adult neoplasms. One of the main reasons for this exclusivity may be that these faulty or delayed processes essentially mirror just two of the fundamental components of physiologic organ development.

Twin studies

The extraordinary opportunity that twins, and occasionally triplets, offer for the investigation of the developmental timing, natural history, and molecular genetics of paediatric leukaemia has recently been reviewed by Greaves.[7] With the help of molecular markers, such as clone-specific IG and TCR gene rearrangements and unique fusion gene sequences, it has been shown that leukaemias in concordant twins have a common clonal origin. The explanation for this intriguing finding is that, at least in twins with a single monochorionic placenta, the pre-leukaemic cells spread from one twin to the other via a shared blood circulation. In other instances, this may occur via vascular anastomoses. However, postnatal latency can vary considerably between twins and the onset of leukaemia can occasionally be delayed by up to 14 years. This observation supports the notion that as yet undetermined factors must cause the final leukaemic transformation during the postnatal period.[5]

Leukaemias

Given the very young age at onset, a prenatal origin of infant leukaemia must of course be expected. Indeed, some cases are even diagnosed neo- or prenatally. However, the surprising insight that we have now gained from an innovative series of 'back-tracking' experiments is that most childhood ALL and AML cases which are diagnosed in the first decade of life are also initiated in utero.[5,32] Even more surprising are the results of sophisticated IG and TCR gene rearrangement studies, which indicate that, except for leukaemias with an MLL/AF4 gene rearrangement, the first transforming hit must take place at a very early stage, i.e. between weeks 7 and 9 of gestation. The only genetically defined subtype for which a prenatal origin has not yet been proved is the more mature form of pre-B ALL with a t(1;19) and an E2A/PBX1 gene rearrangement.[8]

Implications for clinical management

The combined insights obtained from twin studies, Guthrie cards, and umbilical cord blood screening contribute significantly to our understanding of the biologic basis of leukaemias. These analyses have now unequivocally ascertained that childhood leukaemias in general originate from an early prenatal transforming event. Nevertheless, it is still unclear what exactly constitutes this first initiating step. To a large extent, the order in which the further sequences of events take place and how they ultimately lead to the development of these life-threatening diseases is also unknown. Furthermore, preliminary but compelling evidence suggests that concurrently generated presumptive preleukaemic cells coexist with overt leukaemic blasts at diagnosis and that they may survive chemotherapy and occasionally spawn later relapses.[8] These discoveries have significant implications and consequences not only for the design, conduct, and interpretation of molecular genetic epidemiologic studies which examine caus-ality, but also for PCR-based monitoring of MRD in childhood leukaemias.

Finally, the spectacular results of these investigations also provide the basis for risk assess-ment and counselling in cases of twins with asynchronous disease manifestations. This risk may approach 100% for identical monozygotic infant twins who shared a single monochorionic placenta. In parallel with the general decrease in the age-associated incidence rate, it then also declines to approximately 10 per cent in older children[7] (see also Chapter 1). Because the calculated risks are still substantial, clinical surveillance, at least, of the healthy co-twin seems to be justified. However, a more thorough molecular scrutiny is definitely warranted if a co-twin is to be considered as a donor.

Appendix. Websites with further information about haematologic neoplasms and solid tumours

Title/topic	Web address
Human Genome Project	http://www.ornl.gov/TechResources/ Human_Genome/
Human Genome Sequence	http://genome.ucsc.edu/
Cancer Genome Anatomy Project	http://cgap.nci.nih.gov/
Cancer Index	http://www.cancerindex.org/
Online Mendelian Inheritance in Man (OMIM)	http://www.ncbi.nlm.nih.gov/Omim/
Atlas of Genetics and Cytogenetics in Oncology and Haematology	http://www.infobiogen.fr/services/chromcancer/ index.html
Mitelman's Database of Tumor-Associated Cytogenetic Abnormalities	http://cgap.nci.nih.gov/Chromosomes/ Mitelman
Family Cancer Database	http://facd.uicc.org/intro.shtml
Pathways of Life	http://www.biocarta.com/genes/index.asp
Gene Cards	http://bioinfo.weizmann.ac.il/cards/
Human Gene Mutation Database (HGMD)	http://archive.uwcm.ac.uk/uwcm/mg/ hgmd0.html
Human Mutation Databases	http://www.hgmp.mrc.ac.uk/GenomeWeb/ human-gen-db-mutation.html
Universal Mutation Database	http://www.umd.necker.fr/
Fanconi Anemia Mutation Database	http://www.rockefeller.edu/fanconi/mutate/
Gene Tests and GeneClinics	http://www.geneclinics.org/
International Forum for Human Molecular Genetics	http://www.hum-molgen.de
Imprinting	http://www.geneimprint.com/
Webliography for Clinical Geneticist	http://www.faseb.org/genetics/webliog.htm
Molecular Diagnostic Laboratories (EDDNAL)	http://www.eddnal.com/
Links to Genetic Databases	http://www.cdc.gov/genomics/info/ database.htm
Genetics Education Center	http://www.kumc.edu/gec/
Support Groups	http://www.kumc.edu/gec/support/
American Association for Cancer Research	http://www.aacr.org/
American Society of Hematology	http://www.hematology.org
American Society of Human Genetics	http://www.ashg.org/
European Hematology Association	http://www.ehaweb.org/
European Society of Human Genetics	http://www.eshg.org/
European Working Group on Pediatric Myelodysplastic Syndromes (EWOG-MDS)	http://www.ewog-mds.org/
International Society of Paediatric Oncology (SIOP)	http://www.siop.nl/

References

1. **Green DR, Evan GI** (2002). A matter of life and death. *Cancer Cell* 1, 19–30.

2. **Anonymous** (2001). Nature insight: cancer. *Nature* 411, 336–95.

3. **Breivik J** (2001). Don't stop for repairs in a war zone: Darwinian evolution unites genes and environment in cancer development. *Proc Natl Acad Sci USA* 98, 5379–81.

4. **Maris JM, Denny CT** (2002). Focus on embryonal malignancies. *Cancer Cell* 2, 447–50.

5. **Greaves M** (1999). Molecular genetics, natural history and the demise of childhood leukaemia. *Eur J Cancer* 35, 1941–53.

6. **Hanahan D, Weinberg RA** (2000). The hallmarks of cancer. *Cell* 100, 57–70.

7. **Greaves M, Maia AT, Wiemels JL, Ford AM** (2003). Leukemia in twins: lessons in natural history. *Blood*, 102, 2321–33.

8. **Greaves M, Wiemels J** (2003). Origins of chromosome translocations in childhood leukaemia. *Nat Rev Cancer*, 3, 639–49.

9. **Hood L, Galas D** (2003). The digital code of DNA. *Nature* 421, 444–8.

10. **Anonymous** (2000). Nature insight: functional genomics. *Nature* 405, 820–65.

11. **Anonymous** (2003). The double helix—50 years. *Nature* 421, 396–453.

12. **Jones PA, Baylin SB** (2002). The fundamental role of epigenetic events in cancer. *Nat Rev Genet* 3, 415–28.

13. **Steenman M, Westerveld A, Mannens M** (2000). Genetics of Beckwith–Wiedemann syndrome-associated tumors: common genetic pathways. *Genes Chromosom Cancer* 28, 1–13.

14. **Anderson GR, Stoler DL, Brenner BM** (2001). Cancer: the evolved consequence of a destabilized genome. *Bioessays* 23, 1037–46.

15. **Pihan G, Doxsey SJ** (2003). Mutations and aneuploidy: co-conspirators in cancer? *Cancer Cell* 4, 89–94.

16. **Balmain A** (2001). Cancer genetics: from Boveri and Mendel to microarrays. *Nat Rev Cancer* 1, 77–82.

17. **Maser RS, DePinho RA** (2002). Connecting chromosomes, crisis, and cancer. *Science* 297, 565–9.

18. **Perera FP** (1997). Environment and cancer: who are susceptible? *Science* 278, 1068–73.

19. **Huff V** (1998). Wilms tumor genetics. *Am J Med Genet* 79, 260–7.

20. **Garber JE, Offit K** (2005). Hereditary cancer predisposition syndromes. *J Clin Oncol* 23, 276–92.

21. **Albertson DG. Collins C, McCormick F, Gray JW** (2003) Chromosome aberrations in solid tumors. *Nat Genet* 34, 369–76.

22. **Rainis L, Bercovich D, Strehl S, et al.** (2003). Mutations in exon 2 of GATA1 are early events in megakaryocytic malignancies associated with trisomy 21. *Blood*, in press.

23. **Shannon K** (1992). Genetic alterations in leukemia: events on a grand scale. *Blood* 80, 1–2.

24. **Downing JR, Shannon KM** (2002). Acute leukemia: a pediatric perspective. *Cancer Cell* 2, 437–45.

25. **Brodeur GM** (2003). Neuroblastoma: biological insights into a clinical enigma. *Nat Rev Cancer* 3, 203–16.

26. **Knudson AG** (2001). Two genetic hits (more or less) to cancer. *Nat Rev Cancer* 1, 157–62.

27. **Fodde R, Smits R** (2002). Cancer biology. A matter of dosage. *Science* 298, 761–3.

28. **Anonymous** (2002). The chipping forecast. *Nat Genet* 32 (Suppl), 461–552.

29. **Thilly WG** (2003). Have environmental mutagens caused oncomutations in people? *Nat Genet* 34, 255–9.

30. **Reya T, Morrison SJ, Clarke MF, Weissman IL** (2001). Stem cells, cancer, and cancer stem cells. *Nature* 414, 105–11.

31. **Rubin H** (2001). Selected cell and selective microenvironment in neoplastic development. *Cancer Res* 61, 799–807.

32. **Mori H, Colman SM, Xiao Z, et al.** (2002). Chromosome translocations and covert leukemic clones are generated during normal fetal development. *Proc Natl Acad Sci USA* 99, 8242–7.

Chapter 3

Molecular biology of childhood tumours

Rogier Versteeg

The challenge

The past 20 years of clinical cancer management have brought great success: cure rates for many paediatric tumours have reached 80 per cent or higher. This remarkable progress in treatment has been achieved without a significant contribution from the insights obtained in molecular biologic cancer research, although major contributions to prognostic classification have come from cytogenetic identification of chromosomal translocations, particularly in leukaemias and lymphomas. Treatment has been mainly improved by new variations on the classical treatments: cytostatic drugs, radiation, and surgery. However, since the molecular identification of the first oncogene in the late 1970s, basic cancer research has seen an extraordinary development in the understanding of mechanisms which control normal and aberrant cell division. The challenge for the next decennium will be to use these insights to improve cancer treatment further.

Many tumours are still refractory to current therapies. Some tumour types have seen relatively little progress in improving outcome (e.g. neuroblastoma), while other diagnoses still include a small percentage of aggressive and incurable tumours (e.g. Wilms tumour). Diagnostic difficulties persist and current classifications are often insufficiently sensitive to identify high-risk tumours at diagnosis. In addition, it is necessary to spare patients with favourable diagnoses from aggressive therapies which may cause severe side effects during treatment, and from the late effects of the therapy which are now recognized as an increasing problem in survivors of childhood cancer. Can the fundamental insight into the molecular machinery that drives the cancer cell be used to solve these problems?

Several major contributions can be expected in the next few years. These promise significant breakthroughs in treatment and are now moving beyond the stage of speculation. Two particular developments can be highlighted. First, many proteins that cause cancer have been identified. They are mutated forms of normal cellular proteins and there is an opportunity to develop drugs that specifically block these oncogenic proteins. Secondly, new technologies can now analyse the level of expression of all genes in a tumour. This permits the construction of a blueprint for the genetic constitution of a large series of tumours and allows the identification of gene expression patterns that may mark the different clinical and biologic subtypes of a tumour. This approach should facilitate tumour stratification and ultimately offer opportunities for more individualized therapy. Despite such optimism, some caution is also justified. Cancer cells are renowned for their plasticity and their ability to escape from treatment strategies; this may limit the realization of opportunities offered by new technology.

Cancer proteins: general principles

Hundreds of genes and proteins play an essential role in cancer pathogenesis. They contribute to cancer when they are either too active or too inactive. Oncogenes contribute to cancer when they are overactive. This arises, for example, by activating mutations or by mechanisms of overexpression. Tumour suppressor genes normally function to control cell division and homeostasis. When these genes are inactivated, for example by chromosomal defects or mutations, cells can become cancerous. The pathogenesis of cancer is generally considered as a multistep process in which defects in several oncogenes and/or tumour suppressor genes combine to result in uncontrolled cell growth. The oncogenes and tumour suppressor genes so far identified can be categorized in to several main groups according to their function in the cell. Most cancer cells have defects in genes in several functional categories, which include the following: loss of cell cycle control; signal transduction defects; DNA stability control defects; apoptosis defects; metastatic capacity.

Loss of cell cycle control

The most central part of a cancer cell is the machinery that drives cell division. During the G_1 phase, the cell grows and prepares for division. The G_1 phase is followed by the S phase, in which replication of the DNA occurs. The next phase of the cell cycle is the G_2 phase, in which DNA replication is completed and the cell prepares for division, which proceeds in the M phase. After the M phase, cells can either continue cycling by starting a new G_1 phase or enter the resting phase (G_0 phase). The cell cycle is a tightly controlled process, driven by a series of proteins called cyclins and cyclin-dependent kinases (CdKs). When complexed with the appropriate cyclin, CdKs can phosphorylate the Rb protein, which results in the functional activation of proteins of the E2F family and the subsequent activation of the gene transcription program necessary for cell division. The cyclins and CdKs that promote cell division are controlled by a series of small inhibitory proteins called cyclin-dependent kinase inhibitors (CKIs).

Most cancer cells have defective cell cycle machinery. For instance, retinoblastoma is characterized by homozygous defects in the Rb gene (the first tumour suppressor gene that was identified) and the Rb gene is mutated in patients with familial retinoblastoma. Other examples of defects in cell cycle genes include gene amplification of cyclins (e.g. cyclin D1 in breast cancer and, sporadically, in neuroblastoma).

Signal transduction defects

Hundreds of genes in the cell play a role in signal transduction. This is the process by which extracellular signals are received by receptors on the cell membrane and transmitted to the nucleus where they induce transcription programs. Signal transduction plays a role in hundreds of physiologic processes, including regulation of differentiation and cell division. Examples of components of the signal transduction cascade that can play a role in cancer are membrane receptors for extracellular growth factors. These can be mutated in a way which permanently activates the downstream cascade even when no growth factor is bound to the membrane receptors. A well-studied signal transduction pathway that is activated in many tumours is the Wnt–APC pathway (Figure 3.1). This is best understood for its role in colon cancer, but the pathway is also activated in hepatoblastoma. In normal colon, the mucosal crypts harbour rapidly dividing epithelial cells that migrate apically to the villi. Epithelial cells of the villi do not divide, and ultimately die. The Wnt–APC pathway controls the transition of

The Wnt–APC pathway

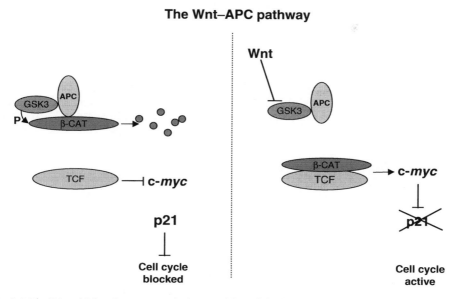

Fig. 3.1 The Wnt–APC pathway controls the transition of dividing cells to non-dividing cells in several tissue types (e.g. colon epithelium). Wnt is an extracellular protein, and when it binds to membrane receptors a signal is transmitted to a complex consisting of the proteins GSK3-β and APC, inactivating the complex and releasing the protein β-catenin (β-CAT). β-Catenin enters the nucleus where it forms a complex with the TCF transcription factor and induces transcription of the c-myc gene. In turn, c-myc transcription silences the gene for the protein p21. As p21 normally blocks the cell cycle, the final result of Wnt induction is activation of the cell cycle.

the rapidly dividing epithelial cells in the crypts to the differentiated non-dividing cells on the villi. The Wnt growth factor is locally produced in the crypts and can activate receptors on the surface of the epithelial cells. As the cells migrate away from the crypts towards the villi, they lose the Wnt signal and start to express p21, resulting in blockage of the cell cycle. Most colon tumours have inactivating mutations in the APC gene which result in the inappropriate release of β-catenin, activation of c-myc and promotion of uncontrolled cell division in the absence of the Wnt signal.

This illustration is an oversimplification as the Wnt–APC pathway involves many more genes, and mutations can arise elsewhere in the pathway. For instance, β-catenin is frequently mutated in hepatoblastoma and, sporadically, in Wilms tumour and medulloblastoma. These mutations prevent the normal breakdown of the β-catenin protein, and accumulation of the protein results in the activation of the cell cycle. Many other signal transduction routes can ultimately activate the cell cycle, but an understanding of the Wnt pathway illustrates how defects in signal transduction can promote uncontrolled cellular growth.

DNA stability control defects

Hundreds of genes in a cell are dedicated to the faithful preservation of the genetic information stored in the DNA. The billions of cells in the body are under the permanent influence of mutagenic events (e.g. sunlight, endogenously produced oxygen radicals, or genotoxic compounds from the environment). Mutations in DNA are detected by a series of specialized proteins which have a direct link to several of the fundamental processes in the cell. When DNA damage is limited, these proteins can stop cell division so that the cell has time to repair defects before they are replicated and irreversibly fixed. In parallel with the signal sent to the cell cycle machinery, this process recruits a series of repair proteins that restore the original DNA sequence. However, when the DNA damage is beyond a certain threshold, the system considers the cell to be beyond repair and drives it into apoptosis (see below). Many cancer cells have defects in the genes that mediate the repair of damaged DNA. Examples are the MSH1 and MSH2 genes that are defective in many colon cancers. When such genes become mutated in a single somatic cell, the cell can accumulate hundreds of other mutations. Some of these mutations may affect oncogenes and/or tumour suppressor genes, which can lead to cancer. Another gene with a central role in repair regulation is p53. The p53 protein is the intermediate between the proteins that identify the DNA defects and the switch that decides whether the affected cells should stop dividing or go into apoptosis. Inactivating mutations of the p53 gene are among the most prevalent defects in tumours and, when present, damage is no longer adequately dealt with, as the cell cycle cannot be stopped.

Apoptosis defects

Each cell has an intrinsic machinery to allow it to commit suicide ('programmed cell death'). The machinery can be triggered by many different stimuli. These stimuli can be physiologic signals, for example in neuronal cells during embryogenesis, or by an attack by T cells that activates the intrinsic apoptotic machinery in virally infected cells. Cells with serious DNA damage or which have aberrant expression of oncogenes are also driven into apoptosis. In general, it is believed that inappropriate combinations of growth-stimulating signals trigger apoptosis as a surveillance mechanism against cancer. Therefore it is not surprising that many tumour cells display defects in their apoptotic machinery. If these are defects that prevent the death of aberrant cells, this will result in their continued proliferation and outgrowth to tumours.

Two main routes to apoptosis have been identified. There is an extrinsic route, activated by extracellular molecules like interferon-γ or TRAIL. These molecules bind to so-called 'death-receptors' which transduce the apopotic signal to the caspase 8 protein. Activated caspase 8 can subsequently activate the so-called 'executioner caspases' which damage cellular proteins and ultimately destroy the chromosomes by fragmenting the DNA. The cell decomposes in a controlled way and is cleaned up by macrophages. There is also an intrinsic route to apoptosis. This route is activated by, for example, extensive DNA damage or inappropriate oncogene activation. Mitochondria play a key role in the activation of the intrinsic route. Pro-apoptotic signals trigger the release of the mitochondrial protein cytochrome c. Outside the mitochondrium, cytochrome c forms a complex with other proteins that triggers the activation of caspase 9. Caspase 9 also activates the executioner caspases, promoting a final process similar to that achieved by the extrinsic route.

Several genes functioning in the apoptosis pathway can be defective in tumours. The *bcl*-2 gene controls the release of cytochrome c from mitochondria in the intrinsic apoptotic pathway. In B-cell lymphoma, the *bcl*-2 gene is permanently activated by a chromosomal translocation (t8;14) and thereby inhibits the release of cytochrome c, blocking the subsequent path to apoptosis. The *bcl*-2 gene is a member of a larger g family of genes that all control cytochrome c release, and many tumours show aberrant expression of this family. The extrinsic route to apoptosis can also be inactivated in tumours. For instance, aggressive neuroblastomas may lack expression of caspase 8 with an inability to progress the apoptotic pathway.

Metastatic capacity

One of the hallmarks of malignant tumours is their metastatic capacity. Until recently, it was assumed that clonal evolution of primary tumours led to subclones with a metastatic capacity. In other words, metastasis was considered as a discrete step in malignant development, resulting from altered gene expression or new mutations. Many genes have been identified that affect the metastatic capacity of tumour cells in experimental settings. However, in human tumours, hardly any mutations have been identified in genes that primarily function to confer a metastatic phenotype. Recent experiments have challenged the concept of clonal selection in the primary tumour and progressive acquisition of metastatic capacity by subclones. This implies that the combination of genes that causes the primary tumour also determines whether the tumour is metastatic or not, and that metastatic capacity may not represent a discrete step in malignant progression.

Is there a fundamental difference between paediatric and adult cancer?

It is an open question whether paediatric tumours have an essentially different mechanism of pathogenesis and progression from adult tumours. The emerging picture is that one or more characteristic genetic aberrations are found in each tumour type, but that they represent variations on the same theme. For instance, although neuroblastoma and medulloblastoma can have amplification of the N-*myc* oncogene, adult small-cell lung tumours can also show the same aberration. The N-*myc* gene is member of a small gene family, which also includes the c-*myc* and L-*myc* genes. The N-*myc* and c-*myc* genes have very similar functions. The c-*myc* gene can also be amplified in small–cell lung cancer, and is also amplified or rearranged in numerous other tumours, including leukaemia. Therefore activation of the *myc* genes cannot be seen as an exclusive property of paediatric tumours. The same holds for activation of cell cycle genes. The cyclin D1 oncogene is amplified or overexpressed in neuroblastoma, and also in several adult tumours. There are certainly aberrations that are specific for some paediatric tumours, like the EWS–FLI translocations in Ewing sarcoma and the PAX–forkhead transloca-tions in rhabdomyosarcoma. However, certain adult tumours also show specific genetic aberrations, and the existence of specific abnormalities in paediatric tumours does not indicate a special biologic characteristic of childhood cancer.

A clear-cut biologic characteristic of paediatric tumours is their peak incidence at an early age and their disappearance after this age. With some exceptions, the adult tumours are of other tissue or cell types, and show an age-related increase in incidence. However, this does not necessarily imply a different biology: both types of tumour stem from rapidly dividing tissues, and the rapid cell division during embryogenesis and infancy gives a window of opportunity for tumours, just as the cumulative number of cell divisions in tissues with a rapid turnover may do in adults (e.g. affecting the epithelial cells of colon, breast, and lung).

Another potential difference between paediatric and adult tumours could lie in aberrations of control genes for embryonal development. Studies of *Drosophila* embryogenesis have identified many genes controlling the differentiation of tissues and organs. These genes appear to be faithfully conserved in humans and many appear to be mutated in human tumours. So far, there is no specific evidence for a prevalence of such genes to be mutated in paediatric cancer, although suggesting that these genes play a role not only in early embryogenesis, but also in the control of cell division and differentiation in adult tissues. For instance, the Wnt–APC pathway is involved not only in the differentiation of early embryonal cell lineages but also in colon epithelium in adults. Accordingly, mutations in the Wnt–APC pathway are found in some paediatric tumours and in some adult tumours.

In conclusion, it is difficult to describe any specific molecular biology of paediatric tumours. All tumour types, adult and paediatric, clearly show genetic aberrations that cause disturbances in a series of major cellular pathways, such as those controlling the cell cycle, apoptosis, signal transduction, and DNA stability. The encouraging consequence is that new drugs developed to specifically inhibit proteins in these pathways may work just as well in tumours at all ages.

Towards protein-specific drugs

The identification of many of the proteins that cause, or contribute to, the malignant transformation of cells has started a huge effort to identify molecules that might specifically inhibit these proteins. Most promising are the so called 'small molecule' drugs. While other approaches like gene therapy, immune therapy or antisense therapy are still experimental, the first small molecules that specifically inhibit the protein products of oncogenes have already successfully entered the therapeutic arena.[1] The best example is imatinib mesylate (STI571, Gleevec™), a small molecule that specifically blocks the activity of the Abelson protein, a tyrosine kinase. The *abl* gene is translocated and activated by the translocation of chromosomes 9 and 22 in chronic myeloid leukaemia (CML) and also in a subset of childhood acute lymphoblastic leukaemia (ALL). Gleevec was developed as a specific inhibitor of the tyrosine kinase activity of the Abelson protein. It is clinically highly successful in the treatment of CML, and trials on high-risk childhood Ph$^+$ ALL are ongoing (see Chapter 5). Unfortunately, a small percentage of patients develop tumour resistance to Gleevec; the Abelson protein is mutated in some of these resistant tumours, and Gleevec is no longer able to inhibit the mutated form. Another form of resistance may result from *de novo* amplification of the *abl* gene in relapsed tumours. Although Gleevec inhibits the tyrosine kinase activity of the Abelson protein, it has also been found to inhibit some related tyrosine kinases, for example the c-Kit tyrosine kinase that plays a central role in gastrointestinal stromal cell tumour (GIST). As tyrosine kinases are members of a large gene family and function in many different cellular processes, Gleevec is currently being tested in a range of tumours, and other drugs are being developed to act against other cell cycle proteins and growth factor receptors.

The development of these new types of cancer drugs is very expensive and it is inevitable that pharmaceutical companies will focus their efforts on the development of drugs for the major types of adult cancer. However, some of these drugs may also hold promise for paediatric tumours, as many of the pathways initially identified as playing a role in one specific cancer are later found to be involved in other tumour types as well. Examples include the Wnt–APC pathway, originally identified in colon cancers but also activated in hepatoblastoma, medulloblastoma and Wilms tumour, and the N-*myc* oncogene, which was originally identified as an amplified oncogene in neuroblastoma but is also amplified in small-cell lung carcinoma. Therefore it will be very important to test drugs developed for adult use in preclinical models of paediatric tumours and in subsequent clinical studies.

It is also possible that some oncogenes are activated only in one paediatric tumour type, but although this might represent a perfect target for a drug, the relatively small number of patients with a specific paediatric tumour is unlikely to encourage efforts to develop drugs for such targets. However, the lesson of Gleevec is that a drug originally developed against one specific protein in one specific tumour may ultimately have a much wider therapeutic spectrum, and on this basis it would be economically more interesting to develop novel drugs directed against proteins known only to cause cancer in children.

How complete is our understanding of oncogenesis?

The functional categories of genes involved in cancer, described above, are relatively imprecise. Hundreds of oncogenes and tumour suppressor genes have been identified and, although most of them can be tentatively placed in one of these functional categories, the complexity of the mechanisms involved precludes the precise characterization of many of them. Each cell type has its own developmental program which is modulated by cues from surrounding tissues. Therefore each tissue can have its specific receptors for these cues and a specific signal transduction cascade that activates or blocks the cell cycle. Thus it is likely that many different signal transduction routes converge on the cell cycle. As a consequence, defects may exist in many different routes, all with the same effect—uncontrolled cell division.

Although many of the basic principles of oncogenesis have been identified in the past 25 years, major elements have probably escaped detection. For example, in neuroblastoma, only the N-*myc* gene (and, to a lesser extent, caspase 8) has been identified as a major mechanism, yet amplification and overexpression of N-*myc* is only found in 20 per cent of neuroblastomas. In the remaining 80 per cent of neuroblastomas, not a single gene has been identified that causes tumorigenesis. However, many structural chromosomal defects have been identified in neuroblastoma, for example extra copies of the long arm of chromosome 17 (17q+) and deletions of long stretches of one copy of chromosome 1(1p del) or chromosomes 4, 11, and 14. This suggests that these chromosomal regions could harbour important genes which might contribute to pathogenesis. Although several candidates for such genes have been proposed, clear identification is awaited. The picture described for neuroblastoma holds for many other childhood tumours. Often only one or two major abnormalities are identified, complemented with impressive series of chromosomal defects with an unknown role in oncogenesis. Much effort is still needed to gain sufficient information to understand the pathogenesis of individual tumours at the molecular level.

Microarrays: a tool for molecular classification of tumours

One of the most far-reaching investigative tools (brought about by work on the Human Genome Project) is genetic profiling by microarray technology. Microarrays can measure the mRNA expression levels of all genes in a tissue or cell line in a single experiment. A microarray consists of thousands of DNA sequences representing human genes which are arranged in a grid on a small solid surface (e.g. a microscope slide). Each array can contain up to 20 000 spots, with each spot representing one gene. Messenger RNA is isolated from a tumour, labelled with a fluorescent dye, and incubated with the array. Homologous mRNA sequences associate with their complementary DNA on the array. Therefore highly expressed mRNAs produce a fluorescent marker at the site of their corresponding gene. The array is scanned with a laser to measure and map the level and distribution of fluorescence, indicating the activity of genes within the tumour. In this way, one experiment, taking only a few days, can assess the expression of 20 000–40 000 human genes.

The application of microarray technology to large series of human tumours describes the gene expression profile of each tumour type in great detail. Sophisticated software can search for patterns in the expression profiles and relate them to the biologic or clinical characteristics of the tumours. For example, studies of a large series of leukaemias have been able to identify expression profiles that discriminate between T-ALL, B-ALL and acute myeloid leukaemia (AML).[2] In other examples, a series of 'small round cell blue tumours' reveal expression profiles which discriminate between neuroblastoma, rhabdomyosarcoma, Ewing sarcoma, and Burkitt lymphoma.[3] These experiments reflect the old clinical insight that tumours of a specific tissue lineage share certain essential characteristics. More important for the clinician is the possibility that this technology could identify prognostic subgroups within a single tumour type. When the clinical course of a series of, for example, 100 tumours analysed by microarray is known, statistical analyses can identify gene sets that may together predict the prognosis of individual patients. As hundreds of genes can be included in these prognostic profiles, the results may be more discriminating than prognosis based on classical analyses. For example, microarray evaluation of a series of medulloblastomas can reliably discriminate between the desmoplastic and classical subtypes and, more importantly, can also identify a gene expression pattern that predicts survival.[4] A similar analysis of a series of leukaemias showed that ALLs with a translocation of the MLL gene, which is known to be a poor prognostic marker, have a gene expression pattern that discriminates them from other ALLs and AMLs and suggests a resemblance to an early haematopoietic progenitor.[5] These tumours were found to have a high expression of the FLT3 gene, a receptor tyrosine kinase. This finding has also opened therapeutic opportunities, as a novel small molecule drug (PKC412) that inhibits the FLT3 kinase activity and could inhibit cell growth was active in a mouse model of MLL-activated tumours.[6]

Microarrays have also been used to identify a set of genes that predict the metastatic potential of tumours. The results of such experiments imply that the gene expression profile of a primary tumour may predict its later metastatic spread (see above), suggesting that metastatic cells do not result from a progressive selection of more aggressive subclones but are similar to the primary tumour cells. Metastatic potential may then be an intrinsic property of the primary tumour. Clinically, this implies that it may become possible to assess the risk of metastasis at first diagnosis.[7]

The predictive power of many microarray analyses should improve with further enhancement at both a technical level and the level of statistical analysis of the complex data generated.

Towards a tailored therapy for each patient: how far in the future?

Microarray technology shows great promise in the prediction of response to therapy. By analysing the expression profiles of a large tumour series, it should be possible to establish whether tumours that respond to a specific therapy have a different expression profile from that seen in non-responding tumours. This could ultimately improve the selection of treatment for individual patients. Array technology will be even more promising when combined with treatment protocols which include innovative target drugs that inhibit specific proteins, such as Gleevec. As these drugs are directed against only one or a few proteins, it should be possible to use the gene expression profile of the tumour from an individual patient to predict, on the basis of gene expression, whether the tumour is likely to respond to treatment with the specific drug. Therefore the availability of rapid screening systems for gene expression profiles of individual tumours, combined with the development of series of novel drugs that can specifically inhibit oncoproteins, raises the hope that individualized therapies may become available in the not too distant future.

References

1. **Smith JK, Mamoon NM, Duhe RJ** (2004). Emerging roles of targeted small molecule protein-tyrosine kinase inhibitors in cancer therapy. *Oncol Res* **14**, 174–225.

2. **Golub TR, Slonim DK, Tamayo P, et al.** (1999). Molecular classification of cancer: class discovery and class prediction by gene expression monitoring. *Science* **286**, 531–7.

3. **Khan J, Wei JS, Ringner M, et al.** (2001). Classification and diagnostic prediction of cancers using gene expression profiling and artificial neural networks. *Nat Med* **7**, 673–9.

4. **Pomeroy SL, Tamayo P, Gaasenbeek M, et al.** (2002). Prediction of central nervous system embryonal tumour outcome based on gene expression. *Nature* **415**, 436–42.

5. **Armstrong SA, Staunton JE, Silverman LB, et al.** (2002). MLL translocations specify a distinct gene expression profile that distinguishes a unique leukaemia. *Nat Genet* **30**, 41–7.

6. **Armstrong SA, Kung AL, Mabon ME, et al.** (2003). Inhibition of FLT3 in MLL. Validation of a therapeutic target identified by gene expression based classification. *Cancer Cell* **3**, 173–83.

7. **van't Veer LJ, Dai H, van de Vijver MJ, et al.** (2002). Gene expression profiling predicts clinical outcome of breast cancer. *Nature* **415**, 530–6.

Chapter 4

The principles of cancer chemotherapy in children

Gilles Vassal and Arnauld Verschuur

Introduction

The majority of malignancies occurring in childhood are sensitive to cytotoxic chemotherapy. This chemosensitivity is generally attributed to the high proliferation rate of childhood malignancies and the capacity of the malignant cells to become apoptotic. Therefore chemotherapy plays a major role in the treatment of paediatric malignancies and contributes to the still improving outcome for the majority of them. However, several malignancies remain refractory to chemotherapy (some intracranial tumours, several metastatic malignancies, some acute leukaemia, some types of soft tissue sarcoma, advanced stages of neuroblastoma, etc.). Moreover, the long-term toxicity of some chemotherapeutic compounds has become obvious during the last decade. Therefore it is necessary to understand the mechanisms of therapeutic failures and long-term toxicity. The unravelling of these mechanisms may lead to the development of novel treatment modalities.

Principles of chemotherapy

In general, a chemotherapy-based strategy aims first at obtaining complete remission and then at eradicating the minimal residual disease (MRD). Several molecular biologic techniques have been developed for the detection of MRD in solid tumours and haematologic malignancies using a (semi)quantitative analysis of tumour-specific and patient-specific gene expression.

In acute lymphoblastic leukaemia (ALL) complete remission is obtained by multi-agent chemotherapy which forms the induction therapy. In addition, intrathecal and intravenous chemotherapy ensures prophylaxis of the central nervous system. According to the protocol and/or patient characteristics, a consolidation or re-induction therapy is applied before the start of maintenance therapy aiming at the eradication of MRD.

In paediatric solid tumours, chemotherapy is adapted to the histologic and/or clinical diagnosis and to the stage of the malignancy. This chemotherapy aims at obtaining regression of the primary tumour in order to facilitate its surgical resection. Moreover, the chemotherapeutic regimen will treat the distant metastases whether they are detectable or not. This preoperative chemotherapy has the advantage of evaluating the chemosensitivity of a particular tumour in a specific patient. It also acts on non-detectable metastases in the earliest stage. Postoperative chemotherapy is essentially required for the treatment of undetectable metastases or MRD. An example of this therapeutic strategy is the treatment of osteosarcoma (see Chapter 19). In other malignancies, surgical removal of the localized primary tumour is followed by chemotherapy, and in some cases radiotherapy, to achieve optimal local control and to treat undetectable distant metastases. An example of this therapeutic strategy is the treatment of medulloblastoma (see Chapter 17).

Chemotherapeutic regimens

Chemotherapy is mostly given in combination regimens of two or more cytotoxic agents. These courses are given sequentially using various combinations to increase the probability of destroying the maximum number of malignant cells. The choice of chemotherapeutic agents depends on several factors such as tumour type, preclinical evidence of *in vitro* cytotoxicity and cellular mechanisms of cytotoxicity of a specific drug, evidence of *in vivo* single-drug activity, and the expected toxicity of the proposed chemotherapy course. Sometimes preclinical data from *in vitro* models or *in vivo* animal models have shown a synergistic effect of two or more compounds. However, most of the standard chemotherapy regimens developed during the last three decades have not been evaluated in paediatric tumour models before their use in children.

Classification of chemotherapeutic agents

There are several classes of anticancer drugs which are defined by their mode of action. In general, drugs of different classes are chosen for combination regimens in order to use different cytotoxic mechanisms to destroy malignant cells. The following classification is used for drugs prescribed in paediatric oncology:

The **antimetabolite compounds** interfere with the synthesis of precursors for DNA and RNA. They can be divided into pyrimidine antimetabolites (cytarabine, gemcitabine, cyclopentenyl cytosine, 5-fluorouracil) and purine antimetabolites (6-thioguanine, 6-mercaptopurine, fludarabine, cladribine, clofarabine). All these drugs inhibit the synthesis of DNA and/or RNA.

The **antifolates** (aminopterin, methotrexate, trimetrexate) form a distinct group of antimetabolites. These drugs inhibit the enzyme dihydrofolate reductase and decrease the synthesis of pyrimidine and purine (deoxy)ribonucleotides, resulting in decreased synthesis of thymidylate (TMP) which is a precursor of DNA.

The **antimicrotubule compounds** include the vinca alkaloids (vincristine, vinorelbine, vinblastine) and the taxanes (paclitaxel, docetaxel). They interfere with the tubulin assembly required for the formation of microtubules which are essential for the cellular architecture, especially during cell replication when they form the mitotic spindle. Microtubules also have a function in intracellular transport, neurotransmission, and signal transduction pathways.

Alkylating agents include a broad spectrum of cytotoxic drugs. The alkylating drugs are able to form covalent bonds between alkyl groups and cellular molecules such as deoxyribonucleotides in DNA. Alkylation alters DNA and its replication. If these DNA lesions are not repaired, the cell dies. The first alkylating agent to be used clinically was mechlorethamine, also known as nitrogen mustard. This drug was derived from the clinical observations of severe lymphopenia after the use of mustard gas in the First World War. Mechlorethamine is still being used for the treatment of Hodgkin lymphoma. Other alkylating agents that have a prominent role in paediatric oncology are cyclophosphamide, ifosfamide, melphalan, busulfan, thiotepa, and nitrosoureas such as carmustine (BCNU) and lomustine (CCNU). All these agents generate cross-links between or within the two DNA strands. The methylating agents, such as procarbazine, dacarbazine (DTIC), and the recent drug temozolomide, alter DNA but do not generate cross-links. The alkylating agents physically alter DNA. They may induce mutations and secondary malignancies such as myelodysplasia.

Platinum compounds have a similar mode of action to the alkylating agents. However, instead of forming a covalent bond between alkyl groups and nucleotides in DNA, the platinum compound acts through an interaction between the platinum atom and DNA, RNA, or proteins. In DNA, the platinum atom covalently binds to two deoxynucleotides, resulting in intrastrand adducts or interstrand cross-links, leading to DNA damage.

Topoisomerase II inhibitors act by interfering with the enzyme topoisomerase II which plays a role in the unfolding of the DNA molecule during DNA replication, transcription, and repair. The classical examples of topoisomerase II inhibitors are the epipodophyllotoxins such as etoposide (VP16) and teniposide (VM26). The anthracyclins, of which doxorubicin, epirubicin, daunorubicin, and idarubicin are well-known examples, form another major class of topoisomerase II inhibitors. The anthracyclins also act through other cytotoxic mechanisms such as DNA intercalation and the production of reactive oxygen radicals. Mitoxantrone is not a classical anthracyclin and acts predominantly through intercalation of DNA strands.

Topoisomerase I inhibitors include the camptothecins such as topotecan and irinotecan (CPT 11). They act through inhibition of the enzyme topoisomerase I which is involved in DNA relaxation. Topoisomerase I inhibitors have recently been shown to have a beneficial antitumour effect in some paediatric solid tumours.[1]

Antitumour antibiotics are bleomycin and dactinomycin. The former acts through the oxidative cleavage of DNA, whereas the latter predominantly acts through binding to DNA, inhibition of RNA and protein synthesis, and inhibition of topoisomerases.

L-**Asparaginase** has a distinct mode of action since it depletes the plasma and intracellular levels of the amino acid asparagine. Since lymphoblasts do not have the capacity to synthethize asparagine because of insufficient activity of the enzyme asparagine synthetase, the drug L-asparaginase has a proven cytotoxic activity in the treatment of ALL.

Some drugs induce differentiation of malignant cells, for example the high doses of retinoic acids used in the treatment of neuroblastoma.

Apoptosis of malignant cells without using the cytotoxic mechanisms summarized above can be achieved by the corticosteroids prednisone, prednisolone, and dexamethasone. They induce apoptosis in ALL cells after binding to the steroid receptors in the cellular membrane. The mechanism through which this leads to apoptosis is being investigated at present

Cytotoxic and targeted drugs developed during the past decade, such as the taxanes (paclitaxel, docetaxel), the topoisomerase I inhibitors (irinotecan, topotecan), temozolomide, and the new platinum compound oxaliplatin, have shown antitumour activity in several adult cancers. These compounds are now in clinical development in paediatric oncology (see Chapter 5). New drugs in clinical development for the haematologic malignancies are the nucleoside analogues fludarabine, cladribine, gemcitabine, cyclopentenyl cytosine, clofarabine, and troxacitabine, and receptor kinase inhibitors such as imatinib.

Toxicity of chemotherapy

Since most chemotherapeutic compounds act on proliferating cells, some normal replicating tissues (bone marrow, gastrointestinal mucosa, and hair follicle bulbs) are at particular risk for toxicity of chemotherapy. Therefore most compounds have a transient toxic effect on these organs. Moreover, some drugs may have a specific toxicity for one or more organs. For example, the anthracyclins are well known for their potential cardiotoxicity. Cisplatinum, and to a lesser extent carboplatin, may be ototoxic and/or nephrotoxic. Methotrexate may be hepatotoxic. In addition, the use of alkylating agents may result in secondary malignancies and impaired fertility in the long term. This latter toxicity depends on the type and cumulative dose of the alkylating agent used and is to a lesser extent dependent on gender. Epipodophyllotoxins may induce secondary myelodysplasia and/or acute myeloblastic leukaemia (AML).

The specific toxicities of the various compounds used in paediatric oncology are listed in Table 4.1. A grading classification for the scoring of toxicity has been developed by the National Cancer Institute [NCI Common Toxicity Criteria (NCI-CTC)] and can be accessed at http:// ctep.cancer.gov/reporting/ctc.html.

Dose intensity

Since the cytotoxic effects of chemotherapy affect both malignant cells and non-malignant physiologically dividing tissues, the toxicity of each compound and each combination should be taken into account. Because the therapeutic window of a chemotherapeutic compound is narrow and there is often a dose–effect relationship, chemotherapy is frequently given at the maximum tolerated dose to obtain the maximum antitumour effect.[2] The concept of dose intensity is defined by the amount of drug administered per unit time. Treatment at high dose intensities has proved to be of benefit in several paediatric tumours, especially Burkitt lymphoma where more than 90 per cent of patients can be cured by intensive combination regimens of relatively short duration (6 months).[3] The concept of dose intensity implies a high probability of severe toxicity (either haematologic or non-haematologic) and requires the shortest intervals possible between sequential chemotherapy courses. Any delay in drug administration decreases the intensity of the administered drugs, leading to a possibly less efficacious treatment. During the last decade, novel treatment modalities (anti-emetic therapy, haematopoietic growth factors) have been developed for supportive care (see Chapter 8) to reduce the toxic side effects of chemotherapy while maintaining its dose intensity.

High-dose chemotherapy

Another step forward for dose intensity is high-dose chemotherapy followed by autologous or allogeneic haematopoietic stem cell transplantation. Several cytotoxic compounds have a linear or almost linear dose–effect relationship. These compounds are suitable for high-dose administration, especially when the toxicity of these drugs is essentially haematologic since the reinfusion of haematopoietic stem cells will ensure effective reconstitution of haematopoiesis after the chemotherapy. Thus the maximum therapeutic effect is obtained and non-haematologic toxicity becomes dose limiting. High-dose chemotherapy strategies are generally applied in situations of very good partial or complete remission in patients with a chemosensitive tumour but a high risk of relapse. The dose–effect relationship increases the probability of destroying residual malignant cells and/or overcoming cellular mechanisms of drug resistance. The most prominent examples of chemotherapeutic agents used for high-dose chemotherapy are the alkylating compounds such as cyclophosphamide, busulfan, melphalan, and thiotepa. In paediatric oncology, high-dose chemotherapy is used in neuroblastoma, Ewing sarcoma, osteosarcoma, medulloblastoma, and relapsed or high-risk leukaemia.[4,5] The quality of haematopoietic stem cell grafts has increased in the last few years, such that such a strategy can sometimes be performed in an ambulatory setting. However, the real value of high-dose treatment strategies in paediatric oncology is still a matter of research and debate.

In the case of allogeneic grafts, especially in acute leukaemia, the immunologic phenomenon of graft versus leukaemia has an additional antitumour effect in addition to the cytotoxic effects of chemotherapy and total body irradiation.

Table 4.1. Specific adverse effects of cytotoxic compounds used in paediatric oncology*

Compound	Short-term side effects	Long-term side effects
Asparaginase	Clotting disorders, anaphylactic reactions, pancreatitis, hyperglycaemia	Unknown
Bleomycin	Fever, malaise, skin rash	Pulmonary fibrosis
Busulfan	Veno-occlusive disease, seizures, hyperpigmentation	Hyperpigmentation, pulmonary fibrosis, fertility disorders
Carboplatin	Ototoxicity, allergic reactions	Ototoxicity
Cisplatin	Renal toxicity, ototoxicity, radiosensitizing	Renal toxicity, ototoxicity
Cyclophosphamide	Haemorrhagic cystitis	Fertility disorders, secondary leukaemia
Cytarabine	Mucositis, rash, conjunctitis, fever, encephalopathy, seizures, pancreatitis	Encephalopathy
Dactinomycin	Jaundice, veno-occlusive disease, radiosensitizing	Unknown
Daunorubicin	Mucositis, cardiomyopathy, radiosensitizing	Cardiomyopathy, secondary leukaemia
Dexamethasone	Mood disorders, increased appetite, Cushingoid appearance, muscular atrophy, bone demineralization, skin disorders	Bone fractures, avascular femoral head necrosis, vertebral flattening, hypocortisolism
Doxorubicin	Mucositis, cardiomyopathy, radiosensitizing	Cardiomyopathy, secondary leukaemia
Epirubicin	Mucositis, cardiomyopathy, radiosensitizing	Cardiomyopathy, secondary leukaemia
Etoposide (VP 16)	Allergic reactions, mucositis	Secondary leukaemia
Fludarabine	Mucositis, fever, pneumonitis, neurotoxicity, hepatitis	Unknown
Idarubicin	Mucositis, cardiomyopathy, radiosensitizing	Cardiomyopathy, secondary leukaemias
Ifosfamide	Haemorrhagic cystitis, tubulopathy, encephalopathy, seizures	Tubular and glomerular toxicity, fertility disorders
Irinotecan	Abdominal pain, diarrhoea, sweating, hyperlacrimation, salivary excess	Unknown
Melphalan	Mucositis, interstitial pneumonitis	Pulmonary fibrosis, fertility disorders
6-Mercaptopurine	Hepatitis	Unknown
Methotrexate	Hepatitis, mucositis, encephalopathy, renal toxicity	Liver fibrosis, encephalopathy
Mitoxantrone	Mucositis, cardiomyopathy	Cardiomyopathy
Prednisolone	Mood disorders, increased appetite, Cushingoid appearance, muscular atrophy, bone demineralization, skin disorders	Bone fractures, avascular femoral head necrosis, vertebral flattening, hypocortisolism
Procarbazine	Allergic reactions, hepatic dysfunction, headache, paraesthesia, hallucinations	Fertility disorders
Teniposide (VM 26)	Allergic reactions, mucositis	Secondary leukaemia
6-Thioguanine	Hepatitis	

Table 4.1. (Continued) Specific adverse effects of cytotoxic compounds used in paediatric oncology*

Compound	Short-term side effects	Long-term side effects
Thiotepa	Headache, encephalopathy, dizziness, allergic reactions, skin rash, fever	Fertility disorders
Topotecan	Mucositis, radiosensitizing	Unknown
Vinblastine	Paraesthesia, neuralgia, sensory disorders, hypertension, Raynaud's phenomenon	Raynaud's phenomenon
Vincristine	Paraesthesia, neuralgia, muscular weakness, sensory disorders, constipation, ileus, abdominal cramps, seizures, SIADH	Neurotoxicity

* The adverse effects are categorized as short-term (days to weeks) and long-term (months to years) side effects. General adverse effects such as bone marrow depression, gastrointestinal toxicity, and alopecia are not included since these side effects are considered as common to all chemotherapy.

Response evaluation

The evaluation of tumour response to treatment is based upon strict criteria of measurements in one, two, or three dimensions of all measurable tumour sites. There is international consensus for documenting response according to WHO or RECIST criteria (Table 4.2). In some tumour types specific response evaluation criteria can be used, as is the case for neuroblastoma where the International Neuroblastoma Response Criteria are generally adopted.

Drug resistance

During the past three decades there has been much preclinical research aimed at unravelling the various mechanisms of drug resistance. Multidrug resistance (MDR) is a well-known mechanism of drug resistance. Several proteins are implicated including MDR1, multidrug resistance proteins 1–8 (MRP), breast cancer resistance protein (BCRP), and lung-resistance-related protein (LRP). High expression of these membrane proteins in tumour cells has been correlated with a poor outcome in some malignancies in paediatric oncology, although the issue

Table 4.2. Methods of response evaluation after chemotherapy

	WHO*	RECIST†
Measurements	Product of two perpendicular diameters; sum of products, in case of multiple lesions	Largest diameter; sum of diameters, in case of multiple lesions
Complete response (CR)	Total regression of any lesion	Total regression of any lesion
Partial response (PR)	≥50% decrease and absence of any new lesion	≥30% decrease and absence of any new lesion
Stable disease (SD)	<50% decrease or <25% increase	<30% decrease or <20% increase
Progressive disease (PD)	≥25% increase or presence of new lesion(s)	≥20% increase or presence of new lesion(s)
Objective response rate	CR + PR	CR + PR

*World Health Organization (1979). *Handbook for Reporting Results of Cancer Treatment*. Geneva: WHO, 48.
†Therasse P, Arbuck SG, Eisenhauer EA, *et al.* (2000). New guidelines to evaluate the response to treatment in solid tumors. European Organization for Research and Treatment of Cancer, National Cancer Institute of the United States, National Cancer Institute of Canada. *J Natl Cancer Inst* **92**, 205–16.

remains controversial. Various preclinical models have been developed to circumvent the MDR-related mechanism of drug resistance. However, clinical trials using MDR blocking agents (verapamil, cyclosporin A, PSC 833) have failed to demonstrate a clinical benefit. Apparently, other cellular mechanisms that are not circumvented by MDR blocking agents also contribute to drug resistance.

Dosing drugs in paediatric oncology

Body surface area

The principle of using body surface area (BSA) for dosing chemotherapeutic compounds in oncology results from pharmacologic research between species and between adults and children. These research data showed that the most reliable method of comparing physiologic variables, such as glomerular filtration rate, cardiac output and basal metabolic rate, between species is by correcting for BSA.[6] Using body weight instead of BSA proved to result in an unreliable interspecies correction of all mechanisms contributing to the clearance and metabolism of drugs. Since the therapeutic window of cytotoxic compounds is generally narrow and cytotoxic drugs are generally prescribed at nearly the maximum tolerated dose, it is common practice in paediatric oncology to prescribe drugs in milligrams per square meter to correct for morphometric variability between patients. Although the use of BSA is controversial in adult oncology, the variation of weight and length is so great in children that the prescription should still be based on BSA in paediatric oncology. Moreover, if cytotoxic drugs are prescribed per square meter, it is easier to determine a starting dose for phase I clinical trials in humans based on the data reported in toxicologic studies in animal models.

The BSA can be calculated using either formulae or nomograms. The gold standard formula was proposed in 1916 by Dubois and Dubois[7] (Table 4.3). Although this formula is very reliable, it is not easy to use. Many other formulae,[8] taking into account either weight and length or weight only, have been validated (Table 4.3).

Chemotherapy in infants

The tolerance to chemotherapy at a given dose is poorer in infants than in older children.[9] Therefore doses should be reduced in infants. Several physiologic mechanisms that contribute to the pharmacokinetics of drugs mature during the first year of life.[10] For instance, the water content of the human body decreases from 75 per cent at birth to 60 per cent at 1 year and 55 per cent in the adult. The content of plasma proteins also changes during the first year of life. Hepatic drug metabolizing enzymes (cytochrome P-450 isoenzymes, UDP glucuronyltransferase, glutathione metabolizing enzymes) acquire their physiologic activity between 6 and 12

Table 4.3. Formulae for calculating body surface area (BSA), body mass index (BMI), and ideal body weight

Dubois' formula	$BSA(m^2) = W^{0.425} \times L^{0.725} \times 0.007184$
Mosteller's formula	$BSA(m^2) = \sqrt{W} \times L/3600$
Formula without using length	$BSA(m^2) = (4W + 7)/(W + 90)$
Body mass index (Quetelet index)	$BMI(kg/m^2) = [W(kg)]/[L(m)]^2$
Lawrence's formula	Ideal body weight (kg) = [length (cm) − 100] − {[length (cm) − 150]/K}

W, body weight (kg; L, body length (cm); $K = 4$ for males and $K = 2$ for females.

Table 4.4. Comparison between dose prescribed in mg/m² and dose prescribed in mg/kg for children

Age	Weight (kg)	BSA (m²)	Calculated dose (mg)		Dose reduction (%)
			For 100 mg/m²	For 3.33 mg/kg	
10 years	30	1	100	100	0
1 year	10	0.46	46	33	28
3 months	6	0.29	29	20	31

months of age. The renal glomerular filtration rate attains values comparable to the adult at the age of 5 months. All these developing clearance mechanisms contribute to a poor tolerance of infants to chemotherapy.

Generally, chemotherapy in infants should be prescribed based on milligrams per kilogram body weight rather than milligrams per square meter since the relationship between body weight and BSA in infants is different from that in older children (Table 4.4 and Fig. 4.1). A dose prescribed in milligrams per square meter in infants leads to a higher dose than a prescription in milligrams per kilogram (Table 4.4). One should be even more cautious when prescribing cytotoxic drugs for very young children (<3 months).

Chemotherapy in obese patients

Obesity is associated with modifications in body composition which may change the pharmacokinetics of the cytotoxic compounds and result in inadequate dosing and increased toxicity.[11] The increased content of fatty tissues will alter the distribution volume of drugs depending on the affinity of the drug for fatty tissues and plasma proteins. Fatty degeneration of liver tissue may also modify the hepatic metabolizing capacities in obese patients. The diagnosis of obesity is defined by an increased body mass index (BMI) according to the Quetelet index (Table 4.3).

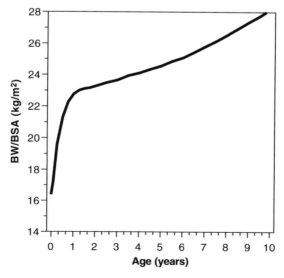

Fig. 4.1 Development of ratio of body weight (BW) to body surface area (BSA) during childhood.

Upper reference values for adults (>18 years) are $23 \, kg/m^2$ in males and $21 \, kg/m^2$ in females. Overweight and obesity are defined by BMI values $> 25 \, kg/m^2$ and $> 30 \, kg/m^2$, respectively. In children the BMI changes with increasing age. Therefore the upper reference values of BMI defining obesity depend on age and sex (Table 4.5).[12]

In order to prescribe cytotoxic drugs appropriately in obese patients it would be necessary to have pharmacokinetic data for a drug in a population of obese patients compared with patients with a normal body composition. However, no such data are available for most cytotoxic compounds. In the absence of such pharmacokinetic data, it is recommended that a cytotoxic compound is prescribed on the basis of the ideal body weight rather than the real body weight. The ideal body weight for adolescents and young adults can be calculated using Lawrence's formula (Table 4.3). In younger children the ideal body weight is determined by the body weight corresponding to the actual length of the patient.[12]

Prescribing chemotherapy in extreme situations

Some patients may require chemotherapy in an acute situation where mechanisms of clearance are failing either because of the malignancy or as a result of previous treatments. For example, there might be renal or hepatic insufficiency resulting in prolonged clearance of a drug and therefore potentially increased toxicity. In such situations, prescribing chemotherapy should be adapted to the patient, taking into account the type of drug used and the mechanisms of clearance that are relevant for that drug. Moreover, the potentially specific toxicity for the affected organ should be taken into account when prescribing a cytotoxic drug. In these extreme situations it might be useful to determine plasma concentrations of the prescribed drugs using a low test dose. Computer models can predict an adjusted dose if clearance is decreased.

For recommendations or dose adaptations in cases of renal or hepatic insufficiency the reader is referred to the handbook *Cancer Chemotherapy and Biotherapy.*[13]

Intrathecal chemotherapy

The volume of the central nervous system is proportionally larger in the young child than in the adolescent and adult and does not correlate with the BSA. A child aged 4–6 years has a central nervous system volume of 80–90 per cent of the adult brain, whereas the adult value of the BSA is not attained until the age of 16–18 years.[14] Thus intrathecal therapy, such as metrotrexate, should be prescribed in an absolute dose (milligrams) depending on the age rather than in milligrams per square meter.

Pharmacogenetics and drug interactions

The metabolic mechanisms of an organism contribute to the clearance of drugs by transforming them to metabolites which facilitate renal or biliary excretion. These metabolites usually have less therapeutic activity than the parent drug, or no therapeutic activity at all, although some may still have a strong cytotoxic effect. Many enzymes are implicated in the biotransformation of drugs; the cytochrome P-450 isoenzymes, the glucuronidation pathways, and detoxifying enzymes implicated in glutathione metabolism are the most relevant. The various enzyme activities influence the plasma concentration of the drugs and thus the concentrations in tumour tissue. It is useful to know the metabolic pathways of drugs in order to identify or prevent drug interactions. Hepatic mechanisms such as CYP450 enzyme induction or enzyme inhibition may alter the effect of a cytotoxic drug dramatically. Phenobarbital, carbamazepine,

Table 4.5. International cut-off points for body mass index for overweight and obesity by sex for ages 2–18 years[12]

Age (years)	Overweight		Obesity	
	Males	**Females**	**Males**	**Females**
2	18.41	18.02	20.09	19.81
2.5	18.13	17.76	19.8	19.55
3	17.89	17.56	19.57	19.36
3.5	17.69	17.4	19.39	19.23
4	17.55	17.28	19.29	19.15
4.5	17.47	17.19	19.26	19.12
5	17.42	17.15	19.3	19.17
5.5	17.45	17.2	19.47	19.34
6	17.55	17.34	19.78	19.65
6.5	17.71	17.53	20.23	20.08
7	17.92	17.75	20.63	20.51
7.5	18.16	18.03	21.09	21.01
8	18.44	18.35	21.6	21.57
8.5	18.76	18.69	22.17	22.18
9	19.1	19.07	22.77	22.81
9.5	19.46	19.45	23.39	23.46
10	19.84	19.86	24	24.11
10.5	20.2	20.29	24.57	24.77
11	20.55	20.74	25.1	25.42
11.5	20.89	21.2	25.58	26.05
12	21.22	21.68	26.02	26.67
12.5	21.56	22.14	26.43	27.24
13	21.91	22.58	26.84	27.76
13.5	22.27	22.98	27.25	28.2
14	22.62	23.34	27.63	28.57
14.5	22.96	23.66	27.98	28.87
15	23.29	23.94	28.3	29.11
15.5	23.6	24.17	28.6	29.29
16	23.9	24.37	28.88	29.43
16.5	24.19	24.54	29.14	29.56
17	24.46	24.7	29.41	29.69
17.5	24.73	24.85	29.7	29.84
18	25	25	30	30

and phenytoin may induce activity of the CYP3A4 and CYP2C9 isoenzymes, and thus may increase the biotransformation and clearance of many cytotoxic drugs.[15] Drugs such as fluconazole, itraconazole and valproic acid may inhibit the activity of a number of CYP isoenzymes, resulting in higher plasma concentrations and potentially more toxicity of cytotoxic drugs metabolized by these isoenzymes. Therefore drug interactions should be taken into account when prescribing chemotherapy and non-cytotoxic drugs.

During the past decade the influences of these pharmacokinetic-modifying enzymes have been revealed and this has led to population-based studies of pharmacogenetics.[16] Genetic polymorphisms of these enzymes may lead to variable phenotypes, resulting in different enzyme activities from patient to patient and thus a modified clearance. An example of such pharmacogenetic variability is encountered in the metabolism of 6-mercaptopurine which is inactivated by the enzyme thiopurine methyltranferase (TPMT).[17]

In this era of insight into the human genome, new genetic polymorphisms of enzymes or receptors will be detected that are implicated in the metabolism of cytotoxic and non-cytotoxic agents. This may lead to patient-adapted prescription of cytotoxic drugs in the future, taking into account the individual genotype and phenotype of clearance mechanisms.

References

1. Vassal G, Doz F, Frappaz D, *et al.* (2003). A phase I study of irinotecan as a 3-week schedule in children with refractory recurrent solid tumours. *J Clin Oncol* 21, 3844–52.
2. Frei E III, Elias A, Wheeler C, Richardson P, Hryniuk W (1998). The relationship between high-dose treatment and combination chemotherapy: the concept of summation dose intensity. *Clin Cancer Res* 4, 2027–37.
3. Patte C, Auperin A, Michon J, *et al.* (2001). The Société Française d'Oncologie Pediatrique LMB89 protocol: highly effective multiagent chemotherapy tailored to the tumor burden and initial response in 561 unselected children with B-cell lymphomas and L3 leukemia. *Blood* 97, 3370–9.
4. Hartmann O (1995). New strategies for the application of high-dose chemotherapy with haematopoietic support in paediatric solid tumours. *Ann Oncol* 6 (Suppl 4), 13–16.
5. Vassal G, Tranchand B, Valteau-Couanet D, *et al.* (2001).Pharmacodynamics of tandem high-dose melphalan with peripheral blood stem cell transplantation in children with neuroblastoma and medulloblastoma. *Bone Marrow Transplant* 27, 471–7.
6. Reilly JJ, Workman P (1993). Normalisation of anti-cancer drug dosage using body weight and surface area: is it worthwhile? A review of theoretical and practical considerations. *Cancer Chemother Pharmacol* 32, 411–18.
7. Dubois D and Dubois EF (1916). A formula to estimate the approximate surface area if height and weight be known. *Arch Int Med* 17, 863–71.
8. Mosteller RD (1987). Simplified calculation of body-surface area. *N Engl J Med* 317, 1098.
9. Jones B, Breslow NE, Takashima J (1984). Toxic deaths in the Second National Wilms' Tumor Study. *J Clin Oncol* 2, 1028–33.
10. McLeod HL, Relling MV, Crom WR, *et al.* (1992). Disposition of antineoplastic agents in the very young child. *Br J Cancer* 18 (Suppl), S23–9.
11. Cheymol G (2000). Effects of obesity on pharmacokinetics: implications for drug therapy. *Clin Pharmacokinet* 39, 215–31.
12. Cole TJ, Bellizzi MC, Flegal KM, Dietz WH (2000). Establishing a standard definition for child overweight and obesity worldwide: international survey. *BMJ* 320, 1240–3.
13. Chabner BA, Longo DL (2001). *Cancer Chemotherapy and Biotherapy. Principles and Practice.* Philadelphia , PA: Lippincott–Williams & Wilkins.

14. **Bleyer WA, Dedrick RL** (1977). Clinical pharmacology of intrathecal methotrexate. I. Pharmacokinetics in nontoxic patients after lumbar injection. *Cancer Treat Rep* **61**, 703–8.

15. **Vecht CJ, Wagner GL, Wilms EB** (2003). Interactions between antiepileptic and chemotherapeutic drugs. *Lancet Neurol* **2**, 404–9.

16. **Boddy AV, Ratain MJ** (1997). Pharmacogenetics in cancer etiology and chemotherapy. *Clin Cancer Res* **3**, 1025–30.

17. **McLeod HL, Krynetski EY, Relling MV, Evans WE** (2000). Genetic polymorphism of thiopurine methyltransferase and its clinical relevance for childhood acute lymphoblastic leukemia. *Leukemia* **14**, 567–72.

Chapter 5

Future trends in cancer chemotherapy

Elizabeth Fox and Peter C. Adamson

Introduction

Despite substantial improvements in survival, the poor treatment outcome for many high-risk patients, coupled with the acute and late effects of current therapy, emphasize the need to develop more targeted and less toxic therapies for children with cancer.

Development of cytotoxic anticancer agents

In order to appreciate the paradigm shift that has occurred in anticancer drug discovery, it is important to understand the history of drug development that formed the foundation of today's successful therapy, which predominantly relies upon the use of cytotoxic agents.

The successful identification of active anti-leukaemia drugs began in the late 1940s, in part through a process of rational drug discovery of antimetabolites.[1,2] As a result of that effort, methotrexate and mercaptopurine remain the cornerstone of acute lymphoblastic leukaemia (ALL) maintenance therapy to this day.[3,4]

Many of the cytotoxic agents in use today were identified through a large-scale screening process carried out at the National Cancer Institute (NCI). The initial screening programme began in 1955 and relied on L1210 and P388 murine leukaemia *in vivo* models. An *in vitro* screening programme for pure compounds and natural products was implemented in 1985, and by 1990 was fully operational as the NCI-60 cell panel. The 60 human tumour cell lines used in this *in vitro* cytotoxicity screening are exclusively adult histologies.[5] Since the NCI-60 panel screen does not include cell lines from paediatric malignancies, its utility for prioritizing new agents for paediatric drug development is limited.[6]

Only a small number of preclinical animal models have been successfully utilized for paediatric drug development. Therefore other criteria have been relied upon in selecting agents for development in paediatric malignancies,[7] including selecting agents with a novel mechanism of action, a unique resistance profile, or an improved toxicity profile. Agents have also been studied because of favourable pharmacologic properties such as good penetration across the blood–brain barrier, improved oral bioavailability, or a new formulation that altered the distribution and toxicity profile. Most commonly, agents that have shown promising activity in early adult trials have been prioritized for paediatric development.

Unfortunately, activity in adult cancers does not necessarily predict for activity in childhood cancers. This has recently been observed with paclitaxel, a taxane that is highly effective in ovarian, breast, non-small-cell lung, and head and neck cancers[8] but has not demonstrated significant activity in a spectrum of paediatric solid tumours.[9,10]

Identification of novel cytotoxic agents for the treatment of childhood tumours continues to be an active area of clinical research. The current status of novel microtubular toxins in paediatric oncology serves as an example of how continued investigation of cytotoxic agents may improve the care of children with cancer.

Microtubular toxins

Microtubules are critical to cell division, intracellular structure, transport, and cell signalling. Before the advent of molecularly targeted therapy, agents that interfered with tubulin function by disrupting the dynamic equilibrium (polymerization and depolymerization) of tubulin were identified as potent anticancer agents[11] (Fig. 5.1) In 1967, the vinca alkaloids, vincristine and vinblastine, were isolated from the periwinkle plant *Catharanthus roseus* and demonstrated cytotoxic activity via inhibition of tubulin polymerization.[12] Vincristine has a broad spectrum of activity in paediatric cancer including ALL, Hodgkin and non-Hodgkin lymphoma, Wilms tumour, rhabdomyosarcoma, Ewing sarcoma, brain tumours, and neuroblastoma. Vinblastine is active in testicular cancer and Hodgkin's disease. Newer microtubular toxins now expand upon this foundation.

Vinorelbine

Vinorelbine, a semisynthetic derivative of vinblastine, has a broad spectrum of cytotoxic activity, may not be cross-resistant to the other vinca alkaloids, and is orally bioavailable. Vinorelbine appears to selectively inhibit mitotic microtubule formation rather than neural axonal microtubule formation and therefore may be less neurotoxic. In 1994, vinorelbine was approved by the US Food and Drug Administration (FDA) for the treatment of non-small-cell

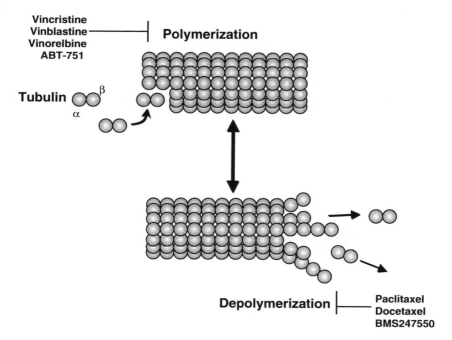

Fig. 5.1 Microtubular toxins. Tubulin, which is composed of α and β subunits, exists in a dynamic equilibrium of polymerization and depolymerization. Microtubulin toxins interfere with microtubule function by disrupting the dynamic equilibrium.

lung cancer in adults. In xenograft models of central nervous system (CNS) malignancies, vinorelbine demonstrated antitumour activity against several adult and paediatric gliomas.[13]

Paediatric phase I and II studies have now been completed. In a paediatric phase I trial of vinorelbine the dose-limiting toxicity was neutropenia and the recommended dose was 33.5 mg/m^2.[14] A Children's Oncology Group (COG) paediatric phase II trial of vinorelbine completed accrual in June 2002. Children with relapsed rhabdomyosarcoma, extraosseous Ewing sarcoma, neuroblastoma, and selected CNS malignancies were treated with i.v. vinorelbine weekly for 6 weeks followed by a 2-week break. Response and toxicity data from this trial are pending. Evidence of activity of vinorelbine in paediatric patients with recurrent sarcoma has been reported in a paediatric trial in Italy in which i.v. vinorelbine 30 mg/m^2 was administered on days 1 and day 8 of a 21-day schedule. Partial responses were observed in six of twelve patients with rhabdomyosarcoma, one of five patients with osteosarcoma, and one of seven patients with Ewing sarcoma.[15]

Taxanes

The taxanes, paclitaxel and docetaxel, inhibit tubulin depolymerization, disrupt the polymerization and depolymerization equilibrium, and thus interfere with microtubule function. As stated above, paclitaxel is active in a variety of adult malignancies but activity has not been demonstrated in paediatric solid tumours. Docetaxel, a semisynthetic taxane, may have activity against selected paediatric solid tumours. Two phase I trials of docetaxel have been completed in children with refractory solid tumours. In the initial trial, docetaxel was administered every 21 days. The MTD was 65 mg/m^2 in heavily pretreated patients and 125 mg/m^2 in less heavily pretreated patients. Dose-limiting toxicity was neutropenia and fatigue.[17] A subsequent study, using the same schedule of docetaxel with granulocyte colony-stimulating factor support, reached an MTD of 185 mg/m^2 with dose-limiting toxicity of desquamating rash and myalgia[18] (Table 5.1) Recently, a phase II study of docetaxel (125 mg/m^2 i.v. every 21 days) in children with refractory solid tumours was completed. Preliminary observations include activity in patients with Ewing sarcoma and osteosarcoma.

Investigational microtubular toxins

Other classes of agents that interfere with microtubule function are being investigated in children with cancer. BMS247550 is an epothilone analogue, a non-taxane microtubule-stabilizing compound, extracted from the fermentation broth of *Sorangium* spp. Epothilones block mitosis, resulting in cell death.[19] BMS247550 has potent cytotoxic activity in paediatric cell lines[20] and is currently being evaluated in a paediatric phase I trial. ABT-751 is a novel orally bioavailable sulfonamide antimitotic agent that binds to the colchicine binding site on

Table 5.1. Dose-limiting toxicities and recommended doses of docetaxel

Patient population	G-CSF	Dose-limiting toxicity	Recommend dose (every 21 days) (mg/m^2)	Reference
Adult	No	Neutropenia	60–100	16
Paediatric (heavily pretreated)	No	Neutropenia, fatigue	65	17
Paediatric (less heavily pretreated)	No	Neutropenia, fatigue	125	17
Paediatric	Yes	Rash, myalgia	185	18

G-CSF, granulocyte colony-stimulating factor.

β-tubulin and inhibits polymerization of microtubules. It has demonstrated a broad spectrum of activity *in vitro* and in xenograft models of human tumours *in vivo* including those that are resistant to paclitaxel, vincristine, and doxorubicin because of the multidrug-resistant phenotype. It was most active in a preclinical murine sarcoma model.[21] The unique binding site for an antimitotic agent, broad spectrum of activity in preclinical studies, and oral bioavailability make ABT-751 a potentially important new agent for evaluation in the paediatric population. A paediatric phase I trial of ABT-751 is being performed.

Molecularly targeted anticancer agents in paediatric oncology

Rapidly accumulating knowledge of the molecular pathogenesis of cancer provides new targets for drug discovery and development resulting in a shift from an empiric random screening of cytotoxic anticancer agents to a more mechanistic target-based approach.

Identification of active molecularly targeted agents often involves high-throughput screening in which large numbers of compounds can be tested for activity as inhibitors or activators of a biologic target. *In vitro* biochemical assays, such as ligand–receptor and protein–protein interactions, or cell-based assays using cell lines or yeast reconstituted with specific targets have been utilized for screening. Specificity, potency, and novel chemical structures are critical factors in screening for lead compounds. Once identified, a lead compound can be optimized and ultimately formulated into a drug.[22]

The clinical development of target-based anticancer drugs may require changes to the traditional clinical trial design and endpoints that have been used for cytotoxic drugs. In the phase I and II setting, the traditional endpoints of toxicity and response may not be appropriate for target-based agents which gain selectivity, in part, in a dose-dependent (concentration-dependent) manner. Traditional endpoints may need to be replaced by biologic or pharmacokinetic endpoints to define the optimal dose and the therapeutic effect of the drug on its target.[23]

Early phase clinical trials of molecularly targeted drugs performed in adults and children must attempt to answer several critical questions. These include the following.[24]

1. Can a sufficient concentration of a drug be achieved safely in blood and in target tumour tissue?
2. Can target inhibition by the agent be demonstrated in the tumour or surrogate tissue?
3. Does target inhibition by the agent result in downstream effects that modulate activity or toxicity?
4. Is the desired biologic effect, such as inhibition of angiogenesis, induction of apoptosis, or inhibition of proliferation or metastasis, observed?

Our increased understanding of the malignant process has identified a spectrum of potential drug targets. Currently, a robust area of drug development is the signal transduction inhibitors, several of which may have a role in the treatment of childhood cancer. Other targets, including the proteosome and histone deacetylase, are actively being pursued as drug targets.

Signal transduction inhibition

Aberrant signal transduction pathways are a hallmark of malignant transformation, tumour initiation, and progression. Numerous agents have been synthesized to target molecules in signal transduction pathways in adult malignancies. Determining the potential role of currently available signal transduction inhibitors for childhood malignancies is an area of ongoing research, with a number of signal transduction inhibitors in early phases of paediatric clinical trials.

Imatinib (Gleevec^{TM})

Imatinib mesylate (STI571, Gleevec™) targets the Bcr–Abl fusion protein, a constitutively activated tyrosine kinase in chronic myelogenous leukaemia (CML). The Bcr–Abl fusion protein is present in 95 per cent of patients with CML, and its tyrosine kinase activity is essential to the malignant transformation in CML. The quest for inhibitors of this tyrosine kinase began in the 1980s using high-throughput screens of chemical libraries. Largely through the research of Dr Brian Druker of The Oregon Health and Science University Cancer Institute, imatinib mesylate was found to inhibit the Bcr–Abl tyrosine kinase as well as the platelet-derived growth factor receptor (PGDF-R) and mutated c-kit in gastrointestinal stromal tumours (GISTs).[25,26] *In vitro* experiments demonstrate that imatinib inhibition of specific tyrosine kinases appears to be concentration dependent[26] (Table 5.2). In 1998, clinical trials with imatinib commenced and the agent received accelerated FDA approval based on response for use in adults with CML in 2001 and GIST in 2002.

A number of paediatric solid tumours are known to over express PDGF-R or c-kit. PDGF-R is expressed on some osteosarcomas, desmoplastic small round blue cell tumours, and synovial cell sarcoma. Some Ewing sarcoma family tumours and neuroblastomas overexpress c-kit or its ligand stem cell factor. Although it is well recognized that expression of protein does not necessarily predict clinical activity of a targeted inhibitor, initial laboratory and paediatric clinical trials of imatinib mesylate are beginning to assess the role of signal transduction inhibitors for children with cancer. A COG phase I trial of imatinib mesylate in paediatric patients with Ph$^+$ leukaemia has been completed; no dose-limiting toxicities were observed and preliminary response rates were similar to those obtained with imatinib in adults with CML. Based in part on this data, imatinib mesylate received FDA approval for the treatment of children with Ph$^+$ CML in May 2003. A COG phase II trial of imatinib in children with refractory or relapsed solid tumours opened in June 2002. In addition to estimating response rates in selected paediatric solid tumours, the trial seeks to determine the time to progression and correlate response to expression of PGDF-R and c-kit in these tumours.

Epidermal growth factor receptor inhibitors

Epidermal growth factor receptor (EGFR) tyrosine kinase is a critical component in the signal transduction cascade related to invasion and metastasis of many tumours.[27] In May 2003, the FDA approved the EGFR inhibitor gefitinib (ZD1839, Iressa^{TM}) for adults with refractory

Table 5.2. Concentration-dependent inhibition of tyrosine kinases by imatinib mesylate

Tyrosine kinase	Imatinib IC$_{50}$ (μM)
Bcr–Abl	0.025
PDGF-R	0.1
c-kit	0.1
Src	>10
Flt-3	>10

IC$_{50}$, concentration achieving 50% inhibition.

non-small-cell lung cancer. A paediatric phase I trial of gefitinib is in progress in the COG. In addition to determining the maximum tolerated dose, toxicity spectrum, and pharmacokinetics in paediatric patients with refractory solid tumours, the expression and activity of EGFR and downstream signalling pathway mediators will be documented and the biologic effects of gefitinib on normal epithelial cells will be studied as pharmacodynamic endpoints. By coupling pharmacokinetic and pharmacodynamic endpoints, this trial aims to determine the optimal biologic dose of gefitinib rather than the maximum tolerated dose of the agent in the paediatric population. A phase I trial of another EGFR inhibitor, OSI-774, is also planned. Since EGRF inhibitors may enhance the cytotoxic effects of standard chemotherapy, OSI-774 will be administered in combination with an alkylating agent (temozolomide) in children with refractory solid tumours.

Farnesyl transferase inhibitors

A number of agents that target *ras* are also being developed for paediatric malignancies. *Ras* genes encode a family of guanosine triphosphate (GTP) binding proteins that play a critical role in the regulation of cell growth and differentiation. Ras proteins are activated by receptor tyrosine kinases on the cell surface and initiate phosphorylation cascades that sequentially activate effectors including Raf-1 and the MAPK pathway, the Rac–Rho pathway, MEK-1 and the JNK pathway, and PI3 kinase. These signal transduction pathways are critical to growth regulation in normal and malignant cells. In order to participate in signal transduction, Ras proteins must be associated with the inner surface of the cell membrane. Membrane association is facilitated by the post-translational addition of a lipid moiety, farnesyl, catalysed by the enzyme farnesyl transferase (FTase) (Fig. 5.2). In normal cells, growth factors bind cell surface receptors causing membrane-bound *ras* to switch from an inactive guanine diphosphate (GDP) bound form to an active GTP-bound form, initiating the signal transduction cascade. In many tumour cells, *ras* is mutated and remains in the active GTP-bound form in the absence of external growth signals. One strategy to inhibit *ras*-mediated signal transduction is to prevent its association with the cell membrane by inhibiting FTase. Two FTase inhibitors are being evaluated in paediatric clinical trials. In studies coordinated by the Paediatric Oncology Branch of the NCI, tipifarnib (R115777, Zarnestra™) is being evaluated in solid tumours, plexiform neurofibroma, and acute leukaemia.[28] In addition to pharmacokinetic studies, pharmacodynamic studies including measurement of FTase activity and inhibition of farnesylation of the protein HDJ-2 in leukaemic blasts or peripheral blood mononuclear cells (PBMCs) from patients are incorporated as surrogate markers of the activity of tipifarnib. A phase I clinical trial of the FTase inhibitor SCH66336 is being conducted for paediatric CNS malignancies by the Paediatric Brain Tumour Consortium.

Vascular endothelial growth factor inhibitors

The growth of solid tumours is dependent, in part, on the tumour's ability to induce the formation of new blood vessels through the process of angiogenesis.[29,30] Tumours secrete proteins, including basic fibroblast growth factor (bFGF) and vascular endothelial growth factor (VEGF), which activate microvascular endothelial cells to proliferate, migrate, and organize into capillary structures.[31] Activated endothelial cells produce cytokines that inhibit cell death (apoptosis) and thus enhance malignant progression.[32] Interaction of growth factors and cytokines from these cells is critical in establishing blood supply to a tumour.

Paediatric solid tumours may be potential targets for anti-angiogenic therapy. Childhood solid tumours can be highly vascular and, compared with adult carcinoma, paediatric sarcomas

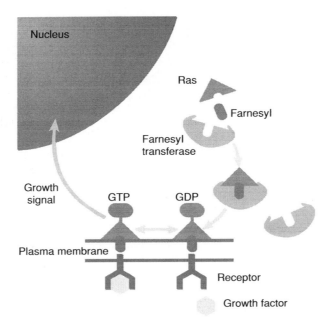

Fig. 5.2 Farnesyl transferase inhibitors. Ras proteins are activated by receptor tyrosine kinases on the cell surface and initiate signal transduction cascades that are critical to cellular growth regulation. To function, Ras proteins must be associated with the inner surface of the cell membrane. Membrane association is facilitated by the addition of a lipid moiety (farnesyl) to Ras by farnesyl transferase. In normal cells, growth factors bind cell surface receptors causing membrane-bound Ras to switch from an inactive GDP-bound form to an active GTP-bound form initiating the signal transduction cascade. In many tumour cells, Ras is mutated and the Ras protein remains in the active GTP-bound form in the absence of external growth signals.

have higher blood flow.[33] Additionally, p53 mutations have been noted in some neuroblastomas, Ewing sarcoma, and osteosarcoma, and since wild-type p53 may induce angiogenesis inhibitors, the loss of p53 gene activity could promote vascularization of paediatric solid tumours.[34]

Many agents, both old and new, can inhibit angiogenesis in laboratory models. Numerous classes of compounds, including small molecules, cytokines, and antibodies, are currently in clinical trials in adults. Selection of agents for clinical trials in paediatric patients requires careful consideration. Small-molecule inhibitors of angiogenesis, including SU5416 and SU6668, showed promising preclinical activity, but did not produce sufficient activity in early adult clinical trials. Development of these agents was discontinued before clinical trials in the paediatric population could be completed. Other agents, including a thrombospondin-1 mimetic and a thalidomide analogue, are currently in phase I clinical trials in adults, and studies in the paediatric population are being considered.

A paediatric phase I trial of the chimeric monoclonal anti-VEGF antibody bevacizumab (Avastin™) will open soon in the COG Phase I Consortium. Bevacizumab has been shown to selectively inhibit VEGF-mediated tumour angiogenesis in laboratory models. In an adult phase I study, bevacizumab was well tolerated and has subsequently shown activity in phase II studies in adults with colorectal cancer.[35,36]

In addition to the promising results from early clinical trials in adults, the decision to move bevacizumab into paediatric clinical trials was supported by studies in paediatric xenograft models including anaplastic Wilms tumour,[37] neuroblastoma,[38] hepatoblastoma, and rhabdomyosarcoma.[39] The paediatric trial of bevacizumab will combine traditional phase I objectives (maximum tolerated dose, toxicities, pharmacokinetics) with measures of potential surrogate antiangiogenic markers including total and free serum VEGF, FGF, ICAM-1, V-CAM-1, and thrombospondin-1.

Other novel agents in development for childhood malignancies

Proteosome inhibitors

Phase I trial designs for molecularly targeted drugs can incorporate both traditional toxicity endpoints and novel methods of measuring target inhibition, as illustrated by the development of the proteosome inhibitor bortezomib (PS-341, Velcade™). Proteosomes are cellular organelles that degrade intracellular proteins and regulate the activity of proteins involved in signal transduction, cell cycle regulation, and metastasis. Bortezomib binds the active site on proteosomes, leading to reversible inhibition of this degradative pathway. No assay is available to measure bortezomib concentrations in plasma. However, a sensitive, specific, and reproducible assay measuring proteosome proteolytic activity in whole blood or PBMCs has been developed to measure the percentage proteosome inhibition by bortezomib in clinical trials. This assay has been used to demonstrate a dose-dependent reversible inhibition of proteosome activity in patients' blood or PBMCs.[40,41] In May 2003, the FDA approved bortezomib for the treatment of multiple myeloma in adults. A phase I trial of bortezomib has been completed in children. As in the clinical trials in adults, percentage proteosome inhibition was used to determine the recommended dose. Clinical trials to combine bortezomib with cytotoxic agents in children with solid tumours and a phase I study in childhood leukaemia are being planned.

Heat shock protein

The ansamycin antibiotics geldanamycin and herbimycin A target the intracellular chaperone heat shock protein 90 (Hsp90). Hsp90 assists proteins, including kinases (Erb-B2, EGFR, Src family kinases, c-Raf-1 and Cdk-4), steroid hormone receptors, and cell cycle and apoptosis mediators, in maintaining stability and conformation. Geldanamycin prevents these proteins from binding the chaperone by competing for the APT binding site on Hsp90. Therefore these proteins are prone to degradation in the presence of geldanamycin.[42] Because of its hepatic toxicity, geldanamycin has limited clinical potential. However, 17-allylamino-17-demethoxygeldanamycin (17AAG), an analogue with reduced liver toxicity, has shown promising clinical activity in adult malignancies and a phase I trial in childhood solid tumours is planned.

Development of drug resistance modifiers in paediatric oncology

Intrinsic or acquired drug resistance poses substantial challenges to treatment in patients with newly diagnosed or recurrent tumours. Our improved understanding of the mechanisms of drug resistance provides possible targets to modulate resistance to chemotherapy.

P-glycoprotein inhibitors

A common mechanism of drug resistance is the multidrug-resistant phenotype (MDR) which is conferred by the presence of P-glycoprotein, a 170-kDa membrane glycoprotein which functions as an energy-dependent drug efflux pump. Chemotherapeutic agents that are substrates for P-glycoprotein include vinca alkaloids, taxanes, anthracyclines, and epipodophyllotoxins. Strategies to block the P-glycoprotein efflux pump in patients have met with limited success, in part due to the use of non-specific competitive inhibitors including cyclosporin or cyclosporin analogues such as valspodar.[43] Recently, agents that specifically block P-glycoprotein have entered clinical trials in adults and paediatric patients with refractory cancers. Tariquidar is a potent inhibitor of basal ATPase activity associated with P-glycoprotein, suggesting that its modulatory effect is derived from inhibition of substrate binding and ATP hydrolyis. *In vitro* tariquidar reverses resistance to doxorubicin, vincristine, and paclitaxel with a potency 10-fold greater than that of the competitive P-glycoprotein inhibitor valspodar. Additionally, tariquidar enhances the cellular accumulation of vinblastine and paxlitaxel in a cell line expressing P-glycoprotein.[44]

A pharmacodynamic assay to determine the function of the P-glycoprotein drug efflux pump has been developed and incorporated into clinical trials of tariquidar in adults and children.[45,46] Lymphocytes (CD56+) which express P-glycoprotein are used as the surrogate tissue. Rhodamine 123 (Rh123), a fluorescent dye and substrate for P-glycoprotein, is added to whole blood collected before and 24 h after the patient receives the P-glycoprotein inhibitor tariquidar. The intracellular accumulation of fluorescent Rh123 in CD56+ lymphocytes is measured using flow cytometry. The percentage inhibition of Rh123 efflux, determined by comparison of the intracellular fluorescence intensity of Rh123 before and after tariquidar administration, increases in a dose-dependent (concentration-dependent) manner.

A phase I trial of tariquidar combined with doxorubicin, vinorelbine, or docetaxel is currently being conducted in paediatric patients with refractory solid tumours. In addition to determining the recommended paediatric dose of tariquidar, the pharmacokinetics of tariquidar alone and in combination with the anticancer agent are being studied, and studies of P-glycoprotein function in surrogate CD56+ lymphocytes and in tumour are being conducted before and after tariquidar administration using $[^{99m}Tc]$sestamibi scanning.

Bcl-2 antisense oligonucleotide

Another strategy being studied in children with cancer is modulation of the expression of the anti-apoptotic protein Bcl-2. Many anticancer agents induce tumour cell death by apoptosis or programmed cell death. The process of apoptosis is regulated by pro-apoptotic and anti-apoptotic proteins. Many tumours, including neuroblastoma, Ewing sarcoma, Wilms tumour, and synovial cell sarcoma, overexpress the anti-apoptotic protein Bcl-2.[47,48] Bcl-2 antisense (G3139, Genasense™) is an oligodeoxynucleotide designed to bind the first six codons of the human Bcl-2 mRNA. Decreasing the expression of Bcl-2 in tumour cells may increase susceptibility to chemotherapy-induced apoptosis.[49] A phase I trial of Bcl-2 antisense in children with relapsed solid tumours, in which Bcl-2 antisense is administered in combination with doxorubicin and cyclophosphamide, is being conducted. The trial aims to determine the dose-limiting toxicities and recommended dose of Bcl-2 antisense, characterize the pharmacokinetics, and assess the biologic activity of Bcl-2 antisense in PBMCs and tumour tissue by determining Bcl-2 and related protein expression.

Conclusion

The principles for rational drug discovery were first demonstrated more than 50 years ago with the development of a number of antimetabolites including methotrexate, 6-MP, and 6-TG. In the past, limitations on our understanding of the malignant process precluded our ability to develop molecularly targeted therapies, and hence we relied predominantly on empiric screening of compounds for non-specific cytotoxic activity. Recently, we have entered an era of anticancer drug development which focuses on the identification of a spectrum of specific targets integral to cellular proliferation and malignant transformation. Certain targets, such as the PDGF-R pathway, may have similar roles in selected adult and paediatric cancers. Other targets, whose functional significance is yet to be identified, may be specific to paediatric malignancies and will present formidable challenges for paediatric drug development.

Target-based chemotherapy holds the promise of selectivity and hope of decreased acute and chronic toxicity. In early clinical trials the aim is to assess the ability of the drug to inhibit the target, determine the relevance of the target to paediatric malignancies, and carefully monitor for toxicities, particularly in agents that may require chronic dosing. For all agents that prove to be active in paediatric malignancies, an additional challenge will be to combine them with currently active regimens to improve overall survival and decrease the toxic side effects of therapy for children with cancer.

References

1. **Heinle RW, Welch AD** (1948). Experiments with pteroylglutamic acid and pteroylglutamic acid deficiency in human leukemia. *J Clin Invest* 27, 539 (**abstr**).

2. **Farber S, Diamond LK, Mercer RD,** *et al.* (1948). Temporary remissions in acute leukemia in children produced by folic acid antagonist, 4-aminopteroyl-glutamic acid (aminoptrin). *N Engl J Med* 238, 787–93.

3. **Goldin A** (1968). Preclinical methodology for the selection of anticancer agents. In: Busch H (ed) *Methods in Cancer Research*, Vol. IV. New York: Academic Press, 193–254.

4. **Elion GB, Hitchings GH** (1965). Metabolic basis for the actions of analogs of purines and pyramidines. *Adv Chemother* 2, 91–177.

5. **Boyd M** (1996). The NCI *in vitro* anticancer drug discovery screen: concept, implementation, and operation, 1985–1995. In: Teicher B (ed) *AntiCancer Drug Development Guide: Preclinical Screening, Clinical Trials, and Approval*. Totowa, NJ: Humana Press, 23–42.

6. **Weitman S, Carlson L, Pratt CB** (1996). New drug development for pediatric oncology. *Invest New Drugs* 14, 1–10.

7. **Houghton P, Adamson PC, Blaney S,** *et al.* (2002). Testing of new agents in childhood cancer preclinical models: meeting summary. *Clin Cancer Res* 8, 3646–57.

8. **Rowinsky E** (1994). Update on the antitumor activity of paclitaxel in clinical trials. *Ann Pharmacother* 28 (Suppl 5), S18–22.

9. **Hurwitz C, Strauss LC, Kepner J,** *et al.* (2001). Paclitaxel for the treatment of progressive or recurrent childhood brain tumors: a Pediatric Oncology Phase II study. *J Pediatr Hematol Oncol* 23, 277–81.

10. **Harris M, Hurwitz C, Sullivan JG, Larsen EC, Pratt CB** (1999). Taxol in pediatric solid tumors: a Pediatric Oncology Group (POG) phase II study (POG 9262). *Proc Am Soc Clin Oncol* 18, abstr 2170.

11. **Dumontet C, Sikic B** (1999). Mechanisms of action and resistance to antitubulin agents: microtubule dynamics, drug transport and cell death. *J Clin Oncol* 17, 1061–70.

12. Johnson IS, Armstrong JG, Gorman M, *et al.* (1967). The vinca alkaloids: a new class of oncolytic agents. *Cancer Res* 23, 1390.

13. Friedman H, Colvin OM, Ludeman SM, *et al.* (1986). Experimental chemotherapy for human medulloblastoma. *Cancer Res* 46, 2827–33.

14. Madden T, Bleyer WA, Hohneker J, Johansen MJ, Wargin W, Reaman G (1995). The pharmacokinetics of vinorelbine (Navelbine) in pediatric cancer patients. *Proc Am Soc Clin Oncol* 30, abstr. 357

15. Casanova M, Ferrari A, Spreafico F, *et al.* (2002). Vinorelbine in previously treated advanced childhood sarcomas: evidence of activity in rhabdomyosarcoma. *Cancer* 94, 3263–8.

16. Cortes JE, Pazdur R (1995). Docetaxel. *J Clin Oncol* 13, 2643–55.

17. Blaney S, Seibel NL, O'Brien M, *et al.* (1997). Phase I trial of docetaxel administered as a 1-hour infusion in children with refractory solid tumors: a collaborative Pediatric Branch, National Cancer Institute and Children's Cancer Group trial. *J Clin Oncol* 15, 1538–43.

18. Seibel N, Blaney SM, O'Brien M, *et al.* (1999). Phase I trial of docetaxel with filgrastim support in pediatric patients with refractory solid tumors: a collaborative Pediatric Oncology Branch, National Cancer Institute and Children's Cancer Group trial. *Clin Cancer Res* 5, 733–7.

19. Bollag D, McQueney P, Zhu J, *et al.* (1995). Epothilones, a new class of microtubule stabilizing agents with a taxol-like mechanism of action. *Cancer Res* 55, 2325–33.

20. Fox E, Stover E, Widemann B, Fojo T, Balis FM (2002). Cytotoxicity of the novel epothilone B analog, BMS247550 in pediatric solid tumor cell lines and comparison with other tubulin binding agents. *Proc Am Assoc Cancer Res*, 43, abstr 3916.

21. Koyanagi N, Nagasu T, Fujita M, *et al.* (1994). *In vivo* tumor growth inhibition produced by a novel sulfonamide, E7010, against rodent and human tumors. *Cancer Res* 54, 1702–6.

22. Broach JR, Thorner J (1996). High-throughput screening for drug discovery. *Nat Genet* 384, 14–16.

23. Fox E, Curt GA, Balis FM (2002). Clinical trial design for target-based therapy. *Oncologist* 7, 401–9.

24. Workman P (2002). Challenges of PK/PD measurements in modern drug development. *Eur J Cancer* 38, 2189–93.

25. Druker BJ (2002). STI571 (Gleevec™) as a paradigm for cancer therapy. *Trends Mol Med* 8 (Suppl), S14–17.

26. Buchdunger E, Cioffi C, Law L, *et al.* (2000). Abl protein–tyrosine kinase inhibitor STI571 inhibits *in vitro* signal transduction mediated by c-kit and platelet derived growth factor receptors. *J Pharmacol Exp Ther* 295, 139–45.

27. Salomon DS, Brandt R, Ciardello F, Normanno N (1995). Epidermal growth factor peptides and their receptors in human malignancies. *Crit Rev Oncol Hematol* 19, 183–232.

28. Widemann BC, Fox E, Goodspeed W, *et al.* (2003). Phase I trial of the farnesyl transferase inhibitor (FTI) R115777 in children with refractory leukemias. *Proc Am Soc Clin Oncol* 22, abstr 3250.

29. Folkman J (1985). Angiogenesis and its inhibitors. *Important Adv Oncol* 1985, 42–62.

30. Kumar S (1980). Angiogenesis and antiangiogenesis. *J Natl Cancer Inst* 64, 683–7.

31. Zetter B (1998). Angiogenesis and tumor metastasis. *Annu Rev Med* 49, 407–24.

32. Rak J, Filmus J, Kerbel RS (1996). Reciprocal paracrine interactions between tumor cells and endothelial cells: the 'angiogenic progression' hypothesis. *Eur J Cancer* 32A, 2438–50.

33. Jain R (1991). Hemodynamic and transport barriers to the treatment of solid tumors. *Int J Radiat Biol* 60, 85–100.

34. Schweigerer L (1995). Antiangiogenesis as a novel therapeutic concept in pediatric oncology. *J Mol Med* 73, 497–508.

35. Gordon MS, Margolin K, Talpaz M, *et al.* (2001). Phase I safety and pharmacokinetic study of recombinant human anti-vascular endothelial growth factor in patients with advanced cancer. *J Clin Oncol* 19, 843–50.

36. **Kabbinavar F, Hurwitz H, Fehrenbacher L, et al.** (2003). Phase II, randomized trial comparing bevacizumab plus fluorouracil (FU)/leucovorin (LV) with FU/LV alone in patients with metastatic colorectal cancer. *J Clin Oncol* 21, 60–5.

37. **Benson AB, Catalano PJ, Meropol NJ, et al.** (2003). Bevacizumab (anti-VEGF) plus FOLFOX4 in previously treated advanced colorectal cancer: an interim toxicity analysis of the Eastern Cooperative Oncology Group Study E3200. *Proc Am Soc Clin Oncol* 22, abstr 975.

38. **Rowe DH, Huang J, Li J, et al.** (2000). Supression of primary tumor growth of a mouse model of human neuroblastoma. *J Pediatr Surg* 35, 977–81.

39. **Gerber HP, Kowalski J, Sherman D, Eberhard DA, Ferrara N** (2000). Complete inhibition of rhabdomyosarcoma xenograft growth and neovascularization requires blockade of both tumor and host vascular endothelial growth factor. *Cancer Res* 6, 6253–8.

40. **Orlowski RZ, Sinchcombe TE, Mitchell BS, et al.** (2002). Phase I trial of the proteosome inhibitor PS341 in patients with refractory hemologic malignancies. *J Clin Oncol* 20, 4420–7.

41. **Aghajanian C, Soignet S, Dizon DS, Pien CS, Adams J, Elliott PJ** (2002). A phase I trial of the novel proteosome inhibitor PS341 in advanced solid malignancies. *Clin Cancer Res* 8, 2505–11.

42. **Neckers L, Schulte TW, Mimnaugh E** (1999). Geldanamycin as a potential anticancer agent: its molecular target and biochemical activity. *Invest New Drugs* 17, 361–73.

43. **Bradshaw DM, Arceci RJ** (1998). Clinical relevance of transmembrane drug efflux as a mechanism of multidrug resistance. *J Clin Oncol* 16, 3674–90.

44. **Martin C, Berridge G, Mistry P, Higgins C, Carlton P, Callaghan R** (1999). The molecular interaction of the high affinity reversal agent XR9576 with P-glycoprotein. *Br J Pharmacol* 128, 403–11.

45. **Witherspoon S, Emerson DL, Kerr BM, Lloyd TL, Dalton WS, Wissel PS** (1996). Flow cytometric assay of modulation of P-glycoprotein function in whole blood by the multidrug resistance inhibitor GG918. *Clin Cancer Res* 2, 7–12.

46. **Stewart A, Steiner J, Mellows G, Laguda B, Norris D, Bevan P** (2000). Phase I trial of XR9576 in healthy volunteers after oral and intravenous administration. *Clin Cancer Res* 6, 4186–91.

47. **Dole M, Nunez G, Merchant AK, et al.** (1994). Bcl-2 inhibits chemotherapy induced apoptosis in neuroblastoma. *Cancer Res* 54, 3253–9.

48. **Re GG, Hazen-Martin DJ, El Bahtimi R, et al.** (1999). Prognostic significance of Bcl-2 in Wilms' tumor and oncogenic potential of Bcl-XL in rare tumor cases. *Int J Cancer* 84, 193–200.

49. **Reed JC** (1995). Bcl-2: prevention of apoptosis as a mechanism of drug resistance. *Hematol Oncol Clin North Am* 9, 451–73.

Chapter 6

Radiotherapy in paediatric oncology

Andreas Schuck

General comments

Requirements

Adequate treatment of malignant disease in children and adolescents can only be provided by an experienced interdisciplinary team including paediatric oncologists, paediatric surgeons, and a radiation oncologist with expertise in the treatment of young patients. Furthermore, there must be close cooperation with diagnostic disciplines (radiology, nuclear medicine, pathology). Paediatric patients with malignant disease should be treated according to national or international protocols for the specific disease. With the introduction of multimodal therapy in the 1970s, considerable improvement was achieved in the treatment of children and adolescents. These results can only be obtained and improved, or achieved with less toxic treatments, if all patients are included in the relevant collaborative protocols. The protocol committees of individual trials usually consist of specialists in each involved medical discipline. The radiation oncologist has two main tasks: recommendation of indications for the use of radiotherapy, radiation doses and fractionation, target volume definitions, and the timing of radiotherapy, and provision of expert advice regarding the treatment of individual patients.

Effect on the tumour and side effects

In most malignant disease in childhood and adolescence, the chance of cure is highest with the primary treatment. In most tumours, relapse is associated with a poor prognosis. This is why the primary treatment of many tumours frequently involves aggressive treatment approaches that may be associated with severe acute and chronic toxicity. Therapy is given in a vulnerable period when patients are growing and developing; this is particularly relevant to the use of radiotherapy. Furthermore, since cure rates have been higher in the last two decades, more patients are developing therapy-associated long-term effects. Decisions regarding the indications for and the extent of radiotherapy involve balancing the expected effect on the tumour against the potential long-term effects of the treatment. This is why age-adapted recommendations are frequently given for very young patients. However, except in prospective clinical trials, the intensity of therapy should not be reduced.

Treatment with sedation or narcosis

Patients who are less than 3 years old generally require deep sedation or anaesthesia to allow a reproducible treatment set-up. This is not usually necessary in older patients. The techniques used for sedation and anaesthesia vary from center to center. It is essential that an experienced anaesthetist monitors the patient during and after treatment.

Malignant tumours

Soft tissue sarcoma

Sarcomas originating from soft tissues form a very heterogenous group of tumours. The most frequent subtype is rhabdomyosarcoma (RMS). Of these chemosensitive tumours, embryonal RMS is generally associated with a favourable prognosis whereas alveolar RMS has a higher relapse rate. Other chemosensitive soft tissue sarcomas include extraosseous Ewing tumours, synovial sarcoma, and undifferentiated sarcoma. There are other soft tissue sarcomas with moderate or no chemosensitivity (non-RMS-like tumours) such as liposarcoma, fibrosarcoma, and malignant rhabdoid tumour. Because of the many histologies and tumour sites, radiotherapy is a complex issue in these diseases and no patient should be treated outside a national or international protocol.

Rhabdomyosarcoma

Risk-adapted chemotherapy is administered in all paediatric patients with RMS. Initial surgical resection is performed if surgery can be complete and not mutilating. In all other cases, delayed surgery is planned after biopsy and the initial courses of chemotherapy.

Local control and survival are improved in all patients with alveolar RMS who receive radiotherapy irrespective of the extent of the initial or delayed surgery, even in patients with initial complete resection.[1] Local relapses are associated with a very poor outcome.

In embryonal RMS, radiotherapy also increases local control after initial or delayed surgery. If no radiotherapy is given, these patients will have a fair chance of cure after local relapse and radiotherapy as salvage treatment.[2] Therefore the decision to use radiotherapy in patients with favourable RMS histology is a balance between improved local control with the use of radiotherapy on the one hand and avoiding radiotherapy with a higher risk that intensive salvage therapy will be necessary on the other hand. The best cure rates have been achieved in the Intergroup Rhabdomyosarcoma Trials (IRS) in the USA with extensive use of radiotherapy.[3] Therefore, as a rule, radiotherapy should be performed in patients with favourable histology who have not had an initial complete resection (IRS groups II and III). In small children with embryonal RMS and in particularly sensitive sites that are associated with a favourable course of the disease (e.g. vaginal RMS), radiotherapy can be omitted when patients are in complete remission following chemotherapy.

Depending on the extent of surgery, histology, and response to chemotherapy, 32–50 Gy are used. In the ICG and CWS trials, hyperfractionated accelerated radiotherapy was given at a dose of 1.6 Gy twice daily. Conventional fractionation was used in the SIOP and IRS groups. The planning target volume is defined as the initial extent of the tumour on MRI plus 2 cm. Areas contaminated during surgery, surgical scars, and drainage sites must be included in the radiation fields. If possible, total coverage of the circumference of extremities should be avoided in order to reduce the risk of lymphoedema.

Extraosseous Ewing tumours, synovial sarcoma, and undifferentiated sarcoma

Radiotherapy is crucial in these types of tumour. It is indicated when initial surgery has not been complete even when further surgery can be performed. Furthermore, radiotherapy may also be given in completely resected tumours with unfavourable characteristics (i.e. >5 cm diameter). Radiotherapy is applied as the only local therapy modality when surgery is not possible. Radiation doses range between 45 and 55 Gy and an additional boost can be given if surgery is not possible. The target volume is defined as the pre-therapeutic tumour extent plus a margin of at least 2 cm.

Non-RMS-like tumours:

Because of the many histological subtypes with differing tumour biology in this group, very limited data are available concerning the role of radiotherapy. It is usually indicated when surgery is incomplete. Furthermore, radiotherapy may also be given in completely resected tumours with unfavourable characteristics (i.e. >5 cm diameter). Radiation doses range between 45 and 60 Gy.

Ewing tumour

The Ewing tumour family consists of Ewing sarcoma, atypical Ewing sarcoma, and primitive neuroectodermal tumours (PNETs). The most frequent tumour sites are the pelvis and the femur. The treatment of Ewing tumours consists of polychemotherapy, surgery, and radiotherapy. Local therapy is performed following biopsy and initial chemotherapy. No randomized trials comparing definitive radiotherapy with definitive surgery have been performed to date. Therefore the superiority of surgery over radiotherapy has not been proved. However, in prospective non-randomized trials, the best local control was achieved when a wide tumour resection was performed. Radiotherapy following or preceding surgery is recommended when only marginal or intralesional resections are possible or in patients who have a poor histological response to initial chemotherapy.[4] Preoperative radiotherapy may be particularly useful when it facilitates function-preserving surgery. Radiotherapy is always necessary for inoperable tumours (e.g. vertebral primaries). Surgical debulking does not improve treatment results and should not be performed. Radiation doses range from 50 to 60 Gy for definitive radiotherapy and from 45 to 55 Gy for pre- or postoperative radiotherapy. Patients treated with a radiation dose ≤40 Gy experience a high local failure rate.[5] In the CESS 86 and EICESS 92 trials, there was no difference in local control and event-free survival between conventional fractionation or a hyperfractionated split course with 1.6 Gy twice daily and a treatment break of about 10 days after 22.4 Gy. Therefore the fractionation seems to be of little or no importance for tumour control.

The planning target volume is defined as the initial tumour extent on MRI with an additional longitudinal margin of 5 cm and lateral margins of 2 cm in long bones. If doses >45 Gy are used, a shrinking field technique is applied. In some patients with an axial tumour site, 5-cm safety margins cannot be used, but a minimum 2-cm safety margin around the initial tumour extent must be allowed. Surgically contaminated areas with scars and drainage sites must be included in the radiation fields. If possible, total coverage of the circumference of extremities should be avoided in order to reduce the risk of lymphoedema.

Good treatment results in patients with lung metastases have been achieved using whole-lung irradiation.[6] Survival in patients who had complete clinical remission in the lung and received an additional 15–20 Gy external beam radiotherapy to both lungs was improved compared with patients who received chemotherapy only. In the ongoing EURO-EWING 99 trial, whole-lung irradiation is randomized against high-dose chemotherapy for these patients.

Patients with initial bone metastases should receive radiotherapy not only at the primary tumour site but also at metastatic bone sites if there are not too many of these. For multiple bone metastases, an individual decision has to be made as to whether only the largest lesions are treated, whether residual metastases shown by functional imaging (positron emission tomography scan after chemotherapy) are treated, or whether radiotherapy is unlikely to improve the outcome.

Osteosarcoma

Osteosarcoma is the most frequent bone tumour in childhood. It usually develops in the epiphyseal region of long bones. The treatment of choice is polychemotherapy and surgical resection of the primary tumour and metastases. Radical surgery is essential for a good prognosis. This tumour has been considered to be radioresistant, and therefore radiotherapy has no role in the treatment of osteosarcoma to date. However, experimental data have shown that the radiosensitivity is equivalent to those of other human tumour cell lines. Furthermore, cure has been reported for patients with inoperable tumours and patients who refused surgery after radiation doses ranging from 50 to 70 Gy. Therefore radiotherapy is indicated for residual tumours with no option for follow-up surgery, for inoperable tumours, and in the palliative treatment of bone metastases. There have also been reports of benefit from adjuvant whole-lung irradiation in patients with initial lung metastases.

2.4 Central nervous system tumours

Central nervous system (CNS) tumours have very different histologies and malignancies. They represent 20 per cent of all malignant diseases in childhood and adolescence and are the largest group of solid tumours.

Medulloblastoma

Medulloblastoma, which is a PNET located in the posterior fossa, is the most frequent brain tumour in children. Tumour dissemination in the cerebrospinal fluid (CSF) is common. Therefore complete tumour resection followed by craniospinal radiotherapy is the treatment of choice. Improved results may be obtained for patients without metastases by the additional use of chemotherapy. In patients aged <4 years, results with surgery and chemotherapy alone for resectable localized tumours are favourable. In this age group, it is justifiable to withhold radiotherapy after complete resection until there is a relapse, therefore avoiding radiation-associated side effects.

In the past, craniospinal irradiation was given with conventional fractionation to a dose of 36 Gy. The posterior fossa was then boosted to a dose of 54 Gy. Single institutional experiences with 24 Gy craniospinal irradiation and a boost to the posterior fossa of up to 54 Gy in conjunction with systemic therapy have shown comparable results.[8] In the ongoing German HIT 2000 trial, the use of hyperfractionation with 1.0 Gy twice daily up to a cumulative dose of 68 Gy in patients with completely resected tumours is being tested with regard to tumour control and late effects. In patients with localized disease, delaying radiotherapy after surgery in favour of chemotherapy was disadvantageous in the random-ized HIT-91 trial. Therefore postoperative radiotherapy should be started as soon as possible. In patients with spinal metastases, the use of chemotherapy after surgery and before radiotherapy was beneficial.

Careful planning of radiotherapy is necessary. It is important that craniospinal irradiation should include the entire compartment of the CSF from the brain down to the cauda equina without gap or overlap. Boost radiation to the posterior fossa must be planned in three dimensions, based on CT and MRI with a three-dimensional conformal approach.

Supratentorial PNET

Treatment is similar to that of infratentorial PNET (medulloblastoma). Craniospinal axis irradiation is followed by a boost to the primary tumour site.

Intracranial germ cell tumours

There are two treatment alternatives for patients with pure germinomas. Craniospinal irradiation with 24–30 Gy can be given followed by a tumour boost to a total dose of 45 Gy. Comparable results have been obtained using systemic therapy combined with involved field radiotherapy to the primary tumour site only.[9]

Patients with secreting germ cell tumours receive chemotherapy followed by involved field radiotherapy to the primary tumour site at a dose of 54 Gy. Craniospinal radiotherapy is only performed when there has been positive CSF cytology.

Ependymoma

Ependymomas develop in the ependyma or lining of the ventricles and the cerebral aqueduct. In two-thirds of cases they are located in the posterior fossa and frequently infiltrate into the cervical spine. In anaplastic tumours arising infratentorially, the risk of CSF dissemination is about 10 per cent. The treatment of choice in malignant ependymoma is complete resection followed by local therapy of at least 54 Gy. No clear benefit has been shown for the use of craniospinal irradiation.[10] Complete tumour resection is essential. Patients who have an incomplete resection have a poor prognosis despite the use of radiotherapy and systemic therapy.

Low-grade glioma

Low-grade gliomas comprise a number of different histologies. The treatment of choice is complete resection. In patients who show no progression after surgery, a wait-and-see policy is followed. When clinical symptoms develop or imaging shows progression, local radiotherapy is given to a dose of 45–55 Gy. External beam therapy is also given when complete tumour resection is not possible and the patient remains symptomatic following biopsy or incomplete resection. In small children, chemotherapy is given first. Delayed radiotherapy is performed when systemic therapy fails.

High-grade glioma

Fortunately, high-grade gliomas are rare in children and adolescents. As in adults, these tumours are characterized by aggressive local growth. The treatment of choice is tumour excision followed by local radiotherapy to 54–60 Gy depending on the age of the patient. So far the additional use of chemotherapy has not improved the results.

Craniopharyngioma

These histologically benign tumours arise in the suprasellar region. Infiltrating local growth is possible, so that vision and hormone production may be affected. Since aggressive resection is associated with a high risk, subtotal resection followed by local radiotherapy at 50–54 Gy is recommended. In young children (<5 years old), the radiation dose can be reduced to 45 Gy. The 10-year survival rate with limited surgery and postoperative radiotherapy is 80–95 per cent.[11]

Neuroblastoma

Neuroblastoma is a disease of early childhood. About 60 per cent of the patients present with initial metastases. Children aged <1 year with dissemination to the skin, liver, and bone marrow have a different prognosis. These tumours are frequently radio- and chemosensitive. Furthermore, spontaneous remission may occur. Therefore a wait-and-see strategy may be appropriate in these patients with favourable prognostic factors.

Although neuroblastomas are radiosensitive, the influence of local radiation on survival is not well defined. Therefore the use of external beam therapy in primary treatment differs in the various ongoing trials. It is used either when there is residual tumour following chemotherapy, [131I]mIBG therapy, and second-look surgery or when patients present with advanced local disease irrespective of response. The radiation dose is 36–40 Gy. The planning target volume consists of the (residual) tumour plus a safety margin of 2 cm. Radiotherapy is also useful in palliative treatment.

Nephroblastoma

Nephroblastomas arise mostly in young children; 80 per cent of the patients are <5 years of age. The primary treatment consists of surgery or initial chemotherapy followed by surgery.[12] The subsequent treatment depends on histology and on lymph node and resection status. Radiotherapy is given for stage II disease and greater. Nephroblastoma is a radiosensitive tumour and doses range from 10 to 30 Gy. The target volume is defined according to tumour extent at diagnosis, the topography of the tumour at surgery, and whether there was tumour spillage during surgery. Radiotherapy to both lungs is performed in selected patients with lung metastases.

Hodgkin disease

As in adults, early tumour stages can be cured with extended field radiotherapy alone. Because of radiation-associated side effects, use of chemotherapy has become general and radiation dose and fields have reduced. No radiotherapy was given to patients treated in the German HD 95 trial when there was a complete remission following chemotherapy. Overall, there was an increased relapse rate with this approach. Patients in complete remission without the use of radiotherapy had a higher relapse rate than those who had residual disease following chemotherapy and who received radiotherapy. Subsequently, it was recommended that radiotherapy should be used for all patients except those in early stage IA, IB and IIA without further risk factors who were in complete remission following chemotherapy. Radiotherapy is essential for patients with a higher stage of disease or known risk factors and in patients with residual disease following chemotherapy. The doses used range from 20 to 35 Gy depending on response to systemic therapy and residual tumour size. The tolerance doses of organs at risk must be considered in treatment planning. Extended field radiotherapy is no longer considered appropriate. Treatment is only given to the lymph node sites initially involved. The incidence of secondary tumours is considerable. The relative risk 15 years after treatment is 15 per cent. The risk of developing second solid tumours increases with time after treatment.[7]

Leukaemia

Leukaemias are the most frequent malignant diseases of childhood. However, the majority of patients can be cured with aggressive systemic therapy.

Historically, the introduction of prophylactic CNS treatment, initially with craniospinal radiation and later with whole-brain radiation alone, resulted in a dramatic reduction of CNS relapses and disease-related mortality. Because of concerns about long-term effects of cranial radiotherapy, mainly neurocognitive effects, its application has been restricted to patients with high-risk acute lymphoblastic leukaemia (ALL), T-ALL, or initial CNS involvement. In all other patients with ALL, CNS prophylaxis is performed with intrathecal and intravenous methotrexate. The radiation dose is usually 12 Gy for prophylactic treatment and 18 Gy for CNS disease.

In acute myelogenous leukaemia (AML), most trials have not shown a benefit using cranial radiotherapy. However, in the German AML-BFM 87 trial, a reduction in bone marrow relapses was observed for patients who received cranial radiotherapy.[13] In the AML-BFM 98 trial, patients were randomized between cranial prophylactic treatment with 12 Gy and 18 Gy.

When there is mediastinal involvement, response to chemotherapy must be evaluated; if residual tumour remains, mediastinal radiation may be given. In most cases with ALL and infiltration of the testes, systemic therapy is adequate. When there is residual tumour, radiotherapy must be considered. Radiation treatment of involved testes is recommended in patients with AML. The doses range from 10 to 24 Gy.

For patients with high-risk ALL or relapse, an allogenic bone marrow or stem cell transplantation is performed. Conditioning is frequently performed with total body irradiation, usually with 12 Gy in six fractions over a period of 3 days. The dose to the lung is reduced to 8 Gy, and some centers reduce the dose given to the kidneys in children to lower the rate of radiation nephropathy.

Radiation-associated toxicity in children and adolescents

Acute side effects are defined as toxicities occuring within 90 days of the start of radiotherapy. They depend on the radiation site, the total dose, the fractionation, the size of treated area, and whether other modalities (surgery, chemotherapy) are given as well. Typical acute side effects in children do not differ from those in adults. They include skin reactions, mucositis, enteritis, epilation, myelosuppression, etc. Most acute side effects are reversible and can be handled with adequate supportive care.

Chronic side effects are defined as reactions occurring or persisting more than 90 days after the start of radiotherapy. Again, they depend on field size and site, total dose, and fractionation, as well as whether further treatment modalities are used. Long-term radiogenic effects are usually irreversible and are more severe the younger the patients are at the time of treatment.

Bone and soft tissue

Radiotherapy results in growth deficits due to damage to chondroblasts. Clinically, a dose of 10–20 Gy results in growth inhibition. Doses above 20 Gy can stop further growth. The extent of the growth deficit depends on the age of the patient at the time of treatment and how much an epiphysis contributes to total growth of the part of the body or the limb. In radiation planning it is essential either to include the growth plate fully in the radiation field or to exclude it entirely if that is possible. A dose gradient through the growth plate results in asymmetric growth and functional deficits. For the same reasons, vertebral bodies should either be fully included in or spared from the treatment.

Hypoplasia in soft tissues can occur after a dose $\geq$20 Gy. In addition to a reduction in volume of the muscles and subcutaneous tissue, fibrosis can occur after higher doses, resulting in limitation of movement.

Testes

Hormonal deficits and impairment of fertility depend on the radiation dose and probably on the age of the patient. Spermatogenesis is very radiosensitive. After a dose of 15 cGy, reversible reduction in the sperm count can occur in adults. Permanent sterilization has been observed after fractionated doses of 1–2 Gy. The application of small fractionated doses is more toxic than a single dose. The dose that results in damage to the germinal epithelia in children is unknown. Shalet et al.[14] observed oligospermia or azoospermia in adulthood in eight of ten patients given testicular doses of 2.7–9.8 Gy during treatment for nephroblastoma in childhood. Young patients with ALL treated with doses of 12 Gy to the testicles and chemotherapy all showed azoospermia after puberty.

Leydig cells are more radioresistant. Normal testosterone levels are observed after 20 Gy of fractionated radiotherapy in adults. Leydig cells in children may be more radiosensitive.

Ovaries

Ionizing radiation results in a reduction in the number of small follicles, inhibition of maturation of the follicle, cortical fibrosis, and capsular atrophy. Inhibition of follicular maturation results in infertility and amenorrhoea. Permanent sterility may be seen in adult women who receive a dose >8 Gy during fractionated radiotherapy. Usually, there is no permanent change in the cell cycle after doses <1.5 Gy. Stillmann et al.[15] evaluated 25 women who received doses of 12–50 Gy to both ovaries when they were <17 years old. Seventeen (68 per cent) of them developed hormonal deficits.

An oophoropexy should be performed in girls who are to receive radiotherapy to the pelvis. The ovaries must be marked with clips to allow identification on radiographic images and therefore facilitate function-conserving radiotherapy.

Offspring

Females who received abdominal radiotherapy and are pregnant are at higher risk for intrauterine death or a child with a low birth weight. The aetiology is not known. Probably it is due to changes in the uterus and pelvis rather than damage to the germinal epithelia. The number of congenital handicaps in live-borns whose father or mother have undergone previous radio- and/or chemotherapy is not increased.[16] There are no clinical data showing that offsping are at higher risk of teratogenesis, although there is an increased incidence of malignancies due to hereditary syndromes.

Central nervous system

The development of the brain is very marked within the first 3 years of life. By the age of 6 years, brain development is almost complete. Therefore radiation-associated side effects are particularly evident in very young children.

Neurocognitive deficits

Neurocognitive deficits have been described after CNS prophylaxis in children with leukaemia. In the past, radiation doses of 18–24 Gy were used. In recent protocols, a dose of 12 Gy is usually given to high-risk patients. There are a large number of retrospective trials evaluating neurocognitive effects in these patients. In the one randomized trial reported,[17] 49 patients were randomized to receive either intrathecal methotrexate and 18 Gy radiotherapy or both intravenous and intrathecal methotrexate. The median follow-up was about 6 years. Patients were evaluated before and after treatment. There was a statistically significant reduction of the full-scale IQ and the verbal IQ for both the chemotherapy only and the chemotherapy plus radiotherapy groups. The total reduction in IQ was <5 per cent in both groups, and the average IQ was within the normal range. Therefore there is a small reduction in intelligence following

CNS prophylactic treatment. It is not clear whether chemotherapy is less toxic than radiother-apy. So far there are no data evaluating patients who have received a dose of 12 Gy.

A dramatic deterioration of IQ can be observed for children <6 years of age treated with craniospinal radiation at higher doses (i.e. for medulloblastoma). The longer the follow-up, the more pronounced these deficits become. Usually, there are no major impairments in older patients.

Thus it is clear that radiation-induced neurocognitive deficits exist after local treatment of brain tumours, but they are difficult to distinguish from tumour- or surgery-related effects.

Cerebral necrosis and myelopathy

The incidence of radiation-induced necrosis in the brain following doses of 50–60 Gy ranges from 0.1 to 5 per cent. The incidence may be influenced by the use of concomitant chemo-therapy.

There is partially contradictory data concerning the risk of developing myelopathy. In adults, the application of 55 Gy is probably associated with a risk of 5 per cent after 5 years. The incidence is influenced by the fractionation schedule and probably by the length of the treated cord segment. It is possible that children have a slightly higher sensitivity.

Endocrine system

The secretion of growth hormone is impaired after a dose of ≥18 Gy to the hypothalamus/hypophysis. The higher the dose, the earlier the deficit is manifest. Further deficits of the hypothalamic–hypophyseal axis (in ACTH, thyrotrophin-releasing hormone, gonadotrophins, and hyperprolactaemia) are observed after doses >40 Gy.

There is a risk of hypothyroidism after doses >20 Gy to the thyroid. In paediatric patients treated for Hodgkin disease at a dose of 30–45 Gy, the rate of hypothyroidism after 5 years has been reported to be as high as 50 per cent.[18]

Lung

Pneumonitis following radiotherapy is a subacute side effect that occurs 1–4 months after treatment. Spontaneous remission is possible but progression to lung fibrosis may occur. When radiotherapy is given to more than a quarter of the lung or at a dose >15 Gy, the incidence of pneumonitis increases. Chemotherapy, particularly with actinomycin D, bleomycin, or busul-fan, can sensitize the lung tissue to radiation. Long-term effects can develop after treatment of very young children because of insufficient formation of alveoli.

Heart

In the past, with the use of high radiation doses for patients with Hodgkin disaese and with coverage of large parts of the heart, acute pericarditis and cardiomyopathy were observed. Today, these are very rare events following radiotherapy alone. Cardiomyopathy occurs mainly with the combined use of anthracyclines. The incidence is dependent on the cumulative dose of anthracycline.

An increased incidence of coronary heart disease has been observed following radiotherapy to the mediastinum. Again, most of the retrospective data come from patients who were treated with high doses. No increase in coronary heart disease is expected following treatment with 25 Gy and conventional fractionation. In an analysis of 635 children with Hodgkin disease, 12 patients died from heart disease; seven of these patients had myocardial infarction. Fatal cardiac events were only observed in patients treated with 42–45 Gy.[19]

Liver

The radiation tolerance of the liver depends on the volume irradiated, the concomitant use of chemotherapy, and the age of the patient. Without the use of chemotherapy, there is a significant risk of radiation-associated hepatopathy at a dose of 30 Gy given to the entire organ with conventional fractionation. With the combined use of chemotherapy and radiotherapy, doses >15 Gy are generally avoided. In the German nephroblastoma trial, changes in liver function were observed in 35 per cent of patients following radiotherapy to the entire liver at doses of 15–30 Gy and concomitant adminstration of actinomycin D and vincristine. Most of these changes were reversible.[20]

Kidneys

There is a significant risk of damage when a dose >25 Gy with conventional fractionation is given to both kidneys. In children, renal damage can occur at a lower dose, particularly if chemotherapy is also used. The risk of nephropathy is reduced if doses to the kidneys are maintained <20 Gy. A temporary increase in blood pressure and urea has been observed after radiotherapy with large fields to the entire abdomen at a dose of 12 Gy.[21] Increased vulnerability of the kidneys after total body irradiation has also been observed in children. In patients with ALL and neuroblastoma surviving for >6 months, fractionated radiotherapy of 12–14 Gy resulted in a nephropathy rate of 41 per cent.

Prospects

There are several important issues in radiotherapy in paediatric oncology that should be considered in the future.

It is essential that radiation-associated toxicities, particularly long-term effects, are studied in the setting of combined treatment modalities in conjuction with surgery and chemotherapy. This will not only allow evaluation of the individual risk for a single patient but provide essential information for the design of future trials.

In tumour entities with good outcome, such as Hodgkin disease, less toxic treatment regimes with reduced radiation doses or smaller planning target volumes can be evaluated in controlled clinical trials. In tumours with a less favourable outcome, such as medulloblastoma, intensification of treatment including radiotherapy must be evaluated in clinical trials to find out whether this results in improved outcome with acceptable toxicities.

The use of modern radiation techniques including three-dimensional treatment planning, intensity modulated radiotherapy, stereotactic radiotherapy, and proton therapy may improve the therapeutic ratio and help to reduce toxicity and increase the antitumour effect.

No patient with a tumour of childhood should be treated outside a national or international clinical trial. The formation of international collaborative groups for single tumour types must be encouraged to allow randomized studies concerning different issues of therapy. Otherwise no real progress can be expected. Furthermore, the treatment must be performed at an experienced center to ensure expertise in the special demands of radiotherapy in paediatric oncology.

References

1. Wolden S, Anderson J, Crist W, *et al.* (1999). Indications for radiotherapy and chemotherapy after complete resection in rhabdomyosarcoma: a report from the Intergroup Rhabdomyosarcoma Studies I to III. *J Clin Oncol* 17, 3468–75.

2. Oberlin O, Rey A, Anderson J, *et al.* (2001). Treatment of orbital rhabdomyosarcoma: survival and late effects of treatment-results of an international workshop. *J Clin Oncol* 19, 197–204.

3. Crist W, Anderson J, Meza J, *et al.* (2001). Intergroup Rhabdomyosarcoma Study—IV: Results of patients with nonmetastatic disease. *J Clin Oncol* 19, 3091–102.

4. Schuck A, Ahrens S, Paulussen M, *et al.* (2003). Local therapy in localized Ewing tumors: results of 1058 patients treated in the CESS 81, CESS 86 and EICESS 92 trials. *Int J Radiat Oncol Biol Phys* 55, 168–77.

5. Arai Y, Kun LE, Brooks T, *et al.* (1991). Ewing's sarcoma: local tumor control and patterns of failure following limited volume radiation therapy. *Int J Radiat Oncol Biol Phys* 21, 1501–8.

6. Paulussen M, Ahrens S, Burdach S, *et al.* (1998). Primary metastatic (stage IV) Ewing tumor: survival analysis of 171 patients from the EICESS studies. *Ann Oncol* 9, 275–81.

7. Wolden S, Lamborn K, Cleary S, *et al.* (1998).Second cancer following pediatric Hodgkin's disease. *J Clin Oncol* 16, 536–44.

8. Packer RJ, Goldwein J, Nicholson HS, *et al.* (1999). Treatment of children with reduced-dose craniospinal radiotherapy and adjuvant chemotherapy: a Children's Cancer Group Study. *J Clin Oncol* 17, 2127–36.

9. Haddock MG, Schild SE, Scheitbauer BW, *et al.* (1997). Radiation therapy for histologically confirmed primary central nervous system germinoma. *Int J Radiat Oncol Biol Phys* 38, 915–23.

10. Merchant TE, Haida T, Wang MH, *et al.* (1997). Anaplastic ependymoma: treatment of pediatric patients with or without craniospinal radiation therapy. *J Neurosurg* 86, 943–9.

11. Rajan B, Ashley S, Gorman C, *et al.* (1993). Craniopharyngioma—long term results following limited surgery and radiotherapy. *Radiother Oncol* 26, 1–10.

12. Coppes MJ, Tournade MF, Lemerle J, *et al.* (1992). Preoperative care of infants with nephroblastoma. Results of SIOP 6. *Cancer* 69, 2721–5.

13. Creutzig U, Ritter J, Zimmermann M, Schellong G (1993). Does cranial irradiation reduce the risk for bone marrow relapse in acute myelogenous leukemia: unexpected results of the childhood acute myelogenous leukemia study BFM-87. *J Clin Oncol* 11, 279–86.

14. Shalet SM, Beardwell CG, Jacobs HS, Pearson D (1978). Testicular function following irradiation of the human prepubertal testis. *Clin Endocrinol* 9, 483–90.

15. Stillman RJ, Schinfeld JS, Schiff I, *et al.* (1981). Ovarian failure in long-term survivors of childhood malignancy. *Am J Obstet Gynecol* 139, 62–6.

16. Aisner J, Wiernik P, Pearl P (1993). Pregnancy outcome in patients treated for Hodgkin's disease. *J Clin Oncol* 11, 507–12.

17. Ochs J, Mulhern R, Fairclough D, *et al.* (1991). Comparison of neuropsychologic functioning and clinical indicators of neurotoxicity in long-term survivors of childhood leukemia given cranial radiation or parenteral methotrexate: a prospective study. *J Clin Oncol*, 145–51.

18. Bhatia S, Ramsay N, Banale J, *et al.* (1996). Thyroid abnormalities after therapy for Hodgkin's disease in childhood. *Oncologist* 1, 62–7.

19. Hancock SL, Donaldson SS, Hoppe RT (1993). Cardiac disease following treatment of Hodgkin's disease in children and adolescence. *J Clin Oncol* 11, 1208–15.

20. Flentje M, Weirich A, Pötter R, Ludwig R (1994). Hepatotoxicity in irradiated nephroblastoma patients during postoperative treatment according to SIOP9/GPOH. *Radiother Oncol* 31, 222–8.

21. Thomas PRM, Tefft M, D'Angio GJ, *et al.* (1988). Acute toxicities associated with radiation in the second National Wilms' Tumor Study. *J Clin Oncol* 6, 1694–8.

Chapter 7

Surgery in paediatric oncology

Helene Martelli

Introduction

The increased survival and decreased morbidity for children with cancer has been one of the most gratifying success stories during the last 30 years. This progress is related to several factors, including the sensitivity of childhood malignant tumours to chemotherapy and the use of a multidisciplinary approach to management. Because of increasingly effective chemotherapy, the role of surgery in the management of childhood cancer has changed considerably from being the only modality available to treat many solid tumours to being one of several therapies which are needed to achieve success. Nowadays, the paediatric surgeon interacts with a multi-disciplinary team of experts including paediatric oncologists, radiologists, pathologists, and radiotherapists. The best outcome will always be achieved by close cooperation between specialists, each clearly understanding the efficacy and limitations of various forms of treat-ment. Therefore the paediatric surgeon should be engaged in the child's management from diagnosis onwards and be aware of all the diagnostic and therapeutic modalities available. Frequently, the paediatric surgeon is the first physician who may suspect a malignant tumour in a child presenting with a palpable mass. Except in emergencies, a thorough consideration of the possible differential diagnoses should be made before any surgical procedure is undertaken, ideally in discussion with the oncology team.

Even if most paediatric solid tumours also require systemic treatment, adequate local therapy remains a major goal and determines the success of therapy in the great majority of tumours. Adequate local therapy is mainly represented by surgery in children, especially infants, but it may include other forms of treatment such as external beam radiotherapy or brachytherapy. Surgical techniques have progressed in recent decades from radical and potentially mutilating interventions to conservative organ-sparing procedures, mainly because of more effective chemotherapy and the development of combined treatments, such as surgery and brachyther-apy, especially in very young children. This has occurred in parallel with a general trend in the treatment of cancer in children of aiming to decrease the intensity of all therapies, with their risk of long-term sequelae, in patients with good prognostic factors, while increasing it in patients with poor prognostic factors. Most malignant tumours are now treated according to multinational clinical trials which include precise guidelines for all the specialists in the oncology team. Theoretically, a paediatric surgeon should not operate on any malignant tumour without being aware of the surgical guidelines in the protocol currently in use for that particular diagnosis.

Surgery may be necessary at different stages during the management of malignant tumours: initially for surgical biopsy or tumour resection (primary excision and re-excision), or after neoadjuvant chemotherapy for secondary resection, or at relapse. Emergency operations are sometimes unavoidable if there is rapid enlargement of the tumour, torsion, or perforation.

The surgeon also has a role in the supportive care of patients, facilitating treatments given by other members of the oncology team or treating complications related to other therapies.

Emergency procedures

Because of the improved accuracy and availability of imaging facilities, the diagnosis of tumour is usually recognized before the first surgical procedure is undertaken. In rare abdominal emergencies, such as intestinal intussusceptions or gonadal torsion, the tumour may not have been diagnosed preoperatively. The surgeon should always try to avoid radical surgery (e.g. right hemicolectomy in a Burkitt lymphoma, cystectomy in a pelvic rhabdomyosarcoma, bilateral oophorectomy, etc.) and only perform a biopsy on such tumours. Sometimes, although a tumour has been diagnosed, the surgeon will need to perform an emergency procedure because of rapid enlargement of the tumour by intratumoral bleeding, or intra-abdominal haemorrhage due to spontaneous or traumatic tumour rupture. Even in such cases, it is desirable to follow protocol requirements and avoid radical surgery.

Biopsy

The acquisition of adequate tissue samples is essential not only for diagnosis but also for prognostic biologic information and evaluation of treatment efficacy during follow-up. Communication with the pathologist before taking the specimen is always good practice.

There are several methods of obtaining tissue specimens:

- fine-needle aspiration cytology
- needle biopsy for a core of tissue (Tru-cut needle biopsy)
- surgical biopsy (incisional or excisional) obtained by open or minimally invasive surgery
- endoscopic biopsy (in specific sites such as bladder or vagina)
- stereotactic biopsy (for brain tumours).

Directed-needle biopsies using ultrasound or CT guidance give better samples than blind biopsies. They may be performed by clinicians or radiologists.

Fine-needle aspiration cytology is rarely used in the diagnosis of paediatric neoplasms because it usually does not provide sufficient material for the necessary investigation. It may sometimes be relevant to confirm clinically suspected regional node involvement.

Needle core biopsies can provide adequate tissue to allow accurate diagnosis of the majority of paediatric neoplasms. At least three cores should be taken to permit adequate studies, including immunohistochemistry. However, the paucity of material frequently makes it difficult for the pathologist to provide detailed information, for example regarding the presence or absence of anaplasia in nephroblastoma or tumour grading in soft tissue sarcoma.

Open surgical biopsies are often necessary, especially in tumours with obvious heterogeneity on initial imaging, in order to obtain a representative sample. Biopsy may be total (excisional) or partial (incisional). In small suspect soft tissue lesions, it is sometimes possible to perform an excisional biopsy with clear margins. In all other situations, biopsy should be incisional. Biopsy incision should be planned so as to allow the biopsy scar to be excised at the time of definitive resection. This is particularly important in bone and soft tissue lesions arising in the limbs or in the trunk or abdominal walls. Biopsies may also be obtained using minimally invasive surgery, i.e. utilizing laparoscopy, thoracoscopy, or mediastinoscopy. These techniques are very useful and may decrease postoperative pain and the duration of postoperative recovery. Nevertheless, the rules of surgical oncology still apply and it is important to avoid tumour spillage in the abdomen or the pleural cavity.

Staging

There is no single uniform staging approach for childhood malignancies and the surgeon needs to be aware of the requirements for staging each tumour type according to current protocols in use in his or her center. Pretreatment staging procedures are mainly based on imaging (ultrasound, CT scanning and/or MRI, scintigraphy) but also, in specific tumours, on biologic markers (α-fetoprotein and human chorionic gonadotrophin in germ cell tumours), cytogenetics, molecular biology (N-*myc* oncogene status in neuroblastoma), etc. Surgery alone is no longer considered as a staging procedure, even in Hodgkin disease, although many staging systems include an assessment of the resectablity of the tumour (for instance that used in the National Wilms Tumor Study (NWTS) in North America, and the International Neuroblastoma Staging System). In hepatic tumours treated with SIOPEL protocols, the PRETEXT staging system (PREtreatment EXTent of the disease) identifies not only the extent of the disease but also the type of resection to be performed.[1]

Primary resection

Primary resection is a surgical procedure performed at diagnosis before any other treatment (chemotherapy or radiotherapy) has been delivered. The aim of primary resection is to achieve complete resection (currently defined as R0: microscopically complete resection) without danger or unnecessary functional compromise. This should be attempted only after careful evaluation of the resectability of the tumour with optimal imaging and discussion with radiologists and oncologists. Extensive 'mutilating' operations should never be considered at primary resection. A 'mutilating' operation is defined as one leading to significant long-term anatomical, functional, or cosmetic impairment, for example orbital exenteration, major resection of the face, pneumonectomy, pelvic exenteration with permanent intestinal or urinary diversion, total cystectomy, total prostatectomy, hysterectomy, limb amputation, or extensive muscular resection.

The first requirement for considering primary resection is to establish the absence of distant metastases. Some localized and potentially resectable tumours are always treated with pre-operative chemotherapy, even if they involve a paired organ. This mainly applies to nephroblastoma in children aged >6 months treated according to the current European protocol (SIOP 2001). The approach is different in North America where patients with localized nephroblastoma may undergo nephrectomy prior to the administration of chemotherapy. In the NWTS, patients are not treated with chemotherapy without histologic confirmation of the malignancy and the surgeon is asked to remove the tumour at diagnosis, define stage by careful evaluation of the liver, the lymph nodes, and the contralateral kidney, and avoid tumour rupture which would mandate postoperative radiotherapy. However, SIOP studies have demonstrated that preoperative chemotherapy can shrink the tumour, downgrade the stage, and reduce the incidence of intraoperative tumour rupture and postoperative complications.[2,3]

Although primary surgical excision may appear to be indicated in some tumours, it may be preferable to stop the attempt and only perform a biopsy rather than to try to remove a mass for which excision would prove to be more invasive than predicted by imaging. Nevertheless, there are certain situations in which primary resection is appropriate.

Localized ovarian or testicular malignant germ cell tumours are often operated on before chemotherapy, sometimes as an emergency procedure following suspicion of torsion. Even in these cases, protocol guidelines should be followed with orchidectomy and high ligation of the cord in testicular tumours, and with salpingo-oophorectomy in ovarian tumours. If the levels of α-fetoprotein and human chorionic gonadotrophin are normal preoperatively, and if the tumour looks benign, well encapsulated, and more cystic than solid, the surgeon should remember that benign teratomas are much more frequent than malignant germ cell tumours and that these should be treated conservatively with tumorectomy and organ preservation.[4,5]

Localized rhabdomyosarcoma (RMS) arising in the paratesticular site, the walls of the trunk, the limbs, or the dome of the bladder may be operated on before chemotherapy if complete resection is feasible without danger or mutilation.

Localized neuroblastoma (abdominal or thoracic) may be operated on before chemotherapy if the surgeon is able to remove the tumour macroscopically without organ impairment and excessive haemorrhage. Factors determining resectability which must be evaluated before surgery are the relationship of the tumour to vessels and neighbouring organs (kidneys, liver, pancreas) and the possibility of intervertebral and intraspinal extension. If the renal pedicle is included in the tumour, the risk of nephrectomy is high and preoperative chemotherapy should be considered.[6,7]

Some adult-type soft tissue sarcomas, with unproven chemosensitivity, may be best operated on at diagnosis if a conservative procedure seems feasible.

Finally, most brain tumours are operated on at diagnosis, sometimes with complete excision, but most frequently with incomplete excision after a debulking procedure. The concept of debulking surgery was introduced about 30 years ago in the treatment of neuroblastoma. When a tumour was not completely resectable, it was thought best to remove as much of the bulk as possible and to treat the residual tumour with chemotherapy or radiotherapy. Nowadays, debulking surgery is not recommended except in brain tumours, since in most primary unresectable tumours preoperative chemotherapy leads to an easier and less dangerous operation and a greater chance of complete resection with a conservative procedure.

Primary reoperation

The aim of primary reoperation is to achieve complete resection (R0) in patients with microscopic (certain or possible) residue before other therapies are given, if this can be done without danger or mutilation. This particular approach is important in RMS and non-RMS soft tissue sarcoma. If a primary marginal excision or excisional biopsy (not recommended) has already been done, or where histologic evaluation is inadequate, primary re-excision should be considered.[8] This applies particularly to trunk, limb, and paratesticular sarcomas. The interval between initial surgical approach and chemotherapy, including primary re-excision, should not exceed 8 weeks.

Secondary operations (after chemotherapy)

Except for some localized tumours (described above) which can benefit from primary surgery, the majority of childhood malignant tumours are operated on after neoadjuvant chemotherapy in order to achieve complete resection (R0) of a residual mass. The intended benefit of preoperative chemotherapy is to reduce the volume and vascularity of the tumour, facilitating complete removal of the tumour with organ preservation, avoiding tumour rupture (except in neuroblastoma where peroperative fragmentation of the tumour has no adverse effect on the outcome), and downstaging the tumour to decrease postoperative treatment.

Secondary operations may be considered either as delayed primary surgery (e.g. in nephroblastoma or hepatoblastoma) or as a second-look procedure for resection of a residual mass after initial chemotherapy (e.g. in RMS or bone tumours). Some tumours, such as osteosarcoma or hepatoblastoma, cannot be cured without complete resection of the local tumour. In other tumours, such as Ewing sarcoma or RMS, adequate local therapy may include a combination of surgery and radiotherapy in order to obtain the best results. In RMS localized in the prostate and/or the bladder neck, the surgical removal of the tumour and the insertion of brachytherapy tubes during the same procedure may be planned with the brachytherapist. This attempt is made to avoid the morbidity of prostatectomy in very young boys.[9,10] The timing of secondary operations should be carefully discussed with the oncologist. For instance, in metastatic neuroblastoma or in patients with stage III neuroblastoma, when the tumour is growing around the major abdominal vessels or in the renal pedicle, resection of the tumour may lead to major complications such as chylous ascites or the need for nephrectomy, and it may be preferable to give further high-dose chemotherapy before surgery, rather than after a long complicated postoperative course or to a child with a single kidney.

Sometimes the patient achieves complete clinical and radiologic remission after initial chemotherapy. In bone tumours, surgical resection (or irradiation if surgery is not feasible) of the bone is necessary even after apparently complete remission. Limbs can be preserved by local excision of the bone tumour and reconstruction with an internal custom-made prosthesis or using bone auto- and allografts. In other tumours, such as RMS, secondary operations for verification of local control do not reliably establish complete histologic remission and are no longer indicated if no tumour is visible clinically, endoscopically, and radiologically.[11]

Surgery for relapse

The surgical procedure at relapse will depend on the treatment used during primary therapy, but mutilating operations may be justified at this stage, particularly if radiotherapy options have already been exhausted. If the tumour was chemosensitive, it is generally preferable to operate after a trial of second-line chemotherapy.

Surgery for metastasis

Surgery for initial or secondary metastasis in the lung, and sometimes in the liver, is justified when the primary tumour is controlled. Good results can be achieved with this approach in osteosarcoma[12] and nephroblastoma.[13] Multiple small peripheral lung metastases can be treated simultaneously by wedge resections, preferably via bilateral thoracotomies rather than midline sternotomy which carries a risk of mediastinitis. Segmentectomy or lobectomy should be reserved for solitary centrally located lung metastases. It is also possible to resect a solitary liver metastasis located in one lobe.

Supportive care

The surgeon has a role in facilitating treatments given by other members of the oncology team. For example, surgeons and/or anaesthetists are frequently asked to insert intravenous devices for chemotherapy or parenteral nutrition (Broviac or Hickman catheters, implantable ports) either percutaneously or surgically.

When radiotherapy is necessary, the surgeon may insert a mesh to displace the bowel out of the radiation field, or displace the ovaries by transposition either to the midline behind the uterus for the inverted field used in Hodgkin disease or to the paracolic areas for external beam radiotherapy or brachytherapy of pelvic tumours. This transposition can be performed using laparoscopic surgery, as in adults.[14]

Organ-sparing surgery

Because of the increasing concern about long-term sequelae in young adults treated for cancer in childhood, the worldwide trend in surgical oncology is to perform organ-sparing surgery. For instance, in nephroblastoma the standard operation for unilateral nephroblastoma is total uretero-nephrectomy. In synchronous bilateral tumours, surgery is planned after tumour reduction with chemotherapy, and nephron-sparing surgery (e.g. partial nephrectomy) is considered, when feasible, to preserve renal function. The risk of very long term consequences of renal hyperfiltration after nephrectomy has led some surgeons to perform partial nephrectomy in unilateral nephroblastoma.[15] This approach is not recommended in the current SIOP and NWTS protocols, except where there are contralateral urologic or nephrologic disorders or in genetic syndromes with an increased risk of Wilms tumour.

Conclusion

Surgery in paediatric oncology has changed considerably in recent years, partly because of progress in surgical and anaesthetic techniques but mainly because of an increasing interest by surgeons in the total management of the patient, with increasing involvement in establishing new multimodality treatment strategies with oncologists and other specialists. This will continue to be the best way to improve the outcome of these children not only in terms of survival, but also in terms of achieving normal life with minimal long-term sequelae.

References

1. Perilongo G, Shafford EA (1999). Liver tumours. *Eur J Cancer* 35, 953–9.
2. Ritchey ML, Kellalis PP, Breslow N, *et al.* (1992). Surgical complications after nephrectomy for Wilms tumour. *Surg Gynecol Obstet* 175, 507–14.
3. Godzinski J, Tournade MF, de Kraker J, *et al.* (1998). Rarity of surgical complications after post-chemotherapy nephrectomy for nephroblastoma. Experience of the International Society of Pediatric Oncology—trial and study SIOP-9 *Eur J Pediatr Surg* 8, 83–6.
4. Valla JS (2001). Testis sparing surgery for benign testicular tumours in children. *J Urol* 165, 2280–3.
5. Cass DL, Hawkins E, Brandt ML, *et al.* (2001) Surgery for ovarian masses in infants, children and adolescents: 102 consecutive patients treated in a 15-year period. *J Pediatr Surg* 36, 693–9.
6. Rubie H, Hartmann O, Michon J, *et al.* (1997) N-*myc* amplification is a major prognostic factor in localized neuroblastoma: results of the French NBL 90 study. *J Clin Oncol* 15, 1171–82.
7. Rubie H, Michon J, Plantaz D, *et al.* (1998) Unresectable neuroblastoma: improved survival after primary chemotherapy including carboplatin-etoposide. *Br J Cancer* 77, 2310–17.
8. Cecchetto G, Guglielmi M, Inserra A, *et al.* (2001). Primary re-excision: the Italian experience in patients with localized soft-tissue sarcomas. *Pediatr Surg Int* 17, 532–4.
9. Haie-Meder C, Breton-Callu C, Oberlin O, *et al.* (2000). Brachytherapy in the treatment of vesico-prostatic rhabdomyosarcomas in children. *Cancer Radiother* 4, 145–9.

10. **Martelli H, Haie-Meder C, Oberlin O** (2003). Conservative surgery + brachytherapy treatment in very young boys with bladder-prostate rhabdomyosarcoma: a single team experience. *Med Pediatr Oncol* **41**, 260.

11. **Godzinski J, Flamant F, Rey A, Praquin MT, Martelli H** (1994). Value of postchemotherapy bioptical verification of complete clinical remission in previously incompletely resected (stage I and II pT3) malignant mesenchymal tumors in children: International Society of Paediatric Oncology 1984 Malignant Mesenchymal Tumour Study. *Med Pediatr Oncol* **22**, 22–6.

12. **Tabone MD, Kalifa C, Rodary C, et al.** (1994). Osteosarcoma recurrences in pediatric patients previously treated with intensive chemotherapy. *J Clin Oncol* **12**, 2614–20.

13. **Godzinski J, Tournade MF, de Kraker J, et al.** (1991). Stage IV nephroblastoma with extrapulmonary metastatic involvement in SIOP 6 and 9 study. *Med Pediatr Oncol* **19**, 371.

14. **Morice P, Castaigne S, Haie-Meder C, et al.** (1998). Laparoscopic ovarian transposition for pelvic malignancies: indications and functional outcome. *Fertil Steril* **70**, 956–60.

15. **Cozzi DA, Schiavetti A, Morini F, Castello MA, Cozzi F** (2001). Nephron sparing surgery for unilateral primary renal tumor in children. *J Pediatr Surg* **36**, 362–5.

Chapter 8

Supportive care during treatment

Marianne van de Wetering

Introduction

Supportive care of the paediatric cancer patient has played an increasingly important role in the management of these critically ill patients. As intensity of primary treatment has escalated so have the side effects such as myelosuppression and infection.[1]

Supportive care has become more than supportive in the role that it has come to play to improve the survival of children and adolescents with cancer. Surgery, radiotherapy, and chemotherapy have led to improvement in survival, but this could not have happened without adequate supportive care.[2]

Prevention of infection

Children receiving treatment for cancer are at increased risk of infection from bacterial, viral, protozoal, and fungal agents. A number of strategies can be applied to reduce the risk of infections.

The environment

If the patient is neutropenic [absolute neutrophil count (ANC) < 500 cells/mm^3] there is an increased risk of acquiring nosocomial infections; it is best to stay away from the hospital-environment. One tries to encourage a normal lifestyle where children continue their school life and hobbies. Teachers should be informed of the situation and asked to tell the parents when contact with viral infections such as varicella or measles has taken place.

The hospital environment

If hospital admission is necessary in a neutropenic phase, these patients will be cared for in single rooms. Handwashing is the most essential preventative measure (in the literature handwashing has consistently been shown to prevent the spread of infection). Contact with people with an active infection should be avoided.

Nutrition and diet

There is no proof of the utility of special measures concerning food products during neutropenia (ANC < 500 cells/mm^3), but it is recommended not to eat raw food, soft cheeses, and 'snack foods'. A healthy diet is important for normal growth of the child and to maintain a healthy immune system.

Invasive procedures

During neutropenia any procedure that can disrupt the normal mucosa or skin barriers (such as dental procedures) should be avoided. Inserting a central venous catheter in children with neutropenia is best done under antibiotic cover.[2]

Selective gut decontamination

Oral non-absorbable and absorbable antibiotics are used to preserve beneficial anaerobic organisms while preventing colonization of the gut by pathogenic aerobic organisms. Usually the combination trimethoprim–sulfamethoxazole (TMP–SMZ) is used. A systematic review pooling data from 56 articles[3] has clearly shown that selective decontamination of the gut is effective in preventing bacteraemia (mainly Gram-negative bacteraemia) during neutropenic episodes. Quinolones are slightly more effective than TMP–SMZ. Newer studies combining quinolones or TMP–SMZ with erythromycin or roxithromycin to decrease Gram-positive bacteraemias have not been shown to give a significant reduction. Based on this systematic review and two other published systematic reviews[4,5] it is recommended that selective gut decontamination should be started 5 days before the expected neutropenia and continued until ANC $> 500/mm^3$.

Fungal prophylaxis

Trials of antifungal prophylaxis have yielded mixed results.[6,7] Evidence was found that oral candidiasis is reduced using drugs that are partially or fully absorbed from the intestinal tract. The partially absorbed drugs (miconazole and clotrimazole) have a better effect than the fully absorbed drugs (fluconazole, itroconazole, ketoconazole) or those that are not absorbed (nystatin, amphotericin, nystatin plus chlorhexidene). Bow et al.[5] performed a meta-analysis which included study regimens using azoles (fluconazole, itraconazole, ketoconazole, and miconazole) or polyenes (intravenous low-dose amphotericin B or the lipid-based formula of amphotericin B), and control regimens. Prophylaxis reduced the use of parenteral antifungal therapy (number needed to treat (NNT) = 10). Furthermore, there was a reduction of superficial fungal infection (NNT = 12) and mortality related to fungal infection (NNT = 52). Overall mortality and the incidence of aspergillosis were unaffected. Antifungal prophylaxis has measurable benefits for patients receiving high-dose chemotherapy, patients undergoing induction therapy for haematologic malignancies, and patients who are expected to have prolonged episodes of neutropenia.

Prevention of *Pneumocystis carinii* pneumonia

Studies by Hughes et al.[8] have clearly demonstrated that TMP–SMZ is highly effective in preventing *Pneumocystis carinii* pneumonia (PCP). All patients with leukaemia, lymphoma, or BMT (allogeneic or autologous) receive prophylaxis. Children with solid tumours who are expected to have prolonged episodes of neutropenia are also advised to use TMP–SMZ as prophylaxis. An alternative to this prophylaxis is aerosolized pentamidine. This has been shown to be effective within the group of HIV patients, but no large studies have been done in oncology patients. Aerosolized pentamidine must be given every 4 weeks.[9,10]

Treatment of infection in children with cancer

The frequency and severity of infection that occurs in the cancer patient depends on a complex interaction of a number of factors of which granulocytopenia is the most important. This is defined as ANC < 500 cells/mm^3. The frequency and severity of infections increase as ANC drops below 100 cells/mm^3. The duration of neutropenia influences the outcome of the infectious episode. Patients with neutropenia for <7 days had a 95 per cent response rate to initial antibiotic therapy compared with a 35 per cent response rate in patients with neutropenia for >15 days.[11–13] Incidence of infection in neutropenic patients is about 10–15 per cent.

The management of febrile neutropenic children with cancer differs because of institutional variations in the spectrum of infections, antimicrobial susceptibility patterns of pathogenic microorganisms, and the underlying aetiology of the neutropenia. The pattern of infective pathogens has changed significantly over time.

Gram-positive organisms are isolated in 15 per cent of febrile episodes and cause 60 per cent of proven bacteraemia, while fungal infections are documented in 2 per cent of all bloodstream infections. Poor outcome has been reported in 7–10 per cent of patients.[11,14] The coagulase-negative staphylococci are the most common Gram-positive organisms, and enterococcal and viridans group streptococcal species are becoming problematic because of increasing antibiotic resistance. The most common Gram-negative organisms are *Escherichia coli*, *Klebsiella* spp, *Serratia* spp, *Proteus* spp, and *Pseudomonas aeruginosa*. Other serious infections emerge with more intensive chemotherapeutic protocols and bone marrow transplantation because of the prolonged severe neutropenia. Infections with fungal organisms such as *Candida* species, *Aspergillus* species, or other opportunistic fungi occur.

In these patients fever is defined as a single temperature $>38.3°C$, or a temperature $>38°C$ for >1 h. In the management the clinician is directed to careful and repeated evaluation of specific signs and symptoms of a focus or type of infection. Lack of neutrophils leads to minimal signs of inflammation at the site of infection. A thorough physical examination is needed, including emphasis on the mucosal membranes, the lungs, the soft tissues, and the central venous catheter.

Laboratory evaluation should include a complete blood count, liver enzymes, renal function, and blood culture (if a central venous catheter is present, a culture should be taken from this). Urine culture, stool culture, and testing for *Clostridium* toxin should only be done if indicated. Routine culture of the cerebrospinal fluid is not recommended unless signs or symptoms of meningitis are present. Chest radiography will only be performed when signs are present which lead to the suspicion that there will be changes on the chest radiograph.

Initial antibiotic therapy

Because the progression of infection in neutropenic patients can be rapid and such patients with early bacterial infections cannot be reliably distinguished from non-infected patients at presentation, empirical antibiotic therapy should be started promptly. The initial goal is to provide broad-spectrum antimicrobial cover for both Gram-negative and Gram-positive organisms. This has generally been achieved by offering a combination of antibiotics, such as a cephalosporin and an aminoglycoside. Monotherapy in the form of carbapenem or meropenem is a reasonable alternative.

Modification of treatment

The therapeutic plan should be reassessed after 3–5 days. If the patient has become afebrile within this period and has a positive blood culture, optimal cover should be provided for that organism but broad-spectrum antibiotic cover should be maintained to prevent breakthrough bacteraemia. Antibiotic treatment should be continued for a minimum of 7 days or until the organism is eradicated. It is not necessary to continue until the neutrophils recover. A group of children can be defined who lack signs of infection, who are afebrile for >48 h, who have ANC > 100 cells/mm³, absolute monocyte count > 100 cells/mm³, and C-reactive protein (CRP) < 90 ng/l, and who are at low risk for complications; these children can have their intravenous treatment stopped after 3 days and oral antibiotics continued (oral cefixime) until day 7.[15] Risk-based therapy has not yet been validated for children. If the patient has persistent fever after 3–5 days of treatment, a careful reassessment should be performed with additional diagnostic tests such as an abdominal ultrasound scan and chest radiograph looking for a focus. If neutrophils are recovering and the child is not septic, the same antibiotics can be continued despite the continuing fever. The second option is to change antibiotics to target anaerobes, *P.aeruginosa*, or other organisms not covered by the original protocol. The third option is to add antifungal agents, especially if one expects neutropenia to be prolonged. The fourth option of stopping all antibiotics on the grounds that fever may be due to the medication as such is not recommended by the CDC guidelines. A summary is given in Figure 8.1.

Treatment of central venous catheter infections

Complications related to the long-term use of central venous catheters are minimized by recommended protocols for catheter placement, dressing, care, administration of solutions, and monitoring.[16] Infectious complications are those that result in infection of the blood-stream and/or device, the subcutaneous pocket, the tunnel, or the exit site. The overall incidence of catheter-related infections is approximately 2 per 1000 catheter days.[17] Treatment of the infected catheter can be successful in more than 80 per cent of documented catheter-related infections. Usually these infections are caused by Gram-positive organisms (mainly coagulase-negative staphylococci). Cover for Gram-negative organisms is necessary until an organism is identified. Treatment failures result from infections with multiple organisms, fungi, *P. aeruginosa*, resistant Gram-negative organisms, and tunnel infections.

In the case of a *Staphylococcus aureus* infection, the treatment should be administered for at least 2–3 weeks if the catheter is left in place as *S.aureus* is associated with a late complication rate of 6.1 per cent. If the catheter is left in place, systemic antibiotics should be administered through the catheter. Cycling antibiotics through each lumen or placing concentrated antibiotics within the locked catheter hub (antibiotic-lock technique)[18] are not widely validated yet, and so cannot be recommended. If antibiotic-lock therapy is given, systemic therapy should be used as well.[18]

Treatment of fever without neutropenia

Good evaluation and physical examination is an absolute necessity. Laboratory evaluation will include a blood count, CRP, and blood culture from the central venous catheter. If there is no central venous catheter, one can wait for the blood culture result before starting antibiotics. If a central venous catheter is present, antibiotics (e.g. amoxicillin or augmentin) can be given orally until the blood culture result is known.

Antiviral drugs

Because of the increased use of high-dose chemotherapy, cellular immunity can be depressed and therefore the chance of acquiring viral infections is increased. The most common viral pathogens affecting the immunocompromised child are the herpesviruses including herpes

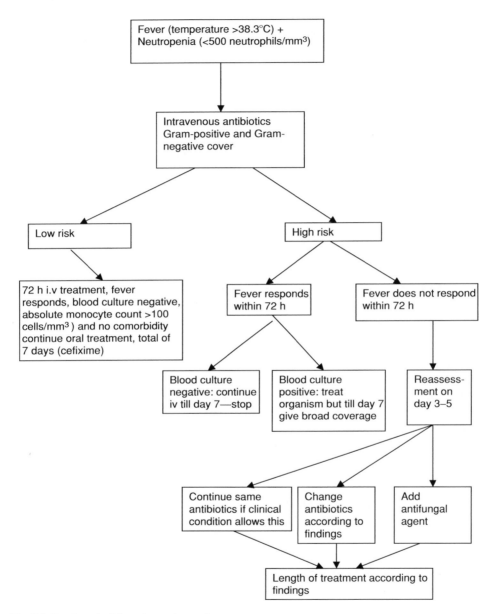

Fig. 8.1 Treatment of fever in neutropenia.

simplex virus (HSV), varicella zoster virus (VZV), cytomegalovirus (CMV), and Epstein–Barr virus (EBV).

Herpesviruses can result in mucosal lesions, skin lesions, and neurologic symptoms. Systemic treatment with aciclovir is needed at a dose of 750 mg/m^2/day divided in three doses intravenously for at least 5 days.

Primary infection with VZV results in chickenpox. In the immunocompromised, severe complications can be seen leading to a fulminating illness with visceral dissemination of the virus. Untreated VZV pneumonitis can be fatal in up to 7 per cent of affected children. Treatment should be systemic with aciclovir or the newer oral drugs such as famciclovir or valaciclovir which show a better oral absorption than aciclovir.

Cytomegalovirus (CMV) can result in fever, rash, hepatosplenomegaly, pneumonia, neuro-logic symptoms, and retinitis. Treatment is with ganciclovir 10 mg/kg/day in two divided doses intravenously or foscarnet. Prolonged courses of therapy are necessary to eradicate the infection.

Respiratory syncytial virus may have a prolonged and more complicated course. Ribavarin may offer therapeutic benefit. Adenovirus is a particular cause of morbidity and sometimes mortality in patients undergoing bone marrow or stem cell transplantation. Therapy is largely supportive.

Haematopoietic colony-stimulating factors

To determine the need for primary administration of colony-stimulating factors (CSFs), it is necessary to decide whether the risk of neutropenia associated with a particular chemotherapy regimen warrants their use.[20] Primary use of CSFs should be reserved for patients expected to have a risk of >40 per cent of experiencing febrile neutropenia. Most children are enrolled in international protocols and the use of CSF will be embedded in the protocol. Secondary prophylactic CSF administration is allowed if previous episodes of neutropenia have led to severe infections or delay or dose reduction of chemotherapy. Again, this is delineated in most paediatric protocols. The recommended CSF dose is 5 μg/kg/day either subcutaneously or intravenously, although pharmacokinetic analysis favours subcutaneous administration. The available data suggest that rounding the dose to the nearest vial size may enhance patient convenience and reduce costs without clinical detriment. Clinical data suggest that CSF should be started 24–72 h after chemotherapy and continued until the neutrophil count is $> 1000/mm^3$ on two occasions. A higher dose of granulocyte colony-stimulating factor has not been recommended because it has not been associated with improved clinical benefit. One exception is in the setting of peripheral blood progenitor cell mobilization where a dose of 10 μg/kg/day has resulted in improved mobilization.[21] Generally, children do not have any side effects from these CSFs. Occasionally a influenza-like illness can be seen, with fever, bone pain, and malaise. Laboratory investigations may show a rise in uric acid, lactate dehydrogenase, and alkaline phosphatase.

Anti-emetics

Nausea and vomiting remain an important concern in cancer treatment. In addition to an adequate pharmacological approach, other techniques, such as relaxation, distraction, and explanation of the procedures, should not be forgotten. Adequate control is usually achieved with the treatment given nowadays. Chemotherapeutic agents are grouped in three classes: low emetogenic (<10 per cent of patients experience nausea and vomiting), moderately emetogenic (50 per cent of patients experience nausea and vomiting), and highly emetogenic (100 per cent of patients experience nausea and vomiting). Medication is adjusted to the degree of emetogenecity.

In low emetogenic chemotherapy, no anti-emetic therapy is needed. Occasionally, agents such as metoclopromide, domperidone, or promethazine can be used. In moderately emetogenic chemotherapy, a serotonin receptor antagonist (usually ondansetron) should be used. If this is not effective alone, corticosteroids should be added. Both drugs will work synergistically. In highly emetogenic chemotherapy, the combination of a serotonin receptor antagonist plus steroids should be used. In this group it is recommended that one of the anti-emetics is continued for 72 h after stopping the chemotherapy (to prevent delayed emesis). A summary of anti-emetics is given in Table 8.1.

It is very important to attempt an aggressive plan at the start of therapy to avoid or minimize the initial experience of nausea, since there is a greater chance of preventing the development of anticipatory nausea and vomiting. If anticipatory vomiting does occur, benzodiazepines are usually effective.

Table 8.1. Anti-emetic agents

Emetogenic potential	Drug	Anti-emetic therapy	Delayed emesis
Low	Bleomycin Busulfan oral Steroids Fludarabine Hydroxyurea Interferon Melfalan oral Mercaptopurine Methotrexate < 50 mg/m^2 Thioguanine Vinblastine Vincristine	None OR Domperidone 0.3 mg/kg oral 4 times daily OR Promethazine 0.5 mg/kg 4 times daily	None
Moderate	Asparaginase Cytarabine < 1 g/m^2 Doxorubicin Etoposide Fluouracil < 1000 mg/m^2 Gemcitabine Methotrexate < 1 g/m^2 Thiotepa Topotecan Cyclofosfamide < 750 mg/m^2 Actinomycin Epirubicin Idarubicin Mitoxantrone < 15 mg/m^2	Ondansetron 15 mg/m^2 3 times daily OR Dexamethasone 5 mg/m^2 3 times daily	None
High	Carboplatin Carmustine Cisplatin Cyclofosfamide < 750 mg/m Cytarabine < 1 g/m^2 Actinomycin Doxorubicin < 60 mg/m^2 Irinotecan Melfalan (i.v.) Methotrexate < 1 g/m^2 Mitoxantrone < 15 mg/m^2 Procarbazine	Ondansetron plus dexamethasone	Continue ondansetron for 72 h after stopping chemotherapy

Newer agents have led to revised anti-emetic guidelines for adults. New serotonin antagonists (palanosetron) and NK-1 antagonists (aprepitant) have improved the effect on both acute and delayed emesis, which is of importance in the high emetogenic group of cytotoxic agents. To date no randomized trials in children have been performed with these new agents.

Radiotherapy can also lead to nausea and vomiting. Therefore it is recommended that a serotonin-receptor antagonist is given about 30 min before the start of radiotherapy.

Obviously the above guidelines are based on the best available evidence. However, discomfort associated with nausea and vomiting is a very subjective experience and therefore treatment should be individualized, allowing the opinions of patients and parents to influence anti-emetic regimens with subsequent courses.[22]

Pain management

Pain in children with cancer may be associated with the diagnosis itself (e.g. bone metastases in children with stage IV neuroblastoma), the treatment (e.g. mucositis during neutropenic episodes), or the procedures that have to be performed (e.g. lumbar puncture, bone marrow aspiration).

The first step in managing pain is to assess its presence accurately. In children <4 years old, the assessment relies on behavioural pain scales, where crying, posture, and facial expression are used to assess pain. Different validated scales are used for children >4 years of age; these include the faces pain rating scale and the word graphic rating scale. It is extremely important that the pain is assessed at regular intervals over the day by parents or nursing staff and the score found is acted on.

Treatment of pain caused by the disease itself or the treatment

The World Health Organization stepladder[23,24] is used as a guideline for adequate treatment of pain (Table 8.2). Its recommendations are as follows

Step 1: acetominophen.
Step 2: mild opioid (tramadol) combined with step 1.
Step 3: opioids (morphine 10 µg/kg/h continuous i.v. or s.c.) combined with step 1.
     The dose of morphine must be increased until adequate pain control is achieved.

If the patient does not achieve adequate pain control with the above stepwise approach, adjuvant therapy should be considered (Table 8.3).

Treatment of pain associated with diagnostic procedures

The main goal during paediatric procedures is to make the child comfortable so that the child and parents will not dread the subsequent procedures. Both pain and anxiety have to be managed to achieve adequate control. In general one must achieve a situation in the treatment room where adequate staff will create a calm environment so that the procedure can be performed rapidly and efficiently.

Sedation is performed in many different ways. The American Academy of Pediatrics[25] and the American Society of Anesthesiology[26] have published guidelines, but these must be individualized to the particular situation for that specific child.

1. For minor procedures such as venepuntures or access to subcutaneous reservoirs, topical anaesthetic cream (Emla®) can be used an hour before the procedure.

Table 8.2. Pain management

Medication	Dose	Remarks
Step 1		
Acetaminophen (paracetamol)	Oral 15 mg/kg 4–6times daily Supplementary 20–30 mg/kg 2–4 times daily	Maximum 4000 mg/day
Naproxen (NSAID)	5 mg/kg 2–3 times daily	Beware of thrombocytopathy
Diclofenac	1–2 mg/kg 3 times daily	
Step 2		
Continue step 1		
Tramadol	>1 year: 1–2 mg/kg 3–4 times daily	Maximum 400 mg/day Weak opioid
Step 3		
Continue step 1		
Morphine solution	0.1–0.3 mg/kg 4–6 times daily	Antagonist: naloxon
Morphine supplement	0.2–0.4 mg/kg 4–6 times daily	0.1 mg/kg i.v. or i.m.
Morphine i.v.	Starting dose 0.01–0.03 mg/kg/h or 0.25 mg/kg/24 h	
Morphine i.v. (PCA)	Bolus: 0.02 mg/kg/10 min Infusion: 0.005 mg/kg/h	
Fentanyl patch: 25, 50, 75 and 100 μg/h	Transdermal, change every 72 h Dose: morphine 90 mg oral equivalent to fentanyl 25 μg/h	Need immediate effect medication first

NSAID, non-steroidal anti-inflammatory drug; PCA, patient-controlled analgesia.
Care has been taken to ensure that the doses are accurate, but the reader should check these carefully.
Readers should also refer to other texts and experienced paediatric pharmacists for further drugs, indications and side effects.

Table 8.3. Adjuvant pharmacological therapy

Drug group	Examples	Dose	Indication
Anxiolytics	Diazepam Oxazepam	0.1–0.2 mg/kg 3–4 times daily <6 years 2.5–10 mg 3–4 times daily >6 years 2.5–15 mg 3–4 times daily	Muscle relaxant
Sedatives	Nitrazepam Temazepam	1–6 years 2.5–5 mg once daily >6 years 5 mg once daily 10–20 mg once daily	
Antidepressants	Amitriptyline	Start dose 0.2–0.5 mg/kg in 2 divided doses; dose can be increased to 3 mg/kg/day	Neuropathic pain
Antiepileptics	Carbamazepine Rivotril	1.5–3 mg/kg; increase to 2.5–5 mg/kg 2–4 times daily	Neuropathic pain and phantom pain
Steroids	Prednisone Dexamethasone	1 mg/kg/day 10 mg/m^2/day	Raised intracranial pressure, brain tumours, severe end-stage tumours

2. For procedures such as bone marrow puncture, conscious sedation can be given. Usually this will consist of midazolam (Versed®) 0.15–0.03 mg/kg rectally 15 min before the procedure or 0.05 mg/kg/i.v. slowly. If the i.v. route is followed, trained anaesthetic personnel should be available as midazolam can produce respiratory depression.
3. Procedures such as bone marrow trephine are always performed under general anaesthesia where airway patency, breathing, and circulation can be assured.

Blood product transfusion

Not only neutropenia but also anaemia and thrombocytopenia can occur as a consequence of chemotherapy or the oncological disorder itself.

Red cell transfusion

It is not necessary to increase the haemoglobin concentration to normal levels. There is no evidence-based level at which transfusion should be carried out, but most centers choose a level of < 4.0 mmol/l (6.5 g/dl) at which to administer red blood cells. If the child is septic or has cardiopulmonary problems, a level of <6.0 mmol/l (9.5 g/dl) is used, and with radiotherapy an even higher level of 7.0 mmol/l (11.5 g/dl) is maintained because of the need for adequate oxygenation during radiotherapy.[1,27] The amount given is 10–15 ml/kg packed red cells in 4–6 h. The product used is leucodepleted (7-log depletion of the number of leucocytes). In this way the chance of HLA sensitization and of infection with prions and cytomegalovirus decreases. The risk of transfusion-related graft-versus-host disease from donor lymphocytes is so small that there is no need to irradiate blood products. The use of irradiated products is only necessary before and after bone marrow transplant until lymphocyte immunity has recovered (6 months after transplant) in the case of severe combined immunodeficiencies and in neonates.[28]

To decrease the need for red blood cell transfusions, erythropoetin (erythropoetic stem cell factor) has been used in trials but is not yet registered for use in children with cancer. First results from randomized controlled trials show that erythropoetin reduces the number of red blood cell transfusions and keeps the mean haemoglobin at a higher level, especially in haematological malignancies.[29]

Platelet transfusions

As a general rule platelet transfusions are indicated if the patient is actively bleeding. Prophylactic platelet transfusions are indicated in septic patients, patients with a known bleeding disorder, and patients undergoing an invasive procedure such as placement of a central venous catheter or lumbar puncture. There is little evidence about the appropriate level for transfusion. In patients with sepsis platelets are kept $> 15 \times 10^9$/liter and for placement of a catheter or lumbar puncture the level will be kept $> 50 \times 10^9$/liter.[30,31] The quantity of platelets transfused is 1 unit/10 kg. Repeated transfusions may lead to allo-immunization, reducing the therapeutic effect of transfused platelets. One can then use single-donor transfusions.

Tumour lysis syndrome

Tumour lysis syndrome (TLS) is a set of complications that can arise from treatment of rapidly proliferating and drug-sensitive neoplasms, mostly haematologic malignancies although it has also been shown in solid tumours. Chemotherapy causes rapid destruction of tumour cells leading to release of intracellular substances into the bloodstream. Metabolic disturbances include hyperuricaemia, hyperphosphataemia, hypocalcaemia, and hyperkalaemia. As a consequence both uric acid crystals and calcium phosphate salts can be formed, precipitating renal failure for which dialysis may be necessary. The primary treatment so far has been allopurinol combined with alkaline hyperhydration. By administering sodium bicarbonate, uric acid can be kept ionized to prevent crystallization in the renal tubules. Allopurinol decreases uric acid production and increases hypoxanthine and xanthine, precursors of uric acid which have a higher solubility in alkaline urine. Since there is pre-existing uric acid and allopurinol cannot break down uric acid, 2–3 days are generally necessary for uric acid levels to decrease after initiation of allopurinol treatment. Clinical trials have now been completed using urate oxidase Uricozyme® or the recombinant form rasburicase (Fasturtec® in Europe and Elitek® in the USA). The primary function of urate oxidase is to catalyse conversion of uric acid to allantoin which is water soluble. Alkalinization is then not necessary, thus facilitating phosphorus excretion. It has been shown that urate oxidase decreased uric acid levels to a greater extent than allopurinol, and the drop in uric acid occurred within 4 h of administration. It is advisable to administer urate oxidase to those patients in whom the risk of TLS is high (Burkitt lymphoma, B-cell leukaemia and haematologic malignancies with a high white cell count). In a randomized prospective multicenter trial it was shown that the risk of developing renal complications requiring dialysis in patients treated with rasburicase was 0.4 per cent. Therefore this is the drug of choice for high-risk groups[32] (Fig. 8. 2).

Vaccinations

Recommendations on vaccination during chemotherapy[33] state that killed or inactivated vaccines do not represent a danger to the immunocompromised host, and as a general rule live attenuated vaccines should be administered at least 6 months after stopping chemotherapy. However, it is well known that the immunogenic response to vaccinations is decreased during

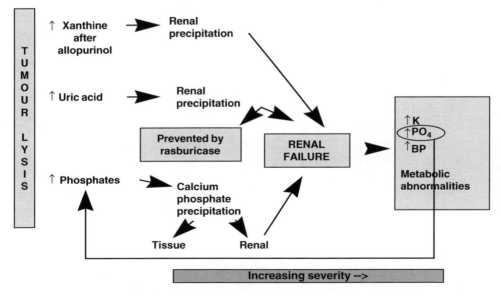

Fig. 8.2 Products of tumour lysis and their disposal.

chemotherapy. This immunogenic response is not zero, which makes it possible to vaccinate with certain vaccines, especially in areas where herd immunity is low. Certain conditions should be met and these include an adequate number of lymphocytes ($> 1000 \times 10^9$/liter), an adequate number of granulocytes ($> 1000 \times 10^9$/liter), and no use of dexamethasone 14 days before and 1 week after vaccination.

Measles–mumps–rubella (MMR) vaccine should not be administered to severely immuno-compromised patients, but if herd immunity for measles is low, single-antigen measles vaccine should be given with the understanding that this should be repeated after stopping chemother-apy. Oral polio vaccine (OPV) should be avoided in immunocompromised patients and even in household contacts. Enhanced inactivated polio vaccine (eIPV) is recommended in these household contacts and can be given to the immunocompromised patient. It is safe and can confer some degree of protection. Diphtheria–tetanus–pertussis (DTP) can be administered to the immunocompromised, including the use of acellular pertussis containing vaccines (DtaP). *Haemophilus influenzae* b conjugate vaccine (Hib) should be administered in those situations where the risk of *H.influenzae* type b is high and in persons with anatomical or functional asplenia or additional sickle cell anaemia. Hepatitis B vaccination should ideally be given after stopping chemotherapy, but in high-risk groups or areas it can be given to the immunocom-promised with a lesser immunogenic response. The vaccine advised under these conditions is Recombivax HB 40 µg/ml. Periodic booster doses are usually necessary following successful immunization, with the timing determined by serologic testing at 12-month intervals.

Special vaccinations during chemotherapy

1. **Influenza vaccination.** A systematic review emphasizing the paucity of data on this vaccine has been published.[34] Serological responses are generally lower than expected in healthy controls. Antibody levels considered protective in healthy individuals may not prevent clinical infection in those with malignant disease. There are no data on protection from clinical infection. The vaccine is well tolerated and therefore it is not contraindicated, but there is no evidence that an adequate degree of protection is achieved.

2. **Varicella zoster vaccination.** As more complications of varicella zoster infection are seen in immunocompromised patients, it would be of great benefit if oncological patients with no detectable antibodies to VZV could receive the vaccine and seroconvert. In the USA, 575 children with leukaemia in remission were immunized in the Varicella Vaccine Collaborative Study.[35] All children were in continuous remission for >1 year and had > 700/mm^3 circulating lymphocytes. Most children stopped chemotherapy for 1 week before and after immunization. It was recommended that steroids were not given for 2 weeks after the immunization. The varicella vaccine was safe, immunogenic, and effective. The major adverse reaction was a varicelliform rash, which in most cases could be treated with oral aciclovir. Seroconversion to VZV occurred in 82 per cent of vaccinees after one dose and in 95 per cent after two doses. In addition, the incidence of clinical reactivation in vaccinated children was lower than in unvaccinated leukaemic children. Varicella vaccine administered under these conditions is extremely beneficial to the leukaemic patient.

3. **Pneumococcal vaccine.** This is recommended for use in patients >2 years of age with increased risk of pneumococcal disease, such as those with splenic dysfunction, anatomical asplenia, or Hodgkin disease, or after radiotherapy to the spleen.

It must be realized that the above are recommendations for vaccination during chemother-apy (Table 8.4). Those patients who have undergone an allogeneic or autologous bone marrow

Table 8.4. Vaccination recommendations during and after chemotherapy

Time related to chemotherapy	Vaccination	Recommendation
During chemotherapy	MMR	Low herd immunity then single Ag–measles vaccine
	OPV	Not allowed; if needed use eIPV
	DTP	Preferable to wait until after stopping chemotherapy
	Hepatitis B	If needed, DTaP; high-risk areas, Recombivax HB
Special vaccinations	Influenza vaccine	Not contraindicated during chemotherapy
		Degree of protection low
		No evidence-based recommendation
	Varicella zoster	Safe and immunogenic in maintenance chemotherapy
		Not registered yet for use in children with cancer
	Pneumococcal vaccine	Splenic dysfunction, Hodgkin, post-radiotherapy (radiation spleen)
After chemotherapy	DTP, MMR, HiB	Restart schedule 6 months after stopping chemotherapy

MMR, measles–mumps–rubella vaccine; OPV, oral polio vaccine; eIPV, enhanced inactivated polio vaccine; DTP, diphtheria–tetanus–pertussis vaccine; DTaP, diphtheria–tetanus–acellular-pertussis vaccine; HiB, *Haemophilus influenzae* B conjugate vaccine.
*Table does not apply to children undergoing an autologous or allogenic BMT

transplant need to be revaccinated with DTP, HiB, and MMR. This must be started 1 year after transplant and the immunogenic response should be measured.

References

1 Ritchey AK (1996) *The Pediatric Oncology Group: Supportive Care Manual.* London: SmithKline Beecham.

2. van de Wetering MD, van Woensel JBM (2003). Prophylactic antibiotics for preventing early central venous catheter Gram positive infections in oncology patients. *Cochrane Database Syst Rev* (2), CD003295.

3. van de Wetering M, Dewitte M, Kremer L, Offringer M, Scholten R, Caron H (2005). Efficacy of profylactic oral antibiotics in neutropenic afebrile oncology patients: Systematic review of randomised controlled trials. *Eur J of Cancer* (in press).

4. Cruciani M, Rampazzo R, Malena M, *et al.* (1996) Prophylaxis with fluoroquinolones for bacterial infections in neutropenic patients: a meta-analysis. *Clin Infect Dis* 23, 795–805.

5. Engels EA, Lau J, Barza M (1998). Efficacy of quinolone prophylaxis in neutropenic cancer patients: a meta-analysis. *J Clin Oncol* 16, 1179–87.

6. Bow EJ, Laverdiere M, Lussier N, Rotstein C, Cheang MS, Ioannou S (2002). Antifungal prophylaxis for severely neutropenic chemotherapy recipients: a meta analysis of randomized-controlled clinical trials. *Cancer* 94, 3230–46.

7. Clarkson JE, Worthington HV, Eden OB (2003). Prevention of oral mucositis or oral candidiasis for patients with cancer receiving chemotherapy. *Cochrane Database Syst Rev* (3), CD000978.

8. Hughes WT, Rivera GK, Schell MJ, Thornton D, Lott L (1987). Successful intermittent chemoprophylaxis for *Pneumocystis carinii* pneumonitis. *N Engl J Med* 316, 1627–32.

9. Vasconcelles MJ, Bernardo MV, King C, Weller EA, Antin JH (2000). Aerosolized pentamidine as *Pneumocystis* prophylaxis after bone marrow transplantation is inferior to other regimens and is associated with decreased survival and an increased risk of other infections. *Biol Blood Marrow Transplant* 6, 35–43.

10. **Weinthal J, Frost JD, Briones G, Cairo MS** (1994). Successful *Pneumocystis carinii* pneumonia prophylaxis using aerosolized pentamidine in children with acute leukemia. *J Clin Oncol* 12, 136–40.

11. **Hughes WT, Armstrong D, Bodey GP, et al.** (2002). 2002 guidelines for the use of antimicrobial agents in neutropenic patients with cancer. *Clin Infect Dis* 34, 730–51.

12. **Pizzo PA** (1999). Fever in immunocompromised patients. *N Engl J Med* 341, 893–900.

13. **Roguin A, Kasis I, Ben Arush MW, Sharon R, Berant M** (1996). Fever and neutropenia in children with malignant disease. *Pediatr Hematol Oncol,* 13, 503–10.

14. **National Comprehensive Cancer Network** (1999). NCCN practice guidelines for fever and neutropenia. *Oncology (Huntingt)* 13, 197–257.

15. **Shenep JL, Flynn PM, Baker DK, et al.** (2001). Oral cefixime is similar to continued intravenous antibiotics in the empirical treatment of febrile neutropenic children with cancer. *Clin Infect Dis* 32, 36–43.

16. **Mermel LA** (2000). Prevention of intravascular catheter-related infections. *Ann Intern Med* 132, 391–402.

17. **Howell PB, Walters PE, Donowitz GR, Farr BM** (1995). Risk factors for infection of adult patients with cancer who have tunnelled central venous catheters. *Cancer* 75, 1367–75.

18. **Krzywda EA, Andris DA, Edmiston CE, Jr., Quebbeman EJ** (1995). Treatment of Hickman catheter sepsis using antibiotic lock technique. *Infect Control Hosp Epidemiol* 16, 596–8.

19. **Mermel LA, Farr BM, Sherertz RJ, et al.** (2001). Guidelines for the management of intravascular catheter-related infections. *Clin Infect Dis* 32, 1249–72.

20. **Ozer H, Armitage JO, Bennett CL, et al.** (2000). 2000 update of recommendations for the use of hematopoietic colony-stimulating factors: evidence-based, clinical practice guidelines. American Society of Clinical Oncology Growth Factors Expert Panel. *J Clin Oncol* 18, 3558–85.

21. **Somlo G, Sniecinski I, Odom-Maryon T, et al.** (1997) Effect of CD34+ selection and various schedules of stem cell reinfusion and granulocyte colony-stimulating factor priming on hematopoietic recovery after high-dose chemotherapy for breast cancer. *Blood* 89, 1521–8.

22. **Gralla RJ, Osoba D, Kris MG, et al.** (1999) Recommendations for the use of antiemetics: evidence-based, clinical practice guidelines. American Society of Clinical Oncology. *J Clin Oncol* 17, 2971–94.

23. **World Health Organization** (2003) *Cancer Pain Relief and Palliative Care.* WHO Tech. Rep. Ser. 804. Geneva: World Health Organization.

24. **Jadad AR, Browman GP** (1995). The WHO analgesic ladder for cancer pain management. Stepping up the quality of its evaluation. *JAMA* 274, 1870–3.

25. **American Academy of Pediatrics Committee on Drugs** (1992). Guidelines for monitoring and management of pediatric patients during and after sedation for diagnostic and therapeutic procedures. *Pediatrics* 89, 1110–15.

26. **American Society of Anesthesiologists Task Force on Sedation and Analgesia by Non-Anesthesiologists** (1996). Practice guidelines for sedation and analgesia by non-anesthesiologists. *Anesthesiology* 84, 459–71.

27. **Hebert PC, Wells G, Blajchman MA, et al.** (1999) A multicenter, randomized, controlled clinical trial of transfusion requirements in critical care. Transfusion Requirements in Critical Care Investigators, Canadian Critical Care Trials Group. *N Engl J Med* 340, 409–17.

28. **Przepiorka D, LeParc GF, Stovall MA, Werch J, Lichtiger B** (1996). Use of irradiated blood components: practice parameter. *Am J Clin Pathol* 106, 6–11.

29. **Rizzo JD, Lichtin AE, Woolf SH, et al.** (2002) Use of epoetin in patients with cancer: evidence-based clinical practice guidelines of the American Society of Clinical Oncology and the American Society of Hematology. *J Clin Oncol* 20, 4083–107.

30. **Gmur J, Burger J, Schanz U, Fehr J, Schaffner A** (1991). Safety of stringent prophylactic platelet transfusion policy for patients with acute leukaemia. *Lancet* **338**, 1223–6.

31. **Heckman KD, Weiner GJ, Davis CS, Strauss RG, Jones MP, Burns CP** (1997). Randomized study of prophylactic platelet transfusion threshold during induction therapy for adult acute leukemia: 10 000/μl versus 20 000/μl. *J Clin Oncol* **15**, 1143–9.

32. **Navolanic PM, Pui CH, Larson RA,** *et al.* (2003) Elitek-rasburicase: an effective means to prevent and treat hyperuricemia associated with tumor lysis syndrome, a Meeting Report, Dallas, Texas, January 2002. *Leukemia* **17**, 499–514.

33. **Anonymous** (1993) Recommendations of the Advisory Committee on Immunization Practices (ACIP): use of vaccines and immune globulins for persons with altered immunocompetence. *MMWR Recomm Rep* **42**, 1–18.

34. **Ring A, Marx G, Steer C, Harper P** (2002). Influenza vaccination and chemotherapy: a shot in the dark? *Support Care Cancer* **10**, 462–5.

35. **LaRussa P, Steinberg S, Gershon AA** (1996). Varicella vaccine for immunocompromised children: results of collaborative studies in the United States and Canada. *J Infect Dis* **174** (Suppl 3), S320–3.

Chapter 9

Psychosocial issues

Bob F. Last and Martha A. Grootenhuis

Introduction

Today approximately two-thirds of children with cancer survive their illness. This also means that one-third of children diagnosed with cancer still die as a result of their illness. Children with cancer generally die because the treatment was not successful after a relapse, or as a consequence of therapy complications. Although chances of survival decrease after a recurrence of the disease, an increasing number of children with relapse do survive, or their lives can be prolonged. Survival rates of children with cancer have increased dramatically in recent decades. In the developed countries about one in every 1000 adults reaching the age of 20 years will be a long-term survivor. This progress in medical care has changed the focus in paediatric psycho-oncology from descriptions of the impact of expectation of death of the child to estimating the impact of living with and after treatment for cancer on the quality of life of the child and the family. The whole family has the difficult task of adjusting to a situation dominated by the stresses of long-lasting uncertainty and uncontrollability. The emotional consequences for the children, parents, siblings, and survivors will be described.

Experiences like hospitalization, undergoing painful medical procedures and multiple oper-ations, or taking medicines affect physical, cognitive, and social–emotional development. Parents are facing the stresses and concerns of raising a child suffering from a disease with an unpredictable course and outcome. How children and parents cope with the disease and its consequences contributes to good or poor adjustment. In the second part of this chapter coping, communication, and child-rearing issues will be discussed as important intermediate factors. Suggestions for support are given in the third section of this chapter. A special section is dedicated to the palliative phase, because this period demands different strengths from the child and the parents.

Emotional reactions

Appraisal

People evaluate the significance of events for their well-being through cognitive appraisal processes. Each specific emotion corresponds to a different appraisal, a different situational meaning structure.[1] Every situation consists of different components. The component which is dominant for a person determines which emotion will arise. Components which are important in the appraisal of the situation for children with cancer and their parents are uncertainty, uncontrollability of the situation, responsibility, restriction of freedom, and the long duration of the situation. **Uncertainty** about the course and outcome of the disease is a condition related to hope and fear. Indications pointing to a remission of the disease contribute to a feeling of hope and trust, while indications of a relapse or recurrence of the disease evoke feelings of fear that all efforts will be unsuccessful. Being confronted with cancer means being confronted with **uncontrollability**, which easily evokes feelings of helplessness. Children and parents cannot influence the disease or the treatment process very much. This is in the hands of doctors and nurses. The child has to undergo many painful medical procedures while parents stand by helplessly. The child is frequently unable to attend school, participate in sports, and/or play with friends. Parents have to make arrangements for work, housekeeping, holidays, support for the siblings, and so on. These **limitations of freedom of action** evoke feelings of frustration and anger. The answer to the question as to who or what is **responsible** for the situation is related to feelings of guilt if the person feels that he or she is to blame, or anger if someone else is to blame. **Long duration** of the threatening situation is associated with feelings of exhaustion and depression if the child or parent does not perceive an end to the suffering.

Children

The family of a child with cancer lives under high emotional distress during the medical treatment of the ill child. Children are faced with repeated invasive medical procedures as part of their treatment or as a method for evaluating the effectiveness of treatment. Frequent visits to the hospital ward are common, especially when the treatment is of long duration or when complications occur. The family is confronted with constant uncertainty regarding the course of the disease and its prognosis, and with changes in the ill child's physical condition, appearance, and behavioural reactions to the illness.

Children differ from adults. From birth until adulthood children are in a process of physical, cognitive, emotional, and social development. In developing their abilities to cope with their environment children are dependent on adults. Together they are in a child-rearing relationship, in which the parents play an important role. Younger children need their parents to cope with basic fears and basic desires and also with the demands of socialization. Older children need their parents in learning to cope with questions related to physical growth, development of personal identity, and difficulties of functioning in peer groups. Children also differ from adults in their understanding and experience of health, illness, and medical care. Depending on the child's developmental level special needs have to be met in the context of the family (parents, siblings) and the wider social environment (friends, school, health care workers).

Improvement in treatment schemes has resulted in a better quality of life during treatment compared with some decades ago. An example is the increase of treatment in day-care centers. Nevertheless, children with cancer experience much physical discomfort during treatment. Feelings of anxiety can easily arise when confronted with painful medical procedures like bone marrow aspiration, lumbar puncture, and venepuncture. Supportive care programmes aimed at preparing children for these procedures have been shown to be effective in reducing negative emotions. Isolation of children (in case of bone marrow transplantation or radio-isotope treatment) can evoke heightened levels of separation anxiety, especially in younger children. In the outpatient treatment period, children with cancer can find it difficult to return to school, which may result in school phobia if proper support is absent. However, studies of emotional functioning of children have not revealed deviant emotional functioning in terms of psychiatric disorders. Like children suffering from a chronic disease, children with cancer tend to develop more submissive and less assertive behaviour.

Since the 1980s, quality of life has been included in studies of the consequences of chronic illness for adults and, more recently, children. The current consensus on the assessment of quality of life is to include at least four domains: physical, cognitive, social, and emotional functioning. Health-related quality of life (HRQoL) refers to the specific impact of an illness, injury, or medical treatment on an individual's quality of life. The effects of childhood cancer and its treatment often increase the child's dependence on his or her parents and other adults and decrease participation in peer- and school-based activities. This could have an adverse effect on the accomplishment of developmental tasks, resulting in an impaired quality of life.

A number of studies have shown implications for quality of life and various areas of functioning when a child is confronted with treatment for cancer. Perhaps one of the major findings is that prophylactic treatment of children with acute lymphoblastic leukaemia (ALL) by cranial radiation affects cognitive development negatively, particularly if this treatment is given at an early age.[2] Many children with cancer experience school-related problems, which create difficulties with academic work as well as jeopardizing social relationships.[3] In many paediatric oncology units part of the intervention programme involves helping children to return to school and to respond to the questions and reactions of others.

Parents

Until the prognosis of childhood cancer improved, studies mainly focused on how parents dealt with the threatened and almost certain loss of their children. Particular emotional reactions for parents were feelings of anger, blame, grief, and guilt. With the increased survival of children with cancer, parents have to deal with the uncertainty and unpredictability of childhood cancer. Many studies have been conducted among parents of children with cancer and different reactions have been reported for different phases of treatment.[4] Researchers who focused on parents of newly diagnosed children, or children who are in treatment, have reported increased emotional distress such as anxiety or depression compared with normal subjects. In longitudinal studies increased negative emotions such as anxiety, depression, insomnia, or somatic and social dysfunctioning are also found shortly after diagnosis. Uncertainty and loneliness were the most frequently reported problems in a study conducted by Van Dongen-Melman et al.[5] Being a mother, low socio-economic status, no religious affiliation, other chronic disease in the family, and concurrent stresses were important risk factors for more emotional problems of parents in this study, and these risk factors have also been reported in other studies. It has been argued that parents of children with cancer are at risk for post-traumatic stress symptoms (PTSS). Highly anxious parents are at particular risk for PTSS and they may benefit from approaches (such as enhancing self-efficacy) that decrease anxiety during and after treatment.[6]

Survivors

Since the introduction of modern therapies (around 1980) more children with cancer are surviving their illness. Therefore the interest in the side effects of cancer treatment in cancer survivors has increased. These side effects include both medical and psychosocial problems that influence the survivors' quality of life. While many survivors have no physical evidence of disease and appear to have made full recoveries, others have to come to terms with the chronic, debilitating, or delayed effects of therapy. All remain at risk for the development of late sequelae of the former disease and/or treatment and of second malignancies. Furthermore, in most cases the life-threatening experience of cancer is never forgotten (see also Chapter 11).

Most research about survivors shows that they function well psychologically. However, some studies report that survivors have lower rates of marriage and parenthood, job discrimination, difficulties in obtaining work, and problems in obtaining health and life insurance, as well as worries about reproductive capacity and/or future health problems in their children. Clinical reports suggest that many survivors of childhood cancer experience fatigue as a long-term effect of their treatment.[7]

Although inconsistent data have been reported across studies, the following factors related to the functioning of survivors have been discussed. Female gender, older age at follow-up, greater number of relapses, presence of severe functional impairment, cranial irradiation, and minority survivors are associated with an increased risk of emotional problems. Survivors of central nervous system tumours and ALL seem to be at risk for educational deficits. The same is true for cranial irradiation and early age at diagnosis. Finally, survivors of bone tumours are more likely to perceive their health as fair or poor, and also report lower physical functioning than controls.

Siblings

When a child is diagnosed with cancer, siblings experience their own distress. They have to adapt to the idea that their brother or sister is ill, to changing roles in the family, and to a sudden decrease in attention from their already overburdened parents. Siblings may be overwhelmed by fear for the health of their brother or sister and by fear for their own health, by guilt for not being sick themselves, by concerns for their parents, and by feelings of isolation, jealousy, anger, and frustration.[8] The siblings of the child with cancer need to adapt to these changes, to additional responsibilities, to a decreased physical and emotional availability of the parents, and to intrusive and conflicting emotions. Whether or not siblings are able to adapt depends on the resilience of the family and the child. There is some evidence for the hypothesis that psychosocial distress is temporary. Although emotional problems diminish over time, siblings may still experience limitations in their social interactions for a longer period. Adolescent girls seem to be especially at risk for internalizing problems.

Coping, communication, and child-rearing issues

Coping

'Coping' is the term used to describe how a person deals with a stressful situation. Lazarus and Folkman[9] define the coping process as 'cognitive and behavioural efforts to manage specific external and/or internal demands that are appraised as taxing or exceeding the resources of a person'. One's perceptions, or cognitive appraisals, are important elements in regulating distress or managing the problem causing the distress. Problem-focused coping involves direct efforts to ameliorate the problem causing the distress, whereas emotion-focused coping is directed towards regulating effects surrounding a stressful experience.[9] People not only have emotions, they also handle them. When a family has to cope with the life-threatening illness of a child, there is little that family members can do to change the situation or exert control over it. Without control, family members have to rely on emotion-focusing coping strategies or cognitive control strategies. The following disease-related cognitive control strategies are often seen in children with cancer and their parents.[10] They can rely on the competence of the medical specialists and keep faith in the treatment regimen (vicarious control). They can try to remain optimistic about the course of the disease and the future and wish for better times (predictive control). Furthermore, they can try to understand the situation in order to gain a sense of control by finding information and sharing feelings with other (interpretative control). Parent's intensive use of the Internet shows the reliance on this control strategy. Apart from information seeking, social support is also an important coping strategy for parents of children with cancer. Social resources can reinterpret the meaning of the situation so that it seems less threatening, or may provide distraction from their concerns.

One of the best-known ways of coping is the use of denial. Individuals facing a life-threatening illness often go through a phase of denial; they try to protect themselves from painful or frightening information related to external reality. Whether denial is a negative force or can be considered as adaptive is a point of controversy. Denial can be useful, but in the long run it can also lead a patient to conceal serious physical complaints. This is the difference between denial of facts and denial of implications. Patients who are able to function effectively and are able to maintain a high degree of optimism, behaviour that may be viewed as denial, can also be viewed, from a cognitive viewpoint, as using 'selective information processing' or considered to be showing healthy denial. The term 'resilience' has been introduced to bridge the gap between the differing viewpoints. It describes the strengths and abilities of patients' and families, who can 'bounce back' from the stress and challenges they face and eliminate, or minimize, negative outcomes.[11] It is the experience of many health care providers that patients or families show the ability to adapt to stress and to be able to cope with a threatening situation. This capacity to keep on going is what is meant by 'being resilient'. This corresponds to the work of Folkman and Moskowitz[12] who stress the importance of positive reappraisal (reframing a situation in a positive light) in coping with a chronic illness.

Communication

Communication about the disease involves two aspects: exchange of information about the disease and exchange of emotions evoked by the situation. To a large extent, communication between child and parents consists of attempts to reduce uncertainty and increase control. Information about the disease can reduce the child's uncertainty. It enables the child to distinguish better between events that are threatening and events that are not. It provides the child with a safety signal and is an important means of achieving control of the situation. The beneficial effects of **open information** on the child's emotional functioning have been shown in various studies.[13] Open information motivates the child to make an (ongoing) effort to endure the highly aversive treatment. Moreover, understanding what is wrong with you can itself provide some sense of control. However, knowing and understanding the facts, given the nature of the situation, is not enough for setting up an effective barrier against the threat. Thus most of the communication concentrates on protection from the arousal of negative emotions evoked by the threat.

In communication between child and parents, it is very striking that protecting oneself is often achieved through protecting the other. Attempts to influence the other's appraisal in order to reduce his or her negative emotions not only involve showing compassion and empathy, but also serve to protect oneself against confrontation with the other's emotions. This is called the **law of double protection**. It is essential for the child to believe that his or her parents are strong; if they can handle the situation, it gives the signal that the threat can be averted. The parents, in turn, need to believe that the child is strong; if the child can handle the situation, it strengthens their confidence that the child will survive. The parents' avoidance of discussing their worries and grief related to the illness prevents the child from thinking about it, and protects the parents from being confronted with the child's emotions. We also find this phenomenon in the child. Not asking questions which might worry the parents, hiding grief, and being brave are attempts at preventing the parents from being distressed and themselves from being overwhelmed by the parents' emotions. The child should not be forced to talk about the disease, but a response should be made to the often subtle hints which children give when they want to talk about the situation. An area of tension exists between the need to control the situation by double protection and the need to share emotions with the other person. If the threatening stimuli and the emotions are too strong to be denied, then the need for sympathy and support becomes dominant. Open communication fulfils this need. Concealing facts which cannot remain hidden from the child strengthens the child's cognition that 'it is too bad to talk about'.

Open information enables the child to discriminate between facts and the implications of those facts. By supplying the facts and simultaneously offering reassurance and hope of a favourable outcome, the child will again be in a position to build up self-protection. Open information is a necessary condition for effective self-protection.

Child-rearing attitude

Parents of children with cancer have a difficult task. They are faced with the threat of a possible loss of their child and have to find a way of coping with the emotions that arise from the situation. Moreover, they have to comfort their child and give him or her the support that is needed during hospitalization and medical treatments which are often painful. It is understandable that most parents tend to be more indulgent and protective to their seriously ill child than they were before the illness was diagnosed. Changes in behaviour as a result of the side effects of treatment (e.g. aggressiveness during periods in which the child is given the drug dexamethasone) can be very difficult for the parents to handle. In general, a more protective attitude is not harmful for the child's development, but over-indulgence without setting limits and structuring the child's behaviour will increase feelings of uncertainty in the child. The same is true for the siblings in the family. The focus of the parents is on the child with cancer and the other children often receive less attention from their parents for a period of time. Parents may have feelings of guilt towards their other children, resulting in an over-indulgent attitude. Alternatively, parents may react more restrictively to their other siblings by changing their child-rearing values since daily worries seem less important. In reaction, the siblings may withdraw themselves from family life. In giving support to the parents one should be aware of these possible changes in child rearing and discuss their problems in this area in an open way.

Support
Guidelines for support

In caring for children with cancer and their families it is helpful to ask three questions on a regular basis.[14]

1. What situational characteristics (uncertainty about the course of the disease, restriction of freedom of action, uncontrollability, or responsibility) are dominating for the child or the parents?
2. Which coping strategies do the child or the parents use and are these strategies (still) effective? In other words, which emotions are dominant?
3. What sources of support are available and do the child and/or parents use these possibilities of social and/or professional support?

In coping with a stressful situation, children and parents use the various control strategies in a specific way. Psychosocial intervention is indicated if control fails and subsequently the child and/or parents need support in rebuilding their defences. At such a moment, the child and/or parents are no longer able to control their emotions themselves and rely on different control strategies. For example, if a child is very scared about the course of the disease, we should look critically at the amount and content of information he or she has about the illness (enhance interpretative control). If the child fears a negative outcome of the disease and shows little confidence in his or her doctor, it may be necessary to give information and enhance faith in the treatment and physician (enhance vicarious control).

An awareness of the developmental and cognitive levels of the child at the time of diagnosis, and the psychologic and situational status of the family, is crucial for providing appropriate interventions. An important guideline in psychosocial preventive care is encouragement of open communication within the family and the wider social environment. It is helpful to ask the child and the parents regularly about their concerns and worries.

In all phases of the disease it may be necessary to refer the child, the parents, or other family members for professional help by a psychologist, social worker, or psychiatrist. Frequent reasons for referral are questions about the cognitive development of the child and school-functioning, difficult behaviour related to side effects of treatment, emotional problems and the need to change ineffective coping strategies, support in reorganizing family life, and financial problems.

Close cooperation between the paediatric oncologist and the psychosocial coworkers is a precondition for effective preventive and supportive psychosocial care. Bereavement follow-up care of parents and siblings, which is an integral part of terminal care, should be integrated into the psychosocial care of families. Continuing improvements in outcomes of cancer therapy and in psychotherapeutic treatment will reduce the psychologic impact and assist with the child and family's adjustment to childhood cancer.

Palliative phase

If the disease cannot be cured the treatment will be focused on palliation. However, in most cases it is not possible to define the terminal period very clearly. Often, the child with cancer is on a sliding slope with worsening prognosis, but the pendulum of hope and fear remains present for a long time. In these circumstances an important role is reserved for the doctor. Giving open information by telling the child and the parents that the treatment is no longer aimed at curing the disease but on palliation of symptoms will bring forward the process of grief and mourning.

After a long period of uncertainty there is now certainty about what can be expected from medical treatment. Research has shown that children with cancer, as early as the age of 4 years, develop a notion of their own mortality based on their experiences with the disease.[13] Their concept of death is linked with their developmental stage: a very young child will perceive death as temporary; in the elementary school period the concept of death develops to a more final separation; from the age of 12 the child knows that death is a universal phenomenon that is related to everything living.[15] In the palliative phase it is important that the child can express his or her thoughts and emotions about the impending death. In this period children need to be reassured that they will not be left alone and they will not endure unnecessary pain. The words that will be used to talk about the meaning of death will depend on the family's beliefs and religion and the age of the child. Some children want to talk specifically about certain wishes, about what they want to do once more, or about the organization of the funeral. Young children may discuss these matters in an indirect way, by making a drawing or by telling a story. In approaching the child it is important to be open to these subtle hints.

For the parents, the message that the child cannot be cured is a shock. Disbelief and the notion that what was feared are becoming reality now often go hand in hand. Thoughts about how the death of their child might come and about the funeral, but also about what fine moments with the child will be missed, evoke feelings of pain and grief. Sometimes parents do not communicate with each other about these thoughts and feelings in order to protect each other.

Often parents fear the way that their child will die. Will my child suffer from needless pain? Will it happen when I am not there? In this period parents are often very irritable. They may be angry not only with the doctor who cannot cure their child, but also with other people in their environment because they are in a condition of heightened irritability with little interest in others. During the child's illness, parents suffer from feelings of guilt. These feelings might arise from perceived shortcomings in meeting the needs of the child, or from questioning whether everything has been done to cure the disease. During these days most parents live in a situation of heightened alertness. They may be very active and want to spend most of the time with the dying child. Sometimes they doubt whether they are strong enough to hold on, especially if other burdensome circumstances are present, such as marital problems, unemployment, health problems in other family members, or financial problems.

For parents, it is important to experience moments of warm closeness and intimacy with the child which they can look back on gratefully later. Many parents describe a change of values in their life. Some goals (e.g. material wishes) become less important, while others, like enjoying family time, are more valued. In many cases these changes in values are long lasting.

In conclusion, it should always be possible for a declining child to die without unnecessary physical pain, fear, or anxiety. It is essential that he or she receives adequate medical, spiritual, and psychologic support, and at no point feels abandoned. Palliative care, in the terminal phase of cancer, should be tailored to the different needs and desires of the child and the family, with the aim of providing the best possible quality of life for the days that remain.

References

1. Frijda NH (1986). *The Emotions*. Cambridge, UK: Cambridge University Press.
2. Jankovic M, Brouwers P, Valsecchi MG, *et al.* (1994). Association of 1800 cGy cranial irradiation with intellectual function in children with acute lymphoblastic leukaemia. ISPACC. International Study Group on Psychosocial Aspects of Childhood Cancer. *Lancet* **344**, 224–7.
3. Eiser E (2001). Cancer. In: Koot HM, Wallander JL (eds) *Quality of Life in Child and Adolescent Illness. Concepts, Methods and Findings*. Hove, UK: Brunner–Routledge, 267–96.
4. Grootenhuis MA, Last BF (1997). Adjustment and coping by parents of children with cancer: a review of the literature. *Support Care Cancer* **5**, 466–84.
5. Van Dongen-Melman JE, Pruyn JF, De Groot A, Koot HM, Hahlen K, Verhulst FC (1995). Late psychosocial consequences for parents of children who survived cancer. *J Pediatr Psychol* **20**, 567–86.
6. Best M, Streisand R, Catania L, Kazak AE (2001). Parental distress during pediatric leukemia and posttraumatic stress symptoms (PTSS) after treatment ends. *J Pediatr Psychol* **26**, 299–307.
7. Langeveld NE, Grootenhuis MA, Voute PA, de Haan RJ, van den Bos C (2003). No excess fatigue in young adult survivors of childhood cancer. *Eur J Cancer* **39**, 204–14
8. Zeltzer LK, Dolgin MJ, Sahler OJ, *et al.* (1996). Sibling adaptation to childhood cancer collaborative study: health outcomes of siblings of children with cancer. *Med Pediatr Oncol* **27**, 98–107.
9. Lazarus RS, Folkman S (1984). *Stress, Appraisal, and Coping*. New York: Springer.

10. **Grootenhuis MA, Last BF** (2001). Children with cancer with different survival perspectives: defensiveness, control strategies, and psychological adjustment. *Psycho-Oncology* **10**, 305–14.

11. **Patterson JM** (1995). Promoting resilience in families experiencing stress. *Pediatr Clin North Am* **42**, 47–63.

12. **Folkman S, Moskowitz JT** (2000). Positive affect and the other side of coping. *Am Psychol* **55**, 647–54.

13. **Van Veldhuizen AM, Last BF** (1991). *Children with Cancer. Communication and Emotions.* Lisse, The Netherlands: Swets & Zeitlinger.

14. **Last BF, Grootenhuis MA** (1998). Emotions, coping and the need for support in families of children with cancer: a model for psychosocial care. *Patient Educ Couns* **33**, 169–79.

15. **Eiser C** (1990). *Chronic Childhood Disease. An Introduction to Psychological Theory and Research.* Cambridge, UK: Cambridge University Press.

Chapter 10

Palliative care

Helen Irving

Introduction

There has been a dramatic improvement in outcome for children with cancer as a consequence of the multidisciplinary approach to care, enrolment of patients in cooperative clinical trials, and advances in the biologic understanding of cancer and mechanisms of drug activity. However, 30 per cent of children still die as a consequence of refractory or relapsed disease and cancer remains the most common medical cause of death in developed countries for children aged between 1 and 19 years. As more children are protected from infectious diseases, cancer also has an increasingly significant role in the developing world. While the focus in cancer care is rightly directed at cure, there is a need to optimize palliative care to enhance quality of life for the child, the family, and the broader community.

Transition to palliative care

Palliative care is defined by the World Health Organization (WHO) as:[1]

> ...the active, total care of patients whose disease, in the light of present medical knowledge, is not responsive to curative treatment. Control of pain, other symptoms and of psychological, social and spiritual problems is paramount...and encompasses ongoing grief and bereavement support...the goal...is achievement of the best quality of life for patients and their families.

This traditional definition implies a precise time point when treatment with curative intent stops and palliative care begins. For many cancers of childhood, there is no definitive point at which the direction of treatment changes. Therefore the transition is more 'fluid' in nature and is directed by the child's illness, the family's wishes, and the physician's understanding of the family and underlying disease. A decision to direct treatment towards palliation is a difficult and gradual process based upon open communication, trust, emotional safety, empowerment of the child and family, and a respect by the physician for the uniqueness of each family.[2]

However, delay in initiation of palliative care can result in crisis-oriented management, loss of opportunity to promote the principles of care, an absence of a framework for proactive interventions or decision-making which may be of benefit to the child and family, and difficulty in providing family support.[3–5] Reasons for delay in the initiation of palliative care come from health professionals and families. A recent survey investigating attitudes and practices among paediatric oncologists regarding end-of-life care found that almost half reported a feeling of failure at the prospect of a patient dying within 6 months.[6]

To optimize care, a more transitional model for the initiation of palliative care will give families more access to supportive care throughout a disease trajectory[7,8] (Fig. 10.1) The American Academy of Paediatrics and the WHO advocate this model such that a child

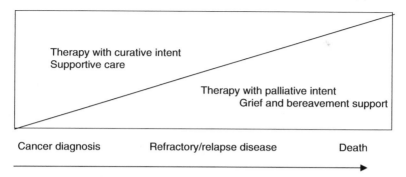

Fig. 10.1 Transitional model of palliative care.

might participate in a phase I trial, for example, while receiving symptom management and support while living with uncertainty and the possibility or probability of death.[9] A recent study in the USA reported that 24 per cent of children who had relapsed or progressive disease entered phase I trials and 38 per cent entered phase II studies. Half received treatment during the last month of life.[10] While it may be reasonable to consider anticancer therapy in the last weeks of life, a clear decision must be made as to the reasoning behind the choice, where hope of cure will be replaced by hope for optimal quality of life and a peaceful and dignified death.[9]

Wherever possible, decision-making should involve the child or adolescent. The ability to make informed choices will depend upon their own life experiences, cognitive ability, and personality, and the family's cultural and religious beliefs. Children experience and understand disease and death differently according to their age, stage of development, and experience with death and illness. Consequently, communication with the child will depend on these factors and should be adaptive.[11] Child preferences and insights may also guide choices and decision-making by families and health professionals. The approach to care must be coordinated by a key worker, should be family centered and flexible, with access to professionals who can provide emotional, physical, spiritual, and psychosocial support to the child and family in a place of their choice.[2,5,9]

Common symptoms and management

Symptom management of a dying child greatly influences the ability of the family and community to cope with a child's death. The approach must be individualized and is outlined in Table 10.1.[2]

Pain management

Cancer pain is a complex mix of physical sensation, agitation, and irritability, and is compounded by anxiety and by psychosocial and cultural factors, as well as by the responses of the child and family to the underlying stage of disease. It is the most frequently experienced symptom in children with cancer, occurring as a result of the cancer itself, treatments, procedures, or incidental causes.[12,13] Aims of management are to relieve pain at rest and during activity, and to ensure comfort during sleep with minimal side effects.

Table 10.1. Approach to symptom management

- ◆ History and assessment
- ◆ Identification of the cause
- ◆ Ongoing communication with the child and family
- ◆ Explanation of symptoms and treatment
- ◆ Establishment of goals of therapy (e.g. pain relief)
- ◆ Implementation of therapy
- ◆ Regular review and modification of treatment as required

Classification of pain

Pain can be classified by its origins and pathway of transmission to the brain into two broad categories, **nociceptive** (somatic and visceral) and **neuropathic**.[14] Invasion of bone and bone marrow is typical of somatic nociceptive pain and is the most common cause of pain in the child with cancer. This pain is typically described as constant and irritating with no paraesthesia. Neuropathic pain is typically associated with burning throbbing sensations and altered sensory perception.[14] Severe pain that is reported after minimal stimuli is sometimes misinterpreted as symptom magnification, but is typical of pain with a neuropathic basis.[15]

Pain assessment

Assessment is dependent upon the child's age, developmental stage, and previous experiences. Obtaining qualitative and quantitative descriptions of pain from very young or non-verbal children can be very difficult. The use of a number of different parameters is necessary for determining location, nature, and severity of pain. Simple observation of the child is very useful. Any change in behaviour may indicate discomfort. Assessment can be enhanced by using of visual analogue tools, including the smiling faces or thermometer scales, and colouring a body outline in different shades[16] (Fig. 10.2).

Treatment

Pain relief is possible for most patients, with >80 per cent of children requiring opioids during the palliative phase of their illness.[5] Medication is generally administered according to the following guidelines.

- ◆ By mouth: oral administration is convenient, non-invasive, and cost effective.
- ◆ By clock: regular scheduling ensures a steady state, reducing the peaks and troughs of on-demand dosing.
- ◆ By ladder: this enables a stepwise approach to treatment[13] (Fig. 10.3).
- ◆ By the individual child: the individualized approach recognizes inter-child variability.[13]

Analgesic agents

Analgesics can be classified into two groups.

Primary analgesics:
   non-opioid and non-steroidal anti-inflammatory drugs
   weak opioids
   strong opioids.

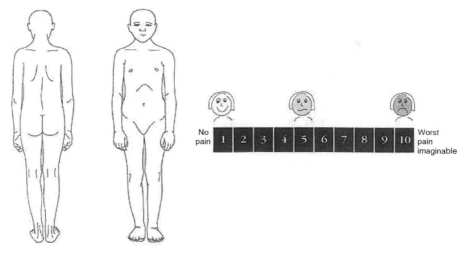

Fig. 10.2 Visual analogue scales and body outline.

Secondary analgesics/adjuvant drugs:
    antidepressants
    anticonvulsants
    corticosteroids.
    Doses and indications are given in Table 10.2.

Primary analgesics The non-steroidal anti-inflammatory drugs (NSAIDs), such as naproxen, ibuprofen, and diclofenac, have an antiprostaglandin activity, suppress inflammation, and reduce pain. Side effects include nausea, gastric irritation, ulceration, and impaired platelet function. They should be used cautiously in children with thrombocytopenia. The Cox-II inhibitors may offer an alternative for children with bleeding diatheses, but further evaluation

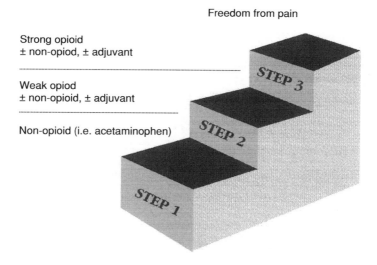

Fig. 10.3 WHO analgesic ladder.

Table 10.2. Common analgesic agents (primary and secondary)

Drug	Dose	Frequency and indication
Acetaminophen	15 mg/kg (oral or rectal)	Every 4–6 h: mild pain, fever
Amitriptyline	0.2–0.5 mg/kg (oral) 1–5 mg/kg/day (oral)	At night: neuropathic pain At night: antidepressant
Carbamazepine	2 mg/kg (oral)	Every 12 h: neuropathic pain
Codeine phosphate	0.5–1 mg/kg (oral)	Every 4 h: mild–moderate pain
Diclofenac	1 mg/kg (oral)	Every 8–12 h: mild pain (NSAID)
Fentanyl	100–400 mg/kg (s.c./i.v.) 2–4 mg/kg/h (s.c./i.v.) 25, 50, 75, 100 mg/h	Bolus: severe pain Infusion, ↑**dose as required** Transdermal patch
Ibuprofen	2.5–10 mg/kg/dose (oral)	Every 6–8 h: mild pain (NSAID)
Methadone	0.1 mg/kg (oral)	Every 4–6 h: severe pain, morphine intolerance
Morphine sulphate	0.3–0.5 mg/kg (oral) 0.1–0.2 mg/kg (s.c./i.v.)	Every 4 h regularly Starting dose, increasing as required ↑**dose as required** Bolus every 4 h, infusion, ↑**dose as required**
Sustained release morphine (MS Contin)	0.9 mg/kg (oral)	Every 12 h, ↑**dose as required**
Naproxen	5–10 mg/kg (oral)	Every 12–24 h; mild pain (NSAID)
Sodium valproate	5–15 mg/kg (oral)	Every 8–12 h; neuropathic pain

Every effort has been made to ensure that the doses are accurate, but the reader is advised to check these carefully. Readers should also refer to palliative care texts and experienced paediatric pharmacists for further drugs, indications and side effects.[2,13,14]

is required. Acetaminophen (paracetamol) has a mild anti-inflammatory effect and is well tolerated.

If pain is not controlled with acetaminophen, a weak opioid such as codeine phosphate can be commenced. However, codeine causes significant constipation and has a ceiling analgesic effect.

Morphine binds selectively to the μ opioid receptor and is available in oral, parenteral, spinal, and rectal preparations. It is readily absorbed orally which is the preferred route of administration. Morphine mixture, in appropriate dosing, provides 4–6 h of analgesia and should be prescribed every 4 h. There is *no* role for on-demand dosing in palliative care, as breakthrough pain is distressing and difficult to control. The dose should be adjusted to that which relieves pain. Incremental increases of 30–50 per cent per dose may be required within 24 h. Once the appropriate 24-h dose of morphine is determined, transfer to controlled release preparations may be possible. Controlled release preparations have a slower onset of action and a longer duration of action. They are available in tablet, granule, or capsule form and can be

Table 10.3. Example of daily morphine dosing and conversion to sustained release morphine for a 15 kg child receiving an initial dose of 0.3 mg/kg

Four-hourly dose	Total 24 h dose	MS Contin dose	Breakthrough dose
5 mg	30 mg	15 mg every 12 h	5 mg

administered twice daily or daily, depending on the formulation. Immediate release morphine should be available to the child for relief of 'breakthrough pain' (Table 10.3). If repeated doses of breakthrough morphine are required, the dose of controlled release morphine should be increased. A continuous subcutaneous/intravenous infusion of morphine is a simple and effective mode of drug delivery if the oral route becomes problematic.

Hydromorphone and oxycodone are analogues of morphine with similar pharmacokinetic and pharmacodynamic properties. Hydromorphone is six times as potent as morphine, and the potency of oxycodone is about three-quarters of that of morphine. These agents can be used if there is sensitivity to morphine.

Methadone is a synthetic long-acting opioid with strong affinity for both μ and δ receptors. It also has antagonist activity at the N-methyl-D-aspartate (NMDA) receptor sites and consequently may have a role in neuropathic pain. It is not generally considered as first-line therapy, but may play a role in children with significant side effects or allergy to morphine. Because of its long half-life, accumulation can occur, leading to sedation. Consequently, the child should be closely monitored for the first few days after initiating methadone or when there is a significant dose increase.[14,15]

Fentanyl is a synthetic opioid that can be given parenterally or via a transdermal patch. Transdermal fentanyl has fewer side effects than morphine; in particular, there is less constipation, nausea, and drowsiness. There is a delay of 12–18 h after patch application before therapeutic levels are reached, and consequently transdermal fentanyl has a limited role in children with rapidly escalating pain. The patches are easily applied, release the drug at a steady rate, and are changed every 72 h. Transdermal fentanyl is most effective in children with relatively stable cancer pain and who require a minimum of 60 mg equivalent of oral morphine daily.[17]

Opioid side effects and precautions for their use All opioids have side effects and constipation is the main problem. Laxatives should always be prescribed whenever opioids are used, unless transdermal fentanyl is used when lower doses or no laxatives at all may be required.[17] Unlike many of the other side effects, tolerance to constipation does not occur. After the administration of breakthrough doses of morphine, drowsiness and nausea can occur, but once a stable dose is achieved these effects become less problematic.

Opioids will cause respiratory depression if given in an inappropriate dose, which is generally above that required for analgesia, or if there is concomitant renal insufficiency or liver failure. The dose of opioid required for analgesia can be close to that which depresses respiration (the double effect), raising concerns about hastening death. However, optimal analgesia and quality of life are of paramount importance and should override these concerns. It is also important to recognize that not all pain can be relieved with morphine alone. For example, neuropathic and muscle pain are often opioid resistant and adjuvant agents or therapies are frequently required to manage pain.

Secondary analgesics Tricyclic antidepressants (TCAs) in low dose are useful for neuropathic pain, particularly painful paraesthesia, peripheral neuropathy, or deafferentation pain. TCAs exert their effect by inhibiting norepinephrine and serotonin uptake, thereby increasing inhibitory neurotransmitter tone at the level of the spinal cord. As well as having a direct analgesic effect, they potentiate opioid analgesia via adrenergic or serotinergic mechanisms. A low dose of amitriptyline at night usually has an effect within 48–72 h.[13,14] The newer selective serotonin-reuptake inhibitors (SSRIs) are ineffective analgesics and should not be substituted for TCAs; however, they may be useful in improving affect and can be used in combination with low-dose TCAs.[15]

Anticonvulsants, such as carbamazepine or sodium valproate, are useful for pain related to nerve infiltration/compression which is often periodic or spasmodic. They have a stabilizing effect on excitable cell membranes and prevent the spread of neuronal excitation.[14] Because of the potential interaction with other agents and the risk of blood dyscrasia with carbamazepine, gabapentin may be useful for neuropathic pain.[15]

Mexiletine, clonidine, nifedipine, and ketamine may also be useful for patients with refractory neuropathic pain. However, they are rarely required in children and are generally used by specialist palliative care physicians.[15]

Low-dose corticosteroids act as anti-inflammatory drugs and can reduce bone pain. However, dosing should be restricted because of potential significant side effects.

Other secondary analgesic drugs include antispasmodics, anxiolytics, and bisphosphonates. Bisphosphonates inhibit bone reabsorption and may be useful for treatment of pain secondary to hypercalcaemia and bony metastases. For example, pamidronate binds irreversibly to bone, resists enzymatic degradation, and inhibits osteoclasts, reducing local synthesis of prostaglandins. Calcitonin is a naturally occurring osteoclast inhibitor and has been used in the adult palliative care setting.[15] However, these drugs are expensive, and bone pain can generally be managed with a combination of opioid and anti-inflammatory drugs or with focal radiotherapy.

Adjuvant therapy Both chemotherapy and radiotherapy can be used for palliation, and radiotherapy in particular can have a potent analgesic effect. One or two fractions are often all that is required, and the effect can be quite rapid. Consequently, the opioid requirement is likely to lessen. Bone-seeking radiopharmaceuticals such as strontium-89 and samarium-153 also effectively reduce bone pain. Eventually, treatment with radiotherapy and chemotherapy is not a viable option, as the disease becomes resistant and the journey from home to treatment center becomes too exhausting for child and family.

Nerve blocks are occasionally indicated in children with well-defined somatic or visceral pain. Spinal opioid therapy and epidural anaesthetics are effective for pelvic pain and often allow a reduction in sedative doses of oral or subcutaneous opioids. Blocks can be temporary, prophylactic, or permanent, and should be placed by experienced anaesthetists.

Complementary therapy Physical therapies such as warmth, cold, touch, and electrical therapy are useful, with touch and massage producing relaxation and stimulation of afferent pathways. Transcutaneous electrical nerve stimulation (TENS) acts by inducing electrical activity in larger afferent fibers, thereby reducing nociceptive pain signals in the dorsal horn of the spinal cord which induce paraesthesia over the painful area. It is useful in treating musculoskeletal and neuralgic pain.

Fear and anxiety will aggravate pain, and good communication with the child and family will assist in management. Simple measures of distraction, play, and music are helpful. Older children and adolescents are also able to learn relaxation techniques and respond well to cognitive therapy which allows them to regain control and pain relief.

Gastrointestinal symptoms

Oral problems

Children who are debilitated, or have poor oral intake or poor oral hygiene, are susceptible to mouth problems. Regular mouth care, tooth cleaning, and mouthwashes are beneficial. Chewing or sucking unsweetened pineapple pieces can also help, as pineapple contains the proteolytic enzyme ananase. Xerostomia or dry mouth is common, and simple measures such as sucking ice, frozen juices, or frozen drinks will moisten the mouth and relieve thirst. Improving mouth care and treating or preventing infection can also reduce mucosal bleeding.

Nausea and vomiting

The most common cause of nausea and vomiting during palliative care is related to opioid use. Other causes include drugs, upper gastrointestinal inflammation, raised intracranial pressure, metabolic disturbances, constipation, and infection. Vomiting is coordinated by the vomiting center in the reticular formation of the medulla and is stimulated by the chemoreceptor trigger zone (CTZ) and by autonomic afferents from the viscera and higher centers. Anti-emetic drugs have different effects upon these sites and the choice of agent is dependent upon the possible aetiology. For example, drug-induced and metabolic anomalies act upon the CTZ, and serotonin antagonists such as ondansetron, haloperidol, prochlorperazine, and metoclopramide will be of benefit. Antacids and H_2 antagonists such as ranitidine will provide relief from gastritis. Disturbances of gastric emptying can be helped with agents that increase emptying such as metoclopramide and domperidone. If raised intracranial pressure is likely, steroids may temporarily alleviate symptoms. Stimulants such as metoclopramide should be avoided in children with possible gut obstruction, as pain and obstruction can be further aggravated. Care should also be taken with phenothiazines in children because of the potential for dystonic reactions.

Constipation

Normal bowel function requires coordination of motility, mucosal transport, and defecation reflexes. When segmental non-propulsive motility predominates, constipation develops. Constipation causes abdominal pain, anorexia, nausea, and vomiting, and when severe it can cause overflow diarrhoea. The aetiology can be divided into the following groups: primary, which is related to intra-abdominal or neurologic pathology; secondary, which is more common and is associated with drugs, particularly opioids; other exacerbating factors, such as electrolyte disturbances, immobility, and poor intake of fluid and fiber.

Assessment is based upon the previous and current pattern of bowel habit, the underlying condition, food and fluid intake, medication, and previous laxative use. Treatment includes general measures such as prevention, encouragement of fluid and fiber intake, enhancing mobility, and laxative treatment. Which laxative to select is based upon cause, patient preference, drug availability, and degree of constipation. Laxatives are classified as lubricants/stool softeners, stimulants/contact, osmotic laxatives, and local rectal applications. As opioids reduce the propulsive movement of the bowel, treatment should aim to stimulate and soften the stool. Naloxone at 10–20 per cent of the morphine dose may have a role in severe opioid-induced constipation.[14] If constipation is well established, suppositories or a small enema will be required to clear the lower bowel before a normal bowel pattern can be established. Large-volume enemas can lead to fluid and electrolyte disturbances, particularly in the debilitated child, and should be avoided.

Diarrhoea

The cause of diarrhoea is usually evident from the history and the underlying condition. Simple measures such as ceasing laxatives, high-fiber foods, and enteric supplements will aid management. Medication is frequently required and loperamide 0.05–0.1 mg/kg (maximum 2 mg) is generally well tolerated and effective. If severe watery/osmotic diarrhoea is suspected, such as can occur with severe gut graft-versus-host disease and in children with HIV infection, subcutaneous octreotide can be helpful. Morphine either orally or subcutaneously will also alleviate diarrhoea.

Anorexia and feeding issues

Anorexia is common in the later stage of the child's illness. Families find this very distressing, and support and explanation is required to assist the family to understand that anorexia is a component of progressive disease. Pain, nausea, oesophagitis and gastritis, constipation, drugs, anxiety, and depression can also contribute. Treatment of reversible conditions and presentation of small simple meals may improve intake. Whether enteral feeding is initiated must be considered on an individual child and family basis, and generally only if the quality of life of the child will be improved by its introduction.

Respiratory symptoms

Dyspnoea

Breathlessness is caused by pulmonary and extrapulmonary conditions. It may be reversible with relatively simple measures, such as oral antibiotics if infection is present and optimizing analgesia when dyspnoea is related to pain. Where anaemia is contributing to dyspnoea, transfusion should be considered. If pleural effusions are symptomatic, drainage can be considered if the general condition allows. However, re-accumulation will occur, and further drainage or interventions should be individually determined. Palliative radiotherapy may reduce mediastinal disease and pulmonary metastases.

Supportive measures Positioning the child in a comfortable and upright position in bed or a chair, increasing air movement with a fan, and improving ventilation in the room by opening windows will aid in the management of dyspnoea. Breathing exercises and relaxation techniques may be beneficial to the older child. Anxiety contributes to the degree of dyspnoea, and so the child and family should be managed in a calm and reassuring manner. Low-dose diazepam (0.04–0.2 mg/kg every 8 h) is often helpful in reducing anxiety. In the terminal phase of illness, midazolam combined with morphine in a subcutaneous infusion is often required to reduce anxiety, agitation, and distress from air hunger.

Bronchodilators If bronchospasm is present or if there is a history of asthma, bronchodilators and corticosteroids may be beneficial. Steroids may also relieve bronchial compression and lymphangitis carcinomatosis.

Opioids Opioids decrease patient awareness of dyspnoea by moderating the reflexive drive to breathe and may also improve the efficiency of breathing and exercise endurance. The role of nebulized morphine is debatable, but it has been shown to be effective for some patients, particularly those receiving morphine for pain relief.[14] Low-dose morphine (2–5 mg) in normal saline is nebulized with air or oxygen and administered every 4 h if a trial has been beneficial to the child. Bronchospasm may occur after the first dose, but responds to bronchodilator therapy.[18] Nebulized fentanyl may cause fewer problems than morphine as it evokes less histamine release, although further studies are required.[15]

Oxygen therapy Oxygen may be helpful in those with metastatic pulmonary or mediastinal disease. Headache, nausea, daytime drowsiness, and confusion may indicate hypoxia, and having oxygen available is reassuring for child and family. The use of oxygen prior to activity may be all that is required. Oxygen should be discontinued if no definite benefit is noted.

Cough

Cough is caused by irritation to receptors in the upper or lower respiratory tract, pleura, pericardium, or diaphragm. Simple measures such as antihistamines or anticholinergic drugs, antibiotics for respiratory infection, and linctus will sooth the throat and reduce irritant dry cough. Suppression of cough with opioids is indicated for distressing dry cough. If a child is already receiving morphine for pain relief, increasing the total dose may be effective. Bronchodilators may ease bronchospasm. Nebulized saline with local anaesthetic agents (lidocaine 2% or bupivicaine 0.25% 5 ml via nebulizer every 4–6 h) can be tried for intractable cough (note that the gag reflex will be anaesthetized and it is recommended that the patient does not eat or drink for 1–2 h after administration).[19]

Excess secretions

Excessive secretions or difficulty in clearing pharyngeal secretions will cause 'rattly' or noisy breathing terminally or in children with brainstem lesions. Positioning will assist with postural drainage of secretions. Anticholinergic drugs, such as hyoscine hydrobromide (0.2–0.4 mg s.c. every 4 h) can be used to reduce the production of secretions. Atropine can also be used but will lead to bradycardia with repeated dosing.

Cheyne–Stokes respiration

In the terminal phase, periodic respiration is common with slowing of breaths and episodes of apnoea. This is distressing for the family, and explanation and reassurance should be given that the child will not be distressed and that this is a normal part of the dying process.

Bleeding and anaemia

Anaemia

Anaemia is frequently seen and decisions regarding blood transfusion should be made on an individual basis depending on the stage, life expectancy, and symptomatology of the child. If anaemia is interfering with the child's activity, transfusion is appropriate. As the disease progresses and the child's activity reduces, anaemia will become less symptomatic and transfusion may not confer any benefit on the child.

Bleeding

Active bleeding is distressing for both the child and the family. Prevention of bleeding with platelet transfusion should be considered for children with thrombocytopenia. As for blood transfusion, the decision to transfuse platelets should be determined on an individual patient basis, discussed with the family, and reviewed periodically. Bruising and petechiae are common but not life threatening, and do not necessarily require treatment. Tranexamic acid (Cyklokapron®) 20 mg/kg every 8 h orally may be given to help stabilize clots that form over a bleeding area, particularly from mucosal surfaces such as gums, mouth, and gut. Thrombin packs and gelfoam may also be helpful. Bleeding from ulcerated areas on the skin or perianally can also be treated with topical 1:1000 epinephrine.[19] Sucralfate dispersed in water-soluble gel can be used topically. If major bleeding occurs when death is imminent, treatment should be directed at calming the family and simple supportive measures. As blood pressure and cardiac output drops, bleeding reduces. Analgesia and sedation should be administered to relieve any distress.

Neurologic symptoms

Anxiety

Fear of the unknown, of potential symptoms, and of suffering will cause anxiety in the child and family. Communicating with the child and family will help allay some fears, but occasionally anxiolytics or antidepressants may be of benefit to the child. Relaxation techniques, distraction, music, meditation, and cognitive therapy may be of benefit for older children.

Seizures

Seizures can occur as a result of metabolic disturbances, intracranial lesions, raised intracranial pressure, and pre-existing epilepsy. Children with epilepsy or previous seizures should continue their usual anticonvulsants. However, control of seizures may be lost if the child is unable to tolerate oral medication and alternative routes or drugs may be required. Diazepam given either intravenously or rectally is an effective anticonvulsant and there is usually a prompt response. Clonazepam may be useful for diazepam-resistant fits. As neither have a prolonged anticonvulsant effect, regular oral or subcutaneous anticonvulsants should be commenced. Midazolam is easily administered subcutaneously in either continuous or bolus dosing (Table 10.4).

Muscle spasm and myoclonus

Muscle spasm can occur as a result of immobility, pain, neuropathic spasm, or cramp. Appropriate analgesia will reduce protective muscle spasm and low-dose diazepam can be considered if muscle spasm itself is causing pain. Encouraging mobility or changing position regularly will reduce spasm and contracture development. Myoclonus is a toxic effect of opioids, but is seen less frequently in children than in adults. Midazolam as a bolus or infusion is usually effective.

Terminal care

Terminal care generally refers to care in the last days or hours of life and is associated with progressive deterioration and changes in physical signs and symptoms. For most children and their families, this care will be home based.[2,4,5,9] Care must be coordinated and flexible

Table 10.4. Management of seizures

Emergency treatment
Diazepam 0.2–0.4 mg/kg i.v. or rectally
OR
Clonazepam 0.5 mg (<10 years) or 1 mg (>10 years) i.v., s.c., or rectally
OR
Midazolam 0.5 mg/kg i.v. or s.c.

Maintenance treatment
Phenytoin 2 mg/kg every 6–12 h
OR
Phenobarbital mg/kg every 12 h
OR
Carbamazepine 2 mg/kg every 8 h

Continuous treatment when oral route is not possible
Diazepam 5 mg (1–5 years) or 10 mg (>5 years) rectally as required
OR
Midazolam 100 mg/kg/h (10–30 mg/24 h) s.c. infusion

with access to 24-h advice from experienced health care professionals. The aims of terminal care are to:

♦ ensure that the child is free from pain and other distressing symptoms
♦ maintain the dignity of the child
♦ neither shorten nor prolong the child's life
♦ prepare and support the family for the child's death.

Generally the child will spend an increasing amount of time sleeping, but restlessness and agitation are common. This may be due to pain, hypoxia, anxiety, nausea, metabolic disturbances, or simple discomfort such as being too hot or too cold. Reassessment and modification of treatment is crucial to alleviate such distress. As death approaches, the child is less likely to tolerate oral medications. Alternative routes such as rectal, transdermal, and subcutaneous will be required. A continuous subcutaneous infusion via a syringe driver is simple to commence and is generally well tolerated, and several drugs can be used in combination. The Graseby syringe driver is a portable battery-operated variable speed driver. It allows subcutaneous infusions of small volumes over periods ranging from 30 min to 50 h.[14] Bolus medications can also be administered. Drugs are generally prepared in normal saline or water for injection. The combination of an analgesic (e.g. morphine) and an anxiolytic (e.g. midazolam) is most common.[2] Morphine dose is calculated based on the current requirement of the child. For example, if the child requires 120 mg oral morphine daily, 40 mg of parenteral morphine will be required for the 24-h period, increased according to the child's needs. Anti-emetics, anticonvulsants, and anticholinergic agents such as hyoscine hydrobromide (30–60 mg/kg/day) or glycopyrrolate (4–8 mg/kg dose) can be added as necessary. The requirements for each child will vary and the prescription should be made on an individual basis and reviewed regularly.

Specific drug notes

Midazolam (0.2–1 mg/kg/day) is an anxiolytic, sedative, and anticonvulsant agent which is suitable for an agitated or distressed child. Additional boluses can also be given. Haloperidol 50–100 mg/kg/day can also be used for agitation and restlessness. It also has an anti-emetic effect and is less sedating than midazolam. Metoclopramide can cause skin reactions, but is generally well tolerated and is an effective anti-emetic. Diazepam, chlorpromazine, and prochlorperazine **should not** be administered subcutaneously as they cause pain and skin reactions at the injection/infusion sites.[2,14]

Total care

Palliative care does not merely involve symptom management. It should include spiritual care, psychosocial support, and ongoing bereavement support. Local resources and cultural background will guide the nature and extent of psychosocial support. It must encompass total care of the child in a culturally sensitive manner and extend to the parents, siblings, grandparents, and friends.

The death of a child is also traumatic for the health professional. In a paediatric oncology palliative care environment, this trauma may be intensified because of the long-term relationship with the child and family, the previous primary focus upon cure, and the prospect of repeated losses associated with deaths of patients who relapse or fail to remit. It is critical that health professionals recognize this stress and employ strategies at both the individual and workplace levels to ensure a healthy professional lifetime. Despite the personal and professional challenges, to be able to assist in the provision of physical, emotional, and spiritual comfort to a dying child and his or her family is one of the most rewarding aspects of medical care.

References

1. **World Health Organisation** (1990). *Cancer Pain Relief and Palliative Care.* WHO Technical Report Series 804. Geneva: World Health Organization.
2. **Irving H, Liebke K, Lockwood L, Noyes M, Pfingst D, Rogers T** (1999). *A Practical Guide to Paediatric Oncology Palliative Care.* Brisbane, Australia: Royal Children's Hospital (Queensland Government Publication).
3. **Hilden JM, Himelstein BP, Freyer DR, Friebert S, Kane JR** (2001). End-of-life care: special issues in pediatric oncology. In: *Improving Palliative Care for Cancer.* Washington, DC: National Cancer Policy Board.
4. **Goldman A** (1996). Home care of the dying child. *J Palliat Care* 12, 16–19.
5. **Goldman A** (1998). *Care of the Dying Child.* Oxford: Oxford University Press.
6. **Hilden JM, Emmanuel EJ, Fairclough DL, *et al.*** (2001). Attitudes and practices among paediatric oncologists regarding end-of-life care: results of the 1998 American Society of Clinical Oncology survey. *J Clin Oncol* 19, 205–12.
7. **Kane JR, Barber RG, Jordan M, Tichenor KT, Camp K** (2000). Supportive/palliative care of children suffering from life-threatening and terminal illness. *Am J Hosp Palliat Care* 17, 165–72.
8. **Frager G** (1999). Paediatric palliative care. In: Joshy SK (ed.) *Palliative Medicine Secrets.* Philadelphia, PA: Hanley & Belfus, 157–73.
9. **Hynson JL, Gillis J, Collins JJ, Irving H, Trethewie S** (2003). The dying child—how is care different? *Med J Aust* 179 (Suppl), S20–2.
10. **Wolfe J, Grier HE, Klar N, *et al.*** (2000). Symptoms and suffering at the end of life in children with cancer. *N Engl J Med* 342, 326–33.
11. **Stevens MM** (1998). Psychological adaptation of the dying child. In: Doyle D, Hanks GWC, MacDonald N (ed.) *Oxford Textbook of Palliative Medicine* (2nd edn). Oxford: Oxford University press, 1046–55.
12. **Miser AW, Dothage JA, Wesley RA, Miser JS** (1987). The prevalence of pain in a pediatric and young adult cancer population. *Pain* 29, 73–83.
13. **World Health Organisation** (1998). *Cancer Pain Relief and Palliative Care in Children.* Geneva: World Health Organization.
14. **Twycross R** (1994). *Pain Relief in Advanced Cancer.* Edinburgh: Churchill Livingstone.
15. **Galloway KS, Yaster M** (2000). Pain and symptom control in terminally ill children. *Pediatr Clin North Am* 47, 711–46.
16. **McGrath, PA.** (1990). *Pain in Children: Nature, Assessment and Treatment.* New York: Guilford Press.
17. **Noyes M, Irving H** (2001). The use of transdermal fentanyl in paediatric oncology palliative care. *Am J Hosp Palliat Care* 18, 333–41.
18. **Chandler S** (1999). Nebulized opioids to treat dyspnea. *Am J Hosp Palliat Care* 16, 418–22
19. **Woodruff R** (1997). *Symptom Control in Advanced Cancer.* Heidelberg, Victoria, Australia: Asperula.

Chapter 11

Late effects of cancer treatment and current protective measures

Meriel E. M. Jenney

Introduction and history

The best protection against the development of late effects following therapy for childhood cancer is to avoid or minimize any damage by therapy in the first place. Where possible, therapy should be reduced by lowering doses of chemotherapeutic agents known to be associated with late adverse effects, or by reducing the dose or field of radiation, minimizing exposure to normal and sensitive tissues, to limit injury. Cure remains paramount, even where concerns of adverse late effects exist. However, as the understanding of the biology of tumours and the risk that individual patients face from their tumours improves, treatment can be delivered with greater confidence to optimize cure rate and at the same time reduce therapy, where possible, to minimize late adverse sequelae.

Some children will inevitably require intensive therapy with predictable late effects, and for them protection means the early identification of problems, prompt intervention, and optimal coordination of ongoing care, often through multidisciplinary support.

This chapter is not an exhaustive list of late effects that occur in different groups of patients. For details of the late effects of therapy the reader can refer to recent texts including that by Wallace and Green.[1] Another important study is the Childhood Cancer Survivors Study (CCSS),[2] which has generated a large body of evidence. This is an epidemiologic study of over 14 000 survivors of childhood cancer in the USA. It provides detailed information relating to the treatment the patients had received and their current health status. Although many of the treatment strategies have changed since the patients within that cohort were treated, it is nonetheless a comprehensive study and the size of the population allows detailed exploration of the long-term impact of different therapies.

Another important group of survivors are those who have undergone bone marrow transplantation. The issues affecting these patients will not be fully discussed in this chapter, and the reader is referred to a recent series of comprehensive reviews of the impact of bone marrow transplantation on both the endocrine[3] and non-endocrine[4,5] late effects that can occur following this procedure.

When considering the evidence base relating to the late effects of therapy for childhood cancer the difficulty in obtaining reliable data systematically must be recognized. Cross-sectional clinical studies of patients can provide important information about the late effects of therapy and have been the backbone of research in this area. However, they are limited by the variation in therapy that many of the patients have received. Other demographic differences such as age at diagnosis, stage of disease, and changes in approach to therapy and provision of supportive care over time may also have an impact on the spectrum and severity of problems seen. Patients treated in a similar way within individual clinical trials are the most valuable source of accurate information about important late effects. There is a need for prospective studies of late effects to be built into ongoing clinical studies, but the late sequelae of therapy can take a long time to develop and follow-up is challenging but costly. Therefore these studies lag behind those of acute clinical therapy.

Protection against late effects is about prevention and intervention. This chapter will explore two themes. First, we consider how the impact of late effects can be minimized through early recognition and, where possible, the use of interventions and additional therapy. Secondly, we explore specific areas where late effects have been recognized and how strategies have been introduced within the treatment setting and clinical trials to minimize long-term toxicity. The importance of coordinating the follow-up of patients in order to optimize ongoing care in a cost-effective way will also be considered. With the steady rise in the numbers of survivors, there is a need to rationalize follow-up strategies and identify how patients can realistically receive ongoing care into the long term.

Predictable late effects: what can be done?

Cardiac complications

If a patient survives >5 years without tumour recurrence, one important cause of late mortality is treatment-related cardiac disease.[6,7] Radiotherapy and anthracycline chemotherapy cause late cardiac dysfunction and have been and continue to be widely used in the treatment of childhood cancer. Many survivors are at some degree of risk. But at how much risk? As echocardiographic and other techniques used to identify abnormalities of cardiac dysfunction improve, many of which may be subclinical, the interpretation and clinical significance of some of these findings, may be debated. Robust evidence relating to the real need for, the frequency, and the appropriate method of follow-up remains elusive.

Cardiac disease is an important cause of morbidity in the general population regardless of prior cancer therapy. Several factors may interact with radiation or anthracycline-related cardiac disease; these include hyperlipidaemia, hypertension, smoking, and obesity, particularly as the age of the population of survivors increases. Appropriate health education is an important aspect of ongoing care and must not be overlooked.

Anthracyclines

Exposure to anthracycline chemotherapy and the use of radiotherapy to the mediastinum, chest, thoracic spine, or whole body are the most important risk factors for the development of cardiac disease in the long term. Exposure to both treatment modalities significantly increases long-term risk, but either therapy alone can lead to late complications. The impact of radiotherapy will be discussed below.

There has been considerable debate about the regimens used for the administration of anthracyclines, in particular the length of infusion (e.g. bolus, 48 h) and the use of cardioprotective agents. There is evidence from a randomized trial that dexrazoxane (cardioxane) has a protective effect against acute injuries.[8] There has been recent reassuring evidence, based on a cohort of patients treated for leukaemia in the UK, demonstrating no association between length of infusion time and later cardiac dysfunction.[9]

Guidelines for follow-up have been based on large retrospective studies of patients and there is a need for prospective assessment of risk factors and the frequency and methods used for follow-up. Those risk factors currently recognized as important are cumulative anthracycline dose, young age at therapy, female gender, and additional radiotherapy (Table 11.1). Subclinical

Table 11.1. Patients at higher risk of cardiotoxicity who may warrant more frequent surveillance

---

- Previously treated for early anthracycline cardiotoxicity
- Total anthracycline dose >250 mg/m^2
- Young age at time of therapy
- Mediastinal, lung, or left chest wall irradiation with anthracycline
- Undertaking isometric exercise (e.g. weightlifting)
- Pregnancy: close monitoring essential
- Patients in puberty or on sex steroid replacement therapy
- Patients on growth hormone therapy
- Patients with congenital heart disease

---

abnormalities of cardiac function have been identified, using echocardiography, in patients following relatively low cumulative doses of anthracyclines. All patients exposed to the agent should have some assessment of cardiac function following therapy. A fractional shortening of <28 per cent is generally regarded as significant in the long term, although other findings such as septal dyskinesia and dysrhythmias may also be important. If significant abnormalities are identified, formal advice regarding limitation of activities should be sought from a cardiologist with an interest in this area. Although aerobic exercise is generally safe and indeed encouraged, there are concerns about patients with known abnormalities undertaking isometric exercise (e.g. weightlifting) and generally this should be avoided in this situation. There are reports of cardiac decompensation during pregnancy, and it is imperative that those girls who have received a higher dose of anthracyclines, particularly at a young age, or who have had additional radiation to the chest are monitored during pregnancy and, if necessary, labour.

The frequency of cardiac evaluation has been difficult to define and varies between international groups, particularly as access to appropriate paediatric or adult cardiology services may also vary. In general, the younger the age at time of therapy and the higher the cumulative dose received, the more frequent is the follow-up. Most cardiologists would reassess patients, even with normal cardiac function, during or at the end of puberty and if clinically significant abnormalities are identified, follow-up would then be more frequent. Cardiac impairment following anthracycline chemotherapy can continue to deteriorate over time. The awareness of potential deterioration during puberty, pregnancy, and isometric exercise is important. Patients and their parents should be fully informed of the risks, and coordination of cardiac follow-up in these settings is essential.

Does early therapy improve outcome?

If there is symptomatic cardiac dysfunction, patients will usually receive appropriate therapy with ACE inhibitors and diuretics with or without digoxin. However, whether early therapy for subclinical dysfunction leads to an improved long-term outcome is unclear. Whether the use of ACE inhibitors in asymptomatic patients with subclinical anthracycline cardiotoxicity is of value remains unproven, although there has been considerable interest in this area. Other measures of cardiac function such as the serum measurement of natriuretic peptides [N-terminal of the propeptide atrial natriuretic peptide (NT-proANP)] are also currently being explored, but their use remains experimental at present.

Radiotherapy

The heart is exposed to radiation within any field involving the mediastinum. However, lung, abdominal, left chest wall, spinal, and total body irradiation may also directly affect the heart and result in late complications. Patients receiving doses $\geq$40 Gy are at greatest risk, as are those who have also received cardiotoxic chemotherapy, such as anthracyclines or high-dose cyclophosphamide, or who were young at the time of radiotherapy. Radiation-induced cardiac disease, particularly coronary vascular disease, has been most commonly reported in survivors of Hodgkin disease. In one large cohort of patients, the relative risk of death due to acute myocardial infarction was 41.5 (95 per cent confidence interval, 18.1–82.1).[10] Cardiomyopathy and valvular disease can also occur. Many patients will be asymptomatic, with symptoms reported to occur 7–39 years following radiotherapy.

Regular clinical evaluation with specific relevance to cardiac complications is clearly very important. Frequency of screening depends on risk factor; the higher the radiation dose and the younger the age at therapy, the greater will be the frequency. Early referral to a cardiologist is strongly recommended if any subclinical abnormality occurs (e.g. prolonged QT interval, cardiac dysfunction, or dysrhythmias). Other factors that predispose to cardiac disease, such as obesity, hyperlipidaemia, and a strong family history, should also be considered and intervention for patients with these additional risk factors may be particularly important. Additional evaluation during pregnancy is also recommended.

Pulmonary complications

Chemotherapy

The frequency of lung complications appears to have fallen over recent years, largely because of a greater understanding of which chemotherapeutic agents cause significant long-term damage and of the impact of radiotherapy which has led to the avoidance of pulmonary complications.

Many patients will have mild abnormalities of pulmonary function; they will be asymptomatic, although on closer questioning some will admit to some exercise intolerance. Formal lung function testing will demonstrate a mild restrictive abnormality (e.g. patients following treatment for acute lymphoblastic leukaemia, Hodgkin disease), but there is no evidence to date that the lung function in these patients deteriorates over time. The pathogenesis of these abnormalities is probably multifactorial, with multi-agent chemotherapy and previous chest infections both playing a part.

However, other patients may be susceptible to significant pulmonary dysfunction (Table 11.2). This may be due to exposure to agents known to lead to significant pulmonary damage,

Table 11.2. Chemotherapy and late lung toxicity

Chemotherapeutic agents	Risk factors	Clinical features
BCNU	Higher cumulative dose Age <5 years at exposure	Fibrosis
Busulphan	High cumulative dose Radiotherapy (avoid)	Pneumonitis Fibrosis
Bleomycin	High O_2 concentrations (avoid on therapy)	Pneumonitis Late effects unknown
Cyclophosphamide	High cumulative dose	Fibrosis
Methotrexate	Hypersensitivity	Late effects uncertain

including fibrosis, or radiotherapy, or a combination of chemotherapy and radiotherapy. The recognition of significant interactions may be critical in the avoidance of major lung toxicity or even death (e.g. the use of busulphan in patients who may receive radiotherapy to the lung).

There is a clear relationship between radiation dose, volume, and risk of radiation pneumonitis with subsequent fibrosis. It is generally accepted that a dose of 14 Gy to one whole lung is safe in the acute setting, but higher doses can only be delivered to part of the lung, as fibrosis is likely to follow. Regular review of pulmonary function is important for patients who have received radiotherapy as there may be a restrictive lung abnormality with or without fibrosis, although there is little therapy available.

Exercise should be encouraged and smoking avoided. The assessment of cardiac function is also important for those with evidence of pulmonary fibrosis who may be at risk of pulmonary hypertension.

Endocrine issues

Bone mineral density

Osteopenia in survivors of childhood cancer is likely to be multifactorial. It has been reported most frequently in survivors of acute lymphoblastic leukaemia but has also been identified in other patients, including those previously treated for brain tumours. The causes of osteopenia are thought to include prior cranial irradiation or direct radiation (spine, total body irradiation), the direct effect of certain chemotherapeutic agents (e.g. chemotherapy for acute lymphoblastic leukaemia, ifosfamide), and steroids. A general reduction in activity both during therapy and even following completion of active treatment (this has been particularly noted in survivors of childhood leukaemia) may also be implicated. It is possible that there is also suboptimal mineralization of bone at critical times such as during puberty. This is an area where intervention may be important.

The treatment of osteopenia (>2.5 SD below mean for age and pubertal status) should be supervised by a clinician with expertise in this area. The use of bisphosphonates is controversial. However, physical activity and regular exercise will help to improve bone mineral density and should be encouraged. Other reasons to encourage exercise include the higher incidence of obesity now recognized in some of these survivors. Nutritional supplementation (e.g. calcium) may confer some benefit.

The assessment of bone mineral density in patients with clinical fractures is clearly important. However, whether survivors of leukaemia should have routine dual-energy X-ray absorptiometry (DEXA) scanning or other imaging is currently a matter of active research interest. It is important to note that the interpretation of DEXA scanning requires correction for size and pubertal status in children in the clinic setting. As osteopenia and osteoporosis become increasingly recognized as an important issue for women in later years, the long-term impact of early osteopenia is as yet unknown and will need careful ongoing evaluation.

Fertility

Perhaps the single most important strategy for preservation of fertility in boys is the facilitation of sperm banking at the time of diagnosis. For many, the impact of therapy on fertility may be unclear, and unless there is an urgent indication for immediate therapy, sperm storage should be encouraged for peripubertal and postpubertal boys.

There are several aspects of therapy for childhood cancer that can lead to impairment of fertility in the long term. In general, boys are more susceptible to late sequelae than girls. They have a greater sensitivity to chemotherapy, particularly alkylating agents. Leydig cell function is preserved to a greater extent than Sertoli cell function. Therefore boys may progress appropriately through puberty, but may nonetheless have inadequate sperm production, with impaired fertility, requiring more detailed investigation. Girls are born with a pool of primordial follicles which potentially can develop, with appropriate hormonal stimulation, into mature oocytes. This pool steadily depletes during childhood and puberty, under normal circumstances to approximately 400 000 by the time of menarche. Cytotoxic chemotherapy and radiotherapy will further deplete this pool and can result in loss of hormone production, lack of ovulation, uterine dysfunction, and a premature menopause. With girls in puberty one can think of harvesting ova from the ovaries before the start of chemotherapy with alkylating agents or before radiotherapy when the ovaries are positioned in the radiotherapy field. Ova banking, as with with sperm banking in boys, may be considered before treatment starts.

Cytotoxic chemotherapy Several chemotherapeutic agents can potentially impair fertility (Table 11.3). There is considerable individual variation in sensitivity to these agents. Most importantly, girls appear to be relatively resistant to the adverse impact of chemotherapy alone, with the exception of alkylating agents, particularly cyclophosphamide in high doses or in combination with other agents known to impair fertility.

Many studies have specifically studied the effects of cyclophosphamide. Interpretation is often difficult, as the impact of other potentially gonadotoxic chemotherapy that may have been received and the age and pubertal status at the time of therapy may also influence long-term fertility potential. Nonetheless it is generally agreed that a cumulative dose of cyclophosphamide $> 7.5\,\mathrm{g/m^2}$ will lead to infertility for boys, but lower doses could also be implicated.

The impact of ifosfamide is less clear. It is similar to cyclophosphamide in its activity but the impact on fertility may be less severe. There are anecdotal reports of pregnancies fathered by boys who have received significant cumulative doses of the agent, but these are not sufficient to be reassuring. It is used with increasing frequency in the treatment of many solid tumours and further definitive information about its impact on fertility is urgently required.

There is evidence that girls receiving alkykating agents (chlorambucil and procarbazine or mustine) as part of a therapeutic regimen for Hodgkin disease will be at risk of early menopause. It is important to inform them of this risk at an appropriate time in terms of their family planning.

Abdominal, pelvic, or total body irradiation is likely to result in impairment of ovarian or testicular function. Furthermore, radiotherapy to the uterus (high-dose pelvic or abdominal irradiation) in childhood may affect uterine distensibility and blood flow and its subsequent potential to accommodate a viable pregnancy. Girls with Wilms tumour or other pelvic sarcomas are at most risk of this problem, and flank irradiation (extending into the pelvis) is particularly associated with low birth weight in subsequent offspring. Limitation of uterine

Table 11.3. Chemotherapeutic agents that can have an adverse impact on fertility

BCNU	Ifosfamide	Chlorambucil
Busulphan	Melphalan	Cytarabine
CCNU	Mustine	Dacarbazine
Cisplatin	Nitrogen mustard	Thiotepa
Cyclophosphamide	Procarbazine	Radiotherapy

distensibility is also an important consideration in the light of new techniques such as embryo transfer which are now becoming available.

Radiotherapy to the brain can also affect fertility indirectly through its effect on the pituitary. High dose (>24 Gy) radiotherapy to the hypothalamus/pituitary (e.g. for brain tumours) may result in delayed puberty, whereas lower doses (>24 Gy) may be associated with precocious puberty, especially in young girls.

Clinical implications A history of primary or secondary amenorrhoea is important, and boys should be asked about potency and nocturnal emissions. Pubertal development should be closely monitored in all patients at risk of late endocrinopathy, particularly in girls who have received radiotherapy to the brain as young children. Where problems are suspected, measurement of FSH and LH, and possibly inhibin, may be helpful, with additional measurement of testosterone in boys and oestradiol in girls. Semen analysis will determine fertile potential for male survivors, although many do not wish to know their fertility status for some time.

The vast majority of patients, particularly girls, need reassurance that they are fertile and indeed should be given or encouraged to seek appropriate contraceptive advice.

Close liaison with, and access to, clinical specialists in fertility is vital to provide appropriate information and access to therapeutic interventions whenever possible. This is also an example where patients of an appropriate age may benefit from attending the clinic without their parents to allow open and honest discussion about important, but sometimes uncomfortable, issues. The timing of these discussions is important and the need for confidentiality must be recognized.

The breast

A field of radiation that includes prepubertal breast tissue may result in significant breast hypoplasia and asymmetry. Girls receiving this therapy are also at an increased risk of second malignancy, which is particularly well recognized in younger women <25 years treated for Hodgkin disease. All female survivors of childhood cancer should be taught breast self-examination and this should be emphasized for those previously exposed to radiotherapy.

Careful monitoring, with appropriate use of mammography or MRI scanning is advised. These examinations are of prime importance in addition to breast self-examination.

The impact of previous radiotherapy on a mother's ability to breast-feed remains unknown, although lactation may be impaired.

Second malignancy

At some stage following completion of therapy, patients need to be informed that they may be at an increased risk of a second cancer. For many this risk is small, although it remains an important cause of late deaths in survivors.[7,11] The greatest risk occurs in those with previous exposure to radiotherapy, when a second malignancy may occur within or on the edge of the radiation field. Exposure to the epipodophyllotoxins (topoisomerase II inhibitors such as VP16 and VM26) and alkylating agents also increases the risk of a second cancer.

Other patients and their families may be at risk if they have a condition known to be associated with an increased risk of malignancy (e.g. Li–Fraumeni syndrome, familial retinoblastoma, or neurofibromatsis type I) (see Chapter 2) These families will need referral for genetic counselling and, for some, ongoing cancer screening.

Patients should be encouraged to take part in any national screening programmes that are available (e.g. cervical or testicular). Breast cancer screening is particularly important, where in addition to breast self-examination and formal clinical breast examination, patients should be advised regarding early mammography. It has been suggested that mammography should commence 8–10 years after radiotherapy to the chest and be undertaken every 1–3 years thereafter (once the patient is >25 years old) depending on risk. Because of the denser breast tissue in younger patients, mammograms may be difficult to interpret. Local policies vary and advice should be taken for patients on an individual basis. Other imaging modalities (e.g. ultrasound and MRI) are currently under evaluation as assessment tools for screening in high-risk patients.

Survivors of childhood cancer should be encouraged to take responsibility for their own health, and advice regarding a healthy lifestyle is important for all survivors. The following should be specifically encouraged:

- avoiding excessive exposure to the sun
- avoid smoking
- healthy diet
- active lifestyle.

Dental issues

The recognition of dental problems is important. They are common following radiotherapy, particularly if it was received at a young age, or given to a relatively high dose (>30 Gy). The development of the tooth or its root may be impaired, with an increase in malocclusion or dental decay. Good oral hygiene and regular dental review should be encouraged, with orthodontic intervention as appropriate. Intensive chemotherapy given at a time of critical development in dentition may also result in the impairment of root development and increased caries.

Hearing

Those at risk of hearing loss will have been exposed to cisplatin or carboplatin (the risk is greater with cisplatin and with higher cumulative doses); the most common impairment is high-tone loss. The risk is increased if the patient has had a high exposure to aminoglycosides. Radiotherapy, particularly to the posterior fossa, can also lead to loss of hearing. If abnormalities are identified, ongoing review is important.

For those at risk of hearing impairment, a pure tone audiogram should be performed at regular intervals throughout treatment, so that the balance of risk and benefit of the chemotherapy can be adequately assessed, and at the end of therapy. For younger children, formal paediatric ENT or audiology assessments should be provided. As children are reviewed in clinic, parents should be specifically questioned about the hearing and speech development of their child with early referral for speech therapy where necessary.

Transfusion-related sequelae

The risk of transfusion-related infection depends on the country where the patient was treated and the screening that was in place at the time of therapy. The screening programmes for hepatitis B, hepatitis C, and HIV vary within Europe and across other countries. Patients should be offered screening whenever appropriate, with referral to specialist care if infection is confirmed.

Splenectomy

Some patients will lose their spleen as a direct result of involvement by the primary tumour (usually lymphoma) and subsequent removal. A greater number will lose splenic function as a result of radiotherapy either to the spleen itself, or following total body irradiation and high-dose conditioning therapy for bone marrow transplant (functional splenectomy). Immuniza-tion is often not possible prior to loss of splenic function, as the patient will have been immunosuppressed at the time of active therapy. Immunization following immune recovery is essential and patients should receive the following:

- pneumococcal vaccine with re-immunization every 5 years
- *Haemophilus influenzae* type b vaccine
- influenza vaccine annually
- new conjugated meningococcal C vaccine.

Long-term antibiotic prophylaxis (penicillin or erythromycin) is strongly recommended, with additional antibiotics available to be used whenever infective symptoms occur or when the patient is travelling. It should be noted that these patients are particularly susceptible to malaria. Care should be taken when travelling to areas endemic for malaria and appropriate chemoprophylaxis should be provided.

Psychosocial issues

Reports of long-term psychologic or adjustment problems in survivors of childhood cancer are conflicting. Many patients adapt extremely well to normal life following therapy, and adjust psychologically and socially as they move through childhood and adolescence into adulthood. However, it is well recognized that some patients are at risk of anxiety and depression in the long term with evidence of post-traumatic stress in some. All patients are at risk of psychologic problems and should be given the opportunity to express their concerns in the clinic setting. More formal consideration of these issues is appropriate for those survivors at greater risk of late adverse psychosocial issues.

A large comparative study of psychosocial outcomes in long-term survivors of acute lym-phoblastic leukaemia and Wilms tumour suggested no increase in rates of psychiatric disorders when compared with a control peer group.[12] However, there was evidence of poorer function-ing in the area of relationships and friendships in the survivors when compared with the control subjects. Poorer coping was associated with lower intellectual ability scores. This is of note, as it mirrors findings in other studies. Although patient selection and study designs vary, some themes persist in the literature relating to the risk factors for problems with long-term psychologic adjustment. Other studies have also suggested that those who have received cranial radiotherapy, particularly at a young age, are at a significantly increased risk of psychologic problems and learning difficulties, and are less likely to marry or be in a long-term relationship.

The diagnosis and its treatment are clearly not the only factors influencing psychologic outcome, and other issues such as family functioning, coping mechanisms, length of follow-up, and premorbid psychologic state may be important.

The complexity of this area should be recognized, and the discussion of issues such as adaptation and coping mechanisms is beyond the scope of this chapter. Nonetheless these issues may be important and the reader is referred to the recent text by Eiser[13] for further details.

Interventions for psychologic sequelae

There is, rightly, a strong focus on the physical late effects of therapy in the clinic setting. However, psychosocial issues and problems should not be overlooked as they may be very amenable to therapy. Timely intervention may make a real difference to long-term outcome, and formal neurologic or psychologic assessment is vital for some. The causes of behavioural problems seen in survivors of childhood cancer are likely to be multifactorial and appropriate supportive therapy should be offered if at all possible.

Educational issues

Ongoing close liaison with education services will also be very important for some patients. Certain specific learning difficulties are known to be associated with previous cranial radiotherapy, and this is recognized as the most important risk factor for educational problems in the long term. Such problems include concentration, visual and spatial awareness, mathematics, and language processing, although any aspect of cognitive functioning may be affected. Prolonged school absence or prolonged hospitalization may adversely affect educational ability in others, again raising the need for formal educational assessment or support.

Early formal assessment for patients with risk factors such as prior cranial radiotherapy, prolonged absence from school, and hearing or visual deficits following therapy is imperative, as subtle problems may be difficult to recognize in the busy classroom setting. It is of particular concern as these patients may be embarrassed and seek to cover up their difficulties; furthermore, children may respond well to additional help with specific learning difficulties. Deficits in educational attainment, social competence, and behaviour can be difficult to predict even when cognitive, sensorimotor, endocrine, and emotional impairments have been documented.

Strategies for minimizing late effects

Minimizing therapy

Significant achievements have been made in the treatment of childhood cancer over the past two decades, despite a remarkable lack of new chemotherapeutic agents or the development of other novel techniques. Much of the progress has been a result of the better understanding of the biology of the disease and, through collaboration and sharing data, analysis of risk factors has led to an ability to stratify patients more appropriately. Those patients who are at a greater risk of relapse can be treated more intensively (with improved supportive care), whilst those with a better prognosis may receive less intensive therapy with fewer late adverse effects. There are a number of examples where a systematic change in therapy has led to a significant fall in the frequency or severity of late effects, such as the omission of cranial radiotherapy as central nervous system prophylaxis in the treatment of acute lymphoblastic leukaemia. Problems with cognitive development and hormonal dysfunction (growth hormone secretion) have been significantly reduced as a result of the change in therapy, although it is possible that the more intensive chemotherapy now used may lead to other late effects.

However, in other situations the balance, or choices, in therapy may be less clear and debate continues about optimizing cure rates whilst limiting late adverse sequelae. Two examples are given below.

Hodgkin disease

Hodgkin disease is one of the clearest examples where the prognosis for the majority of patients with the disease is excellent, yet where there are well-recognized and important late effects of therapy. Chemotherapy and involved field radiotherapy have been the mainstay of treatment for decades. However as the late effects of radiotherapy and the excellent results with chemotherapy alone have been recognized, so the number of patients requiring radiotherapy has fallen and the size of fields used reduced.

The impact of radiotherapy is particularly important for girls, and a dramatic increase in the number with breast cancers was largely responsible for the high incidence of second cancers in survivors of Hodgkin disease (standardized incidence ratio 18.1 [95 per cent confidence interval (CI) 14.3–22.3]), where the estimated actuarial incidence of breast cancer in female survivors with Hodgkin's disease was 35 per cent (CI 17.4–52.6).[14]

Even if radiotherapy can be avoided, other important late effects for patients with Hodgkin disease must be considered, and minimizing the long-term impact of chemotherapy has been also challenging. As previously described, alkylating agents are known to be associated with infertility in boys and early menopause in girls.

Therefore treatment strategies have been developed which attempt to minimize these late effects in a cohort of patients with an excellent prognosis. Radiotherapy is still used for some, but many patients can be treated with chemotherapy alone. In an attempt to reduce the impact of alkylating agents on fertility, new regimens have been introduced which include anthracyclines and avoid some of the alkylating agents. Therefore a different pattern of late effects can be anticipated, with a potentially greater impact on the heart, particularly if radiotherapy for mediastinal disease cannot be avoided.

Whether therapy should be gender based is a matter of debate, and a study in the UK has attempted to give choice to some patients and their families. For example, patients with stage I (neck) disease can be offered a choice of radiotherapy or chemotherapy. This is an interesting question, but whether the families have adequate information to make such a choice, or whether they actually wish to do so, remains to be seen.

Rhabdomyosarcoma

Radiotherapy has been a cornerstone of the treatment of soft tissue sarcomas, including rhabdomyosarcomas, and has been used systematically as a strategy for local disease control, often with surgery. It was then recognized that some patients could be cured without radiotherapy, not just at the very 'good risk' sites (e.g. paratesticular), but also at other sites where the late effects of radiotherapy (e.g. orbit or pelvis) may cause significant morbidity. Different strategies have been developed within different international collaborative groups, and a workshop was convened between these groups to evaluate the relative outcome following the different treatment strategies for one site with a high survival rate, the orbit. The treatment of orbital rhabdomyosarcoma highlights the issue of the philosophical differences in the approach to therapy and the importance of careful risk stratification. The results demonstrated a comparable overall survival for the four international groups participating.[15] However, the event-free survival of those patients who had not received systematic radiotherapy was significantly lower than that of the other groups. These patients went on to receive further chemotherapy and radiotherapy. Nonetheless, this strategy (radiotherapy for selected patients) also demonstrated that approximately 40 per cent of patients could be cured without radiotherapy and its associated late effects.

These examples demonstrate the importance of choices in therapy. Cure remains paramount, but there are some patients currently being overtreated who may be saved late sequelae from both radiotherapy and chemotherapy. Minimizing the numbers that relapse will also be important, as additional chemotherapy and radiotherapy will further increase the burden of late effects.

New strategies

Surgical approaches

Surgery was an important part of cancer therapy long before the introduction of chemotherapy and radiotherapy. It remains a critical part of the management of some malignancies, particularly tumours of the bone, brain, eye, and soft tissues. Surgical techniques have become increasingly sophisticated, and even when major potentially deforming surgery is required, the long-term cosmetic and functional results have dramatically improved. Examples are the endoprosthetic replacement of bone, most commonly used as part of the treatment for osteogenic sarcoma, and laser surgery for retinoblastoma. Reconstructive surgery following surgery or radiotherapy to sites such as the face, bladder, or perineum (vagina) may dramatically improve a patient's quality of life. However, assumptions about the patient's views should not be made. Some will choose to live with their deformity, adapting well even to major facial disfigurement. Others may rate function more highly than the cosmetic result (e.g. amputation versus endoprosthetic replacement). Understanding coping mechanisms and influences on body image are also an important part of optimizing outcome.

Radiotherapy approaches

The avoidance of radiotherapy wherever possible for children >3–5 years of age is the most important strategy in preventing potentially devastating late effects in this age group, as the limitation of the growth of bones and soft tissues and the impact of radiation on the brain is particularly severe in the very young. It is hoped that the use of CT and MRI planning for the treatment of many childhood tumours has dramatically improved the clinician's ability to limit the volume and dose of radiation delivered to normal tissues and therefore minimize long-term damage.

Conformal radiotherapy (i.e. shaping the beam to allow the selective avoidance of important radiosensitive structures) is becoming more sophisticated with intensity-modulated radiotherapy (IMRT), which is a further development in this area. The use of brachytherapy (e.g. for pelvic tumours) is of value in a selected population.

The late effects of radiotherapy are well described elsewhere[16] and relate to the organ exposed to the treatment. Toxicity is related to size (volume) of field and cumulative dose, and the younger the child, the greater the toxicity. Direct tissue damage, inflammation, and fibrosis are most commonly seen. There is also a relationship between radiotherapy exposure and the risk of late second cancers. However, it is important to recognize that as the routine use of radiotherapy for many solid tumours and leukaemias has reduced, so the late effects of more intensive chemotherapeutic regimens may be identified in years to come. Although the avoidance of late effects is important, local control of the disease remains critical and should not be compromised.

Chemotherapy

The acute adverse effects of chemotherapy are well recognized and many strategies are in place to minimize them. This is not the case for late effects, and research in this area has centered on the reduction of late cardiotoxicty. Two strategies have been tried: the use of a cardioprotective agent, cardioxane, and the use of liposomal anthracyclines. Work is ongoing in children at present and data are currently preliminary, although there may be a place for these agents in the future.

The role of the late-effects clinic

For many patients, the model of follow-up in the paediatric oncology clinic by the physicians who originally treated the child is the ideal setting. They are seen in familiar surroundings by medical and nursing staff who have cared for them over a long period of time. However, for others, even if the frequency of follow-up is only on an annual or even biannual basis, hospital attendance may not be necessary or indeed optimal. It can be hard for a child (or the family) to consider themselves 'cured' if they are asked to attend hospital on a regular basis. The attendance itself can perpetuate the perception of an ongoing illness and prevent a full return to normal life. It can be very stressful, even years after therapy has been completed. It may also not be necessary.

The need for some ongoing contact with survivors is clearly very important. If they are not followed up, information about serious late effects, long-term adjustment, and future morbidity will be lost. However, much of this information could be obtained through other models of care and contact between the patient and clinical staff. Work is currently under way exploring different strategies of follow-up. For some, contact with a clinic nurse or the primary care physician, or even a telephone call or questionnaire, may be entirely adequate and less intrusive in the long term.[17] There will be situations where important late effects are newly recognized, and where some asymptomatic patients may benefit from further evaluation. Future access to these patients is clearly important.

The long-term follow-up clinic has a crucial role in a number of ways (Table 11.4):

- ongoing care of those survivors with a high risk of developing late adverse effects of therapy
- monitoring of progression through puberty, particularly if there is a high risk of endocrinopathy
- coordination with other speciality clinics (e.g. cardiology, endocrinology, or neurology)
- provision of information to survivors relating to their own risks and advice regarding lifestyle and responsibility for their own care.

The majority of patients will stay on active follow-up for at least 10 years after diagnosis or until they have completed puberty, whichever is the longer. It is important to remember that the child, not his or her parents, is the patient. There may be very sensitive issues previously unknown to the child (e.g. infertility, second cancer risk) and these should be discussed at an appropriate time, when the patient is ready to receive such information, and in a confidential

Table 11.4. The role of the clinic in long term follow-up

Information	Details and understanding of previous therapy
	Current and future health risks
Observation	Growth
	Obesity
Advice	Lifestyle
	Activity
	Smoking
	Diet
	Sun exposure
	Fertility
	Breast examination
Support	Psychologic
	Coordination with other services
	Specialist services (endocrinology, neurology)
	Transition to adult care
	Education
Independence	Transition from reliance on parental intervention
	Explore issues with patient, not parent

manner. The transition to caring for an adult can be challenging for paediatric doctors and nurses, but the correct handling of this, sometimes difficult, stage can help the survivor to move on to greater independence.

Conclusion

The number of survivors of childhood cancer will continue to rise as survival rates improve. Whilst many important late effects of therapy are recognized and strategies are in place to address them, reliable evidence about the causes of problems and the best way to address them remains scarce. It is even unclear how many of these patients should be reviewed, how frequently, and by whom. However, national and international collaborative groups are currently developing guidelines for the follow-up of survivors. These will be based on available evidence, expert opinion, and good clinical practice in an attempt to provide practical advice and resource for clinicians responsible for these often complex patients. It will always be challenging to undertake clinical research in this area; patients move on not just psychologically, but also physically, and collecting data from cohorts is both costly and time consuming for patients and their carers alike. Nonetheless, we need to learn from these patients as they grow older, and only by following them on into the future will we understand the very-long-term effects of the treatment of childhood cancer, whether risks increase further with age, and what truly are the most cost-effective strategies for their ongoing health care.

References

1. **Wallace H, Green D (eds)** (2003). *Late Effects of Childhood Cancer.* London: Edward Arnold.
2. **Robison LL, Mertens AC, Boice JD et al.** (2002). Study design and cohort characteristics of the Childhood Cancer Survivor Study: a multi-institutional collaborative project. *Med Pediatr Oncol* **38**, 229–39.
3. **Brennan BM. Shalet SM.** (2002)Endocrine late effects after bone marrow transplant. *Br J Haematol* **118**: 58–66.
4. **Leiper AD.** Non-endocrine late complications of bone marrow transplantation in childhood: part I. *Br J Haematol* **118**:3–22, 2002
5. **Leiper AD** (2002). Non-endocrine late complications of bone marrow transplantation in childhood: part II. *Br J Haematol* **118**, 23–43.
6. **Green DM, Hyland A Chung CS, Zevon MA, Hall BC** (1999). Cancer and cardiac mortality among fifteen year survivors of cancer diagnosed during childhood or adolescence. *J Clin Oncol* **17**, 3207–15.
7. **Mertens AC, Yasui Y, Neglia JP, et al.** (2001). Late mortality experience in five-year survivors of childhood and adolescent cancer: the childhood cancer survivor study. *J Clin Oncol* **19**, 3163–72
8. **Wexler LH, Andrich MP, Venzon DB, et al.** Randomized trial of the cardioprotective agentICRF-187 in pediatric sarcoma treated with doxorubicin. *J Clin Oncol* **14**, 362–72.
9. **Levitt GA, Dorup I, Sorensen K, Sullivan I** (2004). Does anthracycline administration by infusion in children affect late cardiotoxicity? *Br J Haematol* **124**, 463–8.
10. **Hancock SL, Donaldson SS, Hoppe RT** (1993). Cardiac disease following treatment of Hodgkin's disease in children and adolescents. *J Clin Oncol* **11**, 1208–15.
11. **Neglia JP, Friedman DL, Yasui Y, et al.** (2001) Second malignant neoplasms in five-year survivors of childhood cancer: childhood cancer survivor study. *J Natl Cancer Inst* **93**, 618–29.
12. **Mackie E, Hill J, Kondryn H, McNally R** (2000). Adult psychosocial outcomes in long-term survivors of acute lymphoblastic leukaemia and Wilms' tumour: a controlled study. *Lancet* **355**, 1310–14.
13. **Eiser C.** *Children with Cancer: Quality of Life.* New York: Lawrence Erlbaum.

14. **Bhatia S, Robison LL, Oberlin O,** *et al.* (1996) Breast cancer and other second neoplasms after childhood Hodgkin's disease. *N Engl J Med* **334**, 745–51.

15. **Oberlin O, Rey A, Anderson J,** *et al.* (2001) Treatment of orbital rhabdomyosarcoma: survival and late effects of treatment—results of an international workshop. *J Clin Oncol* **19**, 197–204.

16. **Halperin EC, Constine LS, Tarbell NJ, Kun LE** (eds) (1999). *Pediatric Radiation Oncology* (3rd edn). Philadelphia, PA: Lippincott–Williams & Wilkins, 457–537.

17. **Wallace WHB, Blacklay A Eiser C,** *et al.* (2001). Developing strategies for long term follow up of survivors of childhood cancer. *BMJ* **323**, 271–4.

Chapter 12

Acute lymphoblastic leukaemia

Kjeld Schmiegelow and Göran Gustafsson

Introduction

Acute lymphoblastic leukaemia (ALL) accounts for 30 per cent of all childhood malignancies. It encompasses a heterogeneous group of biologically and clinically related entities, each with their own characteristic epidemiology, biology, and sensitivity to anticancer agents. Whereas ALL was fatal in the vast majority of patients only 30 years ago, cure is now realistic in ≥75 per cent of patients.[1,2] This impressive success has been obtained by integrating improved understanding of the biology (including cytogenetics and molecular biology) with risk-group-adapted therapy, pharmacology, and supportive care, and not least randomized clinical trials and close international collaboration.[3] This approach has served as a general model for the successful treatment of other childhood cancers.

Epidemiology and aetiology

The annual incidence of ALL in Europe and the USA is 3.5–4.0 per 100 000 children <15 years of age with a male-to-female ratio of 1.2.[4] The risk of developing ALL before the age of 15 years is one in 2000. There is a striking incidence peak at age 2–7 years, where the incidence is as high as 10 per 100 000 children (Fig. 12.1). This peak has implications for the understanding of epidemiology, biology, and effective therapy. It is conspicuously highest in the most developed countries and is higher among White than among Black children, it consists mainly of B-cell precursor leukaemia with the *TEL-AML1* (ETV6-RUNX1) fusion [translocation (t(12;21)(p13;q22)] or a high-hyperdiploid genotype, and the outcome for children aged 2–7 years is superior to that of children in older and younger age groups.

Although a number of risk factors for ALL have been identified, the aetiology and pathogenic mechanisms remain unknown in the vast majority of cases. An increased risk of ALL has been associated with high birth weight (the odds ratio increases by approximately 20 per cent per kilogram), certain congenital syndromes and chromosomal abnormalities (e.g. a 15-fold odds ratio for Down syndrome patients), genetic instability (e.g. ataxia telangiectasia, including *ATM* gene mutation carriers, Fanconi anaemia, and Bloom syndrome), exposure to ionizing radiation, and certain immune deficiencies (e.g. Wiskott–Aldrich syndrome). In addition, some studies have linked the development of ALL to exposure to electromagnetic fields or vitamin K prophylaxis, but others have failed to confirm these associations. Although specific genotypes of certain polymorphic enzymes that may play a role in detoxification or DNA repair processes have been linked to the risk of ALL, the risk of developing ALL is not significantly increased for siblings of children with ALL (except for monozygous twins) despite their common genetic background and environment.[5] Whereas the associations noted above will account for only a small fraction of patients, a growing amount of data indicate that ALL in childhood occurs as a consequence of *in utero* (first hit) genetic aberrations and postnatal

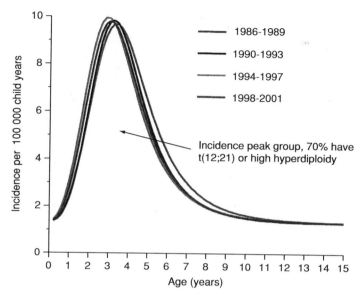

Fig. 12.1 Age-specific incidence rates for 3354 cases of childhood ALL diagnosed in Denmark, Finland, Iceland, Norway, and Sweden between 1982 and 2001. The data can roughly be divided into infant ALL (age <1 year) characterized by a high frequency of 11q23 aberrations, an incidence peak group where 70 per cent or more are cases with t(12;21) translocation or high hyperdiploidy, and a 'base-line' incidence that includes T-cell leukaemia and B-cell precursor ALL without t(12;21) and hyperdiploids.[4]

(second or further hits) abnormal immunologic responses to common childhood infections.[6,7] The latter hypothesis has been supported by computer modelling, space and time cluster analysis, and the finding of an increased risk of ALL with delayed exposure to common childhood infections, population mixing, certain tissue types, and low levels of mannose-binding lectin.[6–8] The prenatal occurrence of leukaemia-associated genetic aberrations, such as translocations t(4;11) or t(12;21), hyperdiploidy, and clonal heavy-chain gene rearrangements, have been convincingly demonstrated by their presence in Guthrie cards for a large proportion of patients who later develop ALL, but even more interestingly they also occur in approximately 1 per cent of healthy newborns.[6,7,9]

Biologic studies

ALL is driven by mutations in a multistep malignant transformation that leads to a deregulated monoclonal expansion of immature lymphoid progenitor cells. Histology, cytochemistry, immunophenotyping, and cytogenetics are crucial for the correct identification of the involved cell lines as well as their stage of cellular maturation. Based on specific morphologic features, the French–American–British (FAB) morphologic classification of the mid-1970s distinguished between L1, L2, and L3 subtypes. Although the small L1 lymphoblasts have a higher chemosensitivity that the somewhat larger and more pleomorphic L2 subtype, the distinction between L1 and L2 subtypes has been surpassed by more informative clinical and biologic factors. In contrast, the FAB L3 subset of ALL remains important as it identifies mature B cells that express immunoglobulin on the cell surface, and which are indistinguishable from the lymphoblasts seen in Burkitt non-Hodgkin lymphoma. The L3 leukaemic cells are larger than those seen in FAB L1 and L2 ALL, they have moderately abundant and deeply basophilic cytoplasm that contains numerous prominent vacuoles, and the nucleus is regular and contains distinct nucleoli.

Immunophenotype

In acute myeloid leukaemia (AML), ALL, and non-Hodgkin lymphomas (defined with respect to ALL by the presence of <25 per cent lymphoblasts in the bone marrow), the malignant cells resemble normal haemopoietic cells. Immunophenotyping by flow cytometry and/or immu-nohistochemistry can be applied to cells from blood, bone marrow, ascites, pleural effusions, cerebrospinal fluid, and lymph node biopsies using monoclonal antibodies directed towards differentiation antigens [cluster of differentiation (CD) antigens] in the nucleus or cytoplasm, or on the cell membrane. Flow cytometry allows rapid analysis of thousands of cells, and in the same run it is possible to determine cell size (forward scatter), granularity (side scatter), and (depending on the technical equipment) two, three, or more different CD antigens by applying different fluorochrome-linked antibodies directed towards these antigens.[10] Since many of the CD antigens are not lineage specific, the immunophenotypic classification is based on the combination of CD antigen expression, and at least 95 per cent of all leukaemias can be classified as lymphoid or myeloid with or without co-expression of myeloid or lymphoid CD antigens (Table 12.1). Less than 5 per cent of all acute leukaemias lack a uniform lymphoid or myeloid pattern and are classified as biphenotypic leukaemias (carrying a combination of markers from different lineages on each malignant cell) or (more rarely) bilineage leukaemias displaying a mixture of two different lineages of malignant cells. Rarely, morphology and cytochemistry, immunophenotyping, and cytogenetic markers fail to determine whether the leukaemia is of lymphoid or myeloid origin. These undifferentiated leukaemias tend to be very resistant to chemotherapy. Weak aberrant expression of myeloid markers is common in ALL [e.g. frequent in t(12;21)-positive ALL], but this feature does not seem to carry prognostic implications.

Determination of the immunophenotype of the leukaemic cells is primarily crucial for the identification of children with mature B-cell ALL, since they need very intensive therapy (see the section on special subsets), and those with T-lineage ALL which is more commonly associated with other known risk factors than B-cell precursor ALL and also needs special treatment considerations (see section on special subsets). Based on the immunophenotyping, ALL can be classified as T-lineage (10 per cent of ALL), B-cell precursor (85–90 per cent of ALL), or mature B-cell disease expressing clonal surface immunoglobulins (2 per cent of ALL). In addition to the mature B-cell leukaemias, B-lineage ALL can be subdivided into pro-B (CD-10 negative), early pre-B, and pre-B (with intracytoplasmic immunoglobulins), but this subdivision is not generally used in the risk group and treatment stratification. Finally, the pattern of CD antigen expression in most cases of childhood ALL is so unique and specific that it can be applied to flow cytometric determination of residual disease in the bone marrow or peripheral blood during therapy, although the sensitivity rarely falls below one leukaemic cell in 10^3-10^4 normal mononuclear cells.[11]

Table 12.1. Characteristics of subsets of childhood ALL

Subset	Frequency of all leukaemias (per cent)	Frequent positive markers	Typical chromosomal abnormalities	Other characteristics compared with B-cell precursor	5-year pEFS (per cent)
B-cell precursor	75	CD10, 19, 22, cy79, HLA-DR, TdT	High-hyperdiploid, t(9;22)(q34;q11), t(1;19)(q23;p13), t(12;21)(p13;q22), dic(9;12)(p11–p12;p12)		75–85
Mature B-cell	2	Surface immunoglobulins, CD19, 20	t(8;14)(q24;q32.2), t(8;22)(q24;q11), t(2;8)(p11–12;q24)	Frequently bulky disease, low WBC, male predominance	80–85
Infants	3	CD19, 22, cy79, HLA-DR (NB usually lacks CD10)	t(4;11)(q21;q23), t(11;19)(q23;p13), other 11q23 aberrations	Very high WBC, frequently CNS disease	50
T-lineage	10	CD2, cy3, 4/8, 5, 7, TCRα/β, TdT	t(11;14)(p13;q11), t(7;v)(q34–36;v)	Older age, higher WBC, mediastinal mass, CNS disease	60–65

CD, clusters of antigens; CNS, central nervous system; cy*, cytoplasmatic; pEFS, probability of event-free survival; TdT, terminal deoxynucleotidyl transferase; v, variable; WBC, white blood cell count at diagnosis.

Cytogenetics

Clonal numerical and structural chromosomal aberrations can be demonstrated in ≥90 per cent of children with ALL (see Chapter 2).[12,13] As far as we know, many of these carry neither pathogenic nor prognostic significance, and probably merely reflect the genomic instability of the malignant clone. Other non-random chromosomal changes are a hallmark for understanding aetiology, biology, and risk stratification, since they correlate with the drug sensitivity of the malignant clone and thus may guide the choice of treatment. The karyotyping is generally done by Giemsa dye (G-band) staining of metaphase chromosome spreads with a resolution of approximately 5–10 Mbp.[12] Although this is a useful method for screening, G-band karyotyping may be hampered by the poor *in vitro* growth of malignant lymphoblasts, the preferential growth of certain subclones, and a lower quality of the banded chromosomes compared with those in AML samples for instance. Even when the technique is successful, some chromosomal translocations are easily overlooked by G-band karyotyping since they involve regions of almost similar size and band staining [e.g. the t(12;21) translocation]. Hence a number of alternative techniques that do not require metaphase spreads have been applied for genomic screening [e.g. high-resolution comparative genomic hybridization (HR-CGH) with a resolution of ∼ 3 Mbp[13]] or to detect specific gene mutations or translocations of prognostic significance. The latter include Southern blot, interphase fluorescence *in situ* hybridization (FISH), and reverse transcriptase polymerase chain reaction (RT-PCR) which detects the chimeric mRNA generated by a chromosomal translocation. Other new techniques used to clarify chromosomal aberrations in malignant cells include spectral karyotyping and spectral colour banding, both of which improve the interpretation of the metaphase chromosomes by chromosome- or band-specific differential colour staining (Chapter 2). Finally, the DNA index or DNA content (ratio of clonal DNA to normal DNA content) quantified by G-band karyotyping or flow cytometry carries prognostic significance. Thus, 3 per cent of children with ALL have a hypodiploid clone (<45 chromosomes, DNA index <0.90–0.95) and a poor prognosis, while 30 per cent have a high-hyperdiploid clone with a modal number (chromosome number of the dominating clone) of >50 chromosomes (median 55) and a favourable outcome.[12] The modal number of 50 represents the antimode of the bimodal distribution of the modal chromosomal number in these leukaemias. The high-hyperdiploid leukaemias, which are most common in the age group 2–7 years (Fig. 12.1), have a very characteristic non-random pattern of trisomies, most commonly involving chromosomes 4, 6, 10, 14, 17, 18, 21, and X. When the modal number exceeds 60–65, a far more random pattern of trisomies emerges. Since the superior prognosis of the high-hyperdiploid cases has been specifically related to the presence of trisomies 4, 10, and 17, interphase FISH techniques to detect these trisomies are applied by the US Children's Oncology Group as part of their risk group classification strategy. An important feature of high-hyperdiploid ALL is the relatively low frequency of chromosomal deletions that involve regions harbouring tumour suppressor genes, and this could be one of the biologic factors determining their prognostic significance.[13] In addition, the favourable prognosis of high-hyperdiploid ALL has been related to a high *in vitro* propensity for apoptosis (programmed cell death), a high *in vitro* sensitivity to antimetabolites, and an increased *in vivo* sensitivity to high-dose methotrexate (HD-MTX).[14] In G-band karyotyping, the DNA index is usually determined by the best growing clone, whereas the DNA index determined by flow cytometry is that of the quantitatively dominating clone even though smaller subclones with hypo- or hyperdiploid DNA indices may be present. The prognostic impact of the presence of such subclones remains to be determined in large clinical studies.

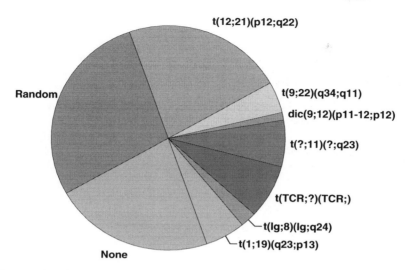

Fig. 12.2 Examples of important and common translocations among children with ALL. Other numerical and structural aberrations are common, but are not shown. The translocations lead to aberrant and dysregulated genes that encode nuclear (most frequently) or cytoplasmic proteins that interfere with the regulatory processes that control cell growth, differentiation, and survival. The translocations are associated with a specific subtype of ALL. The translocations may upregulate proto-oncogenes by placing them under the control of a potent enhancer such as T-cell receptor (T-cell ALL) or immunoglobulin genes (B-cell, commonly Myc oncogene activation (8q24)). Several chimeric fusion genes of prognostic significance have been described. In late (expressing cytoplasmatic immunoglobulins) and early B-lineage precursor (pre-B) leukaemias. The t(9;22) and t(?,11q23) (?, different translocation partners) are found in both myeloid and lymphoid leukaemias, which indicate that malignant events may take place in primitive multilineage stem cells.

The chromosomal translocations affecting regulatory and coding regions involved in cellular growth, differentiation, and survival (Fig. 12.2) are highly significant for our understanding of the pathogenic processes leading to ALL.

t(1;19)

A frequent translocation that identifies a subset of patients with specific treatment requirements is the t(1;19)(q23;p13) translocation, which occurs in 5 per cent of all cases of childhood ALL, especially in the pre-B ALL subset defined by the presence of intracytoplasmatic immunoglobulins. This translocation fuses the *E2A* gene on chromosome 19 with the *PBX1* gene on chromosome 1. Although this translocation was previously found to carry a poor prognosis, intensified induction and consolidation therapy has counteracted this to a large degree.

11q23

The 11q23 aberrations most commonly involve translocations between the very promiscuous *MLL* (mixed-lineage leukaemia) gene located on chromosome region 11q23 and more than 50 different partner genes of which the t(4;11) translocation accounts for approximately 50 per cent.[15] In childhood ALL the 11q23 rearrangements affect ~8 per cent of patients. Patients with t(4;11) and t(11;19) translocations are the youngest (most often infants), tend to have very high white blood cell count (WBC) at diagnosis (median > 180 × 10^9/liter), rarely have T-cell disease, and have a high frequency of central nervous system (CNS) disease at diagnosis. Among infants, any 11q23 abnormality seems related to a poorer outcome, whereas in older children an inferior outcome has primarily been associated with the t(4;11) and t(9;11) translocations. At least for the t(4;11) translocation, stem cell transplantation (SCT) has not been shown to improve survival compared with chemotherapy only.[15]

t(9;22)

The translocation t(9;22)(q34;q11), which can be demonstrated in ~ 3 per cent of ALL cases in children and in 25 per cent of adult cases, fuses the *c-abl* gene on chromosome 9 with the breakpoint cluster region (*bcr*) on chromosome 22. This yields a minor (185 kDa) or major (210 kDa, more commonly seen in chronic myeloid leukaemia) constitutively activated chimeric gene with high expression of a tyrosine-specific protein kinase. Secondary cytogenetic abnormalities are found in two-thirds of the patients. Because of their lower chance of complete remission after induction therapy (80–85 per cent), their high levels of subclinical disease after induction therapy, and their increased risk of relapse, allogeneic SCT from an HLA-matched related or unrelated donor is indicated in first remission.[16] The WBC at diagnosis is negatively correlated with the chances of cure. Patients with a low WBC at diagnosis, aged between 1 and 9 years, and/or with a good response to a 1-week prednisone prephase have a less unfavourable outcome, and a substantial number of such patients can be cured by intensive chemotherapy.[16] The oncogenic protein generated by the t(9;22) translocation can effectively be targeted and blocked by the specific tyrosine kinase inhibitor imatinib mesylate (formerly STI-571). Although it has been shown to be effective in both relapsed and refractory Philadelphia chromosome positive (Ph+) ALL, development of resistance occurs rapidly. The usefulness of this targeted therapy in first-line treatment is uncertain, and several study groups are testing its impact on long-term survival.

t(12;21)

The t(12;21)(p13;q22) translocation fuses the *TEL* gene on chromosome 12 with the *AML1* gene on chromosome 21. This common translocation, which occurs in 25 per cent of cases of B-cell precursor ALL, has been crucial in our understanding of the natural history of childhood ALL. It is a main determinant of the characteristic incidence peak in the age group 2–7 years (the other is high-hyperdiploid ALL), it is associated with a favourable risk grouping (a high WBC at diagnosis or CNS disease is rare), and it confirms that the first genetic aberration(s) in a large proportion of ALL occurs prenatally, since it has been demonstrated not only in the Guthrie cards of children who later develop *TEL–AML1*-positive ALL, but also in 1 per cent of healthy newborns.[6,7,9,17] The vast majority of t(12;21)-positive leukaemias also harbour structural chromosomal changes, e.g. commonly 12p, 6q, and 9p deletions, which include deletions of tumour suppressor genes.[13] Leukaemias with this translocation frequently have a low-level expression of (myeloid) CD13 and CD33 antigens, almost never have a modal number >50, are generally aged 1–10 years, and tend to have late relapses (many of which are extramedullary) with a median time to relapse of 4 years. Following a relapse, they seem to have a better outcome than patients without this translocation, but it is as yet unclear to what extent this reflects patient selection and lack of adjustment for the duration of first remission. Patients with the *TEL–AML1* translocation are more sensitive to L-asparaginase *in vitro* than those who lack the translocation, and some protocols including intensive L-asparaginase therapy have yielded high cure rates for this subset of patients.[18,19]

Microarray studies

Although all the cytogenetic findings discussed above are useful in the risk grouping of children with ALL and offer some hints on the pathogenic mechanisms involved, an even more substantial breakthrough in the mapping of the involved genes and the tumour biology will come from microarray studies in which the expression of thousands of genes can be determined in a single analysis.[20] Although the amount of data generated by these studies is overwhelming and requires extensive and complex bioinformatic analyses, in the coming years we are likely to understand the mechanisms behind disease development, aggressiveness, and drug sensitivity. This will probably have significant impact on our risk classification and treatment approach to childhood ALL.

Clonal immune gene rearrangements

The diversity in the normal immune response towards foreign antigens reflects somatic mutations in the B-cell (immunoglobulin) and T-cell receptor genes. Because of the clonal nature of ALL, quantitatively dominating immune gene rearrangements can be demonstrated by PCR at diagnosis in $\geq$95 per cent of children with ALL.[21] Since the leukaemic cells are degenerate, the clonal immune gene rearrangements are not line specific. Thus T-cell receptor gene rearrangements can be detected in most cases of B-cell precursor ALL. The clonal immune gene rearrangements are useful for diagnosis, since they are rarely found in cases of AML, myelodysplastic syndrome, aplastic anaemia, or non-malignant lymphadenopathies. In addition, they are very specific markers of the malignant lymphoblastic clone, and thus can be used for precise determination of residual bone marrow disease (MRD) during therapy with a detection limit of one malignant cell in 10^4–10^6 normal mononuclear cells (see below).[21,22]

Symptoms and differential diagnosis

At the time of diagnosis, the leukaemic cell burden is of the order of 10^{11}–10^{12} cells (10^9cells $\approx$ 1 g tissue). This immense clonal expansion of lymphoblasts gives rise to bone marrow dysfunction generally with pancytopenia and the classical symptoms of fatigue and pallor (80 per cent), fever (65 per cent), bleeding (50 per cent), enlarged liver and spleen (80 per cent), swollen lymph nodes (40 per cent), bone and joint pains (25 per cent), a thymic mass (10 per cent), and a pattern of symptoms that reflects the organs involved (e.g. breathing difficulties, neurologic symptoms, or renal failure). CNS disease with $>5 \times 10^6$/liter lymphoblasts in the cerebrospinal fluid (CNS-3) or a lower number of unequivocal blasts (CNS-2) are seen in 3–5 per cent of patients. Only some groups have been able to demonstrate an inferior outcome for patients with CNS-2. Except for the presence of a high number of lymphoblasts in a blood smear, none of the presenting clinical and haematologic findings are pathognomonic for childhood ALL, and the presenting clinical picture may occasionally be atypical. Hence a bone marrow examination is warranted in children with prolonged monocytopenia, and should be considered prior to glucocorticosteroid or methotrexate (MTX) therapy of supposed idiopathic thrombocytopenic purpura or rheumatoid arthritis. Most patients are generally well at the time of diagnosis, and the majority of children with ALL have had symptoms for only a few days or weeks, with a trend for the lower risk groups to have a more protracted course of disease. Half of all children with ALL present with a WBC $<10 \times 10^9$/liter, some even without easily detectable lymphoblasts in a blood smear (aleukaemic leukaemia), although PCR amplification of the B- and T-cell receptor genes will demonstrate clonality in the peripheral blood of the vast majority of these 'aleukaemic' patients. Fifteen per cent of all patients have a WBC at diagnosis of $> 50 \times 10^9$/liter. Eighty per cent will have a thrombocyte count $< 100 \times 10^9$/liter, and 85 per cent will have a haemoglobin < 6.0 mmol/l. A thrombocyte count above the upper normal limit is rare in children with ALL and more likely indicates that the patient has an inflammatory disease. Similarly, a high erythrocyte sedimentation rate without a concommitant high C-reactive protein also points towards ALL. Patients who present with high haemoglobin at diagnosis have a somewhat inferior outcome, as this indicates aggressive disease with bone marrow involvement for only a short time period. Other signs of ALL are the indicators of a rapid cell turnover such as high plasma lactate dehydrogenase and high plasma uric acid levels. At diagnosis, some patients are critically ill and may die before or at the initiation of therapy because of septicaemia, severe breathing difficulties (due to a thymic mass, superior vena cava obstruction, or pulmonary leucostasis), CNS disease, or hyperleucocytosis with WBC $> 400 \times 10^9$/liter. Patients with a very high WBC have a risk of disseminated intravascular coagulation, tumour lysis syndrome and electrolyte disturbances, renal failure, and leucostasis with life-threatening breathing difficulties, convulsions, and CNS haemorrhage or thrombosis.

The diagnosis of ALL must be established beyond any doubt. A complete workup is generally much more important than rapidly initiated therapy. Since most cases of ALL are very chemosensitive if given the right therapy, failure to perform the necessary investigations may jeopardize the chances of long-term survival. In addition to the bone marrow biopsy and aspirate for histomorphologic examination, immunophenotyping, and karyotyping, the initial programme must include a full history, performance and neurologic status, lymph node palpation, determination of spleen, liver, and testicular size, skin and mucosal membrane pathology, a chest radiograph to detect an anterior mediastinal mass, full blood counts, determination of blasts in blood and spinal fluid, and basic values such as blood group, immunoglobulins, electrolytes and urate, kidney and liver function tests, and serologic tests for viral infections. CT or MRI of the brain and spinal cord is indicated in cases with signs of CNS disease (e.g. headache and nausea, vision disturbances, cranial or peripheral nerve paresis) or the presence of spinal fluid lymphoblasts.

Juvenile rheumatoid arthritis and infectious mononucleosis may occasionally mimic leukaemia. Other diseases that may cause bone marrow failure and be clinically confused with leukaemia include aplastic anaemia, widely disseminated neuroblastoma, and more rarely Ewing sarcoma, rhabdomyosarcoma, and other anaplastic tumours with bone marrow dissemination. In addition, Epstein–Barr virus, cytomegalovirus, and parvovirus B-19 infections, as well as haemophagocytic or virus-associated lymphohistiocytosis with pancytopenia, may be misinterpreted as leukaemia. Pre-ALL with bone marrow failure, but a level of lymphoblasts in the bone marrow <5 per cent, is a rare condition that occasionally can be precipitated by parvovirus B-19 infection. This condition is more common in girls. PCR amplification of the B- and T-cell receptor gene rearrangements will demonstrate clonality in most of these patients.

Risk stratification

Since childhood ALL consists of a heterogeneous group of distinct biologic subtypes, identical therapy cannot be given to all patients. Approximately 40 per cent of all patients have one or more features that predict a significantly poorer outcome. Identification of these features should be attempted in every patient, since this allows correct risk grouping and the subsequent right choice of treatment intensity. Thus the most important prognostic factor is the treatment itself. Not only will all patients die if deprived of antileukaemic therapy, but specific subsets of ALL differ in their sensitivity to combinations of chemotherapy. An international classification that defines standard-risk patients as those with an age of 1.0–9.9 years and WBC $<50 \times 10^9$/liter and high-risk ALL as all other combinations has been useful for the comparison of treatment results from different study groups.[23] However, each study group needs a risk classification system that reflects its treatment strategy. Although the improvement in risk-adapted therapy has eliminated or reduced the importance of some factors (e.g. haemoglobin and FAB L1 versus L2 morphology), others have proved their robustness across study groups. These include gender, age at diagnosis, the tumour burden, immunophenotype and cytogenetics, and the early response to therapy. As an example, the NOPHO ALL-2000 risk grouping is outlined in Table 12.2.

White blood cells

The leukaemic cell mass at diagnosis, reflected by the WBC and extent of organ involvement, has been the most important prognostic factor for several decades, and is included in treatment stratification by nearly all groups (Fig. 12.3 and Table 12.2).[1] In addition, the significance of many risk factors in univariate analyses reflects their relation to the WBC. Thus WBC is correlated with immunophenotype (lowest in B-precursor ALL), age (lowest in

Table 12.2. Therapy Groups by NOPHO - ALL 2000 protocol for ALL 1.0–14.9 years

Therapy group	Age (years)	Criteria
Standard	<10	WBC < 10 × 10⁹/liter No unfavourable criteria
Intermediate	<10 ≥10 y	WBC 10- < 50 × 10⁹/liter WBC < 50 × 10⁹/liter No unfavourable criteria
Intensive[a]	Any age	WBC 50 to < 200 × 10⁹/liter Hypodiploidy (34–44 chromosomes) t(1;19) T-cell ALL Overt testicular involvement CNS involvement Standard or intermediate at diagnosis with slow response (day 15 M3 or day 29 M2 bone marrow)
Extra-intensive[b]	Any age	WBC ≥ 200 × 10⁹/liter 11q23/MLL rearrangements t(9;22) Hypodiploidy (<34 chromosomes) Day 29 M3 bone marrow

[a]Only patients >5 years at diagnosis with CNS disease, slow response, and/or T-cell disease with mediastinal involvement will receive CNS irradiation.
[b]The extra-intensive arm includes stem cell transplantation in first remission. This is optional for 11q23 aberrations in children aged 2.0–9.9 years.

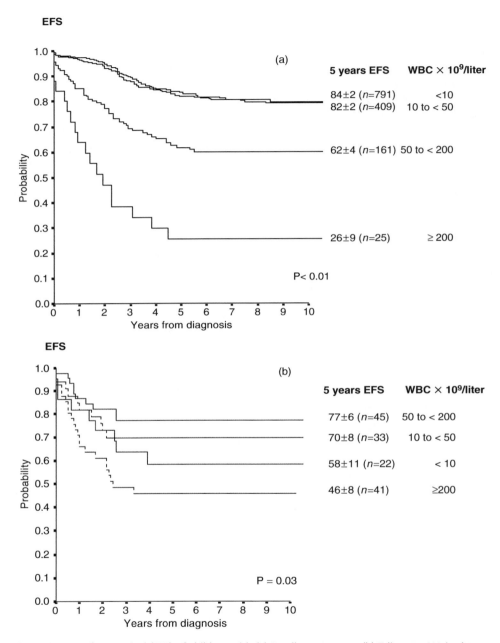

Fig. 12.3 Event-free survival (EFS) of children with (a) B-cell precursor or (b) T-lineage ALL in the NOPHO ALL-92 study. The WBC at diagnosis is one of the strongest prognostic factors, particularly for B-lineage ALL. All T-cell cases received high-risk therapy.

the age group 2–7 years), and cytogenetics (low in high-hyperdiploid and *TEL–AML1-*
positive ALL).

Treatment response

Even when remission is achieved, which is generally the case for 97–98 per cent of all patients,
the rapidity of tumour reduction is a very strong predictor of likelihood of cure. Thus the
prognosis is inferior for patients with $> 1 \times 10^9$/liter lymphoblasts in the peripheral blood
after 7 days exposure to prednisone and one intrathecal (i.t.) dose of MTX, >25 per cent
lymphoblasts in the bone marrow (M3 bone marrow) after 2 weeks of induction therapy, or >5
per cent lymphoblasts in the bone marrow (M2 bone marrow) at the end of induction therapy.
Although these features define a poor risk group of children with ALL, most relapses will
eventually occur among patients who seemingly have responded well to the remission induction treatment. Recently, precise monitoring of the subclinical level of MRD by flow-cytometric
detection of clone-specific patterns of CD antigens or PCR detection of clonal immune gene
rearrangements have emerged as powerful tools to distinguish between the good and poor
responders. Immunologic assays reflect the recognition that nearly all T-cell and most
B-precursor leukaemias have a phenotype (pattern of CD antigens) that is not normally present
in bone marrow. The PCR-based assays identify either the fusion gene transcripts that are
generated by the chromosomal translocations [e.g. t(12;21)] present in 35 per cent of ALL cases
or the junctional regions of the B-cell (immunoglobulin) or T-cell receptor gene rearrangements. The latter are not leukaemia-associated genetic aberrations, but owing to the vast
repertoire of these rearrangements (e.g. 10^{11} for the immunoglobulin heavy chain), the
likelihood of finding non-leukaemic cells with the same rearrangements is extremely low.
Together, the immunologic and PCR-based techniques are applicable in 95 per cent of children
with ALL, and they will probably change our future definition of remission as well as risk
classification. A major pitfall in the quantification of MRD levels based on clonal immune gene
rearrangements is the evolution of subclones that differ both in these gene rearrangements and
in their chemosensitivity. These subclones may go undetected at diagnosis and be responsible
for relapse. However, the variations in the chemosensitivity of subclones seem to be much less
than the variations in their immune gene rearrangement. Thus MRD levels early during
therapy have already become established as a very strong prognostic feature, surpassing even
WBC at diagnosis. Forty per cent of children with ALL will have $< 10^{-4}$–10^{-5} leukaemic cells
in the bone marrow at the end of a 4- to 6-week induction therapy, and these patients will have
a relapse risk of $\leq$5 per cent irrespective of other known risk factors (Fig. 12.4).[21,22] However, it
is not known whether these are the patients who can be cured with the less toxic therapy used in
the 1970s. In contrast, patients who still have $> 10^{-3}$ leukaemic cells in the bone marrow after
several months of therapy will have a 70 per cent risk of subsequent and even very late
relapses.[11,21] So far it is not known whether quantification of low-level residual disease during
therapy will allow control of emerging relapse through treatment intensification. In contrast,
several groups have demonstrated the persistence of leukaemia-associated immune gene
rearrangements at the end of treatment and off-treatment in a substantial number of patients
who continue to remain in remission. These may represent normal cells with the same gene
rearrangements, non-dividing quiescent leukaemic cells, or preleukaemic cells harbouring the
first mutations but lacking the further mutations that lead to overt ALL.[6,9] Consequently, it is
uncertain whether the demonstration of clonal immune gene rearrangements by PCR at the
end of therapy carries prognostic significance.

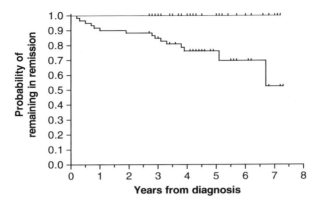

Fig. 12.4 Kaplan–Meier plots for 104 patients treated according to the NOPHO ALL-92 protocol. Patients with day 29 MRD levels $\geq$ 0.01 per cent ($n = 60$, lower curve) and <0.01 per cent ($n = 40$, upper curve) (P = 0.0007); 0.01 per cent is the median level for patients in remission.[22]

Gender

Several reports have demonstrated that after the first 1–2 years of therapy boys have a significantly higher risk of relapse than girls, which is only partially explained by their higher frequency of T-cell disease and lower frequency of high hyperdiploidy. However, beyond offering longer maintenance therapy to boys, few collaborative study groups stratify therapy by gender.

Age

Although modern therapy has reduced the prognostic impact of age at diagnosis (except for infants), most study groups will offer more intensive treatment to children >10 years of age at diagnosis. The poorer outcome for adolescents compared with children <10 years of age reflects a low frequency of translocation t(12;21) and the high-hyperploid karyotype (Fig. 12.1), a lower chemosensitivity,[22] and a lower treatment compliance during oral therapy.

CNS disease

The presence of CNS leukaemia at diagnosis is generally classified as a high risk factor. Although CNS disease requires intensified CNS-directed chemotherapy and/or radiotherapy, it is uncertain whether it is a general feature of more aggressive ALL and thus always justifies more intensive systemic therapy. When high-risk therapy is given, the outcome of these patients is as good as that of other high-risk patients without CNS disease (Fig. 12.5).

Unfortunately, the improvements in outcome during recent decades have been far more pronounced for the lower risk groups, and treatment intensification has had less impact on the cure rates for the higher risk groups (Fig. 12.6).[1] Patients with WBC > 200 × 10⁹/liter at diagnosis, t(4;11) or t(9;22) translocations, a very hypodiploid clone (modal number <34), and those who fail to achieve remission after the first 4 weeks of therapy generally have such a poor outcome that SCT in first remission with a related or matched unrelated donor is a relevant treatment option.[16,24,25] However, it is doubtful whether SCT really improves the long-term survival for some of these subsets of patients at very high risk.[15]

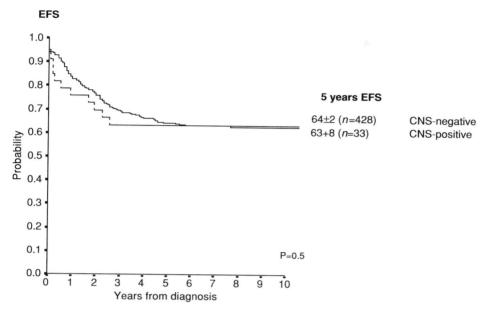

Fig. 12.5 EFS curves for patients with or without CNS disease at diagnosis. All patients received therapy according to the NOPHO ALL-92 protocol.

Therapy

The efficacy of antileukaemic treatment depends on several factors including the dosage (dose and schedule) and pharmacokinetics of the anticancer agents, the chemosensitivity of the leukaemic clone,[14,26] and the tumour cell growth kinetics. Refinements of chemotherapy for childhood ALL have developed immensely over the last decades, and reflect both randomized clinical trials and pharmacokinetic and pharmacodynamic studies. Through the focus on these aspects for every drug used in the treatment of childhood ALL, impressive cure rates have been obtained with the same drugs that were available 30 years ago. Since the leukaemias differ in their chemosensitivity, and as each antileukaemic drug may have a limited tumour-reducing potential, multidrug chemotherapy is necessary to achieve cure, and most protocols will include six to ten anticancer agents. The treatment intensity reflects the risk group assignment based on the combination of clinical presentation and characteristics of the lymphoblasts. Across study groups, the treatment of T-cell and precursor B-cell ALL generally includes four main components (Fig. 12.7):

Induction treatment

A four- to five-drug induction treatment commonly consists of daily prednisolone or dexamethasone, weekly vincristine, repeated doses of L-asparaginase and/or an anthracycline, and i.t. MTX.[1] Whether to use dexamethasone (e.g. 6–10 mg/m^2) or prednisolone (e.g. 60 mg/m^2) depends on the general strategy of the study group. These glucocorticosteroids are among the most powerful antileukaemic drugs. Compared with prednisolone, dexamethasone has higher *in vitro* antileukaemic efficacy, longer half-life, and better CNS penetration, but it is also more

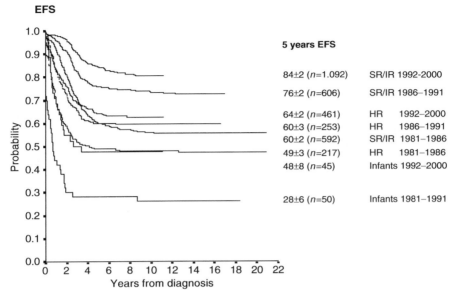

Fig. 12.6 EFS curves for patients treated during three consecutive protocol periods (July 1981–June 1986, July 1986–december 1991, and January 1992–December 2001). Despite some improvement, infants do poorly during all three periods. The improvement in outcome has been most pronounced for children with standard-risk (SR) and intermediate-risk (IR) ALL, whereas the change in EFS is less impressive for children with high-risk (HR) ALL, which includes WBC $\geq$50 $\times$ 10^9/liter, T-cell, mediastinal or CNS, or testicular disease, t(4;11) or t(9;22), or M2/3 bone marrow at treatment day 29.

toxic. Dexamethasone has been shown both to reduce the risk of CNS relapse and to improve the overall event-free survival (EFS). However, dexamethasone has also been suspected of increasing the risk of neurocognitive damage, osteonecrosis, excessive weight, and life-threatening sepsis during induction therapy. Patients with a very high tumour burden at diagnosis (excessively large liver and spleen or WBC $>100 \times 10^9$/liter) may be at risk of tumour lysis syndrome at initiation of therapy and should start pretreatment with reduced doses of prednisolone (e.g. 5 mg/m^2) with subsequent slow increments to standard doses within 3–5 days (depending on the degree of tumour lysis), after which full-dose antileukaemic treatment can be given (see section on supportive care below). Some collaborative groups, including the Berlin–Frankfurt–Münster (BFM), group give all patients a 1-week prednisone prephase with one i.t. dose of MTX. Subsequently, persistence of more than 1×10^9/liter lymphoblasts in peripheral blood will identify a small (10 per cent) subset of patients with a very high probability of remission failure or relapse. As with glucocorticosteroids, the choice of brand of L-asparaginase may also have a significant impact on the cure rate.[27] Thus both pharmacokinetic studies and randomized clinical trials have shown that the longer half-life of the enzyme derived from *Escherichia coli* enzyme improves the EFS compared with that derived from *Erwinia*. Generally, induction therapy will induce morphologic remission (defined as <5 per cent lymphoblasts in the bone marrow) in 99 per cent of children with lower-risk ALL (even

Induction – intermediate intensity

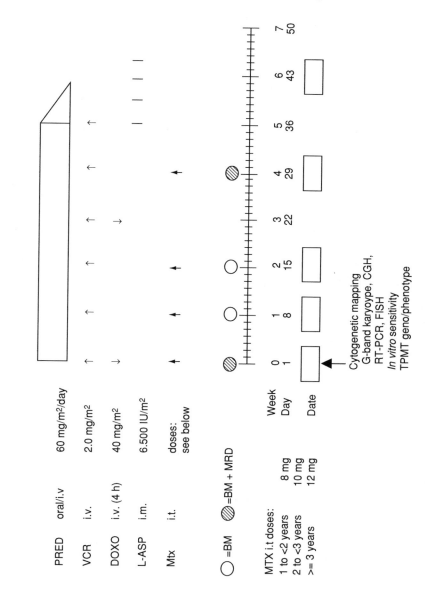

PRED	oral/i.v	60 mg/m²/day
VCR	i.v.	2.0 mg/m²
DOXO	i.v. (4 h)	40 mg/m²
L-ASP	i.m.	6.500 IU/m²
Mtx	i.t.	doses: see below

○ =BM   ◍ =BM + MRD

MTX i.t doses:
1 to <2 years	8 mg
2 to <3 years	10 mg
>= 3 years	12 mg

Week
Day
Date

Cytogenetic mapping
G-band karyoype, CGH,
RT-PCR, FISH
In vitro sensitivity
TPMT geno/phenotype

(b) Consolidation –intermediate intensity

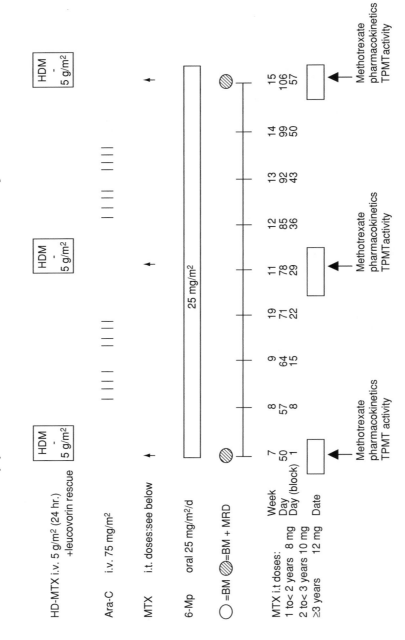

(c) Delayed intensification –intermediate intensity

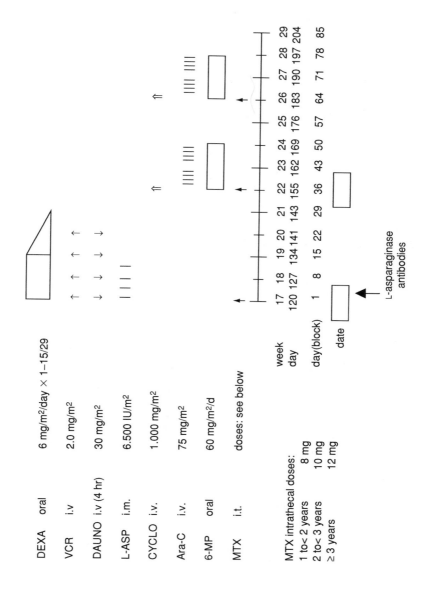

DEXA	oral	6 mg/m²/day × 1–15/29
VCR	i.v	2.0 mg/m²
DAUNO	i.v (4 hr)	30 mg/m²
L-ASP	i.m.	6.500 IU/m²
CYCLO	i.v.	1.000 mg/m²
Ara-C	i.v.	75 mg/m²
6-MP	oral	60 mg/m²/d
MTX	i.t.	doses: see below

MTX intrathecal doses:

1 to< 2 years	8 mg
2 to< 3 years	10 mg
≥ 3 years	12 mg

L-asparaginase
antibodies

(d) MAINTENANCE I – intermediate intensity

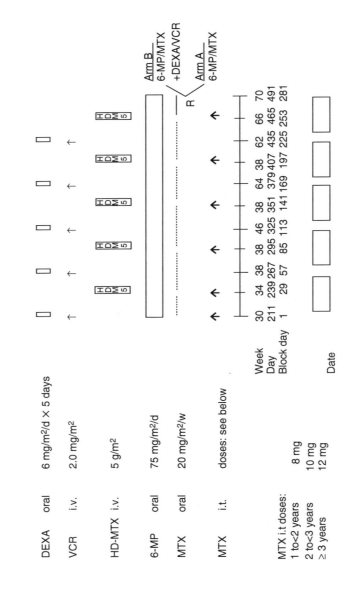

DEXA   oral   6 mg/m²/d × 5 days

VCR   i.v.   2.0 mg/m²

HD-MTX i.v.   5 g/m²

6-MP   oral   75 mg/m²/d

MTX   oral   20 mg/m²/w

MTX   i.t.   doses: see below

MTX i.t doses:

1 to<2 years   8 mg

2 to<3 years   10 mg

≥ 3 years   12 mg

(e) Maintenance II –randomization–intermediate intensity

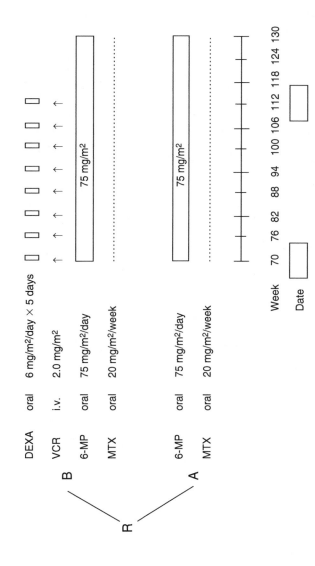

Fig. 12.7 Treatment strategy for children with intermediate-risk B-cell precursor ALL (one-third of all cases; see Table 12.2). Detailed cytogenetic mapping with G-band karyotyping, high-resolution CGH, RT-PCR and/or FISH for certain translocations, and *in vitro* sensitivity studies are performed at diagnosis. Pharmacologic studies of L-asparaginase, HD-MTX, and thiopurines are done routinely. Minimal residual disease measurements by PCR or flow cytometry are made after 1, 2, and 3 months of therapy, prior to randomization, and at the end of therapy.

with relatively low-intensity regimens) and ~95 per cent of the higher-risk patients. Previously the definition of remission also included full haematopoietic recovery, but as therapy has become more intensive, the continuation of therapy will prevent the marrow regenerating up to normal levels. Although failure to achieve remission is a poor prognostic sign, unfortunately the opposite is not the case. Morphologic remission only signifies a reduction of the tumour burden by 2–3 log (with up to 10^9 leukaemic cells left), and eventually most relapses will occur among those patients who were in remission at the end of induction therapy. Thus a high chance of cure can only be obtained by prolonged and intensive post-remission multidrug programmes.

Delayed intensification (re-induction or consolidation) therapy

Delayed intensification (re-induction or consolidation) therapy is administered when remission has been achieved. The post-remission re-intensification or consolidation therapy varies across study groups, but generally includes alkylating agents and/or epipodophyllotoxins, repeated doses of asparaginase, and HD-MTX with or without concurrent thiopurines.[1,2,3,23,28] From the late 1970s onwards, the BFM and other groups have demonstrated the efficacy of a second induction and consolidation treatment with, for example, vincristine, anthracyclines, glucocorticosteroids, and L-asparaginase. Such an intensification (or even double intensification) has been shown to be of benefit for both high-risk and non-high-risk patients. Today, many collaborative groups offer such a second (or even third) induction phase to all patients, while others (such as the NOPHO group) reserve it for the higher-risk patients. The children who are eligible for SCT in first remission should optimally be transplanted within 6–12 months of diagnosis, i.e. as soon as a histocompatible donor has been identified.[24] If a stem cell donor cannot be identified within a year of diagnosis, the advantages of SCT become less obvious for some high-risk groups (e.g. T-cell leukaemia with a WBC $> 200 \times 10^9$/liter at diagnosis or infant ALL) since they are primarily characterized by an increased relapse hazard early in therapy.

CNS-directed therapy

Prior to the introduction of CNS-directed therapy in the 1960s, ≥ 50 per cent of children with ALL would develop a CNS relapse. Today, irradiation and/or HD-MTX and/or Ara-C with i.t. MTX or triple therapy (MTX, Ara-C, and glucocorticosteroids) has reduced the risk of CNS relapse to <5 per cent.[1] At diagnosis, 5 per cent of all children have CNS leukaemia (defined as $>5 \times 10^6$ lymphoblasts/liter), and an even higher number have subclinical involvement. A few studies have indicated that patients with CNS-2 (unequivocal blasts $< 5 \times 10^9$/liter) also have an increased relapse rate, but several groups have failed to confirm this. Even though CNS irradiation is one of the most effective prophylactic and therapeutic modalities for CNS leukaemia, the strategy adopted by many collaborative groups has been to restrict prophylactic cranial irradiation to selected subsets of patients and to reduce the dose to as little as 12 Gy to avoid late effects.[29] Leucoencephalopathy is one of the most worrisome side effects, and the risk is significantly increased if i.v. MTX is given within the first few months after CNS irradiation. On the other hand, the potential neurotoxicity of the intrathecally administered drugs as well as of HD-MTX should not be underestimated, and the frequency and severity of neuropsychologic late effects of high-dose therapy need to be explored thoroughly in future trials. Cranial irradiation can be omitted at least for the low- and average-risk patients, and probably also for the high-risk patients with an M1/M2 marrow on treatment day 7, provided that intensive systemic therapy and/or i.t. MTX (or triple therapy) is given. In the Nordic countries, 10 per cent of the total cohort of patients will receive cranial irradiation (18–24 Gy) in first remission. This includes children with CNS disease at diagnosis and those patients >5 years of age who are in the highest risk groups, since their risk of CNS relapse justifies the neurologic, neuropsychologic, and endocrine late effects induced by irradiation (Table 12.2). The purpose of high-dose chemotherapy is to overcome cellular drug resistance mechanisms or to increase the penetration of the anticancer agent into pharmacologic sanctuaries (such as the CNS). The ratio of CSF to plasma concentration is acceptable for some systemically adminis-tered anticancer agents, such as cyclophosphamide (50 per cent), 6-mercaptopurine (25 per cent), cytarabine (15 per cent), and dexamethasone (15 per cent). In contrast, the ratio is poor for prednisone (<10 per cent), MTX (1–3 per cent), vincristine (<5 per cent), and teniposide (<5 per cent). The pharmacologic barrier to some of these drugs can be overcome by administering high-dose chemotherapy, such as HD-MTX and Ara-C, or by direct adminis-tration of MTX, Ara-C, or glucocorticosteroids into the cerebrospinal fluid. Since the cerebro-spinal fluid volume (and the brain) grows rapidly in early life and reaches close to adult size when the child is ∼3 years of age, the doses of intrathecally administered drugs should be based on the age of the child rather than on the body surface area. Thus for children <1, 1–2, 2–3, and >3 years of age the dose of i.t. MTX will be 6 mg, 8 mg, 10 mg, and 12 mg, respectively. HD-MTX ($1–5\,g/m^2$ with i.t. MTX and leucovorin rescue) is most commonly given together with 6-mercaptopurine because of the synergistic action of these drugs.[28] HD-MTX may reduce the risk of CNS disease, but even more convincingly reduces the risk of bone marrow and testicular failures. At least in the lower dose range of $1–2\,g/m^2$, the interindividual variation in MTX pharmacokinetics may significantly influence the risk of relapse. Thus children with B-lineage ALL who are randomized to receive pharmacokinetically guided doses of MTX during con-solidation therapy to achieve a target plasma drug concentration have a significantly better outcome than those who are treated with dosing based on body surface area.[30]

Maintenance therapy

Following consolidation and re-intensification treatment, maintenance therapy to eradicate low-level residual leukaemia is initiated starting with oral 6-mercaptopurine (6MP) $50–75\,mg/m^2$/day and oral or parenteral MTX $20–40\,mg/m^2$ at 1- to 2-week intervals. Although several studies have shown that ∼50 per cent of patients are cured even if all therapy is truncated at 1 year from diagnosis, it has so far not been possible to identify the patients within each risk group for whom this short treatment is sufficient. Thus maintenance therapy is given until a total duration of therapy of 2–3 years, with the lower-risk groups and boys needing longer therapy. No studies have demonstrated an advantage of extending treatment beyond this duration. During the first year of maintenance therapy (or longer), many study groups give alternate pulses of vincristine–glucocorticosteroid re-inductions, HD-MTX ($2–5\,g/m^2$), or other drug combinations (Fig. 12.7). After cessation of therapy, the relapse rate is 10–20 per cent even if therapy has lasted for more than 2–3 years. Thus the intensifi-cation of antileukaemic therapy over recent decades has had most impact on the risk of relapse during therapy, whereas the risk of relapse after cessation of treatment has changed little. According to most protocols, the doses of 6MP and MTX during maintenance therapy are targeted to maintain a WBC of 1.5×10^9 to $3.0–3.5 \times 10^9$/liter or a low neutrophil count. A neutrophil level $< 2.0 \times 10^9$/liter during maintenance therapy is associated with a superior cure rate, but whether this reflects treatment intensity or the endogenous bone marrow activity is uncertain.[31] A rise in amino transaminase levels is common during MTX–6MP maintenance therapy, but rarely necessitates treatment withdrawal if the liver function parameters (bilirubin and coagulation factors 2, 7, and 10) are normal. A rise in amino transaminase levels primarily reflects the cellular levels of methylated 6MP metabolites, some of which are strong inhibitors of the purine *de novo* synthesis.[32] In addition, the presence of increased amino transaminase levels has been related to a lower risk of relapse.[33] Maintenance therapy has been related to a superior antileukaemic effect if oral MTX and 6MP are given in the evening, but this effect has so far not been explained biologically or pharmacologically.[34] Although interindividual variations in the pharmacokinetics of 6MP and MTX seem to have significant impact on the chances of cure, it remains to be demonstrated that pharmacokinetically guided dose adjustments will improve the cure rate.[31] One of the most important factors that determine the efficacy of 6MP therapy is the genetic polymorphism in the activity of the enzyme thiopurine methyltransferase (TPMT). 6MP primarily exerts its antileukaemic effect through conversion into 6-thioguanine nucleotides (6TGN) that are incorporated into DNA, and TPMT competes with this process by methylating 6MP and some of its metabolites. Because of TPMT mutations, one in 300 patients will be TPMT deficient with very high 6TGN levels and at risk for life-threatening bone marrow suppression unless treated with only 10–20 per cent of the normal 6MP dose. Eleven per cent of all patients will be heterozygous because of mutations in one of the TPMT alleles, and they will have ~50 per cent of the TPMT activity present in wild-type patients. The TPMT-heterozygous patients will experience more bone marrow toxicity when treated with standard 6MP doses, and they will have a reduced risk of relapse but a higher risk of second cancers.[31,35,36] Some studies have indicated that substituting 6MP with 6TGN will improve the EFS (although others have failed to confirm this), but 6TGN therapy also seems to induce a high risk of veno-occlusive disease.

For several decades, standardization of therapy by surface-area-based drug dosing was the mantra. Now the scenario is changing with the availability of new surrogate parameters for predicting tumour response by *in vitro* sensitivity testing,[14,26] precise quantification of residual disease in the blood or bone marrow through PCR or flow cytometric measurements,[11,21,22,37] determination of pharmacogenetic polymorphism (e.g. cytochrome *P*-450, TPMT, and methylenetetrahydrofolate reductase), and options for individual therapeutic drug monitoring.[30,31] Today, many collaborative study groups adapt this biologic approach. An example is the NOPHO ALL-2000 protocol (Fig. 12.7), where detailed cytogenetic mapping and *in vitro* sensitivity studies at diagnosis, pharmacokinetic studies of L-asparaginase, HD-MTX, and thiopurines during consolidation, and re-induction and maintenance therapy combined with PCR or flow-cytometric-based measurements of MRD after 1, 2, and 3 months of therapy allow evaluation of the effect of drug sensitivity and pharmacokinetics on treatment response within well-defined cytogenetic subsets. Such pharmacokinetic–dynamic studies are likely to increase our understanding of treatment failures and to optimize the efficacy of treatment.

Supportive care

Although the impressive improvement in the cure rate of childhood ALL reflects a significant intensification of therapy in recent decades, this has not lead to a parallel increase in the risk of life-threatening complications during therapy.[1,38] Only about 2 per cent of patients will die in first remission because of treatment-related complications. This reflects a comparable impressive improvement in the nursing and supportive care of these patients which includes improved treatment of hyperleucocytosis and tumour lysis syndrome, transfusions of blood products, emphasis on adequate nutrition, better imaging of organs for infections or other complications, improved detection of pathogenic microorganisms in tissue, including blood and lungs, and more effective antimicrobial agents (see Chapter 8).

Hyperleucocytosis and tumour lysis syndrome

Tumour lysis syndrome is a life-threatening complication preferentially seen among cases with mature B-cell ALL or WBC $> 400 \times 10^9$/liter at diagnosis. It is characterized by the triad of hyperkalaemia, hyperphosphataemia, and hyperuricaemia caused by rapid cell lysis, and frequently complicated by hypocalcaemia (with tetany) and renal failure requiring dialysis. It may be present at diagnosis or be precipitated by the introduction of chemotherapy. Thus at diagnosis close monitoring of blood counts, serum electrolytes (not least calcium, potassium, and phosphate), creatinine, uric acid, vital signs including blood pressure, intake/output, and body weight is mandatory. Tumour lysis syndrome should be prevented and treated by intravenous hydration (3000–4500 ml/m^2/24 h), allopurinol (10–15 mg/kg/24 h) or recombinant urate oxidase (e.g. rasburicase 0.2 mg/kg i.v. once daily), urine alkalization to pH 7.0–7.5 with systemic sodium bicarbonate or acetazolamide, and forced diuresis with furosemide (1–2 mg/kg single dose) and/or mannitol 15 g/m^2 at 6-h interval. Dialysis may be indicated by severe hyperkalaemia, hyperphosphataemia with or without symptomatic hypocalcaemia, and falling urinary output with rising creatinine. Although leucopheresis may substantially reduce a very high WBC, it is not known whether this approach improves the survival of patients at risk of tumour lysis syndrome. Treatment with very reduced doses of glucocorticosteroids (e.g. 5 mg/m^2/24 h) should be started when the patient is stabilized, urine pH >7.0, and the urinary output is adequate. In rare life-threatening cases of hyperleucocytosis, the diagnostic workup may occasionally be based on samples of peripheral blood, and cytoreductive therapy may be started before the results of the diagnostic studies are available.

Stem cell transplantation

SCT in first, second, or later remission is a relevant treatment option for certain subsets of ALL, but the definition of these subsets is a moving target which reflects the balance of the likelihood of cure by conventional chemo- and radiotherapy and the risk of SCT-induced morbidity and mortality.[24] At present, the relatively well-established indications for SCT include late remissions (M2/3 bone marrow after conventional induction therapy), t(9;22)-positive ALL, patients with a very high WBC at diagnosis ($> 200 \times 10^9$/liter in the NOPHO ALL-2000 protocol), and patients who relapse within 3 years of diagnosis.[16,24] In contrast, it is uncertain whether children with 11q23-translocation positive ALL (most of whom are infants) will gain from SCT.[15] Patients who are unresponsive to chemotherapy are probably only candidates for SCT as part of clinical trials. The value of SCT in patients with hypodiploid ALL has currently not been established.[3]

As the prophylaxis of and treatment for graft-versus-host disease (GVHD) improves, SCT using unrelated matched donors has become increasingly relevant.[25] Parallel to this development, the donor registries have expanded considerably within the last 5–10 years and now contain HLA information on more than six million potential donors. Since many of the registered donors are of European origin, the chances of finding a good matching donor is especially good for White children, being close to 80–90 per cent. In contrast, there is an unsatisfactory lack of donors from other ethnic groups. Because of the higher availability of unrelated donors and the improvements in tissue-type matching on a genetic level (high-resolution HLA-typing), the percentage of unrelated transplants has increased worldwide, and in many centers unrelated SCT now constitute more than half of the transplants since the benefit of the graft versus leukaemia (GVL) effect outweighs the negative effect of GVHD.

The purpose of SCT is the elimination of the malignant clone by chemotherapy, irradiation, and the alloreactive antileukaemia effect (GVL). Unfortunately, the GVL effect is closely related to donor–recipient incompatibility and, thus to the risk of GVHD. So far attempts to separate the GVL effect and GVHD-induced morbidity have failed. Although T-cell depletion can reduce the risk of acute and chronic GVHD, it increases the risk of graft failure and the relapse rate, and it severely reduces the immune function for a long period. Another alternative is the use of a haplo-identical parent. Although such donors in principle are always available and the graft processing procedures have improved in recent years, there is a significant risk of graft rejection, life-threatening toxicities, and relapse of the leukaemia. Syngeneic HLA-identical twins are not a donor option since they lack both major and minor histocompatability mismatch, and thus also the GVL effect.

Traditionally most transplantations have been performed with bone marrow stem cells. However, in recent years, peripheral stem cells and cord blood stem cells have been used with increasing frequency in children. Bone marrow stem cells cause chronic GVHD less frequently than peripheral stem cells, which on the other hand lead to more rapid engraftment and possibly more GVL effect.

The purposes of the conditioning regimen given in the days before the infusion of stem cells is myeloablation, immunosuppression/ablation to avoid rejection, and reduction of the residual tumour burden. The conditioning regimen most commonly consists of cyclophosphamide (120–200 mg/kg) or VP16 (60 mg/kg) with 12 Gy total body irradiation (TBI) or alternatively busulfan plus cyclophosphamide; the latter is used mainly in children <3–4 years of age because of the risk of TBI-induced leucoencephalopathy. The non-myeloablative conditioning regimens ('mini-transplantation'), which predominantly provide immunoablation, are still not widely used in childhood leukaemia.

The primary causes of death following SCT are recurrence of the leukaemia, viral, bacterial and fungal infections, GVHD, interstitial pneumonia, and multi-organ failure. Although most long-term survivors lead a normal life, a significant fraction of patients are burdened by a varying degree of late effects including second cancers (not least after TBI), endocrinopathies, precocious (most common in girls) or delayed puberty, infertility (predominately after TBI) due to gonadal damage and uterine fibrosis, reduced lung and cardiac function, cataract in at least 20 per cent of the patients within 5 years of TBI, and leucoencephalopathy, which is most common in young children exposed to TBI.

Treatment failures

When the diagnosis has been established and treatment has been initiated, children with ALL are at risk of four different types of treatment failure.

First, 2–3 per cent of all patients fail to achieve remission following a standard induction regimen. These patients are difficult to identify at diagnosis, but features associated with remission failure include older age, T-cell disease with a high WBC at diagnosis, Ph+ ALL, undifferentiated leukaemia, a poor response to a prednisone prephase, and an M3 bone marrow after 2–3 weeks of therapy. Remission may be achieved for some of these patients by treatment intensification by, for example, cyclophosphamide and vincristine, high-dose Ara-C with VP16, intensive relapse protocols, or other established or experimental drug combinations. If remission is achieved, such patients are candidates for allogenic SCT.

Secondly, 2–3 per cent of all patients will die during induction or in remission, most frequently due to leucostasis, bleeding, or opportunistic infections such as Gram-negative septicaemia and *Pneumocystis carinii* pneumonia (see Chapter 8).[1,38]

Thirdly, 1–2 per cent of all patients will develop a second cancer, with a higher risk for those who have received cranial irradiation or epipodophyllotoxins, or who have a TPMT heterozygous phenotype (see section on late effects).

Finally, 15–20 per cent of all children with ALL will develop a bone marrow (15 per cent), CNS (3–5 per cent), testicular (2 per cent), or other focal relapse within the first 5 years after diagnosis. Because of the genetic instability of the cancer cells, subclones may develop with randomly occurring differences in drug sensitivity. The risk of developing chemoresistant subclones is correlated with the tumour burden, and therefore is most likely to occur prior to or during the early phases of therapy. Through the use of anticancer agents, resistant subclones will be selected. The most resistant of these may progress to overt relapse during chemotherapy, whereas the less resistant subclones will recur when therapy is stopped. This supports the clinical observation that recurrent ALL during chemotherapy is generally far more resistant to second-line therapy than relapses that occur after a certain interval from cessation of treatment (Fig. 12.8).

It is unlikely that early morphologic identification of relapses by routine bone marrow or spinal fluid examinations will improve the chances of cure for these patients. However, it remains undetermined whether flow-cytometric- or PCR-based detection of emerging disease reflected by low but increasing MRD levels during treatment or at the end of therapy will allow eradication of such residual disease by intensified chemotherapy.

Previously, the occurrence of relapses more than 5 years after diagnosis was not uncommon, but with modern intensive multidrug chemotherapy such late occurrences are now rare. At relapse, the leukaemia must be explored as extensively as at initial diagnosis, including by morphology and histochemistry, immunophenotyping, karyotyping, and molecular biology. Some biologic features, including the WBC level, are often very similar to the presentation at diagnosis, but cytogenetic evolution is common. Approximately 85–90 per cent of the patients who relapse will achieve a second remission, but less than half of these will be long-term survivors (Fig. 12.8). The prognostic factors at relapse include age <1 year at diagnosis (Fig. 12.8), the duration of first remission, T-cell disease (poor risk), t(12;21) (good risk), extramedullary relapse (good risk), and a low to undetectable MRD level following the first course of relapse therapy (good risk). The outcome is worst for those with T-cell disease (cure rate around 10 per cent) and those who relapse while on therapy, for whom the chance of cure is ≤20 per cent (Fig. 12.8). The small number of patients who develop a bone marrow relapse within the first year of treatment have an extremely poor outcome (Fig. 12.8). In contrast, patients with B-lineage ALL who relapse >3 years from diagnosis have a chance of cure, which may exceed 50 per cent even without SCT. These late recurrences include patients with intermediate chemosensitivity, who will benefit from intensified second-line therapy, patients with poor compliance to oral maintenance therapy, and patients with a true second ALL that has occurred as a consequence of a second hit among the first-hit 'preleukaemic' cells,[9] as has been indicated in cases of t(12;21)-positive relapses. Patients with late relapses tend to have a longer duration of their second remission than those with early relapse, and thus require longer follow-up for judgement of their ultimate outcome.

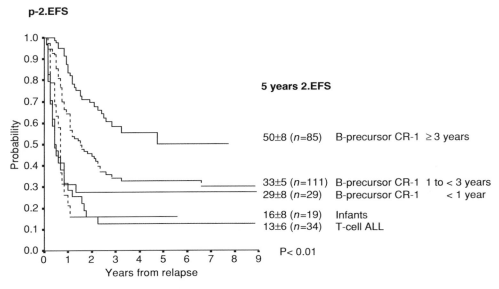

p-2.EFS

5 years 2.EFS

50±8 (*n*=85)	B-precursor CR-1 ≥3 years
33±5 (*n*=111)	B-precursor CR-1 1 to < 3 years
29±8 (*n*=29)	B-precursor CR-1 < 1 year
16±8 (*n*=19)	Infants
13±6 (*n*=34)	T-cell ALL

P< 0.01

Fig. 12.8 Second EFS curves for patients diagnosed between 1992 and 2001 who developed a relapse. Overall the prognosis is very poor for infants and children with T-cell ALL. The prognosis for B-cell precursor ALL is strongly correlated to the duration of first remission.

CNS relapse

The CNS is a well-known sanctuary for leukaemic cells and, before the introduction of CNS-directed therapy in the 1960s, as many as 50 per cent of all patients developed a CNS relapse. With modern therapy this will occur in <5 per cent of patients. Half of these will be combined with other sites of relapse, most often bone marrow, but the remainder will be so-called isolated CNS relapses, although many of these will also have subclinical bone marrow involvement. The risk of CNS relapse seems to be increased in patients with T-cell ALL and additional high-risk features (e.g. a high WBC or a mediastinal mass). In addition, the risk of CNS relapse is increased in patients with > 5 × 10⁶/liter lymphoblasts (CNS-3) at diagnosis, and possibly also in those with a lower number of unequivocal blasts (CNS-2), and this feature has also been associated with traumatic lumbar punctures at diagnosis (> 10 × 10⁶/liter erythrocytes). Only a few groups have been able to demonstrate an inferior outcome for patients with CNS-2. Early combined CNS and bone marrow relapse is most frequently seen in T-cell disease with a high WBC at initial diagnosis, and is associated with a very poor prognosis. Today, most CNS relapses occur during treatment. Later on, CNS recurrences are rare and are most commonly combined with bone marrow relapse. Generally, patients with a CNS relapse should receive craniospinal irradiation, but the radiation dose must be reduced according to CNS irradiation given previously. In addition, all patients must receive intrathecal as well as systemic chemotherapy, which should be at least as intensive as the first-line treatment and should include high-dose therapy. Whether or not to offer SCT will depend on the time of relapse and whether or not it is combined with bone marrow disease.

Testicular relapse

A testicular relapse presents as a non-tender swelling of one or both testes. After the introduction of intensive systemic chemotherapy, and not least HD-MTX, testicular relapses have become rare and now occur in <3 per cent of boys. The testes are probably a pharmacologic sanctuary from where leukaemic cells may seed. Accordingly, patients with combined bone marrow and testicular relapse do better than those with isolated bone marrow relapse, since the former is believed to reflect seeding of chemosensitive leukaemic cells from the testicular sanctuary.[39] In clinically unilateral disease, the affected testis may be removed and the other testis irradiated, whereas in bilateral testicular relapse both testes are irradiated. In addition, intensive systemic chemotherapy is required.

Other sites

More rarely, the recurrence of ALL is located in a lymph node, skin, eye, ovary, kidney, or bone. No standard approaches for these leukaemias exist, but they should always receive intensive systemic chemotherapy followed by oral antimetabolite-based maintenance therapy. Whether or not to offer SCT will depend on the time of their recurrence.

Special subsets

Certain subsets of ALL need special consideration. Some have a very poor prognosis because of inherent chemoresistance and may be eligible for SCT in first remission. Others have a more favourable outcome as long as certain therapeutic precautions are taken (see also the section on cytogenetics).

Down syndrome

Nearly all cancers in children with Down syndrome are leukaemias.[40] Interestingly, the leukaemic clone in >50 per cent of non-Down ALL patients also harbours trisomy 21.[13] Translocation t(12;21)(p13;q22) and high hyperdiploidy (with trisomies 4, 10, and 17) seem to be less common in ALL patients with Down syndrome, but their cure rate is equal to that of non-Down patients without these favourable prognostic genetic aberrations.[41] Leukaemic cells from Down and non-Down patients do not differ in their *in vitro* sensitivity to the most commonly used anticancer drugs. Their risk of severe toxicity following MTX and APA-C therapy is significantly increased, probably because of drug disposition gene dose effects and a propensity for apoptosis.

Infant ALL

It is likely that infant ALL with translocations involving 11q23 reflect *in utero* exposure to carcinogens that interact with the topoisomerase II enzyme.[42] Children aged <1 year at diagnosis are a therapeutic challenge because of their high frequency of adverse clinical features such as hyperleucocytosis and CNS leukaemia at diagnosis. They rarely have a T-cell phenotype, harbour translocations t(9;22) or t(2;21), or have a high-hyperdiploid karyotype. Two-thirds carry chromosomal aberrations that involve the MLL gene at chromosome region 11q23, most frequently t(4;11), have a CD10–N_3 meaning negative immunophenotype, and carry myeloid markers.[15] They are inherently drug resistant, most significantly to prednisolone and L-asparaginase, but have a greater sensitivity to Ara-C compared with children aged 1.5–10 years.[43] It is frequently recommended that doses of anticancer agents to infants should be reduced and calculated by body weight rather than body surface area ($30\,kg = 1\,m^2$). However, a relationship between these dosing principles and systemic drug exposure has not generally been supported by clinical pharmacokinetic studies. The infant leukaemias require intensive ALL-like treatment protocols with inclusion of high-dose Ara-C. It is doubtful whether SCT improves the clinical outcome, at least for the 11q23 aberrant leukaemias.[15] Overall, the prognosis of 11q23 aberrant patients is poor with a cure rate less than 30 per cent (Fig. 12.6), and the outcome is even worse in those aged <6 months. Nearly all relapses occur within 2 years of diagnosis, and the chance of cure once the disease has recurred is poor.

Mature B-cell ALL

This subset, which includes 2 per cent of children with ALL, is characterized by a male predominance (3:1), a median age of 10 years, a median WBC that is similar to that in non-B ALL (although WBC $> 100 \times 10^9$/liter is rare), frequent renal involvement, only moderate hepatosplenomegaly, a normal haemoglobin, and FAB L3 morphology in a less hyperplastic bone marrow compared with what is usually encountered with B-cell precursor ALL. In the vast majority, *c-myc* on chromosome 8 is fused with antigen receptor regulatory sequences either on chromosome 14 in 80 per cent of cases [t(8;14)(q24;q32.3)] or, more rarely, on chromosomes 2 or 22 which leads to a deregulated increased cell proliferation. Previously, mature B-cell ALL (as well as disseminated and/or bulky mature B-cell non-Hodgkin lymphoma) had a very poor outcome, but these patients now have a cure rate of at least 80 per cent with 5–6 months of intensive block therapy that frequently includes HD-MTX, cytarabine, cyclophosphamide, epipodophyllotoxins, glucocorticosteroids, vincristine, and i.t. triple chemotherapy (see Chapter 14). The chance of cure is substantially lower for patients with CNS involvement at diagnosis than for those without this feature. Nearly all relapses occur within the first year of diagnosis, and the outcome after relapse is dismal.

T-lineage ALL

Cases of T-lineage leukaemia differ from B-cell precursor ALL by a higher WBC at diagnosis (median 70.0×10^9 versus 8.0×10^9/liter), predominately male sex (2.4:1), a mediastinal mass (62.1 versus 1.1 per cent), and CNS leukaemia at diagnosis (8 versus 2 per cent). Although the overall risk of relapse for these patients is significantly higher than that of B-precursor ALL, especially during the first 2 years of diagnosis, the impact of WBC at diagnosis on the cure rate is less pronounced than for B-cell precursor ALL (Fig. 12.3). The worse overall outcome primarily reflects the higher frequency of the risk factors discussed earlier. Thus, if adjustment is made for these and intensive therapy for T-lineage leukaemia is applied, the cure rates are very similar to those of B-cell precursor ALL (Fig. 12.3). Compared with B-lineage cell ALL, T-cell disease seems to have a poorer sensitivity to many anticancer drugs and have less propensity for the formation of MTX polyglutamates. HD-MTX $5-8\,g/m^2/24\,h$ to overcome this feature and prolonged use of L-asparaginase seem to improve the outcome of these patients.

Late effects

Even when cure has been obtained, many patients need medical attention for late effects imposed by the leukaemia or its treatment. Those that affect the CNS after CNS irradiation are among the most troublesome and include endocrine disturbances, neuropsychologic deficits (seemingly most prominent in girls), and obesity. Growth hormone replacement may be indicated because of the risk of short stature, and there is no convincing evidence that this treatment increases the risk of relapse. In addition, patients cured of ALL may be at risk of reduced fertility (mostly because of alkylating agents or SCT with TBI), cardiomyopathy (due to high doses of anthracyclines, especially in girls), reduced lung function, osteoporosis, and second cancer. The last of these affects 2–3 per cent of all patients. The most common second cancers are brain tumours, generally related to previous CNS irradiation, especially at a young age, myelodysplastic syndrome, or overt myeloid leukaemia. The risk of second cancers is increased manyfold in children who have undergone SCT with TBI and high doses of alkylating agents. The risks of myelodysplastic syndrome or AML have also been related to intensive exposure to epipodophyllotoxins (the second cancers commonly harbouring 11q23 aberrations) or thiopurine metabolites in patients with TPMT heterozygocity (with a high frequency of monosomy 7 myelodysplastic syndrome or AML).[36] The risk of brain tumours has also been related to a combination of TPMT heterozygocity and CNS irradiation.[35] So far there are no indications of an increased risk of cancers among children of patients cured of childhood ALL.

Palliative chemotherapy

Despite intensive first- and second-line therapy, including allogenic SCT, at least 15 per cent of the patients will eventually die of their disease.[1] These will include patients with B-lineage leukaemia with recurrent late relapses, for whom the disease continues to have some chemosensitivity but still fails to be eradicated. There is no standard approach for these patients, many of whom will have received SCT, and for each case the decision to treat or not to treat demands detailed knowledge of the disease, the previous treatment, the patient, and the family as a whole. For some, a second allogenic SCT with the goal of cure may be a relevant consideration. For others, only palliative care seems reasonable. In the latter case, palliative chemotherapy should not steal the time that is left; in other words, the short survival time gained by intensive treatment should not equal the time spent in hospital. If chemotherapy is chosen, regimens of low toxicity that are applicable on an outpatient basis should be the choice. This may include oral MTX and 6MP/6TG. In selected cases this can be supplemented with vincristine–prednisolone re-inductions, PEG-asparaginase for non-allergic patients, oral cyclophosphamide, and/or even HD-MTX. Some patients with CNS disease may benefit from palliative intrathecal chemotherapy. When to stop all chemotherapy, and even blood transfusions, can only be decided on an individual basis. Both patients and their families will always need other medical and psychosocial support to be able to stay at home, where most parents and patients will choose that the child should die.

Future considerations

In developed countries the cure rate for some subsets of childhood ALL exceeds 90 per cent. Thus it is likely that future therapy programmes will include a reduction of the treatment intensity for patients with favourable cytogenetic aberrations (e.g. high-hyperdiploid ALL), high *in vitro* drug sensitivity, favourable drug metabolism profiles, and/or a low level of residual leukaemia within the first months of therapy.[9–11,21,22,26,30,31] Clinical studies in the 1960s and 1970s showed that a certain proportion of patients can be cured with treatment of very low toxicity (vincristine, steroids, asparaginase, and antimetabolites), and the aforementioned characteristics of good-risk patients indicate that many of these can be identified at diagnosis or during the first months of therapy. In contrast, some patients with adverse cytogenetic findings, high *in vitro* or *in vivo* drug resistance, or who relapse during therapy have such a disappointing prognosis that novel approaches are warranted using new drugs, immune therapy, new SCT procedures, and molecular therapy targeted towards tumour suppressor genes or chimeric proteins generated by chromosomal translocations. To explore the toxicity and efficacy of such approaches extensive multicenter collaboration is warranted, such as that established by the US Children's Oncology Group and the European Consortium for the Cure of Childhood Acute Lymphoblastic Leukaemia.

In addition, there is a global need for the development of easily applied tools for risk group assignment and inexpensive effective chemotherapy that could increase the cure rate of the 80 per cent of children with ALL who live in countries with limited resources.

The attempts to unravel the aetiology and pathogenesis, most notably those headed by Mel Greaves, have yielded promising results in recent years.[6] Ongoing large-scale studies of the frequency of leukaemia-related cytogenetic aberrations among healthy newborns, and the correlation of these results with certain characteristics of their mothers and their *in utero* exposures, as well as epidemiologic studies of factors that influence the disappearance or control of such preleukaemic cells during the first years of life, may within the next 10 years suggest measures by which the occurrence of the most common forms of childhood ALL may be prevented or detected at an early and more easily treated stage.

References

1. **Gustafsson G, Schmiegelow K, Forestier E, et al.** (2000). Improving outcome through two decades in childhood ALL in the Nordic countries: the impact of high-dose methotrexate in the reduction of CNS irradiation. Nordic Society of Pediatric Haematology and Oncology (NOPHO). *Leukemia* 14, 2267–75.
2. **Rubnitz JE, Pui CH** (2003). Recent advances in the treatment and understanding of childhood acute lymphoblastic leukaemia. *Cancer Treat Rev* 29, 31–44.
3. **Gadner H, Haas OA, Masera G, Pui CH, Schrappe M** (2003). 'Ponte di Legno' Working Group - 1. Report on the Fifth International Childhood Acute Lymphoblastic Leukemia Workshop, Vienna, Austria, 29 April–1 May 2002. *Leukemia* 17, 798–803.
4. **Hjalgrim LL, Rostgaard K, Schmiegelow K, et al.** (2003). Age-and sex-specific incidence of childhood leukaemia in the Nordic countries. *J Natl Cancer Inst* 95, 1539–44.
5. **Winther JF, Sankila R, Boice JD, et al.** (2001) Cancer in siblings of children with cancer in the Nordic countries: a population-based cohort study. *Lancet* 358, 711–17.
6. **Greaves M** (2002). Childhood leukaemia. *BMJ* 324, 283–87.
7. **Hjalgrim LL, Madsen HO, Melbye M, et al.** (2002). Presence of clone-specific markers at birth in children with acute lymphoblastic leukaemia. *Br J Cancer* 87, 994–99.
8. **Schmiegelow K, Garred P, Lausen B, Andreassen B, Petersen BL, Madsen HO** (2002). Increased frequency of mannose-binding lectin insufficiency among children with acute lymphoblastic leukemia. *Blood* 100, 3757–60.
9. **Mori H, Colman SM, Xiao Z, et al.** (2002). Chromosome translocations and covert leukemic clones are generated during normal fetal development. *Proc Natl Acad Sci USA* 99, 8242–47.
10. **Szczepanski T, van der Velden VHJ, van Dongen JJM** (2003). Classification systems for acute and chronic leukemias. *Best Pract Res Clin Haematol* 16, 561–82.
11. **Coustan-Smith E, Sancho J, Hancock ML, et al.** (2000). Clinical importance of minimal residual disease in childhood acute lymphoblastic leukemia. *Blood* 96, 2691–96.
12. **Forestier E, Johansson B, Gustafsson G, et al.** (2000). Prognostic impact of karyotypic findings in childhood acute lymphoblastic leukaemia: a Nordic series comparing two treatment periods. For the

Nordic Society of Paediatric Haematology and Oncology (NOPHO) Leukaemia Cytogenetic Study Group. *Br J Haematol* 110, 147–53.

13. **Kristensen TD, Wesenberg F, Jonsson OG, et al.** (2003). High-resolution comparative genomic hybridisation yields a high detection rate of chromosomal aberrations in childhood acute lymphoblastic leukaemia. *Eur J Haematol* 70, 363–72.

14. **Kaspers GJ, Smets LA, Pieters R, Van Zantwijk CH, van Wering ER, Veerman AJ** (1995). Favorable prognosis of hyperdiploid common acute lymphoblastic leukemia may be explained by sensitivity to antimetabolites and other drugs: results of an *in vitro* study. *Blood* 85, 751–56.

15. **Pui CH, Gaynon PS, Boyett JM, et al.** (2002). Outcome of treatment in childhood acute lymphoblastic leukaemia with rearrangements of the 11q23 chromosomal region. *Lancet* 359, 1909–15.

16. **Arico M, Valsecchi MG, Camitta B, et al.** (2000). Outcome of treatment in children with Philadelphia chromosome-positive acute lymphoblastic leukemia. *N Engl J Med* 342, 998–1006.

17. **Rubnitz JE, Downing JR, Pui CH, et al.** (1997). TEL gene rearrangement in acute lymphoblastic leukemia: a new genetic marker with prognostic significance. *J Clin Oncol* 15, 1150–57.

18. **Ramakers-van Woerden NL., Pieters R, Loonen AH, et al.** (2000). TEL/AML1 gene fusion is related to *in vitro* drug sensitivity for L-asparaginase in childhood acute lymphoblastic leukemia. *Blood* 96, 1094–99.

19. **Silverman LB, Gelber RD, Dalton VK, et al.** (2001). Improved outcome for children with acute lymphoblastic leukemia: results of Dana–Farber Consortium Protocol 91-01. *Blood* 97, 1211–18.

20. **Yeoh EJ, Ross ME, Shurtleff SA, et al.** (2002). Classification, subtype discovery, and prediction of outcome in pediatric acute lymphoblastic leukemia by gene expression profiling. *Cancer Cell* 1, 133–43.

21. **Szczepanski T, Orfao A., van der Velden V, San Miguel JF, van Dongen JJ** (2001). Minimal residual disease in leukaemia patients. *Lancet Oncol* 2, 409–17.

22. **Nyvold C, Madsen HO, Ryder LP, et al.** (2002). Precise quantification of minimal residual disease at day 29 allows identification of children with acute lymphoblastic leukaemia and an excellent outcome. *Blood* 99, 1253–58.

23. **Schrappe M, Camitta B, Pui CH, et al.** (2000). Long-term results of large prospective trials in childhood acute lymphoblastic leukaemia. *Leukemia* 14, 2193–94.

24. **Saarinen UM, Mellander L, Nysom K, et al.** (1996). Allogeneic bone marrow transplantation in first remission for children with very high-risk acute lymphoblastic leukaemia: a retrospective case–control study in the Nordic countries. Nordic Society for Pediatric Hematology and Oncology (NOPHO). *Bone Marrow Transplant* 17, 357–63.

25. **Saarinen-Pihkala UM, Gustafsson G, Ringden O, et al** (2001). No disadvantage in outcome of using matched unrelated donors as compared with matched sibling donors for bone marrow transplantation in children with acute lymphoblastic leukaemia in second remission. *J Clin Oncol* 19, 3406–14.

26. **Kaspers GJ, Pieters R, Van Zantwijk CH, van Wering ER, van der Does-van den Berg A, Veerman AJ.** (1998). Prednisolone resistance in childhood acute lymphoblastic leukaemia: *vitro–vivo* correlations and cross-resistance to other drugs. *Blood* 92, 259–66.

27. **Duval M, Suciu S, Ferster A, et al.** (2002). Comparison of *Escherichia coli*-asparaginase with *Erwinia*-asparaginase in the treatment of childhood lymphoid malignancies: results of a randomized European Organisation for Research and Treatment of Cancer-Children's Leukemia Group phase 3 trial. *Blood* 99, 2734–39.

28. **Nygaard U, Schmiegelow K** (2003). Dose reduction of coadministered 6-mercaptopurine decreases myelotoxicity following high-dose methotrexate in childhood leukemia. *Leukemia* 17, 1344–48.

29. **Clarke M, Gaynon P, Hann I, et al.** (2003). CNS-directed therapy for childhood acute lymphoblastic leukemia: Childhood ALL Collaborative Group overview of 43 randomized trials. *J Clin Oncol* 21, 1798–1809.

30. **Evans WE, Relling MV, Rodman JH, Crom WR, Boyett JM, Pui CH** (1998). Conventional compared with individualized chemotherapy for childhood acute lymphoblastic leukemia. *N Engl J Med* 338, 499–505.

31. **Schmiegelow K, Bjork O, Glomstein A, et al.** (2003). Intensification of mercaptopurine/methotrexate maintenance chemotherapy may increase the risk of relapse for some children with acute lymphoblastic leukemia. *J Clin Oncol* 21, 1332–39.

32. **Nygaard U, Toft N, Schmiegelow K** (2004). Methylated metabolites of 6-mercaptopurine are associated with hepatotoxicity in childhood leukaemia. *Clin Pharmacol Ther* 75, 274–81.

33. **Schmiegelow K, Pulczynska M** (1990). Prognostic significance of hepatotoxicity during maintenance chemotherapy for childhood acute lymphoblastic leukaemia. *Br J Cancer* 61, 767–72.

34. **Schmiegelow K, Glomstein A, Kristinsson J, Salmi T, Schroder H, Bjork O** (1997). Impact of morning versus evening schedule for oral methotrexate and 6-mercaptopurine on relapse risk for children with acute lymphoblastic leukemia. Nordic Society for Pediatric Hematology and Oncology (NOPHO). *J Pediatr Hematol Oncol* 19, 102–09.

35. **Relling MV, Rubnitz JE, Rivera GK, et al.** (1999). High incidence of secondary brain tumours after radiotherapy and antimetabolites. *Lancet* 354, 34–39.

36. **Thomsen J, Schroder H, Kristinsson J, et al.** (1999). Possible carcinogenic effect of 6-mercaptopurine on bone marrow stem cells: relation to thiopurine metabolism. *Cancer* 86, 1080–86.

37. **Schmiegelow K, Nyvold C, Seyfarth J, et al.** (2001). Post-induction residual leukemia in childhood acute lymphoblastic leukemia quantified by PCR correlates with *in vitro* prednisolone resistance. *Leukemia* 15, 1066–71.

38. **Wheeler K, Chessells JM, Bailey CC, Richards SM** (1996). Treatment related deaths during induction and in first remission in acute lymphoblastic leukaemia: MRC UKALL X. *Arch Dis Child* 74, 101–07.

39. **Jahnukainen K, Salmi TT, Kristinsson J, Muller J, Madsen B, Gustafsson G** (1998). The clinical indications for identical pathogenesis of isolated and non-isolated testicular relapses in acute lymphoblastic leukaemia. *Acta Paediatr* 87, 638–43.

40. **Hasle H** (2001). Pattern of malignant disorders in individuals with Down's syndrome. *Lancet Oncol* 2, 429–36.

41. **Bassal M, La MK, Whitlock JA, et al.** (2005). Lymphoblast biology and outcome among children with Down syndrome and ALL treated on CCG-1952. *Pediatr Blood Cancer* 44, 21–28.

42. **Alexander FE, Patheal SL, Biondi A, et al.** (2001) Transplacental chemical exposure and risk of infant leukemia with MLL gene fusion. *Cancer Res* 61, 2542–46.

43. **Pieters R, Den Boer ML, Durian M, et al.** (1998) Relation between age, immunophenotype and *in vitro* drug resistance in 395 children with acute lymphoblastic leukemia—implications for treatment of infants. *Leukemia* 12, 1344–48.

Chapter 13

Acute myeloid leukaemia

Brenda Gibson and Geoff Shenton

Introduction

Leukaemia is the most common malignancy in childhood, accounting for 30 per cent of cancer registration in children under the age of 15 years in the USA and Europe. While cancer is the most common cause of death (after accidents) in children, leukaemia, despite its high cure rates, remains the most common cause of cancer-related mortality.

Epidemiology

Acute myeloid leukaemia (AML) accounts for ~20 per cent of leukaemias in childhood and is the seventh most common childhood malignancy. There are ~70 new cases of AML per year in the UK. Data from the National Cancer Institute reported an overall incidence of AML in children of 7.6 per million for the period 1975–1995, with considerable age-related variation. The incidence of AML was found to be highest during the first 2 years of life (12 per million), decreasing to less than 4 per million at around 9 years of age, before increasing again throughout the teenage years to reach an incidence of approximately 8 per million by early adult life. There was no reported significant difference in the sex-adjusted incidence and, unlike acute lymphoblastic leukaemia (ALL), no difference between Black and White ethnic groups, although the incidence was higher in American Hispanic children. Data from the International Association of Cancer Registries reported a marked ethnic variation with the highest rates (14.4 per million) in the Maori population of New Zealand and one of the lowest incidences in the South American countries of Brazil (3.5 per million) and Colombia (1.6/ million). There was also marked geographical variation in subtype, with acute promyelocytic leukaemia being three times more common in Latin than non-Latin countries.

Risk factors for AML

A number of risk factors for the development of AML have been identified. The association is well established for some, such as previous exposure to chemotherapeutic agents, ionizing radiation, and congenital syndromes, but is less so for others.

Down syndrome (trisomy 21) carries a >10-fold increased risk of AML. Neonates with Down syndrome frequently develop a transient clonal megakaryoblastic myeloproliferative disorder that resembles AML and is termed transient abnormal myelopoiesis (TAM). This usually resolves within the first 3 months of life. However, 30 per cent of those affected will go on to develop AML by the age of 3 years. The median age at presentation for AML in Down syndrome is 23 months. Compared with non-Down-syndrome children with AML, Down syndrome patients tend to have lower leucocyte counts, preceding myelodysplasia, megakaryoblastic or undifferentiated AML, and a more favourable outcome. Approximately 10 per cent of all paediatric AML cases occur in children with Down syndrome, and patients with mosaicism are at risk of leukaemia in the affected bone marrow cells. The mechanism of this increased risk has yet to be elucidated, although *GATA1*, a gene involved in regulating survival and maturation of erythroid and megakaryocytic progenitor cells, has been implicated. There is an association with mutations in the *GATA1* gene and megakaryoblastic leukaemia in Down syndrome patients, although the mechanism by which trisomy 21 provides a genetic or molecular environment that promotes leukaemia is unclear.

Fanconi's anaemia and Bloom's syndrome are characterized by increased chromosomal fragility and as a consequence of this are associated with an increased risk of AML. In children with severe congenital neutropenia (Kostman's syndrome), the infection-related mortality has been reduced with the prophylactic use of recombinant granulocyte colony-stimulating factor (rGCSF), whilst an increase in the incidence of AML has been noted in the children who have survived. Patients are reported with mutations in the GCSF receptor, leading to a truncated protein with defective internalization and sustained activation on stimulation with GCSF. This results in an abnormally high proliferative rate in myeloid precursors and a terminal differentiation block.

Neurofibromatosis type I is an autosomal dominant disorder with mutations of the *NF1* gene on chromosome 17. The product of this gene plays a key role in the Ras signalling pathway. Mutations of *NF1* lead to increased levels of activated Ras. Patients have a 20-fold increased risk of developing AML due to mutation of the remaining *NF1* locus.

Other factors, such as maternal alcohol consumption during pregnancy and parental exposure to pesticides and benzene, have been implicated in leukaemogenesis. Further epidemiologic studies should better clarify the contribution of these risk factors to the development of AML.

Presenting features

Children with AML present with signs and symptoms of both failure of normal haematopoiesis and infiltration of extramedullary sites due to expansion of the leukaemic clone. These include pallor, fever, bone pain, anorexia, fatigue, mucosal bleeding, and bruising. Patients are commonly neutropenic at presentation and at increased risk of bacterial infection. Prodromal symptoms may be present from days to weeks before presentation.

Extramedullary infiltration with hepatosplenomegaly and lymphadenopathy is common. Chloromas, collections of leukaemic cells so called because of their greenish appearance, may occur in the skin (leukaemia cutis), soft tissues, gingivae, orbit, or at other sites. Organ infiltration is most common in monocytic/monoblastic leukaemias (FAB type M4 and M5). Chest radiographs may show abnormalities due to leukaemic infiltrates or infection. Central nervous system (CNS) involvement at presentation has been reported in 5–25 per cent of cases. Infants and older children with M4/M5 leukaemia are at particular risk. Chloromas of the nervous system may present as headaches, focal neurologic deficits, cranial nerve palsies, and seizures. The risk of leucostasis involving the lung or brain is greatest when the peripheral blast count is very high ($> 200 \times 10^9$/liter). DIC or hyperfibrinolysis with haemorrhagic complications may be seen in all subtypes of AML, but most commonly in acute promyelocytic leukaemia (FAB type M3) and the M4/M5 subtypes.

Laboratory features

Blood film and blood count

Children commonly present with pancytopenia [low haemoglobin (Hb), white cell count (WCC), and platelet count] and blasts (myeloblasts, monoblasts, or megakaryoblasts) on a peripheral smear. There is usually a normochromic normocytic anaemia and thrombocyto-penia, but in a minority the platelet count may be normal or even high. The peripheral blood cells may show dysplastic features and Auer rods may be present in the myeloid blasts. Pancytopenia without circulating immature cells is common.

Bone marrow appearances

The diagnosis of AML is made by examining the bone marrow, and subtype classification is performed by histochemical staining, flow cytometry, and cytogenetics. It can be difficult or impossible to aspirate bone marrow because of fibrosis or a tightly packed marrow. In this situation of a 'dry tap', a trephine biopsy is necessary for diagnostic purposes and touch preparations of the biopsy specimen may be helpful.

Morphologic assessment is performed on a Romanowsky stained smear. Myeloblasts are larger than lymphoblasts and have more cytoplasm (which often contains a variable number of primary granules). The nucleus may have a number of distinct nucleoli. Auer rods (coales-cences of primary granules) are pathognomic of malignant myeloid blasts (Fig. 13.1). Eryth-roblasts may show grossly abnormal morphology with multinucleate forms, nuclear fragments, and megaloblastic change. Megakaryoblasts are highly polymorphic, ranging from small round cells resembling lymphoblasts to larger more undifferentiated cells which may have cytoplasmic budding.

Cytochemistry

Cytochemical staining provides information on lineage involvement and maturation, and complements the information obtained from the Romanowsky stain and immunophenotyping.

Sudan Black and myeloperoxidase

Myeloperoxidase (MPO) stains the enzyme which is found in the peroxisomes of neutrophilic, eosinophilic, and monocytic cells. The Sudan Black stain non-enzymatically identifies the phospholipid in the membranes of primary and secondary granules. The strength of the reaction generally parallels that of MPO. Monoblasts, when positive, tend to show a fine scattered granular pattern whereas myeloblasts have more localized granular positivity. A positive reaction for Sudan Black is defined as >3 per cent staining.

Esterases

The carboxylic esterases identify granulocytic and monocytic lineage. Chloroacetate esterase is specific for granulocytes and mast cells. Reactivity is due to the presence of several different enzymes in the secondary granules. Myeloblasts are generally negative, with positivity appear-ing as the cells become more differentiated. Non-specific esterase (e.g. α-napthyl butyrate esterase) stains monoblasts, monocytes, and megakaryocytes. Both chloroacetate esterase and non-specific esterase staining can be performed on the same slide (combined esterase).

Immunophenotyping

Panels of monoclonal antibodies detect antigenic determinants on normal and leukaemic myeloid cells. The British Committee for Standards in Haematology (BCSH) recommends a standardized panel of monoclonal antibodies. This includes B-lymphoid (CD79a, CD22, CD19, CD10), T-lymphoid (CD3, CD2), myeloid (CD117, anti MPO, CD13), and non-specific (TdT). If the lineage is not clearly established, a second-line panel of CD33, CD41, CD42, CD61, glycophorin A, and CD7 should be used to clarify lineage. Additional useful markers

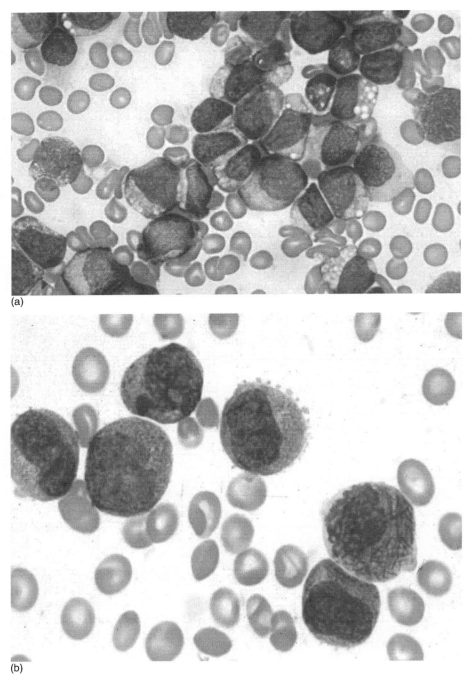

(a)

(b)

Fig. 13.1 (a) Myeloid blasts (FAB type M1); (b) acute promyelocytic leukaemia showing granular blasts and a faggot cell.

Table 13.1. Panel of monoclonal antibodies for the classification of acute leukaemias

Haemopoetic precursors	CD34, HLA-DR, TdT, CD45
Myeloid	CD 13, CD15, CD33, CD117, MPO
Monocytoid	CD11b, CD11c, CD14, CD36, lysozyme
Erythroid	Glycophorin A
Megagakaryoblastic	CD41, CD42, CD61
B-lineage	CD19, CD20, CD22, CD79a
T-lineage	CD2, CD3, CD5, CD7

include HLA-DR and the typically monocytic lineage expressed CD14, CD11, and anti-lysozyme. The BCSH guideline highlights the importance of interpreting the immunophenotype in combination with and not in isolation from the cytochemistry. (Table 13.1).

Immunophenotyping should distinguish between lymphoid and myeloid blast cells in the majority of cases. Difficulty can arise with lymphoblastic leukaemias which express myeloid antigens and with true stem cell leukaemias which show no lineage commitment. Biphenotypic leukaemia can be identified by the coexpression of myeloid and T- or B-lymphoid markers, and diagnosis is dependent on an internationally agreed scoring system.

Classification of AML

For the past 30 years the classification of AML has been based on the French–American–British (FAB) criteria. These attempted to subclassify AML on the basis of the morphologic characteristics and cytochemical staining patterns of bone marrow blast cells. Eight subtypes of AML (M0–M7) are recognized, and the classification has been repeatedly revised to incorporate diagnostic advances, including immunophenotyping and improved cytogenetics. It is now accepted that not only do specific chromosomal rearrangements characterize subtypes, but that it is the genetic change that determines the biology of the leukaemia and the clinical outcome for the patient. In response to these developments the World Health Organization (WHO) has produced a new classification for AML incorporating morphologic, immunophenotypic, genetic, and clinical features. This aims first to define leukaemias that are biologically homogeneous and secondly to be of clinical relevance. AML is classified into four major categories:

♦ AML with recurrent genetic abnormalities
♦ AML with multilineage dysplasia
♦ AML, therapy related
♦ AML, not otherwise categorized.

The WHO classification recognizes factors which are important in predicting the biology of the leukaemic process and, where possible, allocates leukaemias to one of three categories based on specific criteria. Leukaemias which cannot be classified in this manner are grouped together in a fourth category which is based on a modified version of the FAB system (Table 13.2). A number of cytogenetic abnormalities are associated with molecular events which correlate strongly with both response to therapy and outcome, allowing risk stratification of patients with AML. Specific chromosomal abnormalities are associated with a favourable, intermediate, or unfavourable outcome. The translocations inv(16), t(8;21) and t(15;17) are associated with a

Table 13.2. The WHO classification of AML

Acute myeloid leukaemia with recurrent genetic abnormalities
- Acute myeloid leukaemia with t(8;21)(q22;q22); (AML1/ETO)
- Acute myeloid leukaemia with abnormal bone marrow eosinophils, inv(16)(p13q22) or t(16;16)(p13;q22); (CBFβ/MYH11)
- Acute promyelocytic leukaemia with t(15;17)(q22;q12); (PML/RARα) and variants
- Acute myeloid leukaemia with 11q23 (MLL) abnormalities

Acute myeloid leukaemia with multilineage dysplasia
- Following myelodysplastic syndrome or myelodysplastic/myeloproliferative disorder
- Without antecedent myelodysplastic syndrome

Acute myeloid leukaemia and myelodysplastic syndromes, therapy related
- Alkylating agent related
- Topisomerase type II inhibitor related (may include some lymphoid)
- Other types

Acute myeloid leukaemia not otherwise categorized
- Acute myeloid leukaemia minimally differentiated (FAB M0)
- Acute myeloid leukaemia without maturation (FAB M1)
- Acute myeloid leukaemia with maturation (FAB M2)
- Acute myelomonocytic leukaemia (FAB M4)
- Acute monoblastic and monocytic leukaemia (FAB M5)
- Acute erythroid leukaemia (FAB M6)
- Acute megakaryoblastic leukaemia (FAB M7)
- Acute basophilic leukaemia
- Acute panmyelosis with myelofibrosis
- Myeloid sarcoma

Reproduced from R.D. Brunning *et al*. (2001) In E.S. Jaffe *et al*. (eds) *Pathology and Genetics of Tumours of Haemopoetic and Lymphoid Tissues*. *WHO Classification of Tumours*. Lyon: IARC Press.

favourable outcome, whilst -7/del(7q) and -5/del(5q) are seen in AML with myelodysplasia and are associated with an unfavourable outcome. Secondary-therapy-related AML occurring after cytotoxic chemotherapy is recognized as a distinct disease entity.

Prior to the WHO classification the diagnosis of leukaemia required an infiltrate of 30 per cent blasts in the bone marrow, but the revised classification has lowered the requirement to 20 per cent. This followed the recognition that patients with 20–30 per cent blasts in their bone marrow have a similar outcome to those with >30 per cent. Therefore patients with myelo-dysplasia and refractory anaemia with excess blasts in transformation (RAEB-T) are now included within the diagnostic criteria for AML. It must be appreciated that any threshold is arbitrary, and that clinical and other laboratory features must be taken into account when making a diagnosis of AML.

AML with t(8;21)(q22;q22) (*AML1–ETO*)

Occurring in 8–16 per cent of childhood AML, t(8;21) is one of the most common structural abnormalities and is associated with FAB M2 morphology. The blasts are usually large and frequently contain Auer rods. The blasts express myeloid markers (CD13, CD33, MPO) and CD34 is characteristically present. Some patients show weak TdT positivity and coexpression of the lymphoid marker CD19 in a subset of blasts on immunophenotyping.

In t(8;21)(q22;q22), the *AML1* gene (also known as the *RUNX* gene), encoding CBFα, a DNA binding protein, becomes fused with the *ETO* (eight-twenty-one) gene which encodes a zinc-finger transcription factor. The *AML1–ETO* transcript is consistently found in patients with t(8;21), and the disruption of the *AML1* gene is reported to occur within a single intron.

AML with inv(16)(p13q22) or t(16;16)(p13q22); (*CBFβ–MYH11*)

AML with inv(16) occurs in 3–12 per cent of childhood AML. It tends to show monocytic and granulocytic differentiation with an abnormal eosinophil component (M4 with eosinophilia or M4eo). Cases of inv(16)(13q22) have been seen which lack the characteristic eosinophilia. Auer rods may be observed in the myeloblasts and at least 3 per cent show MPO positivity. In addition to myeloid antigens (CD33, CD13, and MPO), the immunophenotype often shows markers of monocytic differentiation (CD14, CD11b, CD11c, CD36, and lysozyme).

The core binding factor β gene is located at 16q22 and encodes half of a heterodimeric transcription factor which is known to bind the enhancers of various leukaemia viruses. The translocation results in the fusion of this gene with the smooth muscle myosin heavy chain (*MYH11*) at 16p13. Occasionally there may be characteristic morphology but without karyotypic evidence of a chromosomal abnormality, and in these cases *CBFβ–MYH11* may be demonstrated by molecular studies.

Acute promyelocytic leukaemia with t(15;17)(q22;q12) (*PML–RARα*) and variants

Acute promyelocytic leukaemia (APL) (FAB subtype M3) is characterized by an arrest of myeloid differentiation at the promyelocyte stage with abnormal proliferation of these cells. It accounts for approximately 4–11 per cent of childhood leukaemias, with significant geographical variations in incidence. There are two subtypes, one characterized by 'typical' hypergranular promyelocytes and the other by 'variant type' hypogranular promyelocytes. The latter subtype is seen in 10–30 per cent of cases of APL.

Patients with APL present with the usual signs and symptoms of pancytopenia. At presentation, APL is more often associated with a severe bleeding diathesis and DIC than other subtypes of AML. This potentially serious complication has been greatly reduced by the use of all-*trans* retinoic acid (ATRA). Correction of the coagulopathy does not completely abrogate the risk of CNS haemorrhage and early death. This complication is more commonly reported in paediatric patients with the M3v subtype. Hypergranular APL usually presents with a lower WCC than other AML subtypes, whilst in variant APL the WCC tends to be very high, with a rapid doubling time.

The diagnosis of APL has traditionally been based on morphology, immunohistochemistry, flow cytometry, and demonstration of the cytogenetic abnormality t(15;17). However, the widespread availability of RT-PCR allows demonstration of the fusion product and rapid confirmation of the diagnosis. Morphologically, classical APL cells are hypergranular promyelocytes containing numerous Auer rods. Characteristic cells containing bundles of Auer rods ('faggot cells') are present in many cases. The cells of APLv have distinct morphology with a paucity or absence of granules and a bi-lobed shape to the nucleus. However, even in APLv a small number of faggot cells or abnormal promyelocyes with clearly visible granules are usually present. By flow cytometry, APL cells are positive for CD33, CD13, and CD9 but negative for HLA-DR, CD34, CD7, CD11b, and CD14. Blasts in APL may also be positive for CD2.

In the majority of cases of APL the t(15;17) can be detected by standard cytogenetics or PCR for the gene transcript. The t(15,17) results in fusion of the retinoic acid receptor α (*RARα*) on 17q12 to the promyelocytic leukaemia (*PML*) gene on 15q22, which is a nuclear regulatory factor. In normal cellular development the *PML*-encoded protein is a component of an intra-nuclear structure which may play a part in mRNA processing. The chimeric *PML–RARα* protein disrupts the formation of this structure, leading to a differentiation block. Treatment with ATRA, a retinoic acid compound, results in selective proteolytic degradation of the *PML–RARα* protein and the promotion of differentiation of APL cells. This leads to differentiation and apoptosis of the malignant cells, and improvement in the associated coagulopathy.

Variant translocations may also be seen in APL and include t(11;17)(q23;q21) in which *RARα* on chromosome 17 fuses with the promyelocytic leukaemia zinc-finger gene (*PLZF*) on chromosome 11, t(5;17)(q23q12) in which the nucleophosmin (*NPM*) gene on chromosome 5 fuses with *RARα*, and t(11;17)(q13;q21) in which the nuclear matrix associated (*NuMA*) gene fuses with *RARα*. The *PLZF–RARα* fusion is particularly important because patients with this translocation are resistant to ATRA.

AML with 11q23 (*MLL*) abnormalities

AML with 11q23 abnormalities is found in 6–11 per cent of childhood leukaemias. The incidence is higher in infants and in secondary-therapy-related AML which has developed after treatment with topoisomerase II inhibitors. Patients may present with DIC and tissue infiltration, the latter especially of skin or gingiva. Morphologically there is a strong association with monocytic and myelomonocytic leukaemias, particularly monoblastic leukaemia.

Molecular studies have shown that the *MLL* gene is a human homologue of the *Drosophila trithorax* gene, a developmental regulator, which is structurally altered in leukaemia-associated translocations. Although the *MLL* gene at 11q23 is involved in a number of translocations with at least 20 different partner chromosomes, the most common in childhood AML are t(9;11) (p21q23) and t(11;19)(q23p13.1)/t(11;19)(q23;13.3). Interestingly t(4,11) is not seen in infants with AML but is common in infant ALL. Molecular techniques have also shown that 11q23 rearrangements may be found more frequently than is seen by conventional cytogenetics alone.

AML with multilineage dysplasia

AML with multilineage dysplasia is an acute leukaemia with >20 per cent blasts in the blood or bone marrow and dysplasia in ≥50 per cent of the cells of at least two or more myeloid cell lines. It may occur *de novo* or following a myelodysplastic disorder. Patients often present with severe pancytopenia. The bone marrow is usually hypercellular with dysgranulopoiesis (hypo-granular and/or abnormally segmented forms), dyserythropoiesis (abnormal nuclear outlines, multinucleate forms, and abnormal haemoglobinization) and dysmegakaryopoiesis (micro-megakaryocytes, monolobular or disparate nuclei). Cytogenetic abnormalities, especially monosomy 7, are seen relatively frequently.

Therapy-related AMLs and myelodysplastic syndromes

AML and myelodysplasia can follow treatment with cytotoxic chemotherapy and/or radiation therapy and are categorized into two main types based on the implicated causative agent. If appropriate, they may be further classified by morphology or cytogenetics with the qualifying term 'therapy related'.

Alkylating agent related AML

This form of treatment-related AML, which usually occurs 5–6 years after exposure to alkylating agents or radiotherapy, arises as a direct result of the mutagenic effect of these agents. Often presenting initially as a myelodysplastic disorder with evidence of isolated or pancytopenias, the disorder progresses through a dysplastic phase with multilineage dysplasia to frank leukaemia. Initially the percentage of marrow blasts may be low (<5 per cent), although a minority of patients present with frank AML.

The marrow morphology reflects the underlying dysplasia with hypolobulated and hypogranular neutrophils and dysplastic erythroid cells. In a minority of cases Auer rods are present. The marrow is usually hypercellular, but hypocellularity and marked marrow fibrosis may be present. Immunophenotyping reflects the heterogeneity of the underlying morphology with blasts constituting only a subpopulation of marrow cells. The blasts are generally CD34 positive and express myeloid markers (CD13, CD33). Aberrant expression of CD56 and/or CD7 may be seen.

There is a high incidence of clonal cytogenetic abnormalities which are similar to those seen in MDS and AML with multilineage dysplasia. These are primarily unbalanced translocations involving chromosomes 5 or 7 and involve the loss of all or part of the long arm of the chromosome. Other chromosomes frequently involved include 1, 4, 12, 14, and 18. Complex chromosomal abnormalities are a common finding.

Topoisomerase II inhibitor related AML

Topoisomerase II induced AML tends to have a shorter latent period than alkylating agent induced AML, with the median presentation ~3 years after exposure. Although the main causative agents are the epipodophyllotoxins etoposide and teniposide, anthracyclines such as doxorubicin and 4-epi-doxorubicin have been implicated. The presentation tends to be with frank AML, although a preceding myelodysplastic phase is sometimes seen.

Morphologically there is usually a significant monocytic component with morphology characteristic of FAB M4 or M5 types, although other FAB types have been reported. The predominant cytogenetic finding is a balanced translocation involving the *MLL* gene (11q23) and this is commonly t(9;11), t(11;19), or t(6;11). Acute lymphoblastic leukaemias have been reported following topisomerase II inhibitors and are usually associated with t(4;11)(q21q23).

Therapy in AML

The survival of children with AML has improved dramatically over the past 30 years and continues to do so (Fig. 13.2).This is in part due to the delivery of increasingly intensive chemotherapy, but equally to improvements in supportive care, including antibacterials, antifungals, growth factors, anti-emetics, and blood product support, which have allowed intensive chemotherapy to be given with less morbidity. Since the introduction of daunorubicin and cytosine arabinoside (Ara-C) in the mid 1970s, treatment has become increasingly intensive and evolved through clinical trials. This has included myeloablative therapy with bone marrow transplantation, and more recently the introduction of newer agents which target leukaemia cells semiselectively. The increase in our understanding of the intracellular pathways in both normal and leukaemic cells has led to the development of agents which can target specific enzymes involved in leukaemogenesis and cell proliferation. The role of immunotherapy is becoming more clearly understood. Advances in therapy have been mirrored by technologic improvements which allow risk stratification and the detection of minimal residual disease. Each new technology and treatment has to be evaluated by clinical trials before its benefit can be accepted.

The aim of treatment of AML is eradication of the malignant clone and restoration of normal haematopoiesis. Paediatric AML is a rare disease, and most children in the developed world are

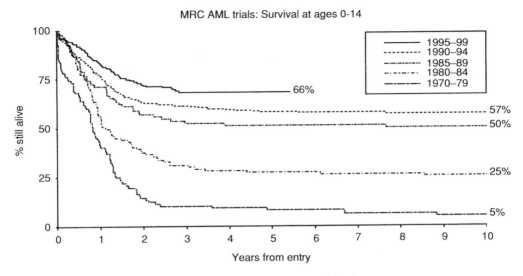

Fig. 13.2 Improvement in AML survival (Medical Research Council data).

treated within clinical trials organized by their national group. National cooperative protocols differ in the choice of drugs, dosages, and scheduling, but generally share the same overall treatment strategy of remission induction and consolidation. The approach to CNS prophylaxis varies between cooperative groups, as does the use of maintenance therapy.

Induction therapy

The aim of induction therapy is to induce a morphologic remission (<5 per cent blasts in bone marrow). However, it is acknowledged that induction treatment influences not only the remission rate but also the disease-free survival (DFS). Induction regimens vary but generally include an anthracycline and Ara-C. This combination chemotherapy is highly myelosuppressive and results in a prolonged period of pancytopenia. Complete remission (CR) rates of 80–90 per cent are now achievable for children with AML; 4–5 per cent of children have resistant disease and a similar number die from infection or haemorrhage before achieving remission.

The UK Medical Research Council (MRC) trials have serially tested the benefit of intensifying chemotherapy by increasing both the number of blocks of treatment and their intensity. Early trials identified DAT 3+10 (daunorubicin, Ara-C, and thioguanine) as superior to previous regimens for remission rates, time to achieve remission, and DFS. MRC AML 10 compared DAT with ADE (Ara-C, daunorubicin, and etoposide) and found no significant difference in the remission rate or DFS (CR rate 89 per cent versus 93 per cent, $P = 0.3$). Therefore the use of etoposide conferred no benefit in monoblastic leukaemia, although benefit had previously been reported. In its subsequent trials, MRC AML 12 and MRC AML 15, the MRC adopted ADE as the standard treatment for children against which other regimens should be tested. It is unlikely that any one regimen of this intensity will prove superior to another, but it is important that trials continue.

The Children's Cancer Group (CCG) in the USA tested the benefit of increasing the intensity of drug scheduling in induction chemotherapy and compared different modalities of post-induction treatment for outcome. The CCG-2891 (1989–1995) trial compared 'standard-timing' induction with a more intensive approach in a randomized manner. Patients in both arms of the study received the standard five-drug regimen DCTER (dexamethasone, Ara-C, 6-thioguanine, etoposide, and daunorubicin). Patients in the intensive arm received a second cycle of therapy after a 6-day rest interval regardless of bone marrow response. Patients randomized to standard timing received a second cycle of treatment depending on their bone marrow findings on day 14 and either preceded immediately to a second cycle or waited for count recovery. There was a significant improvement in outcome for those patients who received intensive-timing induction therapy, regardless of the post-remission therapy they received.

AML BFM-93 compared two different anthracyclines, daunorubicin and idarubicin, in induction. Patients who received idarubicin had significantly better blast cell clearance in the bone marrow on day 15 (17 per cent with >5 per cent blasts versus 31 per cent, $P = 0.01$), but this did not translate into an improved 5-year event-free survival (EFS) or DFS.

The evidence from these and other clinical trials clearly demonstrates the benefit of intensive induction chemotherapy. This has been achieved by choice of drugs, dosage, and scheduling. Induction chemotherapy influences not only the remission rate but also the relapse rate and the DFS. The use of increasingly intensive induction regimens carries the risk of increased treatment-related mortality which must be carefully monitored.

Consolidation therapy

Long-term remission can only be achieved with intensive consolidation chemotherapy. The optimal consolidation therapy is unknown. The benefit of regimens which employ high-dose Ara-C is agreed, but the role of allogeneic and autologous bone marrow transplant (BMT) remains controversial.

Patients entered into the MRC AML-10 trial (1988–1995) received four courses of very intensive chemotherapy. Children with a histocompatible sibling donor were eligible for an allogeneic BMT and those without were randomized to receive a fifth course of high-dose therapy with autologous bone marrow rescue or to stop treatment. Following such intensive chemotherapy, neither matched allografts nor auto-BMT improved overall survival, although both types of transplant were associated with a reduced relapse risk. The benefit from the reduced relapse rate was negated by a higher procedure-related mortality after allogeneic BMT and a better survival from relapse for previously non-autografted patients.

Analysis of data from this trial enabled three prognostic groups to be identified (good, standard, and poor) based on cytogenetics and response to the first block of treatment. Poor-risk patients (20 per cent) were those with >15 per cent blasts in the bone marrow performed after course 1 or adverse cytogenetic abnormalities [−5, −7, del(5q), abn(3q), complex karyotypes]; good risk patients (28 per cent) were those with favourable cytogenetics [t(8,21),t(15,17),inv 16] irrespective of their marrow status after course 1, and all others were standard-risk patients. Five-year overall survival was 82 per cent, 60 per cent, and 22 per cent in the good-, standard-, and poor-risk groups, respectively. Because of these findings, allogeneic BMT was restricted to standard- and poor-risk patients in the subsequent MRC AML 12 trial. ABMT was replaced by an extra block of chemotherapy because of its treatment-related mortality and lack of overall survival benefit.

In the CCG-2891 study, following induction therapy, patients with a matched family donor (MFD) were allocated to allogeneic BMT. All other patients were randomized between autologous bone marrow transplantation or non-marrow ablative chemotherapy which included high-dose Ara-C. There was no significant difference in overall survival between those patients who received chemotherapy or an autologous bone marrow transplant (48 per cent versus 53 per cent, $P = 0.31$). Allogeneic MFD transplant was associated with an improved overall and DFS at 8 years (60 per cent and 55 per cent p 0.02) despite the increase in therapy related mortality, and this was largely due to a reduction in the relapse rate.

In BFM-93 the BFM group investigated the benefit of increasing intensity of consolidation therapy by adding an additional course of high-dose Ara-C with mitozantrone (HAM) for their high-risk patients. The addition of HAM in the high-risk group significantly improved the EFS (51 per cent versus 41 per cent, $P = 0.01$).

The optimal consolidation therapy for children in first CR of AML remains controversial. CCG, BFM, and MRC have shown no benefit for ABMT when compared with intensive chemotherapy. Results for allogeneic BMT in the first CR vary with CCG reporting benefit, and MRC and BFM reporting no benefit. This is in part due to the excellent results achieved with chemotherapy alone, and the benefit for allogeneic BMT maybe less apparent in studies which use very intensive chemotherapy. Whilst allogeneic BMT may reduce the risk of relapse, the results with chemotherapy alone are very encouraging and benefit has to be balanced against transplant-related mortality and long-term sequelae. In current MRC trials allogeneic BMT in the first CR is restricted to patients with unfavourable cytogenetics or a slow and suboptimal response to chemotherapy.

The optimal consolidation chemotherapy is unknown. MRC AML 12 showed no benefit for a fifth block of chemotherapy after four intensive courses, suggesting that there is a ceiling for benefit from chemotherapy.

CNS therapy

Intrathecal chemotherapy with cytosine $\pm$ methotrexate and hydrocortisone has been shown to be effective in preventing CNS relapse for patients with no CNS disease at presentation who are treated on protocols which include high-dose Ara-C. The CCG, Pediatric Oncology Group (POG), and MRC trials which did not include cranial irradiation report very low isolated and combined CNS relapse rates. The BFM group report benefit from CNS irradiation due to a reduction in bone marrow relapse risk. Cranial irradiation, with its associated neurotoxicity, is only justified for patients with CNS disease at presentation.

The role of maintenance therapy in AML

Several studies have investigated whether there is benefit for maintenance therapy in AML. The MRC and CCG-213 studies found no benefit for post-remission maintenance therapy. The LAME 89/91 study failed to show a significant difference in 5-year DFS between those who did and did not receive maintenance treatment, whilst the overall survival was better in the non-maintenance group. This was because of a higher salvage rate following relapse, believed to be due to drug resistance and subsequent treatment failure in those exposed to maintenance therapy. However, the BFM group continue to use maintenance therapy although duration has been reduced from 2 to 1.5 years.

Acute promyelocytic leukaemia

A priority in the treatment of APL is the management of the associated coagulopathy, which can cause significant haemorrhagic problems. It is important to be aware of the potential risk of haemorrhage associated with procedures such as insertion of a Hickman line. Support with platelets, fresh frozen plasma, and cryoprecipitate is commonly required. Various approaches have been employed including maintaining the platelet count $> 50 \times 10^9$/liter and the fibrinogen >0.75–1.0 g/l until the coagulopathy resolves. There is no evidence to support the use of low-dose heparin. The coagulopathy improves with treatment of the leukaemia and the use of ATRA which induces differentiation of the malignant clone.

Studies of RT-PCR for *PML-RARA* transcripts have demonstrated prognostic value in the detection of minimal residual disease during clinical remission in APL. Serial negative PCR after chemotherapy is associated with prolonged remission, whereas patients who remain or revert to PCR positivity after consolidation are likely to relapse. Ongoing studies are assessing whether intervention prior to overt relapse will improve the clinical outcome.

Paediatric patients with relapsed APL usually achieve a second remission with further chemotherapy. The bone marrow is the usual site of relapse, but isolated CNS relapses have been reported. Patients can develop resistance to ATRA therapy, and some of these patients may respond to arsenic trioxide which has been reported to give CR rates of 80–100 per cent. Adult studies suggest that if a second remission is achieved, matched sibling allogeneic BMT or autologous transplant should be considered.

Relapsed and refractory AML

Despite improvements in therapy, about 30 per cent of children with AML still relapse. Children treated on MRC AML 10 who relapsed within 1 year of achieving their first CR had a very poor outlook (overall survival 15 per cent of those treated). Patients with a first CR >1 year fared better [CR 92 per cent; 3-year EFS 60 per cent]. High dose Ara-C alone, or in combination with other agents (anthracycline ± fludarabine) are commonly used to achieve a second remission. The majority of these patients proceed to allogeneic BMT with family or alternative donors. Allogeneic BMT may improve outcome for patients who relapse late. Patients who relapse after allogeneic BMT may benefit from augmentation of the graft versus leukaemia (GVL) effect. This may be achieved by stopping or reducing immunosuppression and by the use of donor lymphocyte infusions, although the latter remains unconfirmed.

Approximately 5 per cent of patients still fail to achieve remission with standard induction chemotherapy. Possible treatment strategies for this group of patients include alternative intensive chemotherapy and the use of novel treatments such as monoclonal antibody therapy. If a remission is achieved, allogeneic transplant from a matched family or unrelated donor is generally recommended, although no definite advantage of this approach has been demonstrated. Failure to achieve remission with salvage therapy is associated with a very poor prognosis, and transplantation in this setting carries a very high procedure-related mortality and little hope of cure.

Infant AML

Infants <12 months of age usually have acute monoblastic or myelomonoblastic AML characterized by hyperleucocytosis and extramedullary involvement. Many patients have 11q23 translocations involving the *MLL* gene. Infant AML has a superior outcome to infant ALL and ~90 per cent can achieve CR with intensive chemotherapy. Studies from the USA and Japan have reported a 3-year EFS of 61–72 per cent, suggesting that many infants with AML can be cured with intensive chemotherapy alone. Matched related donor transplant may be associated with a slightly better EFS but the risk of late effects must be considered.

Minimal residual disease

Relapse remains the main cause of treatment failure in AML and studies suggest that monitoring minimal residual disease (MRD) may be of benefit in identifying those patients at high risk

Table 13.3. Methodologies used in MRD detection

	Approximate percentage of suitable cases	Relative sensitivity	Advantages	Disadvantages
Morphology	100	5×10^{-2}	Routine	Insensitive
Cytogenetics	70	$1{-}5 \times 10^{-2}$	Specific marker Monitors multiple events	Insensitive
FISH	40–60	1×10^{-2}	Specific marker Can be used in interphase	Relatively insensitive
Multiparameter flow cytometry	>50	$10^{-2} - 10^{-4}$	Rapid Relatively sensitive Quantitative	False positive Low frequency of normal cell with leukaemic phenotype Phenotype switch
Molecular (RT-PCR)	Specific fusion gene: 30–40 Other molecular targets: 80–90	$10^{-4} - 10^{-6}$	Highly sensitive Quantitive Automated Rapid Reproducible Allows standardization	False positive due to contamination Reduced sensitivity due to degraded RNA Low mRNA expression Inefficient reverse transcription

Reproduced from J.Yin and K. Tobal (1999) *Br J Haematol* **106**, 578–90.

of relapse. Complete remission is classically defined as the presence of <5 per cent blasts in the bone marrow as assessed by traditional light microscopy. At diagnosis, leukaemic tumour burden may be 10^{12} leukaemic cells, and even at the time of morphologic remission there may still be as many as 10^{10} residual leukaemic cells. Whilst risk stratified treatment based on MRD is common practice in ALL, MRD is less commonly measured in AML and treatment is uniform regardless of the tumour load.

There are currently four main methods for the detection of minimal residual disease (Table 13.3). These are conventional cytogenetics, fluorescence *in situ* hybridization (FISH), multi-parameter flow cytometry, and nucleic-acid-based amplification (PCR).

Emerging therapies

It is likely that there is a ceiling to the benefit that can be achieved from intensive chemotherapy. In addition, the role of BMT may be limited. New agents and technologies are desperately needed. Alternative approaches include monoclonal antibodies such as gemtuzimab (anti CD33 antibody) which targets an epitope highly expressed on many myeloid blasts. Tyrosine kinase inhibitors, which are directed at the fusion products of abnormal genes and drugs and modulate proliferation and apoptosis, are under assessment. Microarray technology and gene profiling will improve understanding of leukaemogenesis and its effect on intracellular pathways. The benefits of these developments require careful assessment in well-designed clinical trials.

Summary

There has been considerable improvement in the survival in AML over the past 30 years, largely because of the high rate of enrollment in clinical trials. With intensive induction chemotherapy

90 per cent of children achieve remission, and with intensive consolidation >60 per cent are long-term survivors. Significant treatment-related mortality, despite improvements in supportive care, suggests that there may be a limit to therapy intensification. Improved understanding of the molecular pathways in AML will allow the development of targeted cytotoxic therapy. It is hoped that combining this with better characterization of prognostic groups will allow optimization of therapy in the future.

Key references and suggested reading

Arceci RJ (2002). Progress and controversies in the treatment of pediatric acute myelogenous leukemia. *Curr Opin Hematol* 9, 353–60.

Bain BJ, Barnett D, Linch D, *et al.* (2002). Revised guidelines on immunophenotyping in acute leukaemias and chronic lymphoproliferative disorders. *Clin Lab Haematol* 24, 1–13.

Brunning RD, Matutes E, Harris NL, *et al.* (2001). Acute myeloid leukaemia. In: Jaffe ES, Harris NL, Stein H, Vardiman JW (eds) *Pathology and Genetics of Tumours of Haemopoetic and Lymphoid Tissues. World Health Organization Classification of Tumours.* Lyon: IARC Press.

Clark JJ, Smith FO, Arceci RJ (2003). Update in childhood acute myeloid leukemia: recent developments in the molecular basis of disease and novel therapies. *Curr Opin Hematol* 10, 31–9.

Creutzig U, Ritter J, Zimmerman D, *et al.* (2001). Improved treatment results in high-risk pediatric acute leukemia patients after intensification with high-dose cytarabine and mitoxantrone: Results of Study Acute Myeloid Leukaemia–Berlin–Frankfurt–Munster 93. *J Clin Oncol* 19, 2705–13.

Gregory J, Feusner J (2003). Acute promyelocytic leukemia in children. *Best Pract Res Clin Haematol* 16, 483–94.

Ishii E, Kawasaki H, Isoyama K, *et al.* (2003). Recent advances in the treatment of infant acute myeloid leukemia. *Leuk Lymphoma* 44, 741–8.

Smith MA, Ries LAG, Gurney JG, *et al.* (1999). Leukemia. In: Ries LAG, Smith MA, Gurney JG, *et al.* (eds) *Cancer Incidence and Survival Among Children and Adolescents: United States SEER Program 1975–1995.* NIH Publication 99–4649. Bethesda, MD: National Cancer Institute, 17–34.

Swirsky DM, Richards SJ (2001). Laboratory diagnosis of acute myeloid leukaemia. *Best Pract Res Clin Haematol* 14, 1–17.

Stevens RF, Hann IM, Wheatley K, Gray RG (1998). Marked improvements in outcome with chemotherapy alone in paediatric acute myeloid leukaemia: Results of the United Kingdom Medical Research Council's 10th AML trial. *Br J Haematol* 101, 130–40.

Webb DKH, Wheatley K, Harrison G, *et al.* (1999). Outcome for children with relapsed acute myeloid leukaemia following initial therapy in the Medical Research Council (MRC) AML 10 trial. *Leukemia* 13, 25–31.

Wheatley K, Creutzig U, Chen AR, *et al.* (2002). Current controversies. Which patients with acute myeloid leukaemia should receive a bone marrow transplantation? *Br J Haematol* 118, 365–84.

Wheatley K, Burnett AK, Goldstone AH, *et al.* (1999). A simple, robust, validated and highly predictive index for the determination of risk-directed therapy in acute myeloid leukaemia derived from the MRC AML 10 trial. United Kingdom Medical Research Council's Adult and Childhood Leukaemia Working Parties. *Br J Haematol* 107, 69–79.

Woods WG, Neudorf S, Gold S, *et al.* (2001). A comparison of allogeneic bone marrow transplantation, autologous bone marrow transplantation, and aggressive chemotherapy in children with acute myeloid leukemia in remission: a report from the Children's Cancer Group. *Blood* 97(1):56–52.

Yin J, Tobal K. (1999). Detection of minimal residual disease in acute myeloid leukaemia: methodologies, clinical and biological significance. *Br J Haematol* 106, 578–590.

Chapter 14

Non-Hodgkin lymphoma

Catherine Patte

Introduction

Lymphomas are a heterogeneous group of malignant proliferations of lymphoid cells at various stages of differentiation and activation. Recent biological studies now allow a better classification.[1] In children, a few subtypes of non-Hodgkin lymphoma (NHL) are seen, predominantly the lymphoblastic and Burkitt types. They are characterized by the predominance of extranodal disease and by very rapid growth and dissemination, especially in the bone marrow and central nervous system (CNS). The prognosis of childhood NHL has changed in the last 20 years as a result of improved understanding of the pathological process and better use of intensive chemotherapeutic regimens.

Epidemiology

NHL has a peak incidence between 7 and 10 years of age, and is uncommon before 2 years of age. There is a male predominance, especially in Burkitt lymphoma, with a ratio of 3:1. An annual incidence of approximately 7 cases per million children makes it the third most common childhood malignancy.

A few familial cases of lymphoid malignancies are observed, without recognized genetic abnormalities. Patients at increased risk of developing NHL include those with congenital immunodeficiency (such as ataxia–telangiectasia or Wiskott–Aldrich syndrome), those with AIDS, and those receiving immunosuppressive therapy (such as after organ transplantation). There is an X-linked lymphoproliferative syndrome characterized by a particular sensitivity to Epstein–Barr virus (EBV) and the occurrence of malignant lymphomas, especially of the Burkitt type, and fatal infectious mononucleosis. Specific geographical areas are also associated with particular types of lymphoma, such as the 'endemic' (African) Burkitt lymphoma.

Aetiology has been particularly linked with EBV after the observation that EBV particles were present in the nucleus of malignant cells in endemic Burkitt lymphoma. Although the virus is known to have transforming and immortalizing properties on B cells *in vitro* and is suspected to have a role in the oncogenic process, evidence of other events is necessary to establish malignancy. Furthermore, primary evidence of viral participation in oncogenesis is rare (EBV is found in only 20 per cent of non-endemic Burkitt lymphoma) and to date no viral particles have been found in childhood T cell lymphoma.

Biology

Histology

The classification of NHL has changed many times over the years and has become clearer with understanding of the differentiation pathways of normal lymphocytes and the explosion of new diagnostic tools (immunophenotyping, cytogenetics, molecular biology, and now gene sequencing). Only four categories of lymphoma are usually encountered in children: Burkitt, lymphoblastic, large B-cell, and anaplastic large cell.[1] Their characteristics are given in Table 14.1. The indicated frequency is an average in Western Europe, which depends on geography. Burkitt lymphoma represents the majority of lymphoma in equatorial Africa and is less frequent in Northern Europe and in Japan. The frequency of large cell lymphomas increases among adolescents.

Microarray technologies, by studying the expression of many genes at once, are very promising, but the implications for diagnosis and prognosis, and their further usefulness in clinical practice, especially in childhood NHL, still have to be demonstrated.

Cytogenetics and molecular biology

Cytogenetic and molecular biological studies have contributed to a better understanding of the fundamental processes in NHL, but have not yet contributed to therapy. In Burkitt lymphoma, tumour cells are characterized by a translocation involving the long arm of chromosome 8, region q24. The majority of cases exhibit the translocation t(8;14)(q24;q32). Variant translocations include t(2;8)(p12;q24) and t(8;22)(q24;q11). In translocation t(8;14), the oncogene c-*myc* moves from its normal position on chromosome 8 and is rearranged with the gene for heavy-chain immunoglobulin, while in the variant translocations c-*myc* remains on chromosome 8, and the κ and λ immunoglobulin light-chain genes translocate from their normal positions on chromosomes 2 and 22, respectively, to a region distal to the c-*myc* oncogene. This results in a transcriptional deregulation of the c-*myc* gene and its overexpression, which is thought to play a crucial role in the genesis and/or maintenance of this malignancy.

In T-cell tumours, chromosomal abnormalities are rarer and more heterogeneous. They can involve chromosome 14, at the locus of the gene for the α chain of the T-cell receptor, or chromosome 7, at the locus of the gene for the β chain of the T-cell receptor.

Clinical features

The clinical presentation of NHL in childhood is varied and depends on the primary site of the disease, the histological subtype, and the extent of the disease.

The abdomen is the most frequent primary site (30–45 per cent of all cases). Intussusception, leading to the discovery of a small resectable abdominal tumour, is a rare presentation; a large and rapidly growing abdominal mass, often associated with ascites, is the usual clinical presentation. Ultrasound scan defines the gut and/or mesenteric mass and any intra-abdominal spread. Laparotomy should be avoided, unless there is an abdominal emergency, and the diagnosis should be made by cytological examination of ascites or percutaneous needle biopsy of the tumour. Cyto/histology shows Burkitt lymphoma in the majority of cases; others are large B-cell.

Mediastinal tumours (25–35 per cent) are typically T-cell lymphoblastic lymphomas (thymic origin), but in rare cases they can be large B-cell (thymic origin) or Burkitt lymphoma (non-thymic origin). Mediastinal compression and/or cervical or axillary lymphadenopathy is an indication for a chest radiograph which will show a mediastinal mass, often associated with pleural or pericardial effusions. Patients are at particular risk of developing respiratory distress which is worsened or provoked by general anaesthesia, which therefore must be avoided. Diagnosis should be made using cytological examination of effusions or bone marrow smears.

Table 14.1. Different types of childhood lymphomas and their biological specifics

	Burkitt (50 per cent)	Lymphoblastic (30 per cent)		Large B-cell (10 per cent)	Anaplastic large cell (10 per cent)
Preferential tumour site	Abdomen Head and neck	Mediastinum (T) Bone, (sub)cutaneous (B)		Abdomen, thymus, bone	Node, skin
Corresponding stage of F cell development	Germinal center	Immature		Germinal center	Mature T-cell
Histology					
Cell size	Medium	Medium		Large	Voluminous
Cytoplasm	Narrow, basophilic with vacuoles	Narrow, pale			Abundant and clear erythrophagocytosis
Nucleus	Round	Sometimes convoluted		Sometimes cleaved, vesicular	Irregular, clear
Nucleoli	Several nucleoli	Poorly discernible		Distinct, often adherent to nuclear membrane	
Chromatin	Coarse and irregular	Finely stippled			Voluminous
FAB equivalent	L3	L1, L2			
Immunophenotyping	CD20+ CD79a+ Sig+	TdT+ B lineage CD19+ CD 79a+ S Ig– cMu–/+	T lineage CD7+ CD2+ CD3c+	CD20+ CD79a+ S Ig +/–	CD30+ EMA+ ALK+ (T or 'null' markers)
	Ki 67+, >95 per cent			bcl6 +/– Ki 67, 60 per cent–90 per cent	
Cytogenetics	t (8;14) (q24;q32) or variant t(2;8) (p11;q24) t(8;22) (q24;q11)	No specific abnormalities Sometimes involvement of T-cell antigen receptor genes (TCR) on chromosome 7(q34) or 14(q11)		Sometimes t(8;14) (q24;q32) der (3)(q27) (bcl6)	t(2;5)(p23;q35) or variant NPM/ALK fusion protein ALK is a tyrosine kinase receptor ALK located on 2p23
Result	Transcriptional deregulation of c-myc			Transcriptional deregulation of bcl6	

If a tumour biopsy is needed, this should be done by percutaneous needle biopsy or mediastinoscopy.

The third most frequent site is the head and neck (10–20 per cent), including Waldeyer's ring and the facial bones, followed by the superficial lymph nodes (5–10 per cent). The remaining 5–10 per cent include tumours that arise from less common sites such as bone, skin, thyroid, orbit, eyelid, kidney, and epidural space. Diagnosis is confirmed by tissue biopsy with immunophenotyping since no particular type of lymphoma is associated with these sites, except Burkitt with facial bones and orbit, especially in endemic Burkitt NHL. Bone lymphoma may be localized, but can be also generalized and is often associated with hypercalcaemia. Kidney lymphoma can be confused with nephroblastoma, but in lymphoma the tumour is frequently bilateral, the infiltration multinodular or diffuse, or renal failure may be present. (Sub)cutaneous lymphoma particularly occurs in young children aged <2 years and is of precursor B-cell phenotype.

Anaplastic large-cell lymphomas have clinical particularities. Nodal involvement, sometimes painful, is characteristic of this disease; other characteristics are frequent skin involvement with inflammatory symptoms in the involved nodes, distant macular lesions, or general skin changes resembling ichthyosis, and frequent generalized symptoms with widely fluctuating fever. A few cases show a 'wax and wane' pattern with previous episode(s) of spontaneous regression.

Initial workup and staging

Diagnosis can be made using biopsy material, including tumour-touch preparations, or cytological examination of effusion fluid or bone marrow smears. Thus surgical procedures can be avoided in diffuse disease. Immunological studies are recommended, preferably obtained on suspended cells from fresh tumours or on frozen sections, but immunohistochemistry on paraffin sections is also of value. Cytogenetic studies are also important. Once the diagnosis of NHL has been made, a speedy assessment of diagnosis, staging, and general evaluation must be performed in order to commence appropriate treatment as soon as possible.

Because of the predominance of extranodal primaries and the unpredictable pattern of spread, the Ann Arbor classification is not suitable for childhood NHL. Several classifications have been proposed, but the system most commonly used is the St Jude staging system (also known as the Murphy system) (Table 14.2). The traditional boundary between leukaemia and lymphoma has been arbitrarily defined as more or less than 25 per cent blast cells in the bone marrow, but this does not correspond to either clinical or biological differences. CNS involvement is defined by the presence of unequivocal malignant cells in a cytocentrifuged specimen of spinal fluid and/or obvious neurological deficits such as cranial nerve palsies. Although not included in the staging system and not a specific marker, lactate dehydrogenase (LDH) level in the serum is a very good indicator of tumour burden and often has a prognostic significance.

Workup procedures are outlined in Table 14.3. Abdominal ultrasonography is adequate to define abdominal disease; CT scanning is not necessary in the primary investigation of extended abdominal and mediastinal disease. Experience with positron emission tomography (PET) scanning in childhood NHL is still at an early stage. It is hoped that this investigation will help to predict active tumour in a residual mass, but its role still needs to be evaluated

Patients often have other problems, such as malnutrition, infection, postsurgical complications, and respiratory and metabolic abnormalities; these may be life threatening or

Table 14.2. St Jude's staging for childhood non-Hodgkin lymphoma

Stage I
- ◆ A single tumour (extranodal) or single anatomical area (nodal) with the exclusion of the mediastinum or abdomen

Stage II
- ◆ A single tumour (extranodal) with regional node involvement
- ◆ Two or more nodal areas on the same side of the diaphragm
- ◆ Two single (extranodal) tumours with or without regional node involvement on the same side of the diaphragm
- ◆ A primary gastrointestinal tract tumour, usually in the ileocoecal area, with or without involvement of associated mesenteric nodes only, grossly completely resected

Stage III
- ◆ Two single tumours (extranodal) on opposite sides of the diaphragm
- ◆ Two or more nodal areas above and below the diaphragm
- ◆ All the primary intrathoracic tumours (mediastinal, pleural, thymic)
- ◆ All extensive primary intra-abdominal disease, unresectable.
- ◆ All paraspinal or epidural tumours, regardless of other tumour site(s)

Stage IV
- ◆ Any of the above with initial CNS and/or bone marrow involvement

compromise the onset of therapy. For example, hypercalcaemia requires treatment as a separate entity. If there is renal failure, its mechanism must be established. It may be uric acid nephropathy, tumour infiltration, or urinary obstruction. In order to start appropriate treatment it is necessary to start hyperhydration promptly. Sometimes dialysis or transcutaneous pyelostomy must be performed to obtain sufficient urine outflow.

The tumour lysis syndrome may be present at diagnosis or develop during treatment. Preventive measures, a diuretic and a 'uricolytic' drug (allopurinol or urate oxidase), must always be instituted. Urate oxidase is preferable in cases of advanced-stage disease. It transforms uric acid into allantoin, which is highly soluble in urine. It has been shown to be more efficient in promptly reducing serum uric acid level, preventing uric acid nephropathy, and

Table 14.3. Initial workup

Mandatory
- ◆ Physical examination
- ◆ Chest and nasopharyngeal radiography
- ◆ Abdominal ultrasonography
- ◆ Two BM aspirations (+ BM biopsies in large-cell NHL)
- ◆ CSF examination
- ◆ Complete blood count
- ◆ LDH, serum electrolytes, BUN, creatinine, uric acid levels

Optional depending on clinical circumstances
- ◆ Bone scan and skeletal survey
- ◆ Local CT scan (head and neck tumours)
- ◆ MRI (CNS disease)
- ◆ Abdominal CT scan (stage I or abdominal stage II)
- ◆ Thoracic CT scan

BM, bone marrow; NHL, non-Hodgkin lymphoma; CSF, cerebrospinal fluid; LDH, lactate dehydrogenase; BUN, blood urea nitrogen.

preserving renal function, allowing better excretion of other cell metabolites such as potassium and phosphorus.[2-4] The recombinant form of urate oxidase is now available. Strict clinical and metabolic monitoring of patients is essential during the lysis phase.

Both the French and the German protocols start with a 'prephase' with low-dose therapy. This generally induces good tumour regression and allows initial problems to be managed without incurring the haematological and mucous complications of the more intensive regimen which commences a week later.

Treatment

Before 1970 only a few localized tumours could be cured by surgery and radiotherapy. Since then, considerable therapeutic improvements have been achieved.

Indications for surgery are very rare. A small localized abdominal tumour may be completely excised in the context of intestinal intussusception. Primary surgical excision or debulking of abdominal, head and neck, or mediastinal tumours should not be attempted. Extensive surgery is uselessly mutilating and is often followed by tumoral regrowth, as well as delaying and possibly complicating chemotherapy. Rarely, abdominal surgery is needed during treatment for complications such as intestinal perforation. At the time of remission evaluation, any residual mass should be removed or widely biopsied for pathological examination to determine whether a complete (no viable cells) or partial remission has been obtained.

Radiotherapy can be efficacious in lymphoma, but this local therapy gives no advantage over chemotherapy alone and adds both immediate and long-term toxicity. Indications for radiotherapy have become very rare. It may be used in some emergency situations, although chemotherapy is often as effective, in a few cases of localized residual tumours, or for CNS-directed therapy (cranial irradiation).

Chemotherapy is the treatment of choice in childhood NHL, which should be considered to be a systemic disease even in the presence of apparently local disease. It must be tailored to the histological subtype and the extent of the disease. CNS prophylaxis is essential in Burkitt and lymphoblastic NHL. It can be given by high dose (HD) methotrexate (MTX) and intrathecal (i.t.) injections of MTX $\pm$ hydrocortisone and cytosine arabinoside (Ara-C).

B-cell lymphomas

Most studies relate to Burkitt lymphoma, but in some recent European studies large B-cell lymphomas were included (where they represent 10–15 per cent of cases). Fractionated cyclophosphamide (CPM), intermediate(ID) MTX or HD-MTX, and Ara-C are the most important drugs in the treatment of Burkitt NHL. Vincristine, adriamycin, etoposide (VP16), ifosfamide, and prednisone are also effective. Drugs are administered in various combinations, but usually as short pulsed courses.

Since 1981, the largest studies have taken place in France (LMB protocols) and Germany (BFM protocols), and as a result of these well-organized multicentre studies there has been considerable improvement in the treatment of B-cell lymphomas.

LMB protocols

The general scheme of the LMB protocols is shown in Figure 14.1. A cytoreductive phase (COP course) with low doses of vincristine, cyclophosphamide, and prednisone is given 1 week before the intensive induction (two consecutive courses of COPAD M) which is based on HD-MTX and fractionated cyclophosphamide. This is followed by two consecutive consolidation

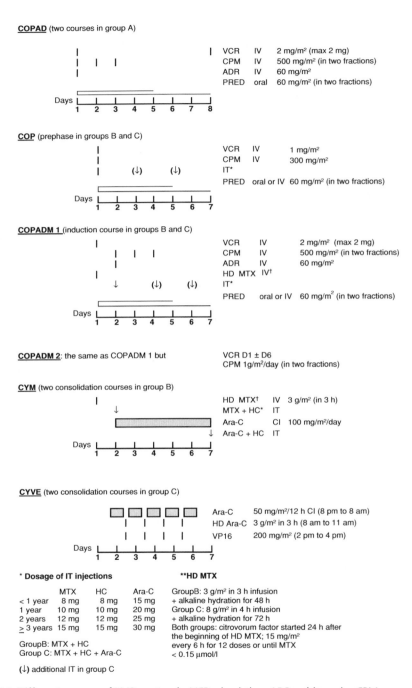

COPAD (two courses in group A)

VCR	IV	2 mg/m² (max 2 mg)
CPM	IV	500 mg/m² (in two fractions)
ADR	IV	60 mg/m²
PRED	oral	60 mg/m² (in two fractions)

Days 1 2 3 4 5 6 7 8

COP (prephase in groups B and C)

VCR	IV	1 mg/m²
CPM	IV	300 mg/m²
IT*		
PRED	oral or IV	60 mg/m² (in two fractions)

Days 1 2 3 4 5 6 7

COPADM 1 (induction course in groups B and C)

VCR	IV	2 mg/m² (max 2 mg)
CPM	IV	500 mg/m² (in two fractions)
ADR	IV	60 mg/m²
HD MTX	IV†	
IT*		
PRED	oral or IV	60 mg/m² (in two fractions)

Days 1 2 3 4 5 6 7

COPADM 2: the same as COPADM 1 but

VCR D1 ± D6
CPM 1g/m²/day (in two fractions)

CYM (two consolidation courses in group B)

HD MTX†	IV	3 g/m² (in 3 h)
MTX + HC*	IT	
Ara-C	CI	100 mg/m²/day
Ara-C + HC	IT	

Days 1 2 3 4 5 6 7

CYVE (two consolidation courses in group C)

Ara-C	50 mg/m²/12 h CI (8 pm to 8 am)
HD Ara-C	3 g/m² in 3 h (8 am to 11 am)
VP16	200 mg/m² (2 pm to 4 pm)

Days 1 2 3 4 5 6 7

* Dosage of IT injections

	MTX	HC	Ara-C
< 1 year	8 mg	8 mg	15 mg
1 year	10 mg	10 mg	20 mg
2 years	12 mg	12 mg	25 mg
≥ 3 years	15 mg	15 mg	30 mg

GroupB: MTX + HC
Group C: MTX + HC + Ara-C

(↓) additional IT in group C

**HD MTX

GroupB: 3 g/m² in 3 h infusion
+ alkaline hydration for 48 h
Group C: 8 g/m² in 4 h infusion
+ alkaline hydration for 72 h
Both groups: citrovorum factor started 24 h after
the beginning of HD MTX; 15 mg/m²
every 6 h for 12 doses or until MTX
< 0.15 µmol/l

Fig. 14.1 Different courses of LMB protocols: VCR, vincristine; ADR, adriamycin; CPM. cyclophosphamide; Pred, prednisone; Ara-C, cytosine arabinoside; MTX, methotrexate; HC, hydrocortisone; CI, continuous infusion.

courses based on Ara-C in continuous infusion. CNS prophylaxis is given by HD-MTX and intrathecal injections. The French Paediatric Oncology Society (SFOP) conducted several consecutive multicentre studies (LMB81, LMB84, LMB86, and LMB89. In the first three studies, designed for advanced stage Burkitt disease, event-free survival (EFS) increased up to 75–90 per cent for CNS-patients, whereas duration of treatment was progressively reduced from 12 to 4 months (randomized LMB84 trial)[5] and toxicity, especially the toxic death rate, decreased as the experience of the investigators increased. CNS prophylaxis with HD-MTX (3 g/m^2 infused for 4 h) and i.t. MTX was effective (CNS relapse rate <2 per cent). It became clear that partial remission (with documented viable cells in the residual mass) at the end of induction could be cured by treatment intensification with autologous bone marrow transplantation, and that the absence of tumour reduction after COP was indicative of a poor prognosis with an EFS of 29 per cent (LMB84). For patients with initial CNS involvement whose EFS was only 19 per cent in the LMB 81 protocol, the pilot LMB 86 study using a higher dose of MTX (8 g/m^2 in 4 h), triple intrathecal injections, and consolidation with continuous infusion and high-dose Ara-C and VP16 (CYVE courses) succeeded in increasing EFS to 75 per cent.

All mature B-cell diseases [Burkitt and large B-cell NHL and acute lymphoblastic leukaemia (ALL)], whatever the stage, were included in the LMB89 study (1989–1996).[6] Patients were stratified into three therapeutic groups: group A (resected stage I and abdominal stage II) received two courses of COPAD (vincristine, cyclophosphamide, adriamycin and prednisone). Group B (patients not eligible for groups A or C) received a 3.5-month treatment identical to the short arm of the LMB84 protocol. Group C (patients with CNS involvement and ALL with $\geq$70 per cent of blasts in bone marrow) received a more intensive treatment similar to that of the LMB86 protocol. Treatment was further intensified for patients who did not respond to COP in group B and any patient with residual viable cells after the consolidation phase. A total of 561 patients were enrolled. Five-year survival was 92.5 per cent [95 per cent confidence interval (CI), 90–94] and EFS was 91 per cent (95 per cent CI, 89–93). EFS was 98 per cent for stages I and II, 91 per cent for stage III, and 87 per cent for stage IV and B-ALL. The outcome was similar in Burkitt and large B-cell disease (EFS of 92 per cent and 89 per cent, respectively). In group B, multivariate analysis of prognostic factors showed that an LDH level more than twice the normal value N (89.5 per cent for LDH $>2N$ versus 95 per cent for LDH $\leq 2N$), no response after COP (EFS, 72 per cent) and age $\geq$15 years were associated with a lower EFS. CNS involvement was the only prognostic factor found in group C (79 per cent for CNS+ versus 90 per cent for CNS$-$).

The next study, FAB LMB96 (May 1996–June 2001), was a randomized international trial with the participation of the SFOP, the UK Children's Cancer Study Group (UKCCSG) and the US Children's Cancer Group (CCG). It was an attempt to reduce treatment further, especially cyclophosphamide dosage, to avoid sterility in boys, to reduce its duration, and to avoid cranial irradiation in patients with initial CNS involvement. Preliminary results indicate that treatment can be reduced further in group B, but not in group C. It also indicates that delay between the two induction courses has a prognostic impact.

BFM protocols

In the four consecutive BFM studies (BFM81, BFM83, BFM86, and BFM90) treatment intensity was progressively increased, treatment duration reduced, and CNS irradiation withdrawn. In the BFM90 study (1990–1995), treatment was stratified into three risk groups (slightly different from those of the French study). It consists of two, four, or six 5-day courses including dexamethasone, MTX $5\,g/m^2$ (or $0.5\,g/m^2$ in the lowest risk group) in 24 h infusion and intrathecal injections in each course, and alternating ifosfamide, cytarabine, and etoposide with cyclophosphamide and doxorubicin. The 6-year EFS was 89 per cent for the whole group of 413 patients, and 97 per cent, 98 per cent, 88 per cent, 73 per cent, and 74 per cent for stage I, stage II, stage III, stage IV, and ALL, respectively.[7]

The most remarkable result is the increase of EFS from ~50 per cent to 80 per cent for patients with stage IV and L3-ALL (BFM86)[8] and those with abdominal stage III and LDH > 500 (BFM90)[7] when MTX was increased from 0.5 to $5\,g/m^2$. In the following BFM 95 study, the duration of the MTX infusion was randomized (24 h versus 4 h). Final data indicate that better results were obtained in the 24-h infusion arm for patients at higher risk.

Other protocols

Other studies have reported interesting results, especially the Pediatric Oncology Group (POG) randomized multicentre trials, and the National Cancer Institute (NCI)[9] and Milan Istituto Nazionaledi Tumori[10] single-centre series. In countries that have limited resources but where Burkitt lymphoma is frequent, therapeutic improvements have also been achieved by adapting therapy to the local environment and by better management of the initial, especially metabolic, problems.

Lymphoblastic lymphomas

Patients with lymphoblastic lymphomas must be treated with protocols similar to those used in high-risk forms of ALL. Most of these lymphomas are T-lineage, but a few are B-lineage. Although their biology is not similar, they are generally treated using the same protocols. The most frequently used protocols were the LSA2L2 or derived protocols, and the non-B BFM[8,11] or derived protocols.

In the BFM protocol, induction (protocol I: prednisone, vincristine, daunorubicin, L-asparaginase followed by cyclophosphamide, Ara-C, and 6-mercaptopurine, and associated with MTX i.t.) is followed by four HD-MTX courses ($5\,g/m^2$ in 24 h infusion) and re-induction (protocol II: same drugs as protocol I, but lower total doses and dexamethasone replacing prednisone). These phases are followed by maintenance with daily 6-mercaptopurine and weekly MTX. Preventive cranial irradiation was progressively reduced and then omitted. In study 90, which enrolled 101 patients, EFS improved to 90 per cent without significant change in the chemotherapy regimen.[11] This might have been due to the long experience of the investigators with the protocol. An international European randomized study based on the BFM scheme is about to start.

Other protocols

Other interesting multicentre studies have been published by the UKCCSG, the POG, and the CCG. In particular, the POG has demonstrated the effectiveness of asparaginase[12] and is demonstrating that of HD-MTX.

Anaplastic large-cell lymphomas (ALCLs)

This disease is rare, and so the largest series include only about 10 patients per year. In the USA, these lymphomas have not been considered as a special entity and were included in the same protocols as the other large cell lymphomas. Interestingly, however, a POG randomized study recently showed that the addition of HD-MTX and Ara-C to the APO regimen was beneficial for large B-cell lymphoma, but not for ALCL. In Europe, ALCL (initially called 'malignant Histiocytosis') has been considered as a specific entity for a long time, and has been generally treated with 'B-cell-like' rather than 'T-cell-like' protocols. Overall survival rate is around 70–80 per cent.[13–15] EFS is often lower, indicating that relapses can be salvaged. Weekly vinblastine has shown its efficacy in relapse.[16] The analysis of the pooled data of the German,[13] French,[14] and UK series indicated that the BFM regimen was at least as effective as the others with lower total doses of drugs, especially cyclophosphamide and adriamycin. It also showed the following poor prognostic factors: mediastinal, visceral (lung, liver, spleen), and skin involvement. This analysis is the basis of the ongoing international European study ALCL 99 which uses the BFM backbone and asks two additional questions.

1. What is the best way of administrating HDMTX: $1 \, g/m^2$ in 24 h infusion with i.t. MTX or $3 \, g/m^2$ in 3 h infusion without i.t. MTX?
2. What is the role of vinblastine as maintenance therapy in higher-risk patients.

The COG is starting a study which also addresses the question of vinblastine.

Questions

What are the indications for high-dose chemotherapy and haematopoietic stem cell transplantation?

The need for high-dose chemotherapy with haematopoietic stem cell transplantation has greatly diminished in parallel with the improvement in survival using intensive conventional regimens. The indications are restricted to some initially poor responders and to relapses which respond to a second-line treatment. However, relapses that occur with the present protocols are more 'resistant' than previously, and finding an effective second-line chemotherapy has become a challenge.

Can granulocyte colony-stimulating factor decrease neutropenia and the related complications?

Most of the polychemotherapy regimens used to treat childhood NHL are intensive and followed by pancytopenia, especially neutropenia. Therefore there was a great deal of hope that granulocyte colony-stimulating factor (GCSF) would decrease the frequency of neutropenia and its related complications. However, three randomized studies performed in childhood NHL, one by the POG in T-lymphoblastic lymphoma,[17] one by the NCI in B-lymphoblastic lymphomas,[9] and one in the SFOP protocols following COPADM courses,[18] did not show any clinical advantage of the use of GCSF. However, these conclusions, which are applicable in the countries where the studies were performed, might be different in other countries where socio-economic context and bacterial environment are different.

Are there other prognostic factors within St Jude staging which could indicate patients requiring more or less treatment?

Since relatively high survival rates have now been reached, the question is raised of how to decrease further treatment intensity without jeopardizing survival rates. To do so, it is necessary to find new prognostic factors.

No-one has yet succeeded in determining the prognostic factors in lymphoblastic lymphoma. Response to corticosteroids at D8, which is such a powerful one in T-ALL, could not be demonstrated in NHL. This might be due in part to the difficulty of finding a measure equivalent to and as simple as 1000 blasts in the blood.

In B-cell disease, the absence of tumour regression 1 week after COP, which is a factor for poor prognosis in the LMB84 study, was taken into account in order to intensify chemotherapy early in subsequent studies. Outcome improved from 22 to 70 per cent in the LMB89 study,[6] but B-cell disease with bad response at day 7 remained among the poor prognostic factors.

Is age a prognostic factor? Age >15 years was found to be prognostic for EFS in the LMB89 study, but not for survival, and the number of patients was small.[6] Age was not prognostic in two small series of both child and adult patients with B-cell NHL at the Istituto Nazionale di Tumori, Milan. Very few data are available on patients between 15 and 20 years because they are treated in different protocols in both paediatric and adult departments, and are often not registered in studies. An effort should be made in the future to clarify this question.

With new technologies, especially DNA microarray, there is hope of identifying biological features that could emerge as independent prognostic factors. However, it should be noted that all therapeutic improvements so far have been obtained independently of understanding the biology of the lymphoma.

Treatment intensity could be further decreased for some patients. This is being done for B-cell resected stage I and abdominal stage II. In the French LMB 89 study these were treated with only two courses of COPAD, and in BFM90 resected tumours were treated with two courses of chemotherapy. Are non-resected stage I and II treated too intensively in LMB group B? However, when treatment is thought not to have immediate life-threatening consequences or long-term sequelae, the rationale behind a further decrease in therapy is debatable.

Are there also groups of patients within the advanced stages for whom treatment could be decreased, knowing that a prognostic factor identified in one study might not be relevant in another? LDH level has generally been recognized as prognostic, especially among stage III patients, but bone marrow involvement, which is prognostic in most studies, was not prognostic in the LMB studies. On the other hand, reducing further treatment might not be so easy. Attempts were made in group C of the FAB LMB96 study and in arms 3 and 4 of BFM95, but interim analyses indicated that both studies should be stopped because of inferior EFS in the experimental arm.

One of the aims of decreasing treatment is to decrease long-term sequelae such as infertility, especially in boys. Cyclophosphamide at a cumulative dose $> 9\,g/m^2$ produces male sterility, and so reaching this dosage should be avoided, at least for patients who have no poor prognostic factors. In fact, it would be preferable not to exceed $5\,g/m^2$ because of individual variation in susceptibility, and the importance of factors such as age at treatment or mode of drug administration remain undetermined.

How should post-transplant B-cell non-Hodgkin lymphoma be managed?

With the development of organ transplantation, there is an awareness of both polyclonal and monoclonal B-cell lymphomas developing in patients profoundly immunosuppressed by immunosuppressive drugs. Such patients, usually recipients of cardiac or renal transplants, may develop 'high-grade' tumours that are histologically indistinguishable from true malignant disease. In some patients there may be a clear viral pathogen, such as EBV, in which case a polyclonal tumour may be demonstrable.

The outcome of these tumours is generally good, and they often resolve spontaneously with reduction or cessation of ciclosporin. However, in a number of patients the disease will be more aggressive and may require therapy. Treatment with monoclonal antibodies such as anti-CD20 is indicated in B-cell lymphoproliferative disease.

What is the place of tumour-specific targeted therapy in B-cell non-Hodgkin lymphoma?

This is a challenge for the coming years. Monoclonal-antibody-targeted therapy for B-cell lymphomas in adults has produced encouraging results. The anti-CD20, rituximab, has been studied in large cohorts of patients. Its efficacy has been proved in follicular lymphoma, and in large B-cell disease in elderly patients in association with chemotherapy. It is now being studied in large B-cell lymphomas in younger adults. Except in post-transplant lymphoproliferative disease, it has not yet been evaluated in paediatric practice. Neither has it been evaluated in Burkitt lymphoma at any age. The therapy seems to have only minor side effects, but it is very expensive. Taking into account the high survival rate now obtained, its place in the treatment of Burkitt lymphoma in children will be difficult to assess. However, it is necessary to evaluate such a specific therapy, knowing that no phase II studies have been performed in this disease.

Summary

Appropriate management at diagnosis of patients with NHL is essential. Prophylaxis and treatment of tumour lysis syndrome is important. Urate oxidase is more effective than allopurinol in reducing uric acid level and preserving renal function.

NHL in children is a fast-growing tumour which disseminates widely, especially in bone marrow and the CNS. Considerable therapeutic improvement has been achieved by prospective multicentre studies. Chemotherapy is the treatment of choice and its modality differs according to the histologic subtype.

Burkitt and large B-cell NHL are treated with intensive pulsed chemotherapy where the most important drugs are cyclophosphamide, HD-MTX, and Ara-C, and the cure rate is 80–90 per cent. The place of rituximab (anti CD20) is not yet determined. Lymphoblastic NHL is treated with intensive semicontinuous and prolonged chemotherapy and the cure rate is 75–90 per cent. In both diseases, CNS prophylaxis is essential and is based on intrathecal injections (MTX ± Ara-C). Cranial irradiation is not necessary. The optimal treatment for ALCL is still under debate. The cure rate is 70–80 per cent.

New tools, such as microarray technology, will tell us more about the biology of these diseases, but prognostic factors identified in one study might not be relevant in another. PET scanning for evaluation of disease extension or of residual masses has yet to be evaluated.

References

1. Jaffe ES, Harris NL, Diebold J, Muller-Hermelink HK (1999). World Health Organization classification of neoplastic diseases of the hematopoietic and lymphoid tissues. A progress report. *Am J Clin Pathol* 111(1 Suppl 1), S8–12.
2. Patte C, Sakiroglu C, Ansoborlo S, et al. (2002). Urate-oxidase in the prevention and treatment of metabolic complications in patients with B-cell lymphoma and leukemia, treated in the Société Française d'Oncologie Pediatrique LMB89 protocol. *Ann Oncol* 13, 789–95.
3. Pui CH, Mahmoud HH, Wiley JM, et al. (2001). Recombinant urate oxidase for the prophylaxis or treatment of hyperuricemia in patients with leukemia or lymphoma. *J Clin Oncol*, 19, 697–704.

4. **Goldman SC, Holcenberg JS, Finklestein JZ, *et al.*** (2001). A randomized comparison between rasburicase and allopurinol in children with lymphoma or leukemia at high risk for tumor lysis. *Blood* 97, 2998–3003.

5. **Patte C, Philip T, Rodary C, *et al.*** (1991). High survival rate in advanced-stage B-cell lymphomas and leukemias without CNS involvement with a short intensive polychemotherapy: results from the French Pediatric Oncology Society of a randomized trial of 216 children. *J Clin Oncol* 9, 123–32.

6. **Patte C, Auperin A, Michon J, *et al.*** (2001). The Société Française d'Oncologie Pédiatrique LMB89 protocol: highly effective multiagent chemotherapy tailored to the tumor burden and initial response in 561 unselected children with B-cell lymphomas and L3 leukemia. *Blood* 97, 3370–9.

7. **Reiter A, Schrappe M, Tiemann M, *et al.*** (1999). Improved treatment results in childhood B-cell neoplasms with tailored intensification of therapy: A report of the Berlin–Frankfurt–Munster Group Trial NHL-BFM 90. *Blood* 94, 3294–306.

8. **Reiter A, Schrappe M, Parwaresch R, *et al.*** (1995). Non-Hodgkin's lymphomas of childhood and adolescence: results of a treatment stratified for biologic subtypes and stage. A report of the Berlin–Frankfurt–Munster Group. *J Clin Oncol* 13, 359–72.

9. **Magrath I, Adde M, Shad A, *et al.*** (1996). Adults and children with small non-cleaved-cell lymphoma have a similar excellent outcome when treated with the same chemotherapy regimen. *J Clin Oncol* 14, 925–34.

10. **Spreafico F, Massimino M, Luksch R, *et al.*** (2002). Intensive, very short-term chemotherapy for advanced Burkitt's lymphoma in children. *J Clin Oncol* 20, 2783–8.

11. **Reiter A, Schrappe M, Ludwig WD, *et al.*** (2000). Intensive ALL-type therapy without local radiotherapy provides a 90 per cent event-free survival for children with T-cell lymphoblastic lymphoma: a BFM group report. *Blood* 95, 416–21.

12. **Amylon MD, Shuster J, Pullen J, *et al.*** (1999). Intensive high-dose asparaginase consolidation improves survival for pediatric patients with T cell acute lymphoblastic leukemia and advanced stage lymphoblastic lymphoma: a Pediatric Oncology Group study. *Leukemia* 13, 335–42.

13. **Reiter A, Schrappe M, Tiemann M, *et al.*** (1994). Successful treatment strategy for Ki-1 anaplastic large-cell lymphoma of childhood: a prospective analysis of 62 patients enrolled in three consecutive Berlin–Frankfurt–Munster group studies. *J Clin Oncol* 12 899–908.

14. **Brugieres L, Deley MC, Pacquement H, A *et al.*** (1998). CD30(+) anaplastic large-cell lymphoma in children: analysis of 82 patients enrolled in two consecutive studies of the French Society of Pediatric Oncology. *Blood* 92, 3591–8.

15. **Seidemann K, Tiemann M, Schrappe M, *et al.*** (2001). Short-pulse B-non-Hodgkin lymphoma-type chemotherapy is efficacious treatment for pediatric anaplastic large cell lymphoma: a report of the Berlin–Frankfurt–Munster Group Trial NHL-BFM 90. *Blood* 97, 3699–706.

16. **Brugieres L, Quartier P, Le Deley MC, *et al.*** (2000). Relapses of childhood anaplastic large-cell lymphoma: treatment results in a series of 41 children. A report from the French Society of Pediatric Oncology. *Ann Oncol* 11, 53–8.

17. **Laver J, Amylon M, Desai S, *et al.*** (1998). Randomized trial of r-metHu granulocyte colony-stimulating factor in an intensive treatment for T-cell leukemia and advanced-stage lymphoblastic lymphoma of childhood: a Pediatric Oncology Group pilot study. *J Clin Oncol* 16, 522–6.

18. **Patte C, Laplanche A, Bertozzi AI, *et al.*** (2002). Granulocyte colony-stimulating factor in induction treatment of children with non-Hodgkin's lymphoma: a randomized study of the French Society of Pediatric Oncology. *J Clin Oncol* 20, 441–8.

Chapter 15

Hodgkin disease

Odile Oberlin

Aetiology, biology, epidemiology, and incidence

Hodgkin, in his first description of the disease subsequently named after him, called it lymphogranuloma malignum, a name which remains appropriate.[1] While the aetiology of Hodgkin disease remains unknown, the biology of the disease confirms neoplastic behaviour. Cytogenetic studies suggest that the Reed–Sternberg cells are the malignant cells in Hodgkin disease. Most authorities believe that these cells originate from activated lymphocytes. With present technical progress in the development of single-cell analysis of Hodgkin/Reed–Sternberg cells, it appears that the majority of these cells may represent a B-cell-derived monoclonal population.[2] There are many possible sources of transformation in Hodgkin cells, including cytogenetic abnormalities, evidence for proto-oncogene involvement, and Epstein–Barr virus (EBV) infection and/or activation. There is now strong evidence linking Hodgkin disease with EBV genomes, and gene products can be detected in Reed–Sternberg cells in a proportion of cases. This proportion is $\sim$ 40 per cent in developed countries, but is much higher in countries such as China, Brazil, Costa Rica, and Kenya.[3,4] The heterogeneity of the clinical and histologic appearances of Hodgkin disease and the multitude of different and controversial cellular markers might be explained by the theory that Hodgkin disease is a group of pathophysiologically associated, but not identical, disease entities. The origin could be the same target cell transformed at different stages of maturation, or there could be several biologically related diseases, each with a different pathogenesis.

The disease has been reported to occur more frequently among young children from developing countries than among those from countries of advanced socio-economic status. Genetic factors are implicated to explain ethnic variations and familial history of Hodgkin disease, with an increased risk of disease among parents, siblings, and identical twins.[5,6] It has been suggested in a number of studies that susceptibility to Hodgkin disease is influenced by the HLA class II region. One of the underlying mechanisms could be the influence of this factor on the immune response to an infectious agent,[7] and detailed HLA studies may help to elucidate the complex variations between populations in the risk of Hodgkin disease and its principal subtypes. An increased incidence is observed in patients with congenital immuno-deficiency such as ataxia–telangectasia.[8]

Age-specific incidence rates reveal a characteristically bimodal curve, with the first peak at age 15–30 years and a second peak at age 45–55 years. Thus, children <15 years of age represent the minority. There is a male predominance in patients aged <10 years. However, during the adolescent peak both sexes are affected equally.[9]

Diagnosis and pathology

Accurate diagnosis of Hodgkin disease can be made only by microscopic examination of one or more tissue specimens. It is best to perform an excisional biopsy of an enlarged lymph node. Definitive diagnosis from extranodal tissue, such as lung or bone marrow, is much more difficult. Needle-aspiration biopsy and frozen section material are not optimal for examining the architecture and stromal cellular pattern of a lymph node. Identification of the characteristic Reed–Sternberg cell, a large multinucleated giant cell with inclusion-like nucleoli, facilitates the diagnosis of Hodgkin disease. However, the presence of these cells alone does not confirm the histological diagnosis, since cells of similar appearance have been found in reactive processes including infectious mononucleosis, phenytoin-induced pseudolymphoma, rubeola, graft versus host disease, and non-Hodgkin lymphoma.

The Rye classification has been replaced by the Revised European–American Lymphoma (REAL) classification in which the nodular lymphocyte predominance subtype is now recognized as a separate entity and distinguished from the classical type Hodgkin lymphoma, which includes lymphocyte-rich, mixed cellularity, and nodular sclerosis subtypes. Lymphocyte depletion has been maintained as an extremely rare subtype, and cases otherwise not subtyped are diagnosed as classical Hodgkin lymphoma, unclassifiable (Table 15.1).[10]

In Europe and the USA, the majority of children present with nodular sclerosis.[11–13] In developing countries, mixed cellularity is more common.[14] Even in Europe and the USA, the distribution of histological subtypes varies with age, with the nodular sclerosis subtype being more common in adolescents and adults than in young children. Conversely, mixed cellularity is more common in young children than in adolescents.

Histological subtypes also correlate with certain patterns of disease. The lymphocyte-predominant type is often associated with localized cervical or inguinal–femoral disease, while the nodular sclerosing subtype commonly presents in the mediastinum. The mixed cellularity and lymphocyte-depletion subtypes often present with advanced stage disease.

Clinical presentation and staging

Painless cervical lymphadenopathy is the most common presenting sign in children with Hodgkin disease, often with a fluctuating course leading to a delay in diagnosis. While 80 per cent of children present with neck disease, only 60 per cent have mediastinal involvement. Fewer than 5 per cent present with disease limited to the upper cervical lymph nodes, above the level of the hyoid bone. The majority of patients present with supradiaphragmatic disease, although subdiaphragmatic presentation does not indicate an unfavourable prognosis. Some

Table 15.1. REAL classifications of Hodgkin disease

REAL classification
A. Classical Hodgkin's disease
Lymphocyte-rich classical
Nodular sclerosing
Mixed cellularity
Lymphocyte depletion
B. Nodular lymphocyte predominant

Table 15.2. Staging classification according to the Cotswold revision of the Ann Arbor definitions

Stages

Stage I: Involvement of a single lymph node region or lymphoid structure (e.g. spleen, thymus, Waldeyer's ring)

Stage II: Involvement of two or more lymph node regions on the same side of the diaphragm (the mediastinum is a single site, hilar lymph nodes are lateralized)

Stage III: Involvement of lymph node regions or structures on both sides of the diaphragm
   III 1: With or without splenic hilar, coeliac, or portal nodes
   III 2: With para-aortic, iliac, mesenteric nodes

Stage IV: Diffuse or disseminated involvement of one or more extranodal organs or tissues, with or without associated lymph node involvement.

General symptoms

A: No symptoms

B: Fever, drenching sweats, weight loss
   Unexplained weight loss >10 % body weight during the 6 months before diagnosis
   Unexplained, persistent, or recurrent fever with temperatures >38°C during the previous month
   Recurrent drenching nights sweats during the previous month

Criteria for 'bulky' disease

Mediastinum widening more than one-third of internal transverse diameter of the thorax at T5/6 level on chest radiograph

≥10 cm maximum dimension of nodal mass

E extension

Involvement of a single extranodal site, contiguous or proximal to known nodal site

---

20–30 per cent of children present with systemic B symptoms, as defined by the Ann Arbor staging criteria of fever over 38°C, drenching night sweats, and an unexplained weight loss of >10 per cent of body weight at the time of presentation. The frequency of these symptoms increases with advanced stage of disease. The staging classification now in use has been defined in the Cotswold report (Table 15.2). It incorporated minor revisions but maintained the anatomically orientated nature of the Ann Arbor classification.

Clinical staging involves careful history-taking and physical examination with special attention to the lymphatic system. If an enlarged lymph node is palpable at a site where involvement would influence staging or treatment, it is a wise policy to biopsy the node to assess involvement. Any suspicious lymph nodes should also be biopsied or treated as if involved. Characteristically, involved lymph nodes are not painful or tender but have a 'rubbery' firmness to palpation, often with a variable growth rate. Although involvement of Waldeyer's ring is infrequent, it may present as symmetric tonsillar enlargement; thus examination of the nasopharynx and oropharynx is important.

Routine laboratory studies involved in the staging of children should include a complete blood count, erythrocyte sedimentation rate, and liver function studies including alkaline phosphatase. Eosinophilia occurs in approximately 15 per cent of patients, while lymphopenia, often a sign of advanced disease, is less common. An elevated erythrocyte sedimentation rate is related to both stage and systemic symptoms, and is an important prognostic indicator as well as a useful marker of disease activity. The alkaline phosphatase level is a non-specific indicator of disease activity and is less useful in children than in adults, since it is characteristically elevated as a function of active growth. However, unusually elevated alkaline phosphatase, with or without symptoms of bone pain, is a signal to evaluate the skeletal system by bone scan. Serum copper, also a non-specific marker of disease activity, is useful as an indicator of relapse, but false-positive evaluations of serum copper have been observed in children with Hodgkin disease secondary to inflammatory disease. Elevated serum levels of interleukin 2 receptor and CD8 antigen correlate with advanced disease, B symptoms, and a poor prognosis.[15,16]

A chest radiograph with posteroanterior and lateral views is the first imaging. A mediastinal mass ratio of greater than one-third of the intrathoracic diameter is generally considered to represent advanced disease, which is optimally treated more aggressively than is limited disease.

Thoracic CT defines the status of intrathoracic lymph node groups (including hila and cardiophrenic angle), lung parenchyma, pericardium, pleura, and chest wall. The major value of CT is in the detection of subtle mediastinal adenopathy in the child with an apparently normal chest radiograph; it is also of value in the child with obvious intrathoracic disease. In $\sim$ 50 per cent of previously untreated patients, disease including pericardial or chest wall invasion, retrocardiac masses, and pulmonary parenchymal involvement is discovered on thoracic CT after having been previously missed on plain film. The value of MRI in the staging of the chest is being evaluated. It appears to be complementary to CT but of less value in assessing the pulmonary parenchyma than is the thoracic CT. Although mediastinal adenopathy is common, hilar adenopathy is less so and rarely appears in the absence of mediastinal adenopathy. Pulmonary and pleural involvement is also uncommon and seldom occurs without mediastinal/hilar disease. Pleural effusions may be commonly seen, but are usually secondary to lymphatic obstruction from large central disease and are rarely cytologically positive for Hodgkin disease. Children present the unique problem of how to differentiate the normal thymus gland from thymic infiltration with Hodgkin disease. Thymic involution secondary to immunosuppressive chemotherapy with subsequent thymic enlargement following cessation of chemotherapy has been observed, and may be mistaken for disease progression.

Optimal imaging studies for subdiaphragmatic and retroperitoneal areas have been a matter of controversy for a long time. Lymphography is useful for detecting involved retroperitoneal lymph nodes, visualizing both size and architecture of these nodes. However, this procedure is technically difficult, requires general anaesthesia in young children, and cannot be performed in patients with massive mediastinal and lung involvement. Abdominopelvic CT scan and ultrasound are easier and less invasive procedures than a lymphogram. The accuracy of current CT scans and ultrasound has progressively improved; they are now more accurate than the lymphogram, providing information not only on all the abdominal nodes, but also on the echogenicity of the spleen and liver.

Radionuclide studies have limited usefulness in Hodgkin disease. Routine liver and spleen scans are not useful. Although gallium scanning is often employed, it has limited accuracy in subdiaphragmatic sites, with true-positive findings (sensitivity) in only $\sim$ 40 per cent of patients. Technetium-99 m bone scanning is helpful in symptomatic children with bone complaints and in those with an unexplained elevation of serum alkaline phosphatase.

Bone marrow biopsies should be performed in all children with systemic symptoms and in those with clinical stage III or IV disease. The bone marrow needle biopsy has a low yield of involvement in children with supradiaphragmatic clinical stage IA and IIA disease. Bone marrow aspiration is not adequate for the staging of Hodgkin disease and is not an alternative to percutaneous needle or open bone marrow biopsy.

Staging laparotomy was the gold standard when radiotherapy was used as a single modality therapy; it was indicated to determine the radiotherapy volumes. However, this procedure became questionable when other treatment options were chosen, such as chemotherapy combined with radiation therapy, and such strategies demonstrated that chemotherapy can control radiologically inapparent disease in the vast majority of patients.

Therapy

Treatment for children with Hodgkin disease may involve radiotherapy, chemotherapy, or combined modality therapy. Many of the guidelines determined from studies in adults may be applied to children, since young age is a favourable prognostic indicator and children fare as well as or better than adults. However, when planning treatment programmes for the paediatric population who are undergoing active growth and development at the time of diagnosis and treatment, practical consideration must be given to tissue development and organ function.

Late consequences of treatment

High-dose large-volume radiotherapy administered to young and prepubescent children is known to result in impairment of soft tissue and bone growth. The growth disturbance is related largely to the age of the child at the time of treatment and the radiation dose administered.[17] The most marked impairment is observed when radiation doses >35 Gy are given to children <13 years old.[18] It appears that doses <25 Gy do not cause the disproportionate standing- and sitting-height abnormalities seen with higher doses. Thus a dose of 25 Gy, in fractions of 1.8–2 Gy, may be a threshold beyond which growth retardation is more likely to occur.

Gonadal toxicity in both boys and girls remains a major problem. Pelvic lymph node irradiation is known to carry a high likelihood of ablating ovarian function. The likelihood of maintaining ovarian function following radiotherapy is directly related to pelvic dose and age at the time of treatment. The younger the girl at the time of treatment, the higher the probability of maintenance of regular menses following therapy. Oophoropexy with appropriate shielding at the time of radiotherapy has allowed the preservation of ovarian function, and normal pregnancies after such a procedure have been reported. The pregnancies have been uncomplicated, the offspring normal, and there has been no increased fetal wastage or spontaneous abortion.

In contrast with girls, the issue of sterility in boys is of much greater severity and requires longer periods of follow-up for accurate assessment. High doses of irradiation to the pelvis, in a standard inverted-Y field, may be associated with transient oligospermia or azoospermia. Testicular shields should be routinely used during pelvic radiotherapy, although they are anatomically difficult to use effectively in prepubertal boys. Testicular injury following combination chemotherapy, specifically mustard, oncovin, procarbazine, and prednisone (MOPP), is more complete than that observed following radiotherapy. There are no data to suggest that the prepubertal testis is in any way protected from the testicular injury that is observed among pubertal boys receiving six cycles of MOPP chemotherapy.[19] However, some data now suggest potential recovery of spermatogenesis 12–15 years after six cycles of MOPP.[20] The adriamycin–bleomycin–vinblastine–DTIC (ABVD) combination appears to carry a lower risk of sterility.[21]

Hypothyroidism, as judged by an elevated level of thyroid-stimulating hormone, is common following mantle irradiation. The incidence of elevated thyroid-stimulating hormone in children with Hodgkin disease is higher than in adults, suggesting a greater sensitivity of the thyroid in the rapidly growing pre-adolescent or adolescent age group. The risk of hypothyroidism appears to be related to radiation dose.[22] Among children who receive neck irradiation of ≤26 Gy, the incidence of hypothyroidism is only 17 per cent compared with 78 per cent incidence among children who receive doses >26 Gy.[23] Children who are chemically or clinically hypothyroid are candidates for thyroid replacement therapy, as the long-term effect of unopposed stimulation of the thyroid gland is unknown, and both thyroid adenomas and thyroid carcinomas are frequently reported among long-term survivors.[24]

Cardiopulmonary complications may be related to both radiotherapy and chemotherapy. Pneumonitis and fibrosis may result from radiation and/or bleomycin, and are dose and volume dependent. While most children are asymptomatic following radiotherapy, echocardiography and pulmonary function or exercise tests reveal that approximately three-quarters have some abnormalities in pulmonary function.[25] In combined modality programmes, pulmonary dysfunction appears to be related more to the chemotherapy dose than the radiotherapy dose.[26] In the Stanford series of children, who received 15–25 Gy and six cycles of ABVD + MOPP, alterations in pulmonary function were observed in as many as 40 per cent of cases, with abnormalities in diffusing capacity in 55 per cent.[27] The Children's Cancer Study Group reported that 9 per cent of children who received 12 courses of ABVD followed by 21 Gy regional radiation developed grade 3 or 4 pulmonary toxicity, largely abnormalities in carbon monoxide diffusing capacity, and that one child died of pulmonary toxicity.[26] The incidence of pericarditis and pancarditis was reported to be as high as 13 per cent in children during the era when high-dose large-volume mantle radiotherapy was used.[28] However, with the more recent use of low doses of mantle radiation to smaller volumes, radiation-related cardiac injury is much reduced. On the other hand, the addition of adriamycin in the ABVD combination may well enhance cardiac injury. In the Stanford series of children receiving only three cycles of ABVD and low-dose radiation, 14 per cent of asymptomatic children had cardiac abnormalities at short-term follow-up, demonstrated by cardiac nuclear-gated angiogram testing.[27] Longer follow-up is certainly necessary, as premature coronary artery disease with coronary fibrosis and accelerated atherogenesis has been observed in long-term survivors of Hodgkin disease. The true risk of cardiac and pulmonary injury following current therapy remains unknown, but may be responsible for late mortality of cured patients.[29]

Second malignant tumours represent a major concern for those who treat children with Hodgkin disease, most of whom will be successfully treated and will have a very long lifespan. Large studies on survivors of childhood Hodgkin disease show that the incidence of any second neoplasm 15 years after diagnosis is 6–8 per cent.[30–33] The Late Effects Study Group (LESG) followed a cohort of 1380 patients treated for Hodgkin disease between 1955 and 1986. They reported that the risk of leukaemia reaches a plateau of 2.8 per cent at 15 years, while the incidence of solid second tumours continues to rise even 25 years after diagnosis. The study demonstrated that the incidence of leukaemias is related to the doses of alkylating agent chemotherapy given. All these studies emphasize the high risk of developing breast cancer. In the LESG study, the estimated cumulative probability approached 35 per cent at 40 years of age. Older age at diagnosis (10–16 years versus. <10 years) and a higher dose of radiation (20–40 Gy versus <20 Gy) were associated with increased risk of breast cancer.[30] This mandates adequate surveillance and screening of this very-high-risk population.

Psychosocial problems among young people with Hodgkin disease include a decline in energy and sexual activity, perception of impaired body image, work-related problems, and difficulties in obtaining health insurance. These problems have received little attention but are extremely important issues for the child who is cured of his or her disease.

Because of the known late effects of both chemotherapy and radiotherapy in children, arguments for the last 15 years have been in favour of single modality treatments to minimize the toxicity of therapy. The different approaches available will be summarized and the advantages of combined modality treatment discussed.

Radiation therapy alone

Even adults, for whom late effects linked to growth do not occur, the choice between radiation therapy alone or combined with chemotherapy in favourable cases continues to be a point of controversy. Several criteria have been defined as indications for combined modality treatment in adults: massive mediastinal mass, B symptoms, the dissemination of Hodgkin lymphoma to three or more lymph node areas, infra-diaphragmatic disease, an elevated erythrocyte sedimentation rate, and mixed cellularity or lymphocyte-depleted subtype. The French EORTC–GELA group demonstrated that three cycles of MOPP and involved field are more effective than subtotal nodal irradiation in adults with favourable supradiaphragmatic clinical stage I–II.[34] Moreover, in this subgroup of patients selected for radiation therapy alone, laparotomy and splenectomy should be included in the staging procedure to delineate the radiation fields, although these procedures have inherent risks. High doses (40–44 Gy) and extended fields, such as subtotal nodal irradiation, are required.

The British experience of radiation alone as a single treatment for stage I showed a 92 per cent overall survival, but 30 per cent of the children relapsed and required salvage chemotherapy.[35] This rate that seems too high considering the results of similar patients treated by a short chemotherapy course and low-dose radiation.[11,36]

Chemotherapy alone or combined modality therapy?

As soon as chemotherapy was proved to be effective, the next question was whether children could be cured without the use of radiation. The rationale for most protocols based on chemotherapy alone was always based on the experience of Olweny et al.[37] in Uganda where radiotherapy machines were not available. On the base of these encouraging results, several teams opted for chemotherapy alone. The earliest chemotherapy-alone studies used 6–12 courses of MOPP or MOPP-like regimens.[38–40] Some trials have excluded patients with large nodal masses[38] or large mediastinum.[35] In all these studies, children received at least four cycles, and generally six or more cycles, of chemotherapy including alkylating agents and procarbazine. In our paediatric and adult experience, six cycles of MOPP induce male sterility in >90 per cent of patients[20,41] as well as an increased risk of secondary leukemia[42] that we consider unjustifiable.

The German–Austrian HD-95 study evaluated the possibility of avoiding radiation therapy in children in complete remission after induction chemotherapy tailored to the stage at diagnosis. In the low-risk group (stage I–IIA), relapse-free survival was similar for irradiated and non-irradiated patients, whereas relapse-free survival was significantly lower in non-irradiated than in irradiated patients at more advanced stages (stages IIB–IV).[43]

There have been three large randomized paediatric trials addressing the question of the efficacy of chemotherapy alone versus chemotherapy combined with radiation therapy.

The US Paediatric Oncology Group (POG) compared four cycles of MOPP plus four cycles of ABVD with or without 21 Gy total or subtotal nodal irradiation in children with stages IIB, IIIA2, IIIB, and IV disease. The event-free survival (EFS) rates of the two arms were not statistically different using an 'intent to treat' analysis.[44] However, when considering the treatment actually delivered, superior results were observed in children treated with chemotherapy plus radiation therapy. Survival was comparable in the two groups (94 per cent and 88 per cent, respectively).[45]

A randomized study was conducted in stage III and IV disease by the US Children's Cancer Group (CCG) comparing MOPP alternating with ABVD for 12 months with ABVD for

6 months followed by 21 Gy irradiation. The EFS rates of the two schedules were similar (87 and 77 per cent).[46] The addition of radiotherapy did not seem to offer a significant advantage over chemotherapy alone. However, it is noteworthy that the children treated by chemotherapy alone in this study received 12 cycles of chemotherapy (six MOPP and six ABVD). The risks of six cycles of MOPP have already been mentioned. Six cycles of ABVD lead to high cumulative doses of adriamycin (300 mg/m²) and bleomycin (120 mg/m²). These doses account for the very high pulmonary toxicity, with one death reported in this study. These results should dissuade physicians from administering so many courses of ABVD in combination with radiation therapy to the mediastinum.[26] The same comments apply to the potential late toxicity of the six cycles of ABVD given in the Dutch study attempting to treat patients with stage I–IV disease by chemotherapy alone.[47]

The CCG investigated whether radiation could be omitted in patients achieving a complete response to chemotherapy. The chemotherapy was stratified according to stage. Children with stages I–III disease were given chlorambucil–vincristine–procarbazine–prednisone (COPP) plus adriamycin–bleomycin–vinblastine (ABV); stage IV patients received additional cytarabine–etoposide combinations. Patients who achieved a complete response after chemotherapy were randomized to receive 21 Gy involved field or no further treatment. There was no difference in the overall survival rates of the two groups, but there was an advantage for the combined modality arm in terms of EFS (92 versus 87 per cent) which was even more impressive with an 'as-treated' analysis (93 versus 85 per cent).[48]

The known late effects of splenectomy, high-dose radiation therapy, and high cumulative doses of chemotherapy and the improved outcome for children treated with combined modality therapy argue in favour of the wide use of combined modality therapy to treat childhood Hodgkin disease. Such an approach would enable a gradual decrease of both radiation therapy and chemotherapy.

Risk-adapted combined modality treatment and prognostic factors for reducing therapy

Reducing the duration of chemotherapy and avoiding MOPP

MOPP chemotherapy was the standard regimen for many years until the effectiveness of ABVD was established, first in patients who had failed MOPP and then as front-line chemotherapy, using six cycles or more in advanced stages. Compared with MOPP, second malignancies and sterility were less common. The predominant adverse effects of ABVD are pulmonary toxicity related to bleomycin and cardiovascular toxicity secondary to adriamycin. The intention was to use a short chemotherapy course, decreasing the number of cycles of MOPP while also diminishing the side effects associated with six cycles of ABVD. In the first French cooperative study, patients with stage I and II disease were randomized and treated with either four cycles of ABVD or two cycles each of MOPP and ABVD. Patients with more advanced stages (IB, IIB, III, and IV) were treated with three cycles each of MOPP and ABVD. Radiation was delivered at a dose of 20 Gy in patients who had a good response to chemotherapy; otherwise the classical 40 Gy dose was used. The conclusion of that study was that, in favourable stages, ABVD alone was equivalent to MOPP combined with ABVD and that chemotherapy followed by 20 Gy radiation was a valid approach in the vast majority of children.[49] The Milan paediatric team corroborated the efficacy of three cycles of ABVD alone combined with low-dose radiation therapy in a non-randomized study.[50]

Even in patients with more advanced disease (stage III), the results of the French studies showed that the number of MOPP + ABVD courses could be reduced from the six used in the MDH82 study to four courses in the MDH90 study without compromising the excellent 96 per cent survival.[49,51]

Using other combinations than MOPP or ABVD

Up to 1985, the German paediatric group used vincristine, prednisone, and procarbazine at MOPP doses, combined with adriamycin (OPPA) and COPP (cycles comparable to MOPP but with cyclophosphamide replacing mustine). In 1985, this group initiated a study to try to eliminate procarbazine. OPPA became OPA, and methotrexate replaced procarbazine in the COPP combination, giving rise to the COMP regimen. Progressions and relapses were significantly higher in advanced stages than in the preceding protocol, and so the study was stopped prematurely on the grounds that a more effective drug was needed to replace procarbazine.[52]

Active drugs which are non-toxic or have acceptable toxicity are few in Hodgkin disease. Data indicated etoposide as a potential alternative, and this drug has been included in the German–Austrian studies in place of procarbazine in OPPA, which became OEPA in the German HD90 study.[12]

Adapting the treatment strategy to the initial response to chemotherapy

The SFOP MDH90 study adopted such a strategy for patients with stage I and II disease. As induction chemotherapy, all were given vinblastine, bleomycin, VP16-etoposide, and prednisone (VBVP) without alkylating agents and doxorubicin. Based on radiological evaluation, patients achieving a good response were given 20 Gy involved field radiation. Poorly responding patients were given one or two additional cycles of OPPA (vincristine, procarbazine, prednisone, and adriamycin–doxorubicin). Radiation therapy dose was decided according to evaluation after OPPA: 20 Gy for good responders and 40 Gy for poor responders. For the 202 patients included in the study, the 5-year survival and EFS were 97 per cent and 91 per cent, respectively. Altogether, 86 per cent of the children were cured with only four courses of VBVP and 20 Gy radiation; 14 per cent received additional OPPA cycles or a higher radiation dose. Significant predictors of worse EFS were nodular sclerosis histology, haemoglobin <10.5 g/dl and the presence of B biological factors.[11]

Identification of factors to select children at low or high risk of relapse

Identification of factors to select children at low or high risk of relapse is of paramount importance to tailor the intensity and duration of treatment.

In the German–Austrian DAL-HD 90 study, significant univariate predictive factors for EFS were nodular sclerosis type 2 histology, presence of B symptoms, number of involved regions, and treatment groups. There was a higher risk for patients with bulky compared with non-bulky disease. In the multiple regression model, only nodular sclerosis type 2 and B symptoms remained strong predictive factors.[53]

Smith et al.[13] developed a prognostic index based on five pretreatment factors associated with poorer disease-free survival on multivariate analysis : male gender, stage IIB–IIB or IV, bulky mediastinal disease; white blood cell count > 13.500/mm^3, and haemoglobin <11.0 /dl.

The Stanford, Dana–Farber and St Jude Children's Research Hospital obtained excellent results (5-year survival and EFS were 99 per cent and 93 per cent, respectively) in a very selective group of patients (clinical stage I and II without bulky disease or B symptoms). Nodular sclerosing histology and number of involved nodes had an impact on the failure rate, and all the failures occurred in patients with this histological subtype.[36] The subgroup of patients treated in this study represents only 34 per cent of the whole cohort of children with Hodgkin disease, in contrast with the French study in which 60 per cent of the children were treated.[11]

The combined modality regimens used in both these studies are not associated with any serious toxicity, which confirms that favourable-risk Hodgkin disease can be cured with therapy which excludes alkylating agents and doxorubicin (in the first study) and etoposide and bleomycin in the second.[11,36]

Poor prognosis Hodgkin disease in childhood

Stage IV disease has the most dismal outcome. As only 8–16 per cent of children have stage IV disease, the absolute number in published series is often small. The results of several studies demonstrate that these patients fare significantly worse than those with less advanced disease. For instance, the EFS of such cases was only 55 per cent in the British study,[54] 61 per cent in the first French study,[49] 67 per cent in the CCG study,[46] and 69 per cent in the Boston series.[55] The German–Austrian group obtained the best results in two consecutive multicentric studies. They were based on surgical staging and chemotherapy with two cycles of OPPA and four cycles of COPP, as previously described. Radiation therapy was given to involved nodes (25 Gy) and involved extra-lymphatic organs (12–15 Gy).[56]

In 1987 an intergroup study for stage IV was initiated within the SIOP group (International Society of Paediatric Oncology), attempting to reproduce the good German results internationally and to limit the radiation dose to 20 Gy after a good response to chemotherapy. The study included 115 children from six countries. The 5-year overall survival was 90 per cent and the disease-free survival was 85 per cent, similar to the 81 per cent observed in the previous German studies. These results confirm that OPPA–COPP chemotherapy followed by 20 Gy is a valid therapeutic approach for stage IV in children.[57]

Patients with refractory or relapsed disease form the second group with a poor prognosis. Attempts have been made to improve the efficacy of chemotherapy by incorporating new drugs into standard regimens or using dose intensification with stem cell rescue.

Etoposide, which has already been mentioned, has been included by several teams in third-line conventional therapy after MOPP and anthracycline-containing regimens. The MIME (methyl GAG, ifosfamide, methotrexate, and etoposide) and MINE [derived from MIME but with an increased dose of ifosfamide and VP16, and vinorelbine (Navelbine)] regimens have yielded response rates of 66 per cent and 75 per cent, respectively, in disease refractory to standard chemotherapy.[58,59]

The relative resistance of tumour cells to cytotoxics can be overcome by administering very high doses of drugs with bone marrow or peripheral stem cell support. Encouraging results have been obtained in adults, with protracted responses in refractory disease. The paediatric experience is limited, as the number of children who enter this high-risk group is small. However, as their outcome is comparable to that of adults, they should be treated according to the same modality. In the Stanford experience, idiopathic lung injury syndrome occurred in 44 per cent of the patients and a quarter of them died from pulmonary failure. The high-dose regimens consisted of cyclophosphamide and etoposide combined with carmustine, chloroethylcyclohexylnitrosurea, or fractionated total body irradiation.[60] Interstitial pneumonitis was also observed in two out of 22 patients[61] and two out of 53 patients[62] in the other two series The toxicity of high-dose regimens remains the major constraint to widening the indications for transplantation in high-risk patients.

An unanswered question: How should one treat lymphocyte-predominant Hodgkin disease?

Lymphocyte-predominant Hodgkin disease (LPHD) is reported to present typically as early stage disease, with slow progression and an excellent outcome with standard therapy.[63,64] In contrast with tumour cells of the classical Hodgkin/Reed–Sternberg type, the tumour cells of LPHD express B-cell antigens such as CD20 and rarely express CD15 or CD30, supporting the fact that LPHD is a malignant B-cell lymphoma of germinal center origin. A tendency towards more secondary non–Hodgkin lymphomas is noted, but this remains equivocal. On the basis of what is proposed for stage I follicular lymphoma, a 'watch and wait' strategy, in which no immediate therapy is given, could be tested for patients who are without residual disease after surgery; the main advantage of this approach is the avoidance of unwanted effects of radiotherapy or chemotherapy. The use of rituximab (anti-CD20 antibody) is attractive, and a phase II study revealed an overall response rate of 100 per cent.[65] Larger studies are warranted to prove the long-term efficacy and tolerability of this therapy. Overall, the question of how to treat such patients, either by reducing treatment intensity or following a 'watch and wait' approach, remains unanswered.

Conclusion

The results of recent studies suggest that the cure rate whose curve was constantly rising between 1960 and 1980 has reached a plateau. Since 1980, efforts have been directed towards curing the disease with a minimal amount of morbidity. Combined modality therapy is clearly a strategy allowing the administration of less toxic truncated chemotherapy and low-dose limited-field radiation therapy. It will be difficult to improve drastically upon the present. The efforts currently deployed to cure patients with chemotherapy without recourse to procarbazine and adriamycin are encouraging in favourable cases.

We hope that during the next decade progress in the field of biology will help us to understand the aetiology and pathogenesis of Hodgkin disease and its apparent heterogeneity, and help us to continue refining therapy at a reduced cost.

References

1. **Wallhauser A** (1933). Hodgkin's disease. *Arkh Patol* 16, 522–62.
2. **Wolf J, Bohlen H, Diehl V** (1996). Report on the biology workshop of the Third International Symposium on Hodgkin's Lymphoma in Cologne 1995. *Ann Oncol* 7 (Suppl 4), 45–7.
3. **Jarrett AF, Armstrong AA, Alexander E** (1996). Epidemiology of EBV and Hodgkin's lymphoma. *Ann Oncol* 7 (Suppl) 4, 5–10.
4. **Weinreb M, Day PJ, Niggli F,** *et al.* (1996). The role of Epstein–Barr virus in Hodgkin's disease from different geographical areas. *Arch Dis Child* 74, 27–31.
5. **Ferraris AM, Racchi O, Rapezzi D, Gaetani GF, Boffetta P** (1997). Familial Hodgkin's disease: a disease of young adulthood? *Ann Hematol* 74, 131–4.
6. **Mack TM, Cozen W, Shibata DK,** *et al.* (1995). Concordance for Hodgkin's disease in identical twins suggesting genetic susceptibility to the young-adult form of the disease. *N Engl J Med* 332, 413–18.
7. **Taylor GM, Gokhale DA, Crowther D,** *et al.* (1999). Further investigation of the role of HLA-DPB1 in adult Hodgkin's disease (HD) suggests an influence on susceptibility to different HD subtypes, *Br J Cancer* 80, 1405–11.
8. **Sandoval C, Swift M** (2003). Hodgkin disease in ataxia–telangiectasia patients with poor outcomes. *Med Pediatr Oncol* 40, 162–6.

9. Cartwright RA, Gurney KA, Moorman AV (2002). Sex ratios and the risks of haematological malignancies, *Br J Haematol* 118, 1071–7.

10. Harris NL, Jaffe ES, Stein H, *et al.* (1994). A revised European–American classification of lymphoid neoplasms: a proposal from the International Lymphoma Study Group. *Blood* 84, 1361–92.

11. Landman-Parker J, Pacquement H, Leblanc T, *et al.* (2000). Localized childhood Hodgkin's disease: response-adapted chemotherapy with etoposide, bleomycin, vinblastine, and prednisone before low-dose radiation therapy-results of the French Society of Pediatric Oncology Study MDH90, *J Clin Oncol* 18, 1500–7.

12. Schellong G, Potter R, Bramswig J, *et al.* (1999). High cure rates and reduced long-term toxicity in pediatric Hodgkin's disease: the German–Austrian multicenter trial DAL-HD-90. The German–Austrian Pediatric Hodgkin's Disease Study Group. *J Clin Oncol* 17, 3736–44.

13. Smith RS, Chen Q, Hudson MM, *et al.* (2003). Prognostic factors for children with Hodgkin's disease treated with combined modality therapy. *J Clin Oncol* 21, 2026–33.

14. Buyukpamukcu M, Atahan L, Caglar M, Kutluk T, Akyuz C, Hazar V (1999). Hodgkin's disease in Turkish children: clinical characteristics and treatment results of 210 patients. *Pediatr Hematol Oncol* 16, 119–29.

15. Nadali G, Tavecchia L, Zanolin E, *et al.* (1998). Serum level of the soluble form of the CD30 molecule identifies patients with Hodgkin's disease at high risk of unfavorable outcome. *Blood* 91, 3011–16.

16. Pui CH, Ip SH, Thompson E, *et al.* (1989). Increased serum CD8 antigen level in childhood Hodgkin's disease relates to advanced stage and poor treatment outcome. *Blood* 73, 209–13.

17. Papadakis V, Tan C, Heller G, Sklar C (1996). Growth and final height after treatment for childhood Hodgkin's disease. *J Pediatr Hematol Oncol* 18, 272–6.

18. Donaldson SS, Kaplan HS (1982). Complications of treatment of Hodgkin's disease in children. *Cancer Treat Rep* 66, 977–89.

19. Heikens J, Behrendt H, Adriaanse R, Berghout A (1996). Irreversible gonadal damage in male survivors of pediatric Hodgkin's disease. *Cancer* 78, 2020–4

20. Ortin TT, Shostak CA, Donaldson SS (1990). Gonadal status and reproductive function following treatment for Hodgkin's disease in childhood: the Stanford experience. *Int J Radiat Oncol Biol Phys* 19, 873–80.

21. Kulkarni SS, Sastry PS, Saikia TK, Parikh PM, Gopal R, Advani SH (1997). Gonadal function following ABVD therapy for Hodgkin's disease. *Am J Clin Oncol* 20, 354–7.

22. Sklar C, Whitton J, Mertens A, *et al.* (2000). Abnormalities of the thyroid in survivors of Hodgkin's disease: data from the Childhood Cancer Survivor Study. *J Clin Endocrinol Metab* 85, 3227–32.

23. Constine LS, Donaldson SS, McDougall IR, Cox RS, Link MP, Kaplan HS (1984). Thyroid dysfunction after radiotherapy in children with Hodgkin's disease. *Cancer* 53, 878–83.

24. Shafford EA, Kingston JE, Healy JC, Webb JA, Plowman PN, Reznek RH (1999). Thyroid nodular disease after radiotherapy to the neck for childhood Hodgkin's disease. *Br J Cancer* 80, 808–14.

25. Kadota RP, Burgert EO Jr, Driscoll DJ, Evans RG, Gilchrist GS (1988). Cardiopulmonary function in long-term survivors of childhood Hodgkin's lymphoma: a pilot study. *Mayo Clin Proc* 63, 362–7.

26. Fryer CJ, Hutchinson RJ, Krailo M, *et al.* (1990). Efficacy and toxicity of 12 courses of ABVD chemotherapy followed by low-dose regional radiation in advanced Hodgkin's disease in children: a report from the Children's Cancer Study Group. *J Clin Oncol* 8, 1971–80.

27. Mefferd JM, Donaldson SS, Link MP (1989). Pediatric Hodgkin's disease: pulmonary, cardiac, and thyroid function following combined modality therapy. *Int J Radiat Oncol Biol Phys* 16, 679–85.

28. Schellong G, Bramswig JH, Hornig-Franz I, Schwarze EW, Potter R, Wannenmacher M (1994). Hodgkin's disease in children: combined modality treatment for stages IA, IB, and IIA. Results in 356 patients of the German–Austrian Pediatric Study Group. *Ann Oncol* 5 (Suppl 2), 113–15.

29. **Hudson MM, Poquette CA, Lee J, et al.** (1998). Increased mortality after successful treatment for Hodgkin's disease. *J Clin Oncol* 16, 3592–600.

30. **Bhatia S, Robison LL, Oberlin O, et al.** (1996). Breast cancer and other second neoplasms after childhood Hodgkin's disease. *N Engl J Med* 334, 745–51.

31. **Metayer C, Lynch CF, Clarke EA, et al.** (2000). Second cancers among long-term survivors of Hodgkin's disease diagnosed in childhood and adolescence. *J Clin Oncol* 18, 2435–43.

32. **Sankila R, Garwicz S, Olsen JH, et al.** (1996). Risk of subsequent malignant neoplasms among 1641 Hodgkin's disease patients diagnosed in childhood and adolescence: a population-based cohort study in the five Nordic countries. Association of the Nordic Cancer Registries and the Nordic Society of Pediatric Hematology and Oncology. *J Clin Oncol* 14, 1442–6.

33. **Shah AB, Hudson MM, Poquette CA, Luo X, Wilimas JA, Kun LE** (1999). Long-term follow-up of patients treated with primary radiotherapy for supradiaphragmatic Hodgkin's disease at St Jude Children's Research Hospital. *Int J Radiat Oncol Biol Phys* 44, 867–77.

34. **Hagenbeek A, Eghbali H, Ferme C, et al.** (2001). Three cycles of MOPP/ABV hybrid and involved-field irradiation is more effective than subtotal nodal irradiation in favorable supradiaphragmatic clinical stages I–II Hodgkin's disease. *Blood* 96, 575a.

35. **Shankar AG, Ashley S, Radford M, Barrett A, Wright D, Pinkerton CR** (1997). Does histology influence outcome in childhood Hodgkin's disease? Results from the United Kingdom Children's Cancer Study Group. *J Clin Oncol* 15, 2622–30.

36. **Donaldson SS, Hudson MM, Lamborn KR, et al.** (2002). VAMP and low-dose, involved-field radiation for children and adolescents with favorable, early-stage Hodgkin's disease: results of a prospective clinical trial. *J Clin Oncol* 20, 3081–7.

37. **Olweny CL, Katongole-Mbidde E, Kiire C, Lwanga SK, Magrath I, Ziegler JL** (1978). Childhood Hodgkin's disease in Uganda: a ten year experience. *Cancer* 42, 787–92.

38. **Behrendt H, Van Bunningen BN, Van Leeuwen EF** (1987). Treatment of Hodgkin's disease in children with or without radiotherapy. *Cancer* 59, 1870–3.

39. **Ekert H, Waters KD, Smith PJ, Toogood I, Mauger D** (1988). Treatment with MOPP or ChlVPP chemotherapy only for all stages of childhood Hodgkin's disease. *J Clin Oncol* 6, 1845–50.

40. **Martin J, Radford M** (1989). Current practice in Hodgkin's disease. The United Kingdom Children's Cancer Study Group. *Cancer Treat Res* 41, 263–9.

41. **Aubier F, Patte C, de Vathaire F, et al.** (1995). Male fertility after chemotherapy during childhood. *Ann Endocrinol (Paris)* 56, 141–2.

42. **Meadows AT, Obringer AC, Marrero O, et al.** (1989). Second malignant neoplasms following childhood Hodgkin's disease: treatment and splenectomy as risk factors. *Med Pediatr Oncol* 17, 477–484

43. **Dörffel W** (2001). The GPOH experience OPPA/OEPA plus COPP in children and adolescents. *Leuk Lymphoma* 42 (Suppl 2), 17.

44. **Weiner MA, Leventhal B, Brecher ML, et al.** (1997). Randomized study of intensive MOPP–ABVD with or without low-dose total-nodal radiation therapy in the treatment of stages IIB, IIIA2, IIIB, and IV Hodgkin's disease in pediatric patients: a Pediatric Oncology Group study. *J Clin Oncol* 15, 2769–79.

45. **Marcus RB, Weiner MA, Chauvenet A** (1998). Radiation in pediatric Hodgkin's disease. In reply. *J Clin Oncol* 16, 392–2.

46. **Hutchinson RJ, Fryer CJ, Davis PC, et al.** (1998). MOPP or radiation in addition to ABVD in the treatment of pathologically staged advanced Hodgkin's disease in children: results of the Children's Cancer Group Phase III Trial. *J Clin Oncol* 16, 897–906.

47. **Behrendt H, Brinkhuis M, Van Leeuwen EF** (1996). Treatment of childhood Hodgkin's disease with ABVD without radiotherapy. *Med Pediatr Oncol* 26, 244–8.

48. **Nachman JB, Sposto R, Herzog P, et al.** (2002). Randomized comparison of low-dose involved-field radiotherapy and no radiotherapy for children with Hodgkin's disease who achieve a complete response to chemotherapy. *J Clin Oncol* **20**, 3765–71.

49. **Oberlin O, Leverger G, Pacquement H, et al.** (1992). Low-dose radiation therapy and reduced chemotherapy in childhood Hodgkin's disease: the experience of the French Society of Pediatric Oncology, *J Clin Oncol* **10**, 1602–8.

50. **Vecchi V, Pileri S, Burnelli R, et al.** (1993). Treatment of pediatric Hodgkin's disease tailored to stage, mediastinal mass, and age. An Italian (AIEOP) multicenter study on 215 patients. *Cancer* **72**, 2049–57.

51. **Pellegrino B, Oberlin O, Leblanc T, et al.** (2002). 2 MOPP + 2 ABVD followed by low dose radiation therapy for children with stage III Hodgkin's lymphoma. *Ann Oncol* **13** (Suppl 2), 30.

52. **Schellong G, Hornig-Franz I, Rath B, et al.** (1994). Reducing radiation dosage to 20–30 Gy in combined chemo-/radiotherapy of Hodgkin's disease in childhood. A report of the cooperative DAL-HD-87 therapy study. *Klin Padiatr* **206**, 253–62.

53. **Dieckmann K, Potter R, Hofmann J, Heinzl H, Wagner W, Schellong G** (2003). Does bulky disease at diagnosis influence outcome in childhood Hodgkin's disease and require higher radiation doses? Results from the German–Austrian Pediatric Multicenter Trial DAL-HD-90. *Int J Radiat Oncol Biol Phys* **56**, 644–52.

54. **Atra A, Higgs E, Capra M, et al.** (2002). ChlVPP chemotherapy in children with stage IV Hodgkin's disease: results of the UKCCSG HD 8201 and HD 9201 studies. *Br J Haematol* **119**, 647–51.

55. **Bader SB, Weinstein H, Mauch P, Silver B, Tarbell NJ** (1993). Pediatric stage IV Hodgkin's disease. Long-term survival. *Cancer* **72**, 249–55.

56. **Schellong G, Bramswig JH, Schwarze EW, Wannenmacher M** (1988). An approach to reduce treatment and invasive staging in childhood Hodgkin's disease: the sequence of the German DAL multicenter studies. *Bull Cancer* **75**, 41–51.

57. **Schellong G, Oberlin O, Vecchi V, et al.** (1998). Stage IV Hodgkin's disease in children: combined modality treatment involving OPPA/COPP chemotherapy. a European study in the International Society of Pediatric Oncology. *Leuk Lymphoma* **29** (Suppl 1), 100.

58. **Ferme C, Bastion Y, Lepage E, et al.** (1995). The MINE regimen as intensive salvage chemotherapy for relapsed and refractory Hodgkin's disease. *Ann Oncol* **6**, 543–9.

59. **Hagemeister FB, Tannir N, McLaughlin P, et al.** (1987). MIME chemotherapy (methyl-GAG, ifosfamide, methotrexate, etoposide) as treatment for recurrent Hodgkin's disease. *J Clin Oncol* **5**, 556–61.

60. **Frankovich J, Donaldson SS, Lee Y, Wong RM, Amylon M, Verneris MR** (2001). High-dose therapy and autologous hematopoietic cell transplantation in children with primary refractory and relapsed Hodgkin's disease: atopy predicts idiopathic diffuse lung injury syndromes. *Biol Blood Marrow Transplant* **7**, 49–57.

61. **Bessa E, Pacquement H, Hartmann O, et al.** (1993). Long term survival of refractory or relapsed Hodgkin's disease treated by high dose chemotherapy with hematopoietic support. *Med Pediatr Oncol* **21**, 552.

62. **Baker KS, Gordon BG, Gross TG, et al.** (1999). Autologous hematopoietic stem-cell transplantation for relapsed or refractory Hodgkin's disease in children and adolescents. *J Clin Oncol* **17**, 825–31.

63. **Diehl V, Sextro M, Franklin J, et al.** (1999). Clinical presentation, course, and prognostic factors in lymphocyte-predominant Hodgkin's disease and lymphocyte-rich classical Hodgkin's disease: report from the European Task Force on Lymphoma Project on Lymphocyte-Predominant Hodgkin's Disease. *J Clin Oncol* **17**, 776–83.

64. **Sandoval C, Venkateswaran L, Billups C, Slim M, Jayabose S, Hudson MM** (2002). Lymphocyte-predominant Hodgkin's disease in children. *J Pediatr Hematol Oncol* **24**, 269–73.

65. **Ekstrand B, Lucas JB, Horowitz S, et al.** (2002). Rituximab in lymphocyte predominant Hodgkins disease (LPHD): results of a phase II trial. *Proc Am Soc Clin Oncol* **21**, 264.

Chapter 16

Langerhans cell histiocytosis

Helmut Gadner and Nicole Grois

Introduction

The term 'histiocytic syndromes' or 'histiocytoses' describes a group of rare and enigmatic syndromes characterized by accumulation and/or proliferation of cells of the mononuclear phagocytic system. This system comprises two groups of immune cells in the tissues: the macrophages as the cardinal phagocytic cells, and the dendritic cells with low phagocytic capacity but highly effective antigen presentation and a potent capability of initiating primary T-lymphocyte responses. Both macrophages and dendritic cells arise from a common CD34+ myeloid precursor cell in the bone marrow. Dendritic cells are primarily situated in connective and lymphoid tissues, as well as in the epithelium; the blood monocytes, which represent the immediate macrophage precursors, transform into tissue-specific macrophages.[1]

In 1997 the Histiocyte Society proposed a new classification of the histiocytic disorders separating those of varied behaviour from those of clearly malignant behaviour.[2] According to this recommendation, histiocytoses are grouped into three classes (Fig. 16.1).

Class I diseases are of dendritic cell origin, with Langerhans cell histiocytosis (LCH) as the most frequent form. Class II disorders, with ordinary histiocytes as lesional cells, include familial haemophagocytic lymphohistiocytosis, infection- or malignancy-associated haemophagocytic syndrome, and sinus histiocytosis with massive lymphadenopathy. Class III embraces truly malignant histiocytic disorders characterized by the presence of histiocytes with malignant features, i.e. acute monocytic leukaemia (FAB M5), and malignant histiocytosis, which is extremely rare since large-cell anaplastic lymphoma has been recognized as a separate non-histiocyte-related entity.

Langerhans cell histiocytosis

Since the first description by Hand in 1893, LCH has remained a poorly understood disorder. The disease comprises a broad spectrum of clinical presentations ranging from spontaneous regression of a solitary lesion to a widespread life-threatening disorder. In the past several synonyms have been used to describe the disease, such as histiocytosis X, eosinophilic granuloma, Hand–Schueller–Christian disease, Abt–Letterer–Siwe disease, etc. Since 1985, 'Langerhans cell histiocytosis' has become the commonly accepted term, acknowledging the central role of the Langerhans cells as the key factor in the various disease forms.[3]

Incidence and epidemiology

LCH can present at any age ranging from the neonatal period to old age. Predominantly young children aged 1–3 years are affected. The incidence in different age groups is about 0.2–1 per 100 000 children per year (median 0.4 per 100 000) with males outnumbering females (ratio

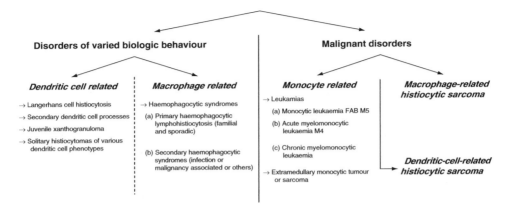

Fig. 16.1 Contemporary classification of histiocytic disorders. Modified from B. E. Favara *et al.* (1997) *Med Pediatr Oncol* **29**, 157–66.

1.7:1). More than a third of children, especially those <2 years old, are prone to 'multisystem' disease with 'organ dysfunction' and no gender preference. The age distribution of LCH manifestations in the paediatric population is illustrated in Figure 16.2.

The disease is essentially sporadic, but has been found associated with congenital anomalies and reported rarely in twins and certain kindreds. In adults, there is some evidence that cigarette smoking plays a key role in the development of pulmonary disease.[2] To date, however, very limited and inconclusive data are available regarding other epidemiologic aspects, i.e. pre- and postnatal risk factors including environmental and genetic risks.[4]

Aetiology and pathogenesis

LCH can be considered as a 'clonal' proliferative neoplasm with highly variable biologic behaviour and clinical severity; however, the question as to what causes the LCH cells to

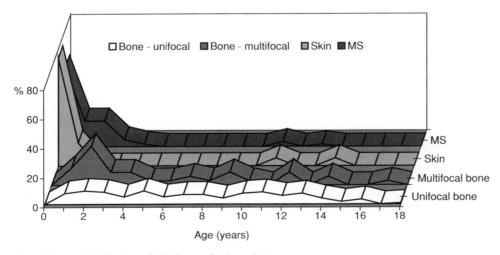

Fig. 16.2 Age distribution of LCH in paediatric patients.

proliferate remains unanswered. Clonality cannot be regarded as a cancer, as there are several examples of inflammatory processes and dermatologic disorders which are clonal but not cancerous.

Viral, immunologic, and genetic causes have been considered for LCH, but so far only hypotheses can be presented. Although viruses might initiate a cytokine cascade leading to a Langerhans cell proliferation, no link between viral infections and LCH has been found. It has also been postulated that LCH is caused by an immunologic dysregulation with a cytokine dysequilibrium ('cytokine storm') derived from an inborn genetic or acquired immune defect. Also, some of the pathologic sequelae of LCH may be explained by the contribution of cytokines such as interleukin 1α (IL-1α) and tumour necrosis factor-α (TNF-α), which enhance osteoclastic activity. The lesional presence of transforming growth factor-β is considered to be related to the evolution of fibrosis in LCH lesions of bone, liver, and lung.[5]

An increasing number of studies recently have demonstrated somatic mutations in LCH, suggesting that a certain genetic instability may be at least a component in the aetiology. These include a loss of heterozygosity in different chromosomal regions of LCH cells, possibly acquired in one or more genes that regulate cell growth, survival, or proliferation, and functional defects in the tumour suppressor gene p53. The association between LCH and other malignancies and, although rarely seen, the documentation of familial cases of LCH also suggest a genetic predisposition.[4]

Another interesting observation in multisystem endstage patients with LCH was the detection of myelodysplastic bone marrow features and the concurrence of LCH with varying degrees of macrophage activation, including fulminant haemophagocytic syndrome. Favara et al.[6] recently hypothesized that LCH might be a final common pathway for several different primary events.

Histopathology

The lesions in LCH consist of an aggregation of dendritic cells of Langerhans type with a variable admixture of other cells (eosinophils, neutrophils, lymphocytes, fibroblasts, and multinucleated giant cells) forming granulomas with proliferative and locally destructive behaviour. The high cellular content of these granulomas decreases gradually, resulting in a xanthomatous and fibrotic pattern. The typical feature of a Langerhans cell (LC) is a 'histiocytic' cell with abundant homogeneous pink cytoplasm in the section stained with haematoxylin and eosin, and a lobulated, 'coffee-bean'-like nucleus. These cells express a number of phenotypic markers, which are also shared by normal LCs and can be demonstrated by immunohistochemistry and electron microscopy.[1]

LCH cells produce a wide variety of cytokines including IL-1, IL-2, IL-3, IL-4, IL-6, IL-8, TNF-α and interferon-γ, which probably reflects the activated state of these cells. Class II MHC molecules and the CD1a complex, together with Birbeck granules, are the most specific markers identifying LCs in tissue specimens. Other markers for LCs are surface ATPase and S-100 protein, but neither of these is cell specific. Activated LCs express the CD4 complex, the IL-2 receptor (IL-2R), and placental alkaline phosphatase (PLAP), which represents a very early transient activation marker. Of further interest is the constitutive expression of the co-stimulatory molecules CD86 and CD80 on LCH cells, and the recently described surface molecule langerin and the actin-binding protein fascin.[4,5]

To avoid difficulties in the distinction of LCH from other histiocytosis syndromes, the histopathologic diagnosis of LCH is based on different confidence levels[3] (Fig. 16.3).

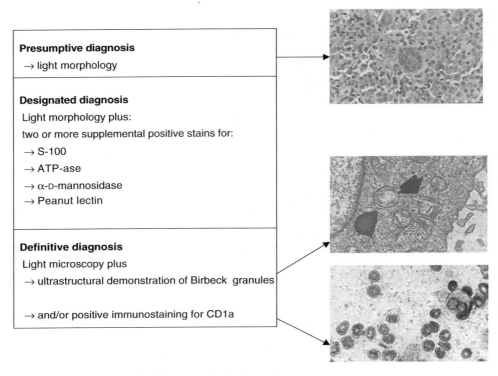

Presumptive diagnosis

→ light morphology

Designated diagnosis

Light morphology plus:

two or more supplemental positive stains for:

→ S-100

→ ATP-ase

→ α-D-mannosidase

→ Peanut lectin

Definitive diagnosis

Light microscopy plus

→ ultrastructural demonstration of Birbeck granules

→ and/or positive immunostaining for CD1a

Fig. 16.3 Confidence levels of histopathologic diagnosis.

Clinical aspects

The clinical manifestations of LCH can range from asymptomatic lesions to significant morbidity depending on the kind and number of organs involved. Almost every organ in the body can be involved, although as yet there are no reports of renal, bladder, gonad, or adrenal involvement. In 'single-system' LCH only one organ/system with localized or multifocal lesions is involved, whereas in 'multisystem' LCH more than one organ/system is affected (Table 16.1).

Bone involvement is found in about 80 per cent of patients. The skull is most frequently affected; other common osseous sites include the vertebrae, long bones, and pelvic bones. Symptoms consist of painful swelling with or without functional impairment. Plain radiography typically shows single or multiple irregularly marginated osteolytic lesions which often appear as a 'punched-out' defect (Fig. 16.4). Pathologic fractures may occur in the weight-bearing bones. In the spine the lytic process can result in compression and collapse of the vertebral body, causing vertebra plana. LCH of the jaws is often associated with hypertrophic gingivitis or 'floating teeth', and proptosis is seen when the orbit is involved. Mastoid or petrous bone lesions may cause persistent otitis with aural discharge, and may lead to hearing impairment.[7,8] Lesions in the craniofacial region (skull base, temporal, zygomatic, sphenoidal and ethmoidal bones, mastoids, orbits, anterior and middle cranial fossa) or spinal column are considered 'special site' diseases as they are often associated with a prominent intracranial or intraspinal soft tissue component which might be difficult to access by local treatment measures.

Table 16.1. Stratification of Langerhans cell hystiocytosis

Single-system disease

Single site
  - ◆ Single bone lesion
  - ◆ Isolated skin disease
  - ◆ Solitary lymph node involvement
  - ◆ Solitary lung disease
  - ◆ Isolated CNS involvement

Multiple site
  - ◆ Multiple bone lesions
  - ◆ Multiple lymph node involvement

Multisystem disease

(multiple organ involvement with or without organ dysfunction)

Risk patients	Any age with involvement of at least one risk organ
Low-risk patients	>2 years old with no risk organ involvement
Risk organs	Liver, lungs, haematopoietic system and spleen

Soft tissue swelling in the adjacent region of a bone lesion caused by extension of the granuloma or local oedema is a common finding, and is not usually considered as a separate organ involvement. Only rarely is an isolated granuloma found in soft tissue. Differential diagnosis of bony disease includes osteomyelitis, bone cysts, aseptic necrosis, and malignant bone tumours.

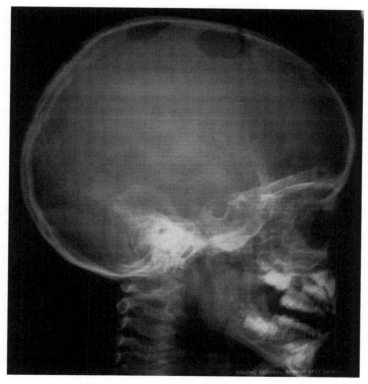

Fig. 16.4 'Punched-out' osteolytic LCH lesions in the skull.

Skin involvement occurs in about 25 per cent of LCH patients, either as single-organ involvement or as part of multisystem disease. Any part of the skin can be affected, including the nails.[9] The lesions may appear as erythematous scaly seborrhoea-like brown to red papules, especially pronounced on the scalp, on the trunk, and in intertriginous zones (behind the ears and in the axillary, inguinal, and perineal areas). These papules may transform into a vesicular–pustular or crusted appearance. Rarely, LCH manifests as a solitary cutaneous or subcutaneous nodule covered by intact skin. Congenital or perinatal occurrence, leaving residual hyperpigmentation of numerous firm nodules which resolve spontaneously within a few months, is known as Hashimoto–Pritzker syndrome. It is often difficult to differentiate LCH from other skin diseases such as mycosis or seborrhoeic or atopic eczema; nodular lesions have to be distinguished from malignant lymphoma or metastatic solid tumours. Localized or disseminated lesions also manifest on the mucous membranes, usually on the buccal mucosa, palate, and gingiva, but also in the gastrointestinal, urogenital, and vaginal tract, presenting as whitish granulomatous plaques that transform into ulcers with a tendency to bleeding.[7,8]

Lymph node involvement may be associated with local disease affecting adjacent skin or bone or may be a part of disseminated disease. The cervical nodes are most frequently involved and, rarely, thymic enlargement may be found. In the case of bone marrow involvement the infiltration with CD1a-positive cells is typically sparse, but their presence is associated with risk of organ involvement and correlates with an unfavourable outcome (unpublished data, LCH Registry, Vienna, Austria). Severe pancytopenia, frequently observed in infants with multisystem disease, is related to bone marrow dysfunction rather than to infiltration, and is usually associated with gross hepatosplenomegaly and a poor prognosis. Splenomegaly is usually seen in very young children with multisystem LCH and may contribute to pancytopenia. To reduce the need for blood transfusion, the removal of the enlarged spleen may be indicated in some cases.[7]

Hepatic enlargement is a common finding in patients with multisystem disease. Infiltration with LCH cells, which are CD1a positive but lack Birbeck granules, as well as massive portal lymphadenomegaly can lead to cholestatic hepatomegaly.[1] Activation of the cellular immune system by cytokines may result in hyperplasia and hypertrophy of Kupffer cells, presenting the histologic picture of sclerosing cholangitis. Ascites and oedema caused by hypoalbuminaemia, often associated with hypocoagulopathy, are clinical signs of liver dysfunction.

Isolated lung involvement occurs more frequently in adolescents and young adults, with >90 per cent of these patients having a history of smoking. In children, pulmonary LCH is usually part of multisystem disease. Clinical signs include tachypnoea with subcostal recession and persistent cough. Respiratory function tests may show a decreased total lung volume and compliance. The radiologic picture consists of diffuse fine interstitial shadowing due to micronodular granulations, which may appear cystic on high-resolution CT. With advancing disease the cysts increase in number and size and form bullae which appear on radiographs as 'honeycomb lungs'. Spontaneous pneumothorax resulting from rupture of superficial bullae may occur. Patients with uncontrolled LCH may develop lung fibrosis. Confirmation of diagnosis is mandatory by finding >5 per cent CD1a-positive cells in the bronchoalveolar lavage fluid or by lung biopsy[10,11] (Fig. 16.5).

Because gastrointestinal involvement seldom produces prominent clinical manifestations, it is often underdiagnosed and its actual frequency is unknown. The most common sign is failure to thrive because of malabsorption. Other symptoms include vomiting, diarrhoea, and protein-losing enteropathy. The diagnosis of gastrointestinal LCH must be supported not only by radiologic evidence of alternating dilated and stenotic segments in the small and large bowel, but also by endoscopic examination and biopsy.[7]

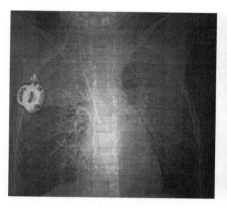
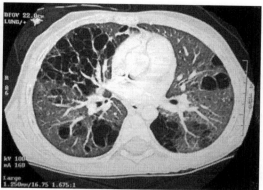

Fig. 16.5 Radiograph and high-resolution CT of the lung in a patient with pulmonary involvement.

Diabetes insipidus is the most common of the endocrinopathies associated with LCH occurring before, simultaneous with, or subsequent to the disease manifestation in other organs. Its incidence varies from 15 to 50 per cent in different studies. It can often be found in patients with extensive disease, lesions of the craniofacial bones, and intracranial tumour extension.[12] Confirmation of the diagnosis by an appropriate water deprivation test and measurement of urinary arginine vasopressin is essential because partial defects occur and may spontaneously remit.[13] A thickening of the hypothalamic–pituitary stalk, absence of the posterior pituitary bright spot, or both can be seen on MRI. Growth failure in children with LCH is commonly reported and appears to have a multifactorial cause. Anterior pituitary function may be compromised, resulting in growth hormone deficiency, hypothyroidism, hypogonadism, and hyperprolactinaemia.[14] Finally, panhypopituitarism may occur, and cranial MRI does not necessarily reveal a hypothalamic mass in these patients. However, persistent cytokine release due to chronic disease, occult gut involvement causing malabsorption, vertebral collapse, and prolonged steroid therapy may also contribute to growth retardation in LCH.

Apart from the common manifestations in the hypothalamic–pituitary axis, virtually all other parts of the central nervous system (CNS) can be affected by LCH, including the following locations in order of frequency: cerebellum, pons, cerebral hemispheres, choroid plexus, basal ganglia, spinal chord, optic tract, and cranial nerves[12] (Fig. 16.6).

Diagnostic procedures

A lesional biopsy is an essential step in obtaining the definitive diagnosis of LCH. In 1987 the Writing Group of the Histiocyte Society outlined an applicable classification of histiocytosis syndromes and standards for histopathologic diagnosis which has been widely accepted.[3] According to this proposal, morphologic, immunohistochemical, and clinical criteria are required for the definitive diagnosis (Fig. 16.3).

In a rare disease like LCH with a highly variable clinical presentation, it is crucial to use uniform guidelines for clinical evaluation and assessment of disease extent. Based on an exact history and a meticulous clinical examination mandatory baseline investigations should be performed in every newly diagnosed patient (Table 16.2), and in selected cases diagnostic procedures are required for specific indications[15] (Table 16.3).

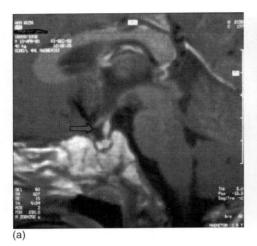
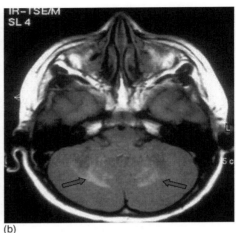

(a) (b)

Fig. 16.6 CNS changes in LCH: (a) infundibular thickening apparent on sagittal brain MRI; (b) axial FLAIR weighted MRI (bilateral hyperintensities in cerebellum).

Table 16.2. Diagnostic guidelines

Clinical evaluation
- Complete history
  Fever, pain, irritability, failure to thrive, nutritional status, loss of appetite, diarrhoea, polydipsia, polyuria, activity level, behavioural changes, neurologic changes
- Complete physical examination
  Measurement of temperature, height, weight, and head circumference, pubertal status, skin and scalp rashes, purpura, bleeding, aural discharge, orbital abnormalities, lymphadenopathies, gum and palatal lesions, dentition, soft tissue swelling, dyspnoea, tachypnoea, intercostal retractions, liver and spleen size, ascites, oedema, jaundice, neurologic examination, papilloedema, cranial nerve abnormalities, cerebellar dysfunction

Laboratory
- Complete blood count
- Liver enzymes and function tests
  Serum glutamic-oxaloacetic transaminase (SGOT), serum glutamate-pyruvate transaminase (SGPT), alkaline phosphatase, bilirubin, total protein, albumin
- Coagulation studies
  Prothrombin time (PT), partial thromboplastin time (PTT), fibrinogen
- Urine osmolality (measurement after overnight water deprivation)

Radiography
- Chest radiograph (posteroanterior and lateral)
- Skeletal radiograph survey

Permanent consequences and late effects

Permanent consequences are defined as any permanent or irreversible physical and/or neuropsychologic sequelae, attributable to the disease itself rather than treatment, which develop at any time during the disease course. The risk of developing permanent consequences correlates with the duration of disease activity and the frequency of reactivations.

Table 16.3. Evaluations upon specific indication

Test	Indication
Bone marrow aspirate and trephine biopsy	Anaemia, leucopenia, or thrombocytopenia
Pulmonary function tests	Abnormal chest radiograph, tachypnoea, intercostal retractions
Lung biopsy, preceded by bronchoalveolar lavage, when available; when diagnostic obviates lung biopsy	Patients with abnormal chest radiograph in whom chemotherapy is being considered to exclude opportunistic infection
Small bowel series and biopsy	Unexplained chronic diarrhoea or failure to thrive, evidence of malabsorption
Liver biopsy	Liver dysfunction, including hypoproteinaemia not due to protein-losing enteropathy, to differentiate active LCH of the liver from cirrhosis
MRI of brain/hypothalamic–pituitary axis with i.v. [Gd]DTPA	Hormonal, visual, or neurologic abnormalities
Panoramic dental radiography of mandible and maxilla, oral surgery consultation	Oral involvement
Endocrine evaluation	Short stature, growth failure, diabetes insipidus, hypothalamic syndromes, galactorrhoea, precocious or delayed puberty; CT or MRI abnormality of hypothalamus/pituitary
Otolaryngology consultation and audiogram	Aural discharge, deafness

In single-system LCH permanent consequences occur in about 33 per cent of the patients, and about 80 per cent of these are related to the site of disease. Patients with initial lesions in the long bones or the spinal column often develop orthopaedic problems or growth failure. If the mastoid, maxilla, or mandible are involved, hearing deficits or tooth loss can occur.[16] The incidence of permanent consequences in patients with multisystem disease varies between 22 and 26 per cent.[17,18] Diabetes insipidus is observed most frequently; others are listed in Figure 16.7.

Endocrinopathies include hypothyroidism, hypogonadism and growth hormone deficiency. Neurologic problems usually associated with neurodegenerative CNS changes consist of hypo- or hyperreflexia, tremor, ataxia, and dysarthria. Convulsions, palsy, and cranial nerve deficits may be seen in patients with intracranial tumorous LCH lesions. Psychosocial and intellectual impairment has also been observed.[12]

Various malignancies have been reported in 5 per cent of long-term survivors of LCH. In a retrospective analysis a high association of malignancy and LCH even without any treatment and, not infrequently, preceding the diagnosis of LCH was recognized.[19] Recently, there has been concern regarding an association of secondary acute myeloid leukemia (sAML) with etoposide administration. However, it has been shown that occurrence of sAML may be linked with high cumulative doses, short intervals, or combination with other topoisomerase-II-inhibiting cytotoxic drugs.[20,21]

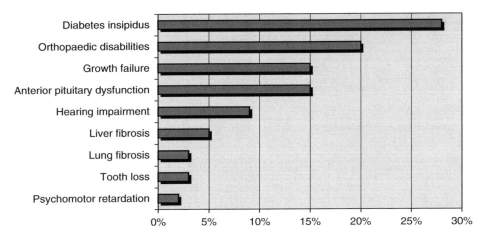

Fig. 16.7 Permanent consequences of LCH: percentage of most frequent sequelae related to the totality of permanent consequences (unpublished data from the LCH Registry, Vienna, Austria).

Current management and prognosis

Background

The course of LCH is highly variable and unpredictable in the individual patient. Spontaneous regression is observed as well as chronic reactivations and, rarely, fulminant lethal courses. The underlying factors responsible for the varying biologic behaviour of LCH are unknown.[18] The lack of knowledge of the pathogenesis of LCH and the failure to establish generally accepted diagnostic criteria have inhibited the development of a rational treatment policy. Therefore the treatment of patients with LCH has varied over the past century according to what was believed to be the cause of the disease. Only with the introduction of new concepts of staging and diagnostic criteria has it become possible to collect sufficiently large numbers of patients to carry out prospective clinical trials.[21] Empirically it has been shown that the treatment of LCH should depend on the extent of the disease, and patients should be stratified as having 'single-system' or 'multisystem' disease (see Table 16.1).

As the disease may follow variable courses, a new definition and assessment of response to a given treatment had to be established. The following criteria were defined by the Histiocyte Society: complete resolution of the disease [no active disease (NAD)], disease regression [active disease (AD-better)], intermediate response with regression of some and reappearance of other lesions (AD-intermediate, mixed) or unchanged disease (AD-intermediate, stable), and progression of the disease (AD-worse).[8,21]

Single-system disease

A solitary bony lesion does not usually require treatment other than curettage at the time of obtaining diagnostic biopsy. Lesions that are painful may respond to intralesional instillation of steroids (crystalline methylprednisolone 75–150 mg), but polyostotic disease may require a short course of systemic therapy. Various systemic regimens have been used including steroids (40 mg/m^2/day), vinblastine (6 mg/m^2/week), etoposide, and methotrexate. Indications for systemic treatment (e.g. prednisone, vinblastine) also include risky locations with imminent spontaneous fracture, spinal cord compression, huge non-resectable tumour mass, and involvement of 'special sites' (craniofacial or vertebral lesions) with impending functional impairment. In bony disease indomethacin ($2 \, mg/m^2/day$) may be an alternative to steroids both for its analgesic effect and as an antiprostaglandin, and recently bisphosphonates have also been recommended. Primary surgical excision of lesions in the craniofacial region or spinal column ('special sites'), beyond a biopsy, is not recommended because of the accompanying prominent intracranial or intraspinal soft tissue component. Although used in only a restricted way during the last decades (because of the risk of late sequelae and secondary malignancy), emergency low-dose radiation (6–12 Gy) should be reserved for critical circumstances (e.g. optic nerve or spinal cord).[8] Patients with solitary bone lesions show a survival rate of 100 per cent; reactivations mostly occur during the first 2 years after diagnosis and are usually restricted to the skeleton.[16]

Connatal LCH confined to skin tends to regress spontaneously within a few months in most of the cases. However, progression to multisystem involvement with fatal outcome may occur, and close observation for a longer follow-up period is mandatory. Erythematous lesions usually respond to topical steroids. In severe persisting or progressing skin involvement a topical 20 per cent solution of nitrogen mustard or psoralen–ultraviolet A (PUVA) photochemotherapy may be useful, but can be recommended only for short-term therapy because of concern about possible carcinogenicity. In severe resistant skin disease mild systemic steroid therapy with or without vinca alkaloids is needed. This therapy should also be used if multiple enlarged or bulky lymph nodes are present.[8,21] Surgical excision is the treatment of choice for skin nodules and isolated lymph node involvement, with a cure rate of nearly 100 per cent.[16]

In young children, isolated lung involvement should be treated with chemotherapy according to protocols for multisystem patients. As in adults, it is essential that adolescents refrain from smoking, and mild systemic therapy with steroids with or without vinblastine can be effective.[11] There are anecdotal reports of a positive effect of ciclosporin A and bisphosphonates in progressing disease.[22]

Active LCH mass lesions in the CNS have been shown to respond to conventional LCH chemotherapy. The choice of therapy depends on the individual case and possible pretreatment. A beneficial effect of combined chemotherapy [prednisone, vinblastine, etoposide, and 2-chlorodeoxyadenosine (2-CdA)] has been reported.[23] Radiotherapy or systemic therapy are usually unable to restore pituitary function, and hormone replacement therapy is required.[13,24] No specific therapy can yet be recommended for neurodegenerative CNS disease.

Multisystem disease

Two major approaches to the treatment of multisystem disease have existed for the last 20 years: a conservative approach with treatment used only during disease exacerbations (single-center study),[18] and an intensive chemotherapy induction followed by treatment (two large cooperative clinical trials, the Italian AIEOP-CNR-HX 83 study[25] and the German–Austrian DAL-HX 83/90 study[17]). Surprisingly, the overall mortality was about 20 per cent in both the conservative and the aggressive treatment approaches. In contrast, the incidence of disease-related late sequelae was 67 per cent in the conservative treatment and only 33 per cent in the DAL-HX studies. The low incidence of disease reactivations in the DAL-HX studies (overall 23 per cent) provided evidence that effective treatment may beneficially influence the natural course of the disease.

The aim of the first international randomized chemotherapy trial (LCH I), initiated by the Histiocyte Society in 1991, was to compare the efficacy of monotherapy with vinblastine and etoposide with respect to the course of the disease and outcome.[26] No significant difference was found between the two treatment arms. In the next international trial (LCH II) the effect of continuous oral prednisone combined with vinblastine with or without the addition of etoposide was compared in a randomized way in severely affected multisystem disease patients. A new stratification system was adopted, distinguishing between 'risk' patients with involvement of 'risk organs' like liver, spleen, lungs, or haematopoietic system, or age <2 years, and 'low-risk' patients without involvement of such organs and age >2 years.[8] Risk patients were eligible for randomization between the two-drug and the three-drug arm, low-risk patients received initial treatment according to the two-drug arm only, and all patients went on continuation therapy with 6-mercaptopurine and prednisone–vinblastine pulses. Treatment duration was limited to 24 weeks as in LCH I.

The results in the low-risk group were satisfying, with 89 per cent responders at week 6 and no fatalities. No statistical difference with respect to initial response, survival, and reactivation-free survival was found between the two treatment arms in risk patients. However, it was shown that patients with involvement of risk organs, who did not show disease regression by weeks 6 or 12 of therapy, had a high risk of poor outcome and mortality. Notably, all the patients who died in the LCH I and LCH II studies had involvement of at least one risk organ, irrespective of age. Therefore it seems justified to regard risk organ involvement and response to initial treatment as the most important prognostic factors, whereas age <2 years did not prove to be of independent prognostic importance. Interestingly, the overall probability of survival of the multisystem patients did not differ significantly between the DAL-HX, LCH I, and LCH II studies, and was ~80 per cent. This indicates that there is a therapy-resistant 'high-risk' population of ~20 per cent of the multisystem patients who cannot be rescued by standard treatment. When the results were compared with those of the DAL-HX studies, there was a clear superiority of therapy given for 1 year, with respect to the rate of reactivations, over treatment for 6 months.[27]

The third international randomized trial (LCH-III) was started in April 2001 (www.histio.org/society) (Fig. 16.8). Patients are stratified into three groups: multisystem risk patients (patients with involvement of one or more risk organs), multisystem low-risk patients (patients with multiple organs involved but without involvement of risk organs), and patients with single-system 'multifocal bone disease' or localized 'special site' involvement (craniofacial or vertebral lesions). Risk patients are randomized between two different treatment arms including prednisone, vinblastine, and 6-mercaptopurine with or without methotrexate. Initial treatment consists of one or two courses depending on response and is followed by continuation therapy (treatment duration, 12 months). Treatment for low-risk patients includes prednisone and vinblastine; the overall duration of therapy for this patient group is 6 or 12 months as randomly assigned. Patients with multifocal bone disease or special site involvement are treated with prednisone and vinblastine for 24 weeks.

Resistant disease

Patients who do not respond to initial treatment are considered to have a high risk of mortality (~75 per cent). Ciclosporin A has been suggested as an alternative treatment approach. However, convincing data are lacking, especially for patients with advanced chemotherapy-resistant multisystem disease. Regarding the role of bone marrow transplantation only scanty and inconsistent data are available. Regimen-related mortality in these studies is high;[22] only recently the application of intensity reduced conditioning showed promising results.[29] Other studies report on the successful treatment of LCH with interferon-α, anti-CD1a and anti-TNF-α antibodies, but further investigation is necessary.[8,21,28]). The use of 2-CdA and 2'-deoxycoformycin has recently appeared to be successful in refractory LCH.[23] According to

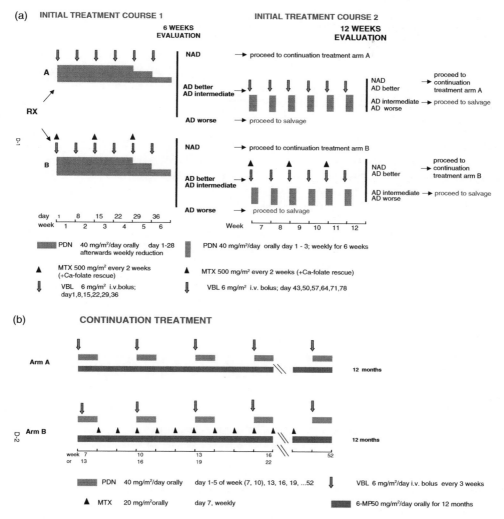

Fig. 16.8 LCH-III protocol: (a) initial treatment plan for risk patients; (b) protocol continuation treatment plan for risk patients. PDN, prednisone; MTX, methotrexate; VBL, vinblastine; 6-MP, 6-mercaptopurine.

salvage treatment protocol of the Histiocyte Society, 2-CdA is given as monotherapy (5 mg/m^2 2-CdA daily for 5 days at intervals of 3–4 weeks; two, four or six courses) to non-responding multisystem patients or patients with recurrent disease was not convincing.[23] A new salvage approach including 2-CdA combined with cytarabinoside is in progress.[30]

References

1. **Schmitz L, Favara BE** (1998). Nosology and pathology of Langerhans cell histiocytosis. *Hematol Oncol Clin North Am* 12, 221–46.

2. **Favara BE, Feller AC, Pauli M, et al.** (1997). Contemporary classification of histiocytic disorders. The WHO Committee on Histiocytic/Reticulum Cell Proliferations. Reclassification Working Group of the Histiocyte Society. *Med Pediatr Oncol* **29**, 157–66.

3. **Writing Group of the Histiocyte Society** (1987). Histiocytosis syndromes in children. *Lancet* **i**, 208–9.

4. **Arceci RJ, Longley BJ, Emanuel PD** (2002). Atypical cellular disorders. *Hematology (Am Soc Hematol Educ Program)*, 297–314.

5. **Willman CL, McClain KL** (1998). An update on clonality, cytokines, and viral etiology in Langerhans cell histiocytosis. *Hematol Oncol Clin North Am* **12**, 407–16.

6. **Favara BE, Jaffe R, Egeler RM** (2002). Macrophage activation and hemophagocytic syndrome in Langerhans cell histiocytosis: report of 30 cases. *Pediatr Dev Pathol* **5**, 130–40.

7. **Egeler RM, D'Angio GJ** (1995). Langerhans cell histiocytosis. *J Pediatr* **127**, 1–11.

8. **Gadner H, Grois N** (2004). Langerhans cell histiocytosis. Pinkerton R, Plowman RN, Pieters R. *Pediatric Oncology 3rd edition*, 469–483.

9. **Munn S, Chu AC** (1998). Langerhans cell histiocytosis of the skin. *Hematol Oncol Clin North Am* **12**, 269–86.

10. **McClain KL, Gonzalez JM, Jonkers R, et al.** (2002). Need for a cooperative study: Pulmonary Langerhans cell histiocytosis and its management in adults. *Med Pediatr Oncol* **39**, 35–9.

11. **Vassallo R, Ryu JH, Colby TV, et al.** (2000). Pulmonary Langerhans'-cell histiocytosis. *N Engl J Med* **342**, 1969–78.

12. **Prayer D, Grois N, Prosch H, et al.** (2004). MR imaging presentation of interacranial disease associated with Langerhans cell histiocytosis. *Am J Neuroradiol* **25**, 880–1.

13. **Broadbent V, Pritchard J** (1997). Diabetes insipidus associated with Langerhans cell histiocytosis: is it reversible? *Med Pediatr Oncol* **28**, 289–93.

14. **Nanduri VR, Bareille P, Pritchard J, et al.** (2000). Growth and endocrine disorders in multisystem Langerhans' cell histiocytosis. *Clin Endocrinol (Oxf)* **53**, 509–15.

15. **Writing Group of the Histiocyte Society** (1989). Histiocytosis syndromes in children: II. Approach to the clinical and laboratory evaluation of children with Langerhans cell histiocytosis. *Med Pediatr Oncol* **17**, 492–5.

16. **Titgemeyer C, Grois N, Minkov M, et al.** (2001). Pattern and course of single-system disease in Langerhans cell histiocytosis data from the DAL-HX 83- and 90-study. *Med Pediatr Oncol* **37**, 108–14.

17. **Gadner H, Heitger A, Grois N, et al.** (1994). Treatment strategy for disseminated Langerhans cell histiocytosis. DAL HX-83 Study Group. *Med Pediatr Oncol* **23**, 72–80.

18. **McLelland J, Broadbent V, Yeomans E, et al.** (1990). Langerhans cell histiocytosis: the case for conservative treatment. *Arch Dis Child* **65**, 301–3.

19. **Egeler RM, Neglia JP, Arico M, et al.** (1998). The relation of Langerhans cell histiocytosis to acute leukemia, lymphomas, and other solid tumors. The LCH-Malignancy Study Group of the Histiocyte Society. *Hematol Oncol Clin North Am* **12**, 369–78.

20. **Haupt R, Fears TR, Heise A, et al.** (1997). Risk of secondary leukemia after treatment with etoposide (VP-16) for Langerhans' cell histiocytosis in Italian and Austrian–German populations. *Int J Cancer* **71**, 9–13.

21. **Ladisch S, Gadner H** (1994). Treatment of Langerhans cell histiocytosis—evolution and current approaches. *Br J Cancer* **23** (Suppl), S41–6.

22. **Minkov M, Grois N, Broadbent V, et al.** (1999). Cyclosporine A therapy for multisystem Langerhans cell histiocytosis. *Med Pediatr Oncol* **33**, 482–5.

23. **Weitzman S, Wayne AS, Arceci R, et al.** (1999). Nucleoside analogues in the therapy of Langerhans cell histiocytosis: a survey of members of the Histiocyte Society and review of the literature. *Med Pediatr Oncol* **33**, 476–81.

24. Howell SJ, Wilton P, Shalet SM (1998). Growth hormone replacement in patients with Langerhan's cell histiocytosis. *Arch Dis Child* 78, 469–73.

25. Ceci A, De Terlizzi M, Colella R, *et al.* (1993). Langerhans cell histiocytosis in childhood: results from the Italian Cooperative AIEOP-CNR-H.X '83 study. *Med Pediatr Oncol* 21, 259–64.

26. Gadner H, Grois N, Arico M, *et al.* (2001). A randomized trial of treatment for multisystem Langerhans' cell histiocytosis. *J Pediatr* 138, 728–34.

27. Minkov M, Grois N, Heitger A, *et al.* (2002). Response to initial treatment: an important prognostic predictor in multisystem Langerhans cell histiocytosis. *Med Pediatr Oncol* 39, 581–5.

28. Henter JI, Karlen J, Calming U, *et al.* (2001). Successful treatment of Langerhans-cell histiocytosis with etanercept. *N Engl J Med* 345, 1577–8.

29 Steiner M, Matthes-Martin S, Attarbaschi A, *et al.* (2005). Improved outcome of treatment-resistant high-risk Langerhans cell histiocytosis after allogeneic stem cell transplantation with reduced-intensity conditioning. *Bone Marrow Transplant* 6, (in press)

30 Bernhard F, Thomas C, Bertrand Y, *et al.* (2005). Report of multicenter pilot study of 2-CdA and Ara -C combined chemotherapy in refractory Langerhans cell histiocytosis with haematological dysfunctions. *Eur J Cancer* (in press) (accepted for publication Nov. 2004).

Chapter 17

Tumours of the central nervous system

R.Pötter, T. Czech, K. Dieckmann, I. Slavc,
D. Wimberger-Prayer, and H. Budka

Introduction

Tumours of the central nervous system (CNS) constitute the most common solid tumour in children (2.7 per 100 000 children annually), and therefore contribute to a major part of daily practice in paediatric oncology. Brain tumours are very heterogeneous with regard to tissue, location, pattern of spread, clinical picture, natural history, and age of occurrence (from the neonatal period to adolescence). As significant progress has been achieved and is developing in the different areas of diagnosis and treatment, adequate clinical management and follow-up now involves an interdisciplinary paediatric neuro-onocology team (neuropaediatrician, paediatric oncologist, neurosurgeon, radiotherapist, neuropathologist, neuroradiologist, and psychologist). Management decisions for childhood brain tumours should be based exclusively on such a team approach, in which the different members must be familiar with all the available knowledge, experience, and developments in their respective fields.[1] The goal of brain tumour therapy is to achieve cure while avoiding unacceptable long-term sequelae.

Modern neurosurgery remains the mainstay of treatment for most brain tumours, followed by modern brain radiotherapy as the most important adjuvant procedure in a large number of patients.[2] Over the past decade chemotherapy has been shown to be clearly beneficial for patients with medulloblastoma and high-grade glioma.[3,4]

Tumour classification and histologic diagnosis

Progress in our understanding of the molecular basis of neoplastic development may lead to molecular tumour diagnosis in the future. At present, however, descriptive classification by histologic examination remains pivotal for the appropriate management of CNS tumours. Since location and cellular differentiation are the basis of this diagnostic system, tumour classification has remained 'histogenetic'. The most recent edition of the WHO Classification of tumours of the nervous system[5] lists 127 entities, reflecting the remarkable variety of cellular constituents of the CNS. Theoretically, all types might develop in children. However, the number of tumour types which are of special importance in children is significantly smaller (Table 17.1). The majority of paediatric CNS tumours are of only five types: medulloblastoma, pilocytic astrocytoma, diffuse astrocytoma, ependymoma, and craniopharyngioma.

As with their counterparts in adults, CNS tumours in childhood have important properties which differ from those of tumours at other sites, but profoundly influence their behaviour:

- many are highly invasive, even when histologically of low malignancy
- many are heterogeneous in composition with areas of mixed tumour type and differing malignancy (special attention is necessary in stereotactic biopsies)

Table 17.1. Histologic CNS tumour types of particular importance in children: most frequent age and site, WHO grade, and approximate percentage of all brain tumours in children

Tumour type	Most frequent site	Percentage of all brain tumours[a]	WHO grade	Most frequent age
Pilocytic astrocytoma	Cerebellum	12–18	I	Childhood and adolescence
	Hypothalamus, optic pathways	4–8		
Subependymal giant cell astrocytoma	Foramen of Munro region (usually in tuberous sclerosis)		I	Childhood, adolescence
Diffuse astrocytoma (low grade)	Cerebral hemispheres	8–20	II	Adolescence, young adults
Pleomorphic xanthoastrocytoma	Brainstem	3–6		Childhood
	Superficial cerebral hemispheres		II	Late childhood, adolescence
Anaplastic astrocytoma, glioblastoma	Cerebral hemispheres	6–12	III, IV	All ages
	Brainstem	3–9		Childhood
Oligodendroglioma, mixed glioma	Cerebral hemisphere	2–7	II, III	Adolescence, young adults
	Anaplastic oligodendroglioma			
Ependymoma, anaplastic ependymoma	Lateral and third ventricles	2–5	II, III	Childhood and adolescence
	Fourth ventricle	4–8		
Choroid plexus papilloma, choroid plexus carcinoma	Lateral and fourth ventricles	2–4	I, IV	Infancy, childhood
Gangliocytoma, ganglioglioma	Temporal lobe	1–5	I	Childhood and adolescence
Desmoplastic infantile ganglioglioma	Superficial cerebral hemispheres			
	Desmoplastic cerebral astrocytoma of infancy		I	Infancy
Dysembryoplastic neuroepithelial tumour	Temporal lobe		I	Childhood to young adults
Central neurocytoma	Lateral ventricles		I	Adolescence, young adults
Pinecytoma, pineoblastoma	Pineal region		II–IV	Childhood to young adults
	Parenchymal tumour of intermediate differentiation			

(Continued)

Table 17.1. (Continued) Histologic CNS tumour types of particular importance in children: most frequent age and site, WHO grade, and approximate percentage of all brain tumours in children

Tumour type	Most frequent site	Percentage of all brain tumours[a]	WHO grade	Most frequent age
Neuroblastoma	Cerebral hemispheres		IV	Infancy and childhood
Ependymoblastoma	Lateral and fourth ventricles		IV	Infancy and childhood
Medulloblastoma	Cerebellum	20–25	IV	Infancy and childhood
Other primitive neuroectodermal tumours	Whole neuroaxis	1–5	IV	Infancy and childhood
Atypical teratoid/rhabdoid tumour	Infra- and supratentorial		IV	Infancy and childhood
Germ cell tumours	Pineal region especially germinoma and teratoma	0.5–2	I–IV	Infancy and childhood
	Hypothalamus	1–2		
Colloid cyst of third ventricle	Foramen of Munro region		I	Adolescence, young adults
Craniopharyngioma	(Supra)sellar	6–9	I	Adolescence
Meningioma	Supratentorial	1–2	I	All ages
Pituitary adenoma	(Supra)sellar	0.5–2.5	I	Adolescence

[a]Percentages in children modified from Pollack;[6] some entities were not individually listed.
Data from Pollack.[6]

+ many are notorious for spreading to CSF pathways, thus enabling CSF seeding even in low-grade tumours
+ tumours may progress from low to high grade, most prominently in diffuse astrocytomas.

Most CNS tumour types occur preferentially in specific age-groups and at specific sites (Table 17.1). Nevertheless, exceptions to these rules must be kept in mind. Compared with tumours in adults, the posterior fossa site is over-represented (about half of all paediatric CNS tumours occur at this site). However, the distribution depends upon age: during the first year of life and in adolescence, supratentorial tumours are more frequent than those in infratentorial sites, which predominate during childhood. Spinal cord tumours are rare in children. Many CNS tumours in the young age group occur near the midline, suggesting a developmental aspect to their origin.

Histologic grading of malignancy according to the WHO indicates how a given tumour type usually behaves on a four-point scale (Table 17.1). Again, exceptions may occur. In general, histologic malignancy is judged according to cellularity, pleomorphism, nuclear atypia, mitotic activity, invasiveness and metastasis, anaplasia (cellular differentiation), and secondary features such as necrosis and neovascularity. However, some of these items do not have the same meaning in all tumour types. It is important to separate pilocytic astrocytoma, which is the most frequent glioma of childhood and usually has an excellent prognosis, from the much less favourable diffuse astrocytomas.

The impact of modern morphologic techniques, with immunocytochemistry as an indispensable tool, on a refined histogenetic classification of CNS tumours cannot be overemphasized. Information on biologic tumour properties, such as proliferation, can also be obtained. While CNS tumour proliferation indices generally reflect the malignancy scale of the present classification system, proliferation on its own has not yet been shown to be of decisive prognostic importance. Thus it is the combined consideration of distinct features of the histologic examination (tumour type, grade of malignancy, growth pattern, proliferative activity, etc.), which will provide the maximum relevant information for further management and therapy of an individual tumour patient.

The concept of the primitive neuroectodermal tumour

In Bailey and Cushing's original histogenetic tumour classification, tumour morphology was considered to mirror specific stages of normal neural tissue development. Since then, highly undifferentiated neural neoplasms have been considered as 'embryonal', with the medulloblastoma as the most important clinicpathologic entity. More recently, the unifying concept of the primitive neuroectodermal tumour (PNET) was proposed to encompass all types of undifferentiated or primitive small-celled neural neoplasms with a potential for multiple differentiation (neuronal, glial, ependymal, pineal, etc.), irrespective of their site of origin. The PNET concept has become generally accepted and has entered the present WHO classification of embryonal tumours in a somewhat hybrid format. The distinct clinicopathologic tumour entities with traditional terminology such as the medulloepithelioma, medulloblastoma, and ependymoblastoma are retained in addition to PNETs in supratentorial presentations. Thus PNET may be used as a general term for all types of densely cellular ('blue-celled'), primitive, or 'embryonal' neural tumours. Whenever possible, however, further delineation as medulloblastoma etc. should be given. Confusingly, 'PNET' (*peripheral* neuroectodermal tumour) is sometimes used to designate a peripheral nervous system tumour with similarities to Ewing sarcoma.

'New' CNS tumour entities of childhood

In addition to earlier accepted PNETs and the long list of traditional tumour entities, the more recent editions of the WHO classification (1997 and 2000) include a number of recently recognized tumour entities, including some that usually present in childhood.[5] The now well-established pleomorphic xanthoastrocytoma is a predominantly extracerebral growth with pleomorphic, lipidized astrocytes and a generally, but not universally, favourable prognosis. The desmoplastic infantile ganglioglioma and its variant, the desmoplastic cerebral astrocytoma of infancy, are usually very large tumours presenting during the first 2 years of life. The dysembryoplastic neuroepithelial tumour usually presents in a temporal location with long-standing complex partial seizures; it features a mixed glioneuronal population in a mucinous matrix, distributed in characteristic multiple cortical nodules. The central neurocytoma is almost invariably an intraventricular tumour of the lateral ventricle, and has been misdiagnosed for decades as oligodendroglioma or ependymoma; its prognosis is mostly, but not always, favourable. The pineal parenchymal tumour of intermediate differentiation has a variable clinical behaviour and constitutes about 10 per cent of all pineal parenchymal tumours. An important new addition to the group of embryonal tumours is the atypical teratoid/rhabdoid tumour which constitutes 2.1 per cent of a group of primary CNS tumours of children. It manifests more frequently infratentorially than supratentorially with a histology of rhabdoid cells (large eosinophilic cell bodies with eccentric nucleus), with or without PNET-like areas, epithelial or mesenchymal structures, and a complex immunocytochemical expression of glial, neuronal, epithelial, mesenchymal, and muscle proteins. Most patients die within a year of diagnosis.

Molecular biology

Over the past two decades, work in the field of molecular neuro-oncology has evolved from being largely descriptive in nature to the implication of specific genes and the functional analysis of their role in the evolution of the malignant process. Cytogenetic and molecular techniques have resulted in the cloning of the retinoblastoma, the neurofibromatosis type 1 and type 2 genes, and the characterization of the molecular physiology of the *TP53* gene as well as genes involved in the inherited genetic disorders discussed below. These efforts will help to improve understanding of the many and complex pathways that lead to tumour initiation and progression, and to guide therapeutic strategies.

The most common and sometimes the only structural abnormality seen in medulloblastoma is an isochromosome 17q [i(17q)] present in approximately 50 per cent of cases. This finding implicates the presence of a tumour suppressor gene on 17p, which is important in tumour development. So far, a number of genes on 17p have been eliminated as candidates for this locus, including *TP53*.

Recently, two independent groups in Boston and Philadelphia found in retrospective studies of medulloblastomas that high neurotrophin receptor TrkC mRNA expression is a powerful independent predictor of a favourable clinical outcome in medulloblastoma patients.[7,8] In addition, independent studies in Göttingen and Philadelphia identified low proto-oncogene *MYC* (c-*myc*) mRNA expression as a second independent predictor of a favourable survival outcome.[9,10] *MYC* mRNA expression was found to range widely and did not correlate with the presence of *MYC* gene amplification in medulloblastoma cell lines or primary tumours.

Other biologic prognostic indicators include increased expression levels of the neuregulin receptors ErbB2 and ErbB4,[11] which were found to be highly correlated with poor outcome.

Pomeroy *et al.*[12] recently extended these findings by demonstrating that predictors based on microarray gene expression profiles can predict clinical outcome with high statistical significance. Using oligonucleotide microarray-based gene expression profiling to monitor the expression of over 6800 genes in the tumours of children with medulloblastoma, 5–20 marker gene predictors were found to be accurate outcome predictors, performing significantly better than clinical staging.

Other studies have examined the functional role of genes implicated in glioma malignancy and investigated the mechanisms of their dysregulation in the generation of the malignant phenotype. These studies suggest that there are at least two pathways that lead to glioblastoma in adults. The first pathway involves progression from a diffuse astrocytoma to an anaplastic astrocytoma to a glioblastoma multiforme. An early event in this progression is loss of the short arm of chromosome 17 in combination with an inactivating mutation in the retained copy of *TP53*. Later events in this pathway may involve alterations of genes on chromosome 9, 19, and 22. The second pathway suggests the formation of a *de novo* glioblastoma, rather than progression from a lower-grade tumour, and involves loss of heterozygosity on chromosome 10. Chromosome 10 loss, but not 17p loss, is often associated with amplification and rearrangement of the epidermal growth factor receptor gene, resulting in increased cell proliferation.

Interestingly, work on paediatric astrocytomas suggests that the genes involved are different. In contrast with glioblastoma multiforme in adults, paediatric glioblastomas generally lack *EGFR*, *MDM2* and/or *CDK4* gene amplification, and chromosome 10 deletions are rare.[13] Taken together, these observations imply that the pathways leading to the development of malignant astrocytomas in children may differ significantly from those involved in adults, which may in part account for the somewhat better prognosis of such lesions in children. The only paediatric tumour that exhibits many of the same chromosomal abnormalities as the adult tumours is brainstem glioma, perhaps explaining its dismal prognosis.[14]

Epidemiology

CNS tumours represent the second most frequent malignancy and the most common type of solid tumour in children <16 years of age. The annual incidence rate for all CNS tumours combined is approximately 2.5 cases per 100 000 children annually, with astroglial tumours accounting for 60.9 per cent and neuroectodermal tumours for 23.9 per cent.[15] Approximately 8 per cent of these children are ≤2 years of age at the time of diagnosis.[16]

There are still no identifiable predisposing or aetiologic factors for the majority of children with brain tumours. However, in a small group of children the occurrence of primary CNS tumours is associated with certain hereditary and congenital diseases such as the neurocutaneous syndromes and the Li–Fraumeni syndrome. The best known of these is neurofibromatosis type I, in which there is a high incidence of visual pathway gliomas and other glial tumours. The hallmark of neurofibromatosis type II is the development of bilateral vestibular Schwannomas. In tuberous sclerosis, subependymal giant cell and other glial tumours may develop. In patients with von Hippel–Lindau syndrome, cerebellar haemangioblastoma, pheochromocytoma, renal cell carcinoma, and retinal tumours have been observed. Medulloblastoma and other malignancies may occur in association with the autosomal dominant nevoid basal cell carcinoma syndrome (Gorlin–Goltz syndrome) as well as Turcot's syndrome and ataxia–telangectasia. The most common CNS tumour in individuals with Li–Fraumeni syndrom is astrocytoma. Pineoblastomas can be seen in some cases of familial bilateral retinoblastoma.

Another confirmed aetiology for brain tumours in children is exposure to ionizing therapeutic radiation.

Clinical presentation

The signs and symptoms of neurologic dysfunction in a child with a brain tumour are various and depend more on age, premorbid developmental level, and site of origin than history. Brain tumours may cause neurologic impairment directly, by infiltrating or compressing normal CNS structures, or indirectly, by causing obstruction of cerebrospinal fluid (CSF) flow and increased intracranial pressure (ICP). The latter is responsible for the 'classic' triad of ICP—morning headache, vomiting, and visual disturbances. When present, these symptoms strongly suggest a rapidly growing midline or posterior fossa tumour. More commonly, the initial signs of ICP are more subtle, subacute, non-specific, and non-localizing. In school-age children, slowly developing ICP may be accompanied by declining academic performance, fatigue, changes in affect, energy level, motivation, personality, and behaviour, and complaints of vague intermittent headaches. In the first few years of life, irritability, anorexia, and developmental delay, with later regression of intellectual and motor abilities, are frequently early signs of ICP.

Infratentorial tumours (brainstem and cerebellar) commonly present with deficits of balance or brainstem function (truncal steadiness, extremity coordination and gait, cranial nerve function). Nystagmus and gaze palsy alone, or more likely in combination with deficits of cranial nerves V, VII, and IX, strongly suggest invasion of the brainstem. Head tilt may be a presenting sign.

Supratentorial tumours may cause a variety of signs and symptoms, depending on the size and location of the tumour. The most common presenting complaint is headache, followed secondly by seizures. Upper motor neuron signs such as hemiparesis, hyper-reflexia, and clonus, as well as associated sensory loss, may also be present.

Anorexia, bulimia, weight loss or gain, somnolence, mood swings, failure to thrive, diabetes insipidus, sexual precocity, or delayed puberty may be non-specific or suggest hypothalamic or pituitary dysfunction. Tumours of the region of the hypothalamus may also cause visual loss due to compression of the optic chiasm or the optic nerve.

Diagnosis and investigation

The advent of MRI has greatly altered the pre- and postoperative evaluation of children with brain tumours. Multiplanar imaging is extremely helpful in determining the exact extent of the tumour and its relationship to surrounding normal structures. The importance of CT is restricted to the proof of calcifications or associated bone destruction. The administration of paramagnetic resonance contrast agents, such as gadolinium diethylenetriaminepentaacetic acid (DTPA) in MRI studies and iodinated contrast agents with CT, have been proved to identify tumours and metastatic disease in brain and spine more accurately.[17] In addition to MRI, magnetic resonance spectroscopy (MRS) has been shown to be helpful in differential diagnosis, management, and prognostication of brain tumours (Fig. 17.1). Positron emission tomography (PET) and single photon emission computed tomography (SPECT) are functional imaging tools which are increasingly used.

Sonography is the appropriate first investigation in children with open fontanelles. The children do not have to be sedated or transferred to an imaging center, sections can be obtained

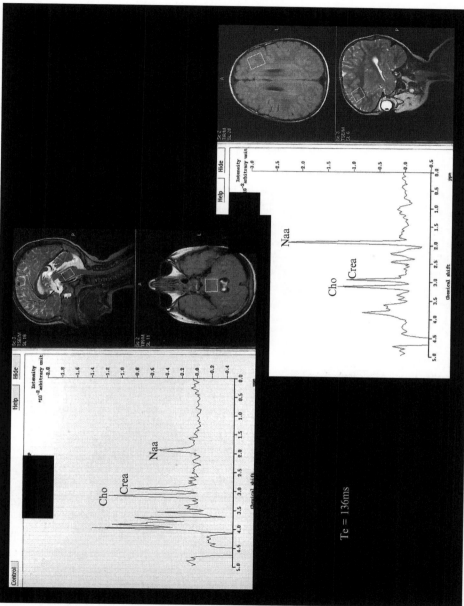

Fig. 17.1 Magnetic resonance spectra of a brainstem tumour and a cerebral glioma. The distribution and intensity of the different substances [choline (Cho), creatine (Crea), and *N*- acetyl aspartate (Naa)] are characteristic of the malignancy of the tissue. The pattern of the brainstem lesion indicates high malignancy; that of the cerebral glioma indicates low malignancy.

in a variety of orientations, and examinations can be repeated frequently. However, if a tumour is diagnosed by ultrasound, MRI or, if this is not available, CT is required for additional information.

Angiography is usually not needed unless a highly vascular lesion is suspected or a vascular malformation cannot be ruled out by non-invasive studies. In most cases, MR angiography, combined with a perfusion study, is sufficient to answer these questions.

Spinal imaging

Leptomeningeal metastases may affect the entire neuroaxis and necessitate evaluation of both the brain and the spinal cord. MRI has become the imaging method of choice as it has been shown to be clearly superior to myelography or CT myelography. When a brain tumour which is particularly prone to spinal seeding is diagnosed, MRI of the spine must be done before surgery of the primary tumour; otherwise postoperative reactive meningeal enhancement may mimic tumour involvement.

Postoperative imaging assessment

Surveillance imaging of the CNS at predetermined intervals is used to document the extent of tumour resection, to assess the tumour response to adjuvant treatment, to detect recurrence, and to evaluate the complications of treatment. The first contrast-enhanced postoperative MRI or CT scan should be scheduled within 72 h of surgery; within this period, enhancing structures are due to residual disease and not to therapy-related blood–brain barrier disruption. Consecutive scans can then be reliably compared with this 'baseline'study. However, distinction between residual tumour and post-therapeutic effects can also be made by means of MRS.

Treatment modalities

Neurosurgical treatment

Surgical intervention remains the mainstay of the diagnostic and therapeutic management of primary brain tumours. The goals of the surgery are:

- to establish a tissue diagnosis
- to excise or reduce the tumour volume and the mass effect
- potentially to cure the disease.

Completeness of surgical excision is the most important prognostic factor. Accurate histologic classification of a tumour is crucial for planning further therapy and determining prognosis. MRI- and CT-guided stereotactic biopsy is used as a first step in selected cases of thalamic and basal ganglia tumours, multifocal lesions, and radiologically diffusely infiltrating lesions without significant mass effect.

Most paediatric neurosurgeons prefer open craniotomy to stereotactic biopsy in the majority of children, even when only a subtotal resection is anticipated preoperatively. As the expanding mass or resulting hydrocephalus leads to raised ICP, with the risk of herniation through either the tentorial notch or the foramen magnum, prompt and effective cytoreduction can be lifesaving, even when the tumour is only subtotally resected.

After acquisition of diagnostic imaging results, the child is prepared for surgery by first managing the most urgent symptomatic problems. This includes steroid administration to relieve accompanying brain oedema, and anticonvulsive treatment if indicated in supratentorial hemispheric tumours. In patients who present with hydrocephalus, a CSF shunt should be avoided. Endoscopic third ventriculostomy is the procedure of choice in obstructing hydrocephalus. If removal of the mass is anticipated, the decision about third ventriculostomy can be made after surgery, as permanent hydrocephalus occurs in only 25–30 per cent of all patients with posterior fossa tumours and hydrocephalus.

The safety and efficacy of surgery has improved because of advances in surgical techniques, progress in neuroimaging, and developments in neuroanesthesia and paediatric critical care.

Consideration of the anatomical location of the tumour as visualized by MRI [Fig. 17.2(a)], the knowledge of the possibilities for postoperative adjuvant therapy depending on tumour type (determined by frozen section and smear), the age of the patient, and ultimately the intraoperative findings will determine surgical aggressiveness. Surgery alone is increasingly able to cure some paediatric brain tumours or to keep them in extended remission. Tumours that invade deep grey nuclei, such as the hypothalamus, thalamus, or basal ganglia in the dominant hemisphere, tumours in eloquent cortical areas, and tumours that are intrinsic to the brainstem can often not be totally resected without significant risk of devastating neurologic sequelae. Technical adjuncts allowing safer and more complete resection of radiologically well-defined tumours include intraoperative ultrasound, frameless stereotactic techniques allowing

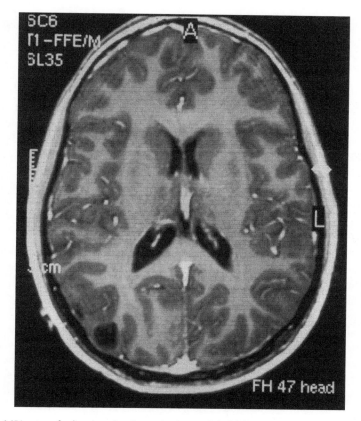

Fig. 17.2 (a) MRI scan of a low-grade glioma in the occipital lobe.   (Continued)

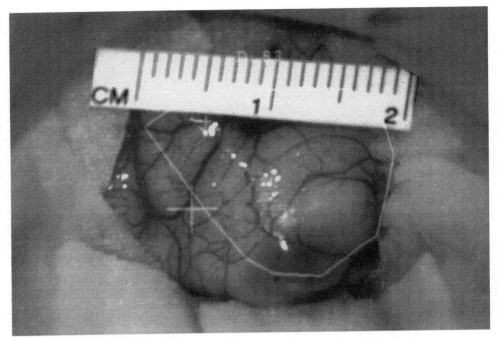

Fig. 17.2 (Continued) (b) The exposed cortex over the tumour with the contour of the lesion projected onto the operative site through a stereotactic surgical microscope.

interactive 3D-image-guided procedures [Fig.17.2(b)], and neurophysiologic monitoring of cortical, subcortical, and cranial nerve function.[18] The Cavitron ultrasonic aspirator (CUSA) enables the removal of firm tumours while minimizing injury to surrounding structures. The surgical laser is advocated by some as helpful, especially in dealing with intrinsic spinal cord tumours.

Endoscopy may also assist the microsurgical procedure in evaluating the completeness of a resection, and offer alternatives for biopsy, or even resection, of intraventricular masses.

Radiotherapy

Radiotherapy has been known to be an effective modality in the treatment of childhood brain tumours for decades. Nevertheless, local control and survival, in particular in aggressive and invasive tumours, still need to be significantly improved. On the other hand, late side effects related to radiotherapy have been recognized more clearly with the increase in numbers and follow-up of long-term survivors.[19,20]

Current treatment policies, including radiotherapy, therefore aim to increase the therapeutic ratio by different means: minimizing side effects by limiting the indications for radiotherapy for good-prognosis tumours (e.g. low-grade astrocytomas accessible by modern neurosurgical techniques), postponing or avoiding radiotherapy in very young children (e.g. ependymoma, medulloblastoma), dose reduction in radiosensitive tumours (e.g. craniospinal irradiation in germ cell tumours), volume reduction through better adaptation of the treated volume to the target (e.g. circumscribed low-grade tumours), improving local control by improving the quality of radiotherapy (e.g. medulloblastoma), or dose escalation using modern radiotherapy techniques (e.g. stereotactic irradiation, intensity-modulated radiotherapy) in the case of less radiosensitive tumours (e.g. high-grade glioma, ependymoma).

Radiation-related side effects in CNS radiotherapy are generally related to total dose, fractionation of dose, radiation volume, area of CNS irradiated, and the age of the child at the time of treatment.

With advances in neurologic and biologic imaging (MRI, MRS, SPECT, PET), target definition for radiotherapy has improved or will improve considerably in the future in nearly all CNS tumours. With the integration of sectional, functional, and biologic imaging tools into 3D treatment-planning procedures and 'conformal radiotherapy' techniques (using multiple individually shaped fields), the treated volume can be more adequately tailored to the target volume. Thus, in conformal radiotherapy, the high-dose irradiation of normal brain tissue can be reduced, without jeopardizing treatment results, provided that target definition has been correct. Conformal radiotherapy techniques based on 3D treatment planning have become general clinical practice in the majority of advanced radiotherapy departments in recent years, in particular for brain tumours.

A precondition for such precision radiotherapy is immobilization of the patient, which only permits minimal variations throughout the planning procedure and the whole course of fractionated radiotherapy. A variety of custom-made immobilization devices are available and should be in common use for the treatment of childhood brain tumours.

One of the most difficult procedures is craniospinal irradiation (CSI), in which children are treated in a prone position using an individually adapted fixation system (e.g. a plaster immobilization device) for the head and the spinal axis. Detailed quality assurance procedures are necessary and should be performed at regular intervals (e.g. weekly) during the treatment course to check the accuracy of the treatment set-up.

Major technical advances in dose-delivery systems have been the introduction of stereotactic radiotherapy and intensity-modulated radiotherapy. The advantage of these techniques, which use multiple radiation fields or arcs, is the steep fall-off of radiation dose in all directions outside the treated volume. By using this technique, small tumours (up to ~4 cm in diameter) directly adjacent to critical structures can be treated with high radiation doses with reduced radiation-related morbidity. In future, stereotactic irradiation and intensity-modulated radio-therapy, in combination with biologic imaging, may allow a highly focused dose escalation with better local control. The efficacy of 3D conformal proton radiotherapy with its very steep fall-off in dose (Bragg peak) has been demonstrated for low-grade tumours (e.g. large optic pathway tumours) in some specialized centers. With growing availability of proton treatment facilities, this most conformal radiotherapy will be increasingly used in paediatric brain tumours as well.

Image-guided stereotactic low-dose-rate interstitial and intracavitary brain radiotherapy with different isotopes (e.g. ^{125}I, ^{192}Ir, ^{90}Y, ^{32}P) has been in use in some specialist centers and may be indicated in specific situations in slowly proliferating well-circumscribed lesions. However, great experience is necessary to handle these techniques adequately, and as the results reported so far are not clearly superior, they should only be used in experienced hands and in prospective clinical protocols.

Chemotherapy

Progress in the chemotherapy of brain tumours has lagged behind that of other neoplasms of childhood. Reasons for this include problems unique to the treatment of tumours of the CNS.

Special aspects of brain tumours

One cause of ineffectiveness of certain chemotherapeutic agents is the blood–brain/CSF barrier. While the role of this barrier is questionable in some tumours, such as medulloblastoma, it appears to be a more important issue in diffuse infiltrating gliomas as it is often difficult to deliver adequate concentrations of drugs to the periphery of the tumour. In addition, many brain tumours have a low mitotic index and thus a reduced susceptibility to cell cycle specific drugs. Another obstacle is brain tumour heterogeneity. Each entity has its own biologic characteristics, including cellular mechanisms within the tumour that are responsible for the ability to retain a chemotherapeutic agent or to repair drug-induced damage. A further problem is the tendency of paediatric malignant brain tumours to spread throughout the nervous system early during the course of disease. Therefore cytocidal drug levels must be obtained in the tumour tissue, brain parenchyma, and CSF.

Role of chemotherapy in brain tumours

Over the past decade chemotherapy has been shown to be clearly beneficial for medulloblastoma and high-grade glioma, and patients who received chemotherapy in addition to surgery and radiotherapy experienced better survival rates.

However, in paediatric neuro-oncology the use of chemotherapy is not limited to trying to improve survival. Given the long-term toxicities associated with whole-brain and/or neuraxis irradiation in children, chemotherapy is also used to delay and possibly replace some of the radiotherapy otherwise needed. In fact, in some patients, the need for radiotherapy has been eliminated by the use of chemotherapy. Chemotherapy is now widely used for infants and young children with malignant brain tumours and for patients with low-grade tumours that are not surgically resectable.

Chemotherapeutic agents and drug-delivery strategies utilized in brain tumours

Significant response rates have been reported for a number of chemotherapeutic agents. These include vincristine, procarbazine, the nitrosoureas BCNU and CCNU, etoposide, cisplatin, carboplatin, cyclophosphamide, ifosfamide, methotrexate, and temozolomide. As for most childhood cancers, multi-agent chemotherapy is utilized in brain tumours to improve efficacy and reduce the likelihood of resistance. Another strategy to improve the response rate of poor-prognosis CNS tumours is high-dose chemotherapy with autologous stem cell rescue. Early reports in both newly diagnosed and recurrent CNS tumours have shown some encouraging results for subgroups of patients, and new trials have begun in several centers.

Strategies to overcome problems posed by the blood–brain/CSF barrier

As many brain tumours will spread throughout the CSF, future design of brain tumour protocols may include administration of a drug directly into the spinal fluid. The intrathecal route offers significant therapeutic advantage for molecules too large to pass through the blood–brain barrier and may avoid systemic toxicity.

The steep dose–response curve of bifunctional alkylating agents, coupled with their known activity against a variety of paediatric brain tumours, suggest the need for strategies to achieve high levels of these drugs in the CSF. Recent trials have demonstrated that agents such as mafosfamide, a preactivated cyclophosphamide derivative, can be safely administered into the CSF and may produce responses in leptomeningeal neoplasia. Intratumoral administration of chemotherapeutic agents is also undergoing investigation as a new modality to improve drug delivery to the tumour.

Since it does not appear that surgery or radiotherapy alone will improve the cure rate of brain tumours in the near future, the search must continue to identify new and better agents and to develop more effective delivery mechanisms for these agents. It is hoped that eventually better understanding of the molecular genetics and biology of brain tumours will translate into new treatments, including immunotherapy, gene therapy, and the use of anti-angiogenesis factors and second-messenger inhibitors.

Specific management

Low-grade gliomas

Low-grade gliomas account for ~40 per cent of all childhood brain tumours and comprise a heterogenous group with regard to histologic subtype, anatomical location, and biologic behaviour.[21] Childhood cancer registries assume a systematic under-reporting of these neoplasms which is partially due to the limited patient referral to centers of tertiary care.[22] Although most children with low-grade gliomas already have an excellent prognosis, a proportion of these children will have recurrences following resection or experience progression following incomplete tumour removal or biopsy. Therefore the International Consortium of Low-Grade Glioma Research developed a protocol (SIOP–LGG 2003) which offers a comprehensive treatment strategy for all children and adolescents who are affected by a low-grade glioma arising in any part of the CNS. Results of the preceding SIOP–LGG trial, as well as from national trials and reports in the literature, form the basis of the recommendations and the randomized part(s) of the study.

Cerebellar astrocytomas

Cerebellar astrocytomas carry a more favourable prognosis than most other brain tumours.[23] The majority are histologically benign, slow-growing, well-circumscribed, and often cystic lesions which involve the vermis and cerebellar hemispheres with approximately equal frequency. Invasion of the cerebellar peduncles or brainstem may occur. The goal in the treatment of these tumours is gross total resection. If achieved, a cure rate of nearly 100 per cent is expected. However, in some children, total removal may be impossible or hazardous due to brainstem involvement or perioperative complications. Although subtotal resection may allow an extended period of disease control in these patients, a significant percentage of lesions ultimately progress and require additional therapy. At present, the role of radiotherapy after incomplete resection remains unclear. In the absence of convincing data favouring the routine use of radiotherapy, many groups defer it until there is evidence of progressive disease that is surgically unresectable. Early experience at some institutions with radiosurgery and stereotactic radiotherapy for the treatment of focal areas of tumour recurrence suggests that this modality is useful in managing small areas of unresectable disease in critical locations.

Gliomas of the optic pathway

Most gliomas of the optic pathways occur during the first 5 years of life and are low-grade pilocytic astrocytoma. These tumours are associated with neurofibromatosis (NF-1) in 15–20 per cent of patients. Clinical symptoms depend on the location along the optic pathway, and include exophthalmos, decrease in visual acuity, disk pallor, visual field changes, endocrine dysfunction, and the diencephalic syndrome. The behaviour of these tumours is highly variable and unpredictable. Large tumours may remain stable for years, while initially small chiasmatic tumours may show rapid disease progression.

Management strategies for visual pathway gliomas include observation, chemotherapy, radiotherapy, surgery, and various combinations of these modalities. The time for intervention and choice of treatment modality have to be considered carefully. The risks of treatment-related side effects, such as optic nerve injury, vasculopathy, and endocrinopathy, have to be weighed against irreversible symptoms of tumour progression, leading to deterioration of visual and endocrine function.

Children without evidence of tumour growth after diagnosis are followed by MRI and neurodevelopmental, ophthalmologic, and endocrinologic examinations. When tumour progression is diagnosed, therapeutic intervention should be considered.

Unilateral optic nerve gliomas without chiasmal involvement may be cured by resection of the affected optic nerve. An alternative approach which conserves the optic nerve is conformal stereotactic radiotherapy. Tumours involving the chiasm and hypothalamic tumours are treated by a combined approach including surgery, radiotherapy, and chemotherapy.

Neurosurgical intervention aims at tissue diagnosis, resection of exophytic tumour extensions, drainage of tumour cysts, and decompression of the optic nerve.

The role of chemotherapy for the treatment of young children with progressive symptomatic tumours can be considered fairly well established in terms of achieving tumour responses and prolonged progression-free survival, and delaying the need for radiotherapy.[24–26] According to SIOP–LGG 2003, children <8 years of age with visual pathway tumours and without NF-1 will be randomized to receive standard induction chemotherapy with vincristine and carboplatin or intensified induction chemotherapy with vincristine, carboplatin and etoposide. In older children (≥8 years) radiotherapy is the preferred first adjuvant therapy. Children affected by NF-1 are particularly prone to developing vasculopathies and should be treated with chemotherapy at all ages.

Local radiotherapy is performed by applying radiation doses of 40–50 Gy with highly focused conformal and stereotactic techniques to limit irradiation of uninvolved tissues, where possible. If there is tumour progression during or after chemotherapy, local radiotherapy remains the treatment of choice.

Low-grade brainstem gliomas

Low-grade tumours of the brainstem are typically 'focal' and can be differentiated from the prognostically unfavourable diffuse tumours by MRI. They make up ∼ 20 per cent of tumours in this location and can be further classified on the basis of their topography and growth pattern. Clinical symptoms depend on location and tumour size, and often consist of cranial nerve deficits, long tract signs, and ataxia, whereas symptoms of hydrocephalus are present in the dorsally exophytic tumours of the pons and medulla filling the fourth ventricle and are the typical presentation of tectal tumours. This subgroup of midbrain tumours of the quadrigeminal plate with obstructive hydrocephalus usually has an indolent course, and treating the hydrocephalus with an endoscopic third ventriculostomy without histologic confirmation is considered appropriate. The histology of the focal tumours of the brainstem is mostly that of a low-grade lesion and includes astrocytoma grade 2, pilocytic astroytoma grade 1, and ganglioglioma. Rapidly progressing symptoms in a patient with a focal tumour on MRI are suggestive of a high-grade tumour (e.g. PNET).

Surgical resection should be discussed for focal low-grade tumours which can be reached without unacceptable morbidity. While complete resection is possible in selected cases, the residual disease may remain stable without need for adjuvant therapy even with partial resection.[27] In the case of progression or non-resectability with severe symptoms, chemotherapy should be considered according to current trials. An interesting alternative is (stereotactic) conformal radiotherapy which is being investigated in some centers.

Supratentorial low-grade gliomas

Low-grade gliomas comprise a heterogeneous group with regard to histologic subtype, anatomical location, and biologic behaviour.

Roughly half of supratentorial low-grade gliomas are located in the cerebral hemispheres, and the remainder occur in the deep midline structures of the diencephalon and basal ganglia. Pilocytic and diffuse astrocytomas are the most frequently encountered gliomas, although other variants, such as the ganglioglioma, pleomorphic xanthoastrocytoma, and oligodendroglioma, must also be considered in the differential diagnosis. Surgical excision remains the primary therapy for the majority of these low-grade gliomas. Since at least 50 per cent of children with low-grade gliomas of the cerebral hemispheres present with seizures, the goal of surgery includes the alleviation of an associated seizure disorder, when intractable. It is now possible to target the operative approach to a subcortical lesion or a superficial lesion that is located within 'eloquent' cortex by using a combination of functional studies and stereotactic localization. Provided that a total excision can be achieved, no further therapy is warranted. Conservative management with routine imaging follow-up is appropriate for those lesions that are incompletely resected as childhood tumours rarely progress histologically to more malignant lesions. Reoperation is necessary if recurrence is documented, and radiotherapy is utilized for those lesions that are incompletely resected following recurrence.[18]

Unitl recently, thalamic astrocytomas were considered to be largely unresectable. However, with the implementation of computer-assisted stereotactic approaches, perioperative morbidity and mortality have dropped substantially, and near-complete resection has become an attainable goal in many children with pilocytic, low-grade, and cystic astrocytomas. In such cases, adjuvant therapy can often be deferred. For patients in whom a subtotal resection is performed to avoid the risk of incurring neurologic deficit, long-term disease-free survival can occur with certain indolent low-grade astrocytomas which correspond histologically to pilocytic astrocytoma of the cerebellum or optic pathway. Adjuvant therapy, either radiation (e.g. stereotactic procedures) or chemotherapy, is utilized in those cases of low-grade lesions that are unresectable and have documented disease progression.

High-grade gliomas

Anaplastic astrocytoma and glioblastoma

Most malignant gliomas, other than brainstem gliomas, are supratentorial in location and are among the most difficult tumours to treat in children. With a combination of surgery and irradiation, the median survival for children with malignant gliomas is only 9 months. In a randomized Children's Cancer Support Group trial (1985–1990), a multidrug regimen ('eight in one') was tested against CCNU, vincristine, and prednisone which had been evaluated in the first trial (1976–1981). No difference was detected. However, both groups had outcomes superior to standard irradiation and surgery. Five-year-survival for anaplastic astrocytoma and glioblastoma was 42 per cent and 27 per cent, respectively, for patients with >90 per cent resection, compared with only 14 per cent and 4 per cent, respectively, with less resection. However, it remains uncertain whether this survival advantage is a direct result of surgery, or merely reflects the fact that certain tumours, by virtue of their less aggressive growth characteristics or more favourable location, are amenable to more extensive resection.[28]

In Germany children with high-grade gliomas are treated according to recently proposed prospective cohort studies (HIT-GBM-D 2003). All patients receive simultaneous radio-chemotherapy consisting of external beam therapy (54–59 Gy) and cisplatin, ifosfamide, etoposide, and vincristine followed by maintenance therapy with CCNU, vincristine, and prednisone, a combination which has shown efficacy in the earlier trials mentioned above. In one of the two treatment arms patients receive high-dose methotrexate before radiotherapy. Survival rates of the prior HIT GBM trials (A, B, C) for patients with completely resected supratentorial high-grade gliomas were 48 per cent after 5 years. For patients in whom the tumour could not be resected the 3-year survival was only 3 per cent (J. Wolff *et al.*, unpublished data).

High-grade brainstem glioma

Approximately 80 per cent of tumours arising in the brainstem are diffuse intrinsic lesions which mostly carry an unfavourable prognosis. They can be distinguished from the favourable glioma by their typical diffuse growth pattern as seen on MRI. As a rule, there is no need for histologic confirmation by stereotactic biopsy if the clinical presentation and the MRI findings are characteristic, even though stereotactic procedures now carry a low risk of morbidity.

Clinical symptoms often consist of deficits in cranial nerves V–IX, long tract signs, and ataxia, and depend on location and tumour size. A short duration of symptoms (e.g. 1 month) and diffuse infiltration on MRI indicate a high grade of malignancy and an unfavourable prognosis.

Radiotherapy remains the standard treatment for diffuse intrinsic brainstem tumours as surgery is not an option in the majority of patients. The target is the macroscopic lesion on MRI (T1 weighted with contrast medium) with a safety margin. Although the majority of patients (~ 70 per cent) show a significant improvement in neurologic status following such treatment, the prognosis is very poor. The median time to disease progression is of the order of 5–6 months, the median survival time is <1 year, and survival at 2 years and beyond is <10 per cent. These findings have led to dose-escalation studies with hyperfractionation (55–78 Gy, 1.2 Gy twice daily) by the Paediatric Oncology Group (POG), the Children's Cancer Group (CCG), the University College of San Francisco (UCSF), and the Children's Hospital of Philadelphia (CHOP). No clear survival advantage could be proved in this relatively large cohort of children. High doses (>72 Gy) led to more radiation-related brain damage (e.g. intralesional necrosis). Results of further (randomized) trials (e.g. POG) have to be awaited before recommendation of any aggressive hyperfractionated high-dose radiotherapy for standard treatment.[29] In the POG trial survival for patients treated with hyperfractionated radiotherapy plus cisplatin was worse than for patients receiving the same radiotherapy alone.[30]

The principles of chemotherapy are identical to the protocols described above for glioblastoma.

Medulloblastoma

Medulloblastoma, the most frequent malignant paediatric brain tumour, is a distinctive embryonal brain tumour originating in the posterior fossa, locally infiltrating in the brainstem or the fourth ventricle, or growing continuously along the cerebrospinal pathway. Tumour cell dissemination into the CSF is detected at diagnosis in a quarter of the patients.

The diagnosis of medulloblastoma is usually suspected from preoperative MRI. Dissemination via the CSF must be investigated by MRI and CSF cytology before starting postoperative therapy. A surgically based staging system attempts to classify tumour stage (T1–T4) (location, volume, and extension into neighbourhood structures), and stage of metastatic disease (M0–M4). Disease classified as T1–T3a M0 is regarded as early stage (favourable), and T3b–4 is regarded as locally advanced high stage (unfavourable).

Some prognostic factors are commonly described in series dealing with medulloblastoma. The most significant adverse factor is CSF spread at diagnosis (M1) and presence of macroscopic metastatic disease (M2–M4). Further important prognostic factors are the age of the child, with worse outcome in young children (<2 years), and tumour resectability, which is correlated with local stage.

Surgery and postoperative radiotherapy are the standard treatments, but nowadays chemotherapy also plays an important role for all patients. In patients with low and average risk disease the use of chemotherapy has allowed a reduction in the dose of radiotherapy to the craniospinal axis and appears to have brought about a significant improvement in disease-free and overall survival. Patients with high-risk disease now fare better with combined chemo- and radiotherapy.[4]

Surgery aims at total tumour removal, which can now be achieved in the vast majority of cases (including 'near-total' removal). However, in general, no major surgery-related permanent neurologic deficits are acceptable.

After surgery a 'posterior fossa syndrome' (e.g. truncal ataxia, cerebellar mutism) may occur. This may be transient but may also take months to remit. Its presence should not delay postoperative treatment.[31]

Postoperative CSI with 35 Gy (less in low risk patients with chemotherapy) and an additional field to the posterior fossa with a total dose >50 Gy using 1.6–1.8 Gy per fraction is currently the gold standard for cure of medulloblastoma. New studies with hyperfractionated radiotherapy have attempted to increase the dose to the tumour region up to a high total dose without increasing the risk for late effects. A dose of 1 Gy twice daily to the whole cerebrospinal target, CSI up to 24–36 Gy, and a local dose up to 68–72Gy are being evaluated in different studies.[32,33]

There is some controversy about the adequate dose for prophylactic irradiation (spinal and supratentorial). In series with a final outcome of >50 per cent 5-year survival, the most frequently reported doses have been about 35 Gy. In favourable cases, radiation dose reduction alone (without additional chemotherapy) has led to inferior results with early isolated neuraxis relapse and lower 5-year event-free and overall survival than standard irradiation (36 Gy).[34] In disseminated disease the standard dose of 36 Gy is suboptimal; therefore the CSI dose should be increased to 40 Gy, with additional boost doses of up to 45–50 Gy.[35] Careful design of target volumes is mandatory (CSI and posterior fossa boost), based on all the information available (e.g. surgical and histopathologic reports, MRI) and on institutional experience. CSI is one of the most complicated radiation treatment techniques in a young child. Poor results may be due to inadequate radiation treatment planning and performance, and therefore great care should be taken with this treatment.

Medulloblastoma is a chemosensitive tumour. Chemotherapy (platinum, vincristine, CCNU, alkylating agents) is becoming increasingly accepted as standard in all patients with medulloblastoma during first-line treatment. Five-year progression-free survival rates are better after combined chemo- and radiotherapy than after radiotherapy alone. Many trials are currently

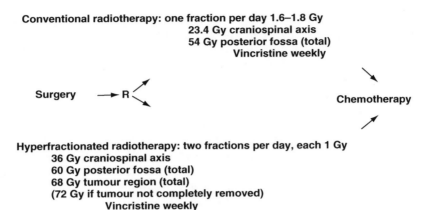

Conventional radiotherapy: one fraction per day 1.6–1.8 Gy
23.4 Gy craniospinal axis
54 Gy posterior fossa (total)
Vincristine weekly

Surgery —→ R

Chemotherapy

Hyperfractionated radiotherapy: two fractions per day, each 1 Gy
36 Gy craniospinal axis
60 Gy posterior fossa (total)
68 Gy tumour region (total)
(72 Gy if tumour not completely removed)
Vincristine weekly

<u>Chemotherapy</u>

1. **Weekly chemotherapy during radiotherapy**
    Vincristine 1.5 mg/m² (max. 2mg) bolus injection

2. **Eight chemotherapy cycles after radiotherapy with 4-week interval**
    Cisplatin 70 mg/m² i.v. infusion over 6 h   Day 1
    CCNU 75 mg/m² oral   Day 1
    Vincristine 1.5 mg/m² i.v. bolus injection   Days 1, 8, 15

Fig. 17.3 Design of medulloblastoma HIT 2000 trial for tumours without metastasis.

under way, trying to clarify chemotherapy schedules and the timing of their delivery within a combined treatment approach (CCG, POG, SIOP, GPOH, and CHOP). The current HIT 2000 protocol for medulloblastoma without metastasis is shown in Figure 17.3. Bone marrow or stem cell transplantation with high-dose chemotherapy is a treatment option for high-risk patients.

In various series, survival rates ranging from 50 to 70 per cent at 5 years, and from 30 to 60 per cent at 10 years, have been reported after surgery and radiotherapy. Single institutions even report survival rates of ∼80 per cent at 5 years.[1,36]

PNETs

PNETs arising in the supratentorial region are associated with a different outcome, even when treatment similar to that given for medulloblastoma is used. These tumours often occur between birth and 5 years. They are found predominantly in the cerebral hemispheres, most commonly in the frontal and temporal lobes. On imaging, they may appear as well-circumscribed masses, but there is often widespread microscopic extension. Glial, neuronal, or ependymal differentiation may be seen. Leptomeningeal spread is uncommon compared with medulloblastoma and is less frequent at presentation than with medulloblastoma. Patients present with non-specific signs of raised intracranial pressure, seizures, or motor impairment. Investigations should include imaging of the whole ventricular system and spine to exclude seeding. Surgical resection is often difficult because of their size and position. Craniospinal irradiation has been recommended, but results in progression-free survival rates of only 30 per cent. Chemotherapy follows the guidelines for medulloblastoma.

Ependymoma

Ependymomas arise from ependymal cells lining the ventricles and the central canal of the spinal cord. Nearly two-thirds occur in the infratentorial compartment. Anaplastic tumours tend to be more common in the posterior fossa than in the supratentorial region of young children. Tumour cells in the CSF are described in 5–15 per cent of patients; the rate of drop metastases is higher in anaplastic ependymoma. Prognostic factors are the age of the patient, tumour location, tumour stage, histology, extent of resection, and radiation dose.

MRI of the brain and spinal cord at the time of diagnosis are mandatory for optimal treatment planning. Surgery, radiotherapy, and chemotherapy are used in treatment. Surgery is the most effective treatment, but is rarely curative. There are three indications for surgery: for tumour resection at diagnosis, for resection of residual disease after adjuvant therapy, and for resection of a relapse, usually at the primary site. The primary goal is to remove the tumour totally and re-establish CSF flow. If significant morbidity is to be avoided, total removal is often not possible in posterior fossa tumours because of the specific growth pattern of ependymomas with invasion of the fourth ventricular floor and encasement of lower cranial nerves and regional arteries.

Although the role of postoperative radiotherapy is well established, there are many controversies regarding the appropriate extent of radiotherapy. Currently, local postoperative radiotherapy (55 Gy, 1.8–2 Gy per fraction) to the primary tumour site with broad margins (>2 cm) is considered appropriate not only for low-grade and all supratentorial ependymoma but also for anaplastic infratentorial ependymomas. CSI is the standard basic treatment only for disseminated tumours.[19] At present, local dose escalation is being prospectively evaluated if there is postoperative residual disease.

The role of chemotherapy is unclear. In current clinical trials, chemotherapy with vincristine, cisplatin, etoposide, and cyclophosphamide is being investigated. There seems to be an indication for children aged <3 years, but neither the St Jude study nor 'Baby POG' has shown improved long-term outcome.

Overall, 5-year survival rates, mostly after combination treatment, range from 28 to 60 per cent depending on prognostic factors.[1,36] The frequent local recurrence (within 18–24 months of diagnosis) is almost always incurable. Nevertheless, local palliative treatment procedures may improve symptoms for the limited life expectancy (Fig. 12.4).

Choroid plexus neoplasms

Choroid plexus neoplasms occur in all age groups but represent 10–20 per cent of brain tumours seen in children during the first year of life. They more commonly arise in the lateral ventricles in children and are capable of secreting CSF. The dominant presenting feature are signs and symptoms of raised intracranial pressure. Papillomas and carcinomas are capable of leptomeningeal dissemination.

The treatment of benign choroid plexus papillomas is total surgical excision, which is usually curative. Because of the haemorrhagic tendency of the tumour, operative mortality still remains high. A more aggressive and anaplastic tumour, the choroid plexus carcinoma, accounts for 10–20 per cent of choroid plexus neoplasms. The likelihood of achieving gross total resection is less in this tumour because of local invasion, and therefore the likelihood of cure is limited.

A pilot study evaluating the feasibility of an intercontinental phase III chemotherapy study for patients with choroid plexus tumours is active (CPT-2000). According to this protocol, patients with choroid plexus papilloma will be followed without adjuvant treatment and

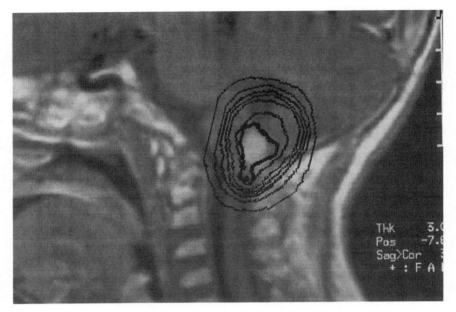

Fig. 17.4 Recurrence of ependymoma: distribution of radiation dose from stereotactic radiotherapy using multiple arcs.

reoperated on if there is recurrence. Patients in whom further surgical resection is impossible and patients with choroid plexus carcinoma are randomized between a carboplatin-based and a cyclophosphamide-based protocol. Both arms will also include vincristine and VP16. Since the majority of patients are infants, they will not receive irradiation. However, irradiation will be given in both treatment arms after the second block of chemotherapy to patients >3 years of age.

Pineal tumours and germ cell tumours

Tumours arising in the region of the pineal gland are rare, and can be classified into three groups: germ cell tumours, pineal parenchymal tumours, and gliomas.

Primary CNS germ cell tumours (40–65 per cent of all pineal tumours) mainly arise in the pineal or suprasellar region. Their incidence is substantially higher in Japan than in Western countries. Their peak age incidence is in the second or third decades of life. Germ cell tumours are pathologically heterogeneous, reflecting varied cell types of origin. At least half to two-thirds are pure germinomas. The remaining patients have non-germinomatous tumours, which may be classified, depending upon their predominant constituent cell type(s), into embryonal carcinoma, endodermal sinus (or yolk-sac) tumour, choriocarcinoma, malignant teratoma, or malignant mixed germ cell tumours. The histologic appearance of these tumours is identical to similar tumours occurring outside the CNS. Rare patients are found with immature or mature teratomas without any malignant germ cell elements.

Once the presence of a pineal region mass has been demonstrated radiographically, CSF and serum should be examined for tumour markers such as α-fetoprotein (AFP) and the β subunit of human chorionic gonadotrophin (β-HCG), which are produced by intracranial yolk-sac tumours and choriocarcinoma, respectively. This is important, because in patients with significant marker elevation (β-HCG > 50 IU 1^{-1}; AFP > 25 ng ml^{-1}), surgery is not necessary to establish a tissue diagnosis before starting therapy. In all other patients, however, a histologically verified diagnosis is mandatory. Benign teratomas are often surgically completely resectable, and thereby cured. Leptomeningeal seeding may be present in patients with malignant germ cell tumours, and spinal MRI and CSF cytology are required for clinical staging.

For pure germinomas, radiotherapy alone leads to cure rates of up to 100 per cent (e.g. GPOH trial[32]). However, dose (40–50 Gy local treatment and 22–35 Gy CSI) and volume remain issues of debate. Some groups (e.g. SFOP) use platinum-based multidrug regimens in combination with local radiotherapy and achieve slightly worse results.

Non-germinomatous germ cell tumours are rarely cured with radiotherapy alone, and the addition of platinum-based chemotherapy is essential. Preoperative chemotherapy has been shown to be effective in facilitating complete resection of large or infiltrating tumours and in diminishing the risk of a primary operation. However, local radiotherapy is important for local control, even in patients with complete response to chemotherapy.

Pineal parenchymal tumours consist of pineoblastomas and pineocytomas. Pineoblastomas develop in the younger patient and are PNETs. The high malignancy suggests that the approach to treatment should be similar to medulloblastoma and include aggressive resection, CSI with a local boost, and chemotherapy. Pure pineocytomas are slower-growing, relatively well-circumscribed masses, and have a benign course. Complete surgical removal represents the definitive treatment. Careful evaluation of the histology must exclude malignant components revealing a mixed tumour, which should be treated according to its most malignant part.[1]

Craniopharyngiomas

Craniopharyngiomas are histologically benign tumours originating in the sellar and suprasellar area from embryonic squamous cell rests of the pharyngeal–hypophyseal duct. Their macroscopic and neuroradiologic appearance is of a cystic, solid, or mixed-mass lesion, typically with calcifications. Since they are slow-growing tumours, they may reach large sizes before they become symptomatic, with endocrine dysfunction, visual problems, or signs of ICP with obstructive hydrocephalus in ~30 per cent.

The best management of craniopharyngioma in children remains controversial. Treatment options for this tumour include microsurgery, fractionated conformal radiotherapy, stereotactic procedures, intracavitary radiotherapy, and intracavitary chemotherapy.

Surgery is performed with either an attempt at radical total removal or more conservatively, if necessary followed by radiotherapy. Total removal is possible in 60–90 per cent of cases. However, even in these recent series, recurrence rates between 7 and 34 per cent are reported, with an average of 23 per cent, and major morbidity remains a concern even in experienced hands. Morbidity relates not only to a deterioration of visual and pituitary function, but even more importantly to complex and severe cognitive and neurobehavioural disturbances. If the tumour is totally removed, no further immediate treatment is indicated.[37]

Recurrence is treated by reoperation followed by radiotherapy, or by radiotherapy alone. As ~70 per cent of patients with partial resection will show tumour progression, these patients should be irradiated using conformal or stereotactic techniques (55–60 Gy). Occasionally, radiation will be deferred in a young child, but these patients require close follow-up. With a definitely lower mortality and morbidity, the long-term tumour control with this combined approach compares well with initial aggressive total resection alone, with ~ 20 per cent recurrent tumour growth.

Intracavitary radiotherapy with ^{32}P or ^{90}Y in experienced centers has given excellent results in monocystic tumours. Intracystic application of bleomycin has not only been shown to facilitate subsequent resection due to fibrosis of the capsule, but can also lead to shrinkage and long-term control.

Intramedullary spinal cord tumours

Spinal cord tumours account for only 3–6 per cent of primary CNS tumours in children. Of intramedullary tumours, up to 60 per cent are astrocytomas and 20–30 per cent are ependymomas. Oligodendrogliomas and gangliogliomas are less frequent. In general, these tumours are well-differentiated low-grade tumours, with only 10 per cent having high-grade or anaplastic features. The tumours may be focal or extend to involve multiple segments. The most common symptom is local pain along the spinal axis, alteration of a previously normal gait, and other signs of spinal cord malfunction occurring later in the course of the disease. Hydrocephalus may complicate the clinical picture in as many as 15 per cent of patients with spinal cord tumours.

Surgery for diagnosis and resection, if possible, is mandatory. Complete surgical resections are difficult in astrocytomas and appear to be possible more frequently in ependymomas which tend to have a clearer cleavage plane. Postoperative orthopaedic follow-up and monitoring for spinal deformity are important.

No controlled trial of radiation or chemotherapy has been carried out for intramedullary tumours, and evidence for their usefulness has to be inferred from the treatment of similar tumours in other CNS sites, such as cranial low-grade glioma and ependymomas. If radiotherapy is performed, it is targeted to the tumour region, with a total dose of 40–50 Gy, and seems to improve functional recovery.

The overall survival rates of low-grade astrocytomas with various degrees of resection and postoperative radiation therapy are 66–70 per cent at 5 years and 55 per cent at 10 years. Local recurrence rates as high as 33–86 per cent have been reported. In ependymomas, survival rates, depending on the amount of resection, vary from 50 to 100 per cent at 5 years and 50 to 70 per cent at 10 years.[38]

In the rare anaplastic or high-grade tumours, postoperative total neuraxis irradiation and adjuvant chemotherapy are recommended. However, patients usually succumb to their disease because of local progression or dissemination along CSF pathways.

Management of brain tumours in very young children

Brain tumours in infants and very young children have unique properties with regard to clinical presentation, anatomical location, histology, and prognosis that distinguish them from brain tumours occurring in the older child. By the time of diagnosis, most tumours in infants are quite large.

Delay in diagnosis occurs, in part, because the infant skull can expand to accommodate raised ICP, hence masking for some time the typical signs and symptoms associated with a mass lesion. Infants may present with failure to thrive (despite good appetite and food intake), endocrinopathies, developmental delay, vomiting, decreased visual acuity, and nystagmus accompanied by expanding head circumference.

Historically, infants with brain tumours have had the worst prognosis of any age group. Although delay in diagnosis, tumour type and size, and the tendency for early dissemination may be important factors, the poor outcome probably reflects the limitations of treatment.

Surgery is more difficult in the young child because of tumour size, the fragility of the immature brain, and problems related to neuroanaesthesia. In addition, radiation is known to be very toxic in this age group. Therefore, the dose is routinely reduced by at least 10–20 per cent. This reduced dose is probably inadequate for tumour control. Nevertheless, even with reduced radiation dose, major long-term effects, including learning disabilities, mental retardation, endocrinopathies, leucoencephalopathy, and vasculopathy, are to be expected in a significant number of patients. These concerns have resulted in interest in delaying or eliminating radiation in this young population by using postoperative chemotherapy.

The largest study of prolonged postoperative chemotherapy and delayed radiation in infants with brain tumours has come from the POG.[39] A total of 198 children aged <3 years with malignant brain tumours were treated with a combination of cyclophosphamide, vincristine, cisplatin, and VP16. Brainstem gliomas and pineoblastomas showed little or no response. The 5-year progression-free survival was 30 per cent and the overall 5-year survival was 39.4 per cent, which compared favourably with historical controls using standard postoperative radiation. Except for ependymomas, which tended to progress after several years, most failures occurred during the first 6 months of chemotherapy. While studies over the past decade have clearly confirmed that medulloblastomas are chemosensitive and that even leptomeningeal disease can be effectively treated at times, the POG data on ependymomas suggest that these tumours are chemosensitive but not chemocurable. Therefore, unlike young children with good-risk medulloblastoma, i.e. those who have had a gross tumour resection and no metastases, from whom radiation can be withheld, radiation may be deferred but usually cannot be eliminated in children with ependymoma. However, it is hoped that radiation-induced neurotoxicity to the hypothalamus–pituitary region, temporal lobes, and auditory apparatus can be reduced by the use of focal conformal radiation techniques, thereby potentially limiting the damage to growth, hearing, and cognition.

Another approach to prevent the need for craniospinal irradiation that deserves further evaluation is the use of high-dose chemotherapy with either autologous bone marrow transplant or stem cell rescue.

Late effects in children treated for brain tumours

As 5- and 10-year survival rates of children with CNS tumours have increased, so has concern over late effects of treatment. Many long-term survivors have intellectual, endocrine, and neurologic deficits that lead to significant social handicaps as well as diminished quality of life. Damage to the CNS from several sources may play a role in these deficits. Direct destruction of normal brain tissue by tumour, as well as surgical trauma, may cause some degree of irreversible neurologic damage. Likewise, chemotherapy, especially in combination with radiation, appears capable of inducing encephalopathy. However, it is radiation therapy that has been implicated as the main cause of adverse long-term sequelae, particularly intellectual impairment. Some reports suggest that most children receiving whole-brain radiation have some form of cognitive deficit in various intelligence quotients, visual/perceptual skills, learning abilities, and adaptive behaviour. Prospective controlled studies have found a younger age at diagnosis, radiotherapy, methotrexate chemotherapy, tumour location, and time interval to testing to be important and related to a high risk of subsequent cognitive deficits.[40,41] Dose, fractionation, and volume of radiation influence the development of these deficits, with more severe sequelae occurring at higher doses and larger volumes.[19] Only recently, vasculopathies and multiple cerebral cavernomas have been described as relevant late effects of radiotherapy.[42,43] Thus, current cooperative group studies are treating infants and very young children with brain tumours with prolonged postoperative chemotherapy in an attempt either to delay or to eliminate cranial radiation entirely.

Detailed studies have revealed a wide range of endocrine dysfunction following cranial irradiation which includes the hypothalamic–pituitary region. The most common impairment is growth failure due to growth hormone deficiency.[1] Although growth hormone replacement therapy will improve longitudinal growth, it has not been as effective as in children with idiopathic growth hormone deficiency. Another factor contributing to decreased growth is spinal irradiation. The younger the child at the time of spinal irradiation, the more severe are the adverse effects on vertebral body growth.

Hypothyroidism may also occur, and if not corrected may lead to poor linear growth, learning difficulties, and lethargy. Evaluation of thyroxine and thyroid-stimulating hormone function will allow early treatment of this problem. Gonadal dysfunction has only recently been reported in children with brain tumours. Radiation to the sacral spine and a number of cytotoxic drugs, particularly alkylating agents, are associated with gonadal damage and can cause ovarian failure, oligospermia, or azoospermia in these patients. As more chemotherapy is used and the patients are followed longer, it is likely that a much higher incidence of these side effects will be noted. Thus several risk factors need to be addressed by future studies, and careful planning of drug–radiation combinations is essential to maximize survival while reducing long-term local and systemic sequelae. Therefore it is of paramount importance that these children remain under long-term surveillance so that problems are anticipated and therapeutic strategies instituted as early as possible (see also Chapter 7). Secondary tumours have been observed, but exact data are lacking.

References

1. **Cohen ME, Duffner PK** (eds) (1994). *Brain Tumours in Children. Principles of Diagnosis and Treatment* (2nd edn). New York: Raven Press, 127–46, 177–201, 219–39, 329–46, 455–81.

2. **Thomas DGT, Graham DI** (eds) (1995). *Malignant Brain Tumours*. New York: Springer-Verlag.

3. **Sposto R, Ertel IJ, Jenkin RD, et al.** (1989). The effectiveness of chemotherapy for treatment of high grade astrocytoma in children: results of a randomized trial. A report from the Children's Cancer Study Group. *J Neurooncol* 7, 165–77.

4. **Freeman CR, Taylor RE, Kortmann RD, Carrie C** (2002). Radiotherapy for medulloblastoma in children: a perspective on current international clinical research efforts. *Med Pediatr Oncol* 39, 99–108.

5. **Kleihues P, Cavenee WK** (eds) (2000). *Pathology and Genetics of Tumours of the Nervous System*. Lyon: IARC.

6. **Pollack IF** (1994). Brain tumours in children. *N Engl J Med* 331, 1500–7.

7. **Segal RA, Goumnerova LC, Kwon YK, et al.** (1994). Expression of the neurotrophin receptor trkC is linked to a favorable outcome in medulloblastoma. *Proc Natl Acad Sci USA* 91,12867–71.

8. **Grotzer MA, Janss AJ, Fung K-M, et al.** (2000). TrkC expression predicts good clinical outcome in primitive neuroectodermal brain tumors. *J Clin Oncol* 18, 1027–35.

9. **Herms J, Neidt I, Lüscher B, et al.** (2000). c-*myc* expression in medulloblastoma and its prognostic value. *Int J Cancer* 89, 395–402.

10. **Grotzer MA, Hogarty MD, Janss AJ, et al.** (2001). MYC messenger RNA expression predicts survival outcome in childhood primitive neuroectodermal tumor/medulloblastoma. *Clin Cancer Res* 7, 2425–33.

11. **Gilbertson RJ, Perry RH, Kelly PJ,** *et al.* (1997). Prognostic significance of HER2 and HER4 coexpression in childhood medulloblastoma. *Cancer Res* 57, 3272–80.

12. **Pomeroy SL, Tamayo P, Gaasenbeck M,** *et al.* (2002). Prediction of central nervous system embryonal tumour outcome based on gene expression. *Nature* 415, 436–42.

13. **Kraus JA, Felsberg J, Tonn JC,** *et al.* (2002). Molecular genetic analysis of the *TP53, PTEN, CDKN2A, EGFR, CDK4* and *MDM2* tumour-associated genes in supratentorial primitive neuroectodermal tumours and glioblastoma of childhood. *Neuropathol Appl Neurobiol* 28, 325–33.

14. **Raffel C** (1996). Molecular biology of paediatric gliomas. *J Neurooncol* 28, 121–8.

15. **Gurney JG, Severson RK, Davis S, Robison LL** (1995). Incidence of cancer in children in the United States. *Cancer* 75, 2187–95.

16. **Koos WT, Miller MH** (1971). *Intracranial Tumors of Infants and Children.* Stuttgart: Thieme, 14–22.

17. **Barkovoch AJ** (1993). Paediatric neuroimaging. *Contemporary Neuroimaging* (2nd edn), Vol 1. New York: Raven Press.

18. **Berger MS** (1996). The impact of technical adjuncts in the surgical management of cerebral hemispheric low-grade gliomas of childhood. *J Neurooncol* 28, 129–55.

19. **Halperin EC, Constine LE, Tarbell NJ, Kun LE** (1994). *Paediatric Radiation Oncology* (2nd edn). New York: Raven Press, 40–139.

20. **Kun L** (1994). Principles of radiotherapy. In: Cohen ME, Duffner PK (eds) *Brain Tumours in Children. Principles of Diagnosis and Treatment,* (2nd edn). New York: Raven Press, 95–116.

21. **Kaatsch P, Rickert CH, Kühl J,** *et al.* (2001). Population-based epidemiologic data on brain tumors in German children. *Cancer* 92, 3155–64.

22. **Michaelis J, Kaletsch U, Kaatsch P** (2000). Epidemiology of childhood brain tumors. *Zentralbl Neurochir* 61, 80–7.

23. **Campbell JW, Pollack IF** (1996). Cerebellar astrocytoma in children. *J Neurooncol* 28, 223–32.

24. **Janss AJ, Grundy R, Cnaan A,** *et al.* (1995). Optic pathway and hypothalamic/chiasmatic gliomas in children younger than age 5 years with a 6-year follow-up. *Cancer* 75,1051–9.

25. **Packer RJ, Ater J, Allen J,** *et al.* (1997). Carboplatin and vincristine chemotherapy for children with newly diagnosed progressive low grade gliomas. *J Neurosurg* 86, 747–54.

26. **Prados MD, Edwards MSB, Rabbitt J,** *et al.* (1997). Treatment of pediatric low grade gliomas with a nitrosourea-based multiagent chemotherapy regimen. *J Neurooncol* 32, 235–41.

27. **Walker DA, Punt JAG, Sokal M** (1999). Clinical management of brain stem glioma. *Arch Dis Child* 80, 558–64.

28. **Lyden DC, Mason WP, Finlay JL** (1996). The expanding role of chemotherapy for supratentorial malignant gliomas. *J Neurooncol* 28, 185–91.

29. **Heideman RL, Packer J, Albright LA,** *et al.* (1997). Tumours of the central nervous system. In: Pizzo PA, Poplack DG (eds) *Principles and Practice of Paediatric Oncology* (3rd edn) Philadelphia, PA: JB Lippincott, 633–98.

30. **Freeman CR, Kepner J, Kun LE,** *et al.* (2000). A detrimental effect of combined chemotherapy-radiotherapy approach in children with diffuse intrinsic brain stem gliomas. *Int J Radiat Oncol Biol Phys* 47, 561–4.

31. **Sutton LN, Phillips PC, Molloy PT** (1996). Surgical management of medullo-blastoma. *J Neurooncol* 29, 9–21.

32. **Kortmann RD, Kuhl J, Timmermann B,** *et al.* (2001). Current and future strategies in interdisciplinary treatment of medulloblastomas, supratentorial PNET (primitive neuroectodermal tumors) and intracranial germ cell tumors in childhood. *Strahlenther Onkol* 177, 447–61.

33. **Prados MD, Wara W, Edwards MS,** *et al.* (1996). Treatment of high-risk medulloblastoma and other primitive neuroectodermal tumors with reduced dose craniospinal radiation therapy and multi-agent nitrosourea-based chemotherapy. *Pediatr Neurosurg* 25, 174–81.

34. **Thomas PR, Deutsch M, Kepner JL, *et al.*** (2002). Low-stage medulloblastoma: final analysis of trial comparing standard-dose with reduced-dose neuroaxis irradiation. *J Clin Oncol* **18**, 3004–11.
35. **Jenkin D** (1996). The radiation treatment of medulloblastoma. *J Neurooncol* **29**, 45–54.
36. **Kaye AH, Laws ER Jr (eds)** (1995). *Brain Tumours.* Edinburgh: Churchill Livingstone, 493–504, 561–74, 665–671.
37. **Epstein FJ, Handler MH (eds)** (1991). Craniopharyngioma: the answer. *Paediatr Neurosurg* **21** (Suppl 1), 1–130.
38. **Epstein FJ, Constantini S** (1995). Spinal cord tumours of childhood. In Pang D (ed)*Disorders of the Pediatric Spine.* New York: Raven Press, 371–88.
39. **Duffner PK, Horowitz ME, Krischer JP, *et al.*** (1999). The treatment of malignant brain tumors in infants and very young children: an update of the Pediatric Oncology Group experience. *Neuro-oncology,* **1**, 152–61.
40. **Radcliffe J, Bunin GR, Sutton LN, *et al.*** (1994). Cognitive deficits in long-term survivors of childhood medulloblastoma and other non-cortical tumors: age-dependent effects of whole brain irradiation. *Int J Dev Neurosci* **12**, 327–34.
41. **Mulhern RK, Reddick WE, Palmer SL, *et al.*** (1999). Neurocognitive deficits in medulloblastoma survivors and white matter loss. *Ann Neurol* **46**, 834–41.
42. **Siffert J, Allen JC** (2000). Late effects of therapy of thalamic and hypothalamic tumors in childhhood: vascular, neurobehavioural and neoplastic. *Pediatr Neurosurg* **33**, 105–11.
43. **Heckl S, Aschoff A, Kunze S** (2002). Radiation-induced cavernous hemangiomas of the brain: a late effect predominantly in children. *Cancer* **94**, 3285–91.

Chapter 18

Soft tissue sarcoma

Gianni Bisogno and Christophe Bergeron

Introduction

Soft tissue sarcomas comprises a heterogeneous group of tumours derived from mesenchymal cells. As these cells normally mature into muscle, fibrous structures, fat, etc., the different histiotypes of soft tissue sarcomas are designated according to the line of differentiation that can be recognized in the tumour. Soft tissue sarcomas comprise ~8 per cent of all paediatric malignancies. Rhabdomyosarcoma (RMS) is the most common subtype in the first two decades of life, accounting for ~60–70 per cent of these diagnoses. RMS is rare in adults and arises before the age of 6 years in two-thirds of cases. Non-rhabdomyosarcoma soft tissue sarcomas (NRSTSs) comprise 20–30 per cent of all sarcomas in children and have a histology similar to that of adult sarcomas. The most common NRSTSs seen in children include synovial sarcoma, fibrosarcoma, and malignant peripheral nerve sheath tumour.

Rhabdomyosarcoma

Rhabdomyosarcoma can develop in any anatomic location of the body where mesenchymal tissue other than bone is present, and it can spread to the lungs, bone marrow, bones, lymph nodes, and other sites. The most common primary sites are the head and neck (40 per cent), genitourinary sites (20 per cent), and extremities (20 per cent). The strong chemosensitivity of RMS has been proved by the studies promoted by cooperative groups from North America and Europe, and the current approach to treatment includes a variable combination of chemotherapy, surgery, and radiotherapy. A number of prognostic factors have been identified, and defining the therapeutic strategy according to these factors creates complexity. The comparison between the results reported by the main international collaborative groups (IRS, SIOP, CWS, ICG)[1] is complicated by the use of different staging systems. However, recent collaboration between these groups has begun to resolve some of these difficulties, and agreement has been found on a standard approach to the criteria used for staging[1] and the pathologic classification.[2]

Aetiology

Rhabdomyosarcoma cannot be simply considered as a cancer arising from skeletal muscle; it is more appropriate to define it as a tumour derived from primitive mesenchyme and exhibiting a profound tendency towards myogenesis. Disease aetiology is unclear, but an association with familial cancer risk in both the Li–Fraumeni syndrome and neurofibromatosis type 1 has created interest in possible genetic causal factors. Additional aetiologic theories may emerge from data suggesting links between RMS and various environmental factors although no consistent relationships have been proved.

Pathology and biology

Rhabdomyosarcoma is characterized by a greater or lesser degree of myogenic differentiation, a feature that results from biologic forces related to aberrant transcription signals and the resultant production of myogenic proteins.[3] Classically, RMS is histologically distinguished into two main forms: embryonal (which accounts for ~80 per cent of all RMS) and alveolar subtypes (15–20 per cent of RMS). A third form, pleomorphic RMS, is described in adults but almost never encountered in children and no longer forms part of the paediatric classification.

Desmin and muscle-specific actin are relatively sensitive immunohistochemical markers, but they are also expressed by a variety of cells other than rhabdomyoblasts and detection of muscle transcription factors such as MyoD and myogenin is the most sensitive diagnostic indication. Other technologies, particularly the molecular genetic detection of the expression of myogenic transcription factors (e.g. *MYF* genes from the MyoD protein family) and the presence of cytogenetic abnormalities representing abnormal fusion genes, are likely to become increasingly important in clarifying the diagnosis of RMS, in distinguishing it from other soft tissue or small round cell tumours, and in confirming histologic subtype. Most alveolar RMSs display a t(2,13)(q35;q14) translocation, with genetic breakpoints which result in the fusion of genes *PAX3* and *FKHR*, or, less frequently, a variant t(1,13)(p36;q14) translocation with fusion of genes *PAX7* and *FKHR*, whilst many embryonal RMSs exhibit a loss of heterozygosity at chromosome 11p.[3]

Embryonal rhabdomyosarcoma

Embryonal rhabdomyosarcoma, described by Bérard in 1894 as 'tumeur embryonnaire du muscle strié' is characterized by a spindle or spindle and round cell tumour by a loose myxoid or dense collagenous stroma. Rhabdomyoblastic differentiation is expressed by the presence of strap-like cells, but cellularity, pleomorphism, and the number of mitoses vary considerably. Cross-striations are seen in more differentiated forms, and ultrastructural examination with electron microscopy demonstrates the presence of features such as sarcomeric Z bands and thin and thick filaments. The botryoid subtype is typically found at vaginal or nasopharyngeal sites where tumour grows into organ cavities. It is histologically similar to embryonal RMS with the additional feature of a condensed layer of tumour cells under the overlying mucosa, the so-called cambium layer. The spindle cell variant presents as either a collagen-poor leiomyomatous form or a collagen-rich form with a storiform pattern arising in paratesticular locations. Distinction from other forms of soft tissue sarcoma relies on the presence of well-differentiated rhabdomyoblasts in the spindle cell population.

Alveolar rhabdomyosarcoma

Alveolar rhabdomyosarcoma was first described by Riopelle and Theriault in 1956. Classically, this form displays an alveolar architecture, i.e. well-defined alveolar-like spaces separated by thick collagenous bands and lined with round tumour cells showing variable myogenic features. It is now generally accepted that the percentage of cells showing an alveolar pattern is unimportant and that even a focal presence is sufficient to justify the diagnosis. However, attention has also been paid to the cytologic features of alveolar RMS which are distinct from embryonal RMS, and a diagnosis of alveolar RMS can be made in the absence of an overt alveolar pattern when characteristic cytologic features are present. This is the basis for the diagnosis of the so-called solid alveolar variant.

International Classification of Rhabdomyosarcoma

Recently, pathologists from the major international soft tissue sarcoma groups published a consensus for a new International Classification of Rhabdomyosarcoma (ICR).[2] This has been tested in multivariate analysis and shown to be strongly predictive of survival in addition to established clinical risk factors. Three risk groups have been identified:

- superior prognosis: botryoid and spindle cell RMS
- intermediate prognosis: embryonal RMS
- poor prognosis: alveolar RMS (including the solid variant).

This classification system should now be used by all pathologists and cooperative groups in order to provide comparability between and within multi-institutional studies (Table 18.1). However, there remain areas of uncertainty, particularly with tumours that do not demonstrate clear cytologic evidence for myogenic differentiation (undifferentiated sarcoma) or cannot be adequately classified (sarcoma, not otherwise specified). There are also tumours, such as those with rhabdoid features, where it is not clear whether they form a distinct and separate group or represent morphologic variants of the major subtypes.

Clinical presentation and diagnosis

RMS is encountered at almost all anatomic sites, although the head and neck and genitourinary locations are the most common (Fig. 18.1). Presentation is strongly influenced by site. For example, tumours within the orbit tend to present early with obvious displacement of the globe and are rarely associated with regional lymph node or distant metastatic spread (Fig 18.2), whilst tumours in the nasopharynx may result in a relatively long history of nasal discharge and obstruction and frequently involve local extension to the base of the skull or the posterior aspect of the orbits with the potential for associated cranial nerve palsies or visual loss (Fig. 18.3). The definition of certain head and neck sites as 'parameningeal' relates to the risk of direct tumour extension into the meninges and beyond. Such tumours carry a risk of intracranial extension and, in some cases, involvement of the cerebrospinal fluid (CSF). Tumours within the genitourinary tract may present with urinary obstruction in bladder and prostate sites (Fig. 18.4), as a scrotal mass (paratesticular), or as a vaginal polyp or discharge

Table 18.1. Classifications of rhabdomyosarcoma: comparison of different systems

Horn-Enterine (1958)	SIOP (Caillaud, 1989)	NCI (Tsokos 1992)	International (Newton 1995)
Embryonal	Embryonal Dense, well differentiated Dense, poorly differentiated Not otherwise specified	Embryonal Leiomyomatous	Embryonal Spindle cell
Botryoid	Loose, non-botryoid Loose, botryoid	Botryoid Pleomorphic embryonal	Botryoid
Alveolar	Alveolar	Alveolar Solid variant	Alveolar (includes solid variant)
Pleomorphic	Pleomorphic	Pleomorphic	RMS, not otherwise specified Sarcoma, not otherwise specified Undifferentiated sarcoma

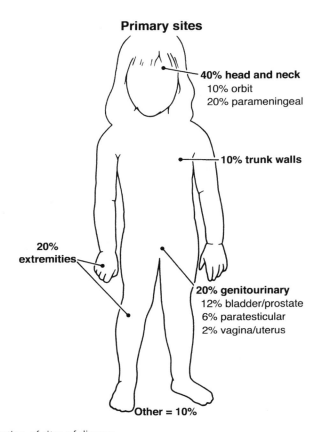

Fig. 18.1 Distribution of sites of disease.

(vaginal and uterine tumours). Elsewhere, presentation is usually associated with the development of a mass, and the child is often not unwell unless there is metastatic disease. In rare cases,
widespread metastatic disease is encountered without clear evidence of a primary tumour and
the diagnosis is confirmed by bone marrow examination.

Diagnostic and staging investigations must include adequate imaging of the primary site (CT
or MRI) and accurate assessment of sites of potential metastatic spread (lung, bone, and bone
marrow). The CSF should be sampled in the case of parameningeal tumours. The involvement
of regional lymph nodes depends on the primary site, and the frequency with which positive
lymph node spread is reported also depends on the manner in which this is investigated. This
remains a source of some controversy and, for example, the strategies promoted by the North
American Intergroup Rhabdomyosarcoma Study (IRS) Group have encouraged greater systematic use of surgicopathologic lymph node assessment than in European (particularly SIOP)
studies, in which clinical and radiologic evaluation has always been the standard approach.

Diagnosis must be confirmed histologically. Although needle biopsy may be the simplest
approach favoured by some clinicians, it has the disadvantage of limiting tissue available
for conventional histologic examination, including immunohistochemistry, and may restrict
access to fresh and frozen tissue for cytogenetic and molecular genetic investigation, both of
which may be of considerable importance in guiding diagnosis in difficult cases. Therefore open

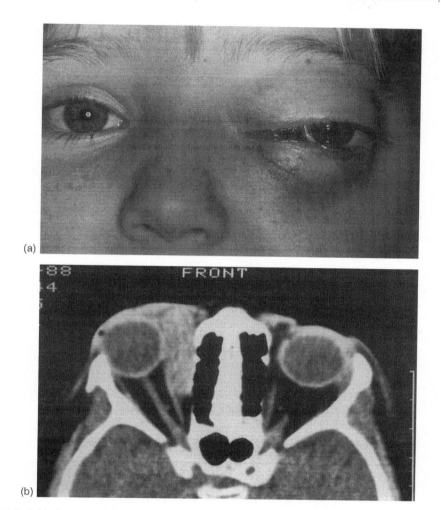

Fig. 18.2 Orbital tumour: (a) clinical presentation with proptosis and deviation of globe. (b) CT scan shows a large anteromedial soft tissue mass without bone erosion.

biopsy is frequently preferred and, when possible, should be undertaken at an oncology center where optimal use of diagnostic material can be achieved and the initial surgical approach determined by the multidisciplinary team responsible for the child's subsequent treatment. As site is such an important determinant of prognosis and treatment strategy, classification by site has been standardized by international agreement into seven major groups (Table 18.2).[4]

Treatment

Chemotherapy, which became an option in the 1970s, has proved efficient for the treatment of RMS, contributing to the remarkable increase in survival of such patients from ~25 to 70 per cent. Advances in surgery and radiotherapy have paralleled those of chemotherapy.

The multidisciplinary clinical management of RMS promotes systemic treatment for both local and metastatic lesions, with further local treatment using surgery and/or radiotherapy. As

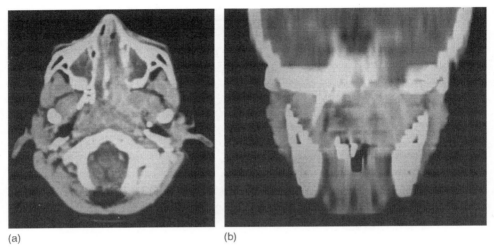

(a)   (b)

Fig. 18.3 Nasopharyngeal tumour: (a) CT scan showing a large soft tissue mass filling the nasopharynx and nasal cavities with destruction of the pterygoid plate; (b) CT scan reconstruction showing tumour extension through the base of skull.

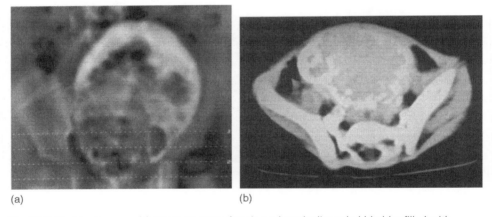

(a)   (b)

Fig. 18.4 Bladder tumour: (a) CT scanogram showing a hugely distended bladder filled with lobulated tumour; (b) cross-sectional CT image showing a lobulated tumour filling the bladder and outlined by contrast excretion into surrounding urine.

RMS often occurs in young children, the treatment strategy must balance the best chance of cure with the lightest possible burden of therapy in order to decrease sequelae and risk to future health. Treatment strategies are based on the prognostic factors developed over the past 20 years.

Prognostic factors

Histology It is now clear that alveolar RMS conveys a poorer prognosis than the embryonal subtype. This was apparent in the early IRS and SIOP trials and confirmed by results of the IRS IV study which showed 88 per cent relapse-free survival in embryonal RMS compared with 66 per cent in alveolar disease.[5]

Table 18.2. Definition of sites of involvement in childhood rhabdomyosarcoma

Favourable
Head and neck
Orbit
Non-parameningeal
Genitourinary
Non-bladder, non-prostate[a]
Unfavourable
Head and neck
Parameningeal[b]
Genitourinary
Bladder, prostate
Limbs
Other[c]

[a]Genitourinary non-bladder, non-prostate sites include paratesticular, vaginal, and uterine tumours.
[b]Parameningeal sites include nasopharynx, nasal cavity, paranasal sinuses, middle ear, mastoid, pterygoid fossa, and any non-parameningeal site with extension into a parameningeal position (e.g. orbital tumour extending intracranially into ethmoid sinus).
[c]Other sites include: trunk, chest and abdominal walls, intra abdominal, intrapelvic, perineal, and paravertebral tumours.

Site Site of disease has long been shown to be of prognostic value, both in North American and European studies. International consensus associates good prognosis with orbit, non-bladder prostate genitourinary, and non-parameningeal head and neck disease sites; all other sites are considered to have poor prognosis (Table 18.2).

Stage Ever since 1972, North American teams have favoured a classification of rhabdomyosarcomas into four groups, taking into account the extent of the initial surgical excision and the spread of the tumour to local tissues and/or the lymph nodes [IRS Grouping System (Table 18.3)]. The same approach has been used in Europe by the German and Italian cooperative groups, whereas centers associated in the SIOP group chose to use a tumour, nodes, and metastases

Table 18.3. IRS Clinical Grouping System

Group	Description of disease
I	Localized disease, completely resected
	(a) confined to organ or muscle of origin
	(b) infiltration outside organ or muscle of origin
	Regional nodes not involved
II	Compromised or regional resection of three types:
	(a) grossly resected tumours with microscopic residual disease; no evidence of regional lymph node involvement
	(b) regional disease, completely resected, in which nodes may be involved and/or extension of tumour into an adjacent organ but with no microscopic residual disease
	(c) regional disease with involved nodes, grossly resected, but with evidence of microscopic residual disease
III	Incomplete resection or biopsy only with gross (macroscopic) residual disease
IV	Distant metastases present at diagnosis

Table 18.4. SIOP pretreatment clinical (TNM) staging

Stage	TNM characteristics		
I	T1a, T1b	N0, NX	M0
II	T2a, T2b	N0, NX	M0
III	Any T	N1	M0
IV	Any T	Any N	M1

T = primary tumour
T0	No evidence of primary tumour
T1	Tumour confined to the organ or tissue of origin
	T1a Tumour ≤5 cm in its greatest dimension
	T1b Tumour >5 cm in its greatest dimension
T2	Tumours involving one or more contiguous organs or tissues or with adjacent malignant effusion, or multiple tumours in the same organ
	T2a Tumour ≤5 cm in its greatest dimension
	T2b Tumour >5 cm in its greatest dimension

N = regional lymph nodes (see Table 18.6)
N0	No evidence of regional lymph node involvement
N1	Evidence of regional lymph node involvement

M = distant metastases
M0	No evidence of distant metastases
M1	Evidence of distant metastases

(TNM) classification relying on the clinical description of the disease before (Table 18.4) and after (Table 18.5) initial surgery (Figs 18.5 and 18.6). The distinction between these classification systems has made the comparison of results difficult. However, collaboration between the groups has clarified the importance of pre- and postsurgical stage in prognostic significance.

Age The IRS IV study demonstrated that three age groups could be associated with prognosis in localized RMS: <1 year, 1–9 years, and >10 years of age.[5] This also applies to subgroups of patients: the IRS III and IV trials demonstrated that age >10 years was a factor of poor prognosis in paratesticular RMS and identical results were obtained from the SIOP MMT 84 and MMT 89 studies.[6] Age is also predictive of prognosis in metastatic RMS with a poorer survival associated with age >10 years.

It is important to note that factors predictive of prognosis (histology, postsurgery stage, lymph node involvement, tumour size, and patient age) are often interdependent (Fig. 18.7): limb tumours are generally of the alveolar type, whereas vaginal or bladder RMSs are known to be botryoid, and paratesticular RMSs more frequently present the spindle cell variants. It is also well known that alveolar subtypes tend to spread more frequently to both regional nodes and distant metastatic sites. Finally, the status after surgery (complete microscopic surgical excision, incomplete microscopic excision, gross residual tumour) is strongly determined by the site of the disease.

Therapeutic strategy

Both North American and European groups determine treatment strategy according to disease histology (alveolar versus non-alveolar), postsurgical status, IRS Group, disease site (favourable versus unfavourable), tumour size, and age.

Table 18.5. SIOP postsurgical histopathologic (pTNM) classification

pT = primary tumour	
pT0	No evidence of tumour found on histological examination of specimen
pT1	Tumour limited to organ or tissue of origin Excision complete and margins histologically free
pT2	Tumour with invasion beyond the organ or tissue of origin Excision complete and margins histologically free
pT3	Tumour with or without invasion beyond the organ or tissue of origin Excision incomplete
pT3a	Evidence of microscopic residual tumour
pT3b	Evidence of macroscopic residual tumour or biopsy only
pT3c	Adjacent malignant effusion regardless of the size
pN = regional lymph nodes	
pN0	No evidence of tumour found on histologic examination of regional lymph nodes
pN1	Evidence of invasion of regional lymph nodes
pN1a	Evidence of invasion of regional lymph nodes Involved nodes considered to be completely resected
pN1b	Evidence of invasion of regional lymph nodes Involved nodes considered to be completely resected

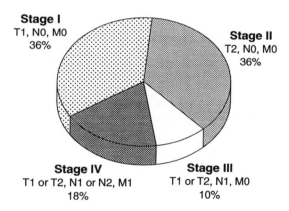

Stage I
T1, N0, M0
36%

Stage II
T2, N0, M0
36%

Stage IV
T1 or T2, N1 or N2, M1
18%

Stage III
T1 or T2, N1, M0
10%

Fig. 18.5 Pie chart showing distribution of clinical (TNM) stages at diagnosis.

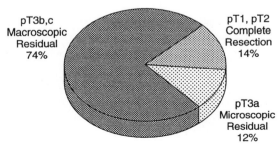

pT3b,c
Macroscopic
Residual
74%

pT1, pT2
Complete
Resection
14%

pT3a
Microscopic
Residual
12%

Fig. 18.6 Pie chart showing the distribution of postsurgical stages (pTNM) before chemotherapy.

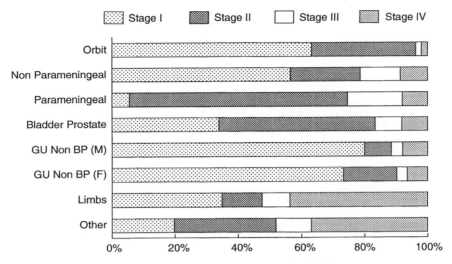

Fig. 18.7 Histogram showing the relationship between site and clinical stage.

Distinct risk groups can be defined:

♦ low-risk RMS with an average of 90 per cent event-free survival (EFS) at 5 years
♦ intermediate-risk RMS with 60–80 per cent survival
♦ high-risk RMS with <60 per cent survival
♦ very-high-risk RMS with <40 per cent survival.

Local tumour control is central to the possibility of cure for patients with non-metastatic disease. Controversies here relate to the method and timing of local treatment, and, more specifically, to the place of radiotherapy in guaranteeing local control for patients who appear to achieve complete remission with chemotherapy with or without surgery. This represents an important philosophical difference between the SIOP MMT studies and those of the IRS Group and, to some extent, of the German and Italian Cooperative groups. Local relapse rates are higher in the SIOP studies than those experienced elsewhere, although the SIOP experience has also made it clear that a significant number of patients who relapse may be cured with alternative treatment.[7] In the context of such differences in approach to local treatment, overall survival rather than disease-free or progression-free survival may become the most important criterion for measuring outcome. However, the 'cost' of survival must take into account the predicted late effects of treatment and the total burden of therapy experienced by an individual patient. This must include an assessment of all the treatments necessary to cure the child, including those used after relapse.

Surgery Primary tumour resection should be undertaken only if there is no evidence of metastatic disease and the tumour can be excised with good margins without danger, functional impairment, or mutilation. If this is not possible, a diagnostic biopsy is required. An attempt at surgical resection which leaves microscopic residual disease makes treatment decisions more complicated because the patient is unassessable for the efficacy of chemotherapy and may still require further local treatment. Primary re-excision (i.e. a second surgical resection before chemotherapy) may be worthwhile in a minority of cases if there is confidence that clear margins of excision can be achieved without functional or cosmetic disadvantage.[8] This applies particularly to trunk, limb, and paratesticular tumours. Histological assessment of tumour margins is not always consistent with the surgical findings because of the diffuse infiltration of some tumours into adjacent tissues.

The importance of surgical evaluation of lymph nodes at diagnosis is controversial. Clinically and radiologically suspicious nodes should be sampled (fine-needle aspiration may be a useful technique in such circumstances), but radical lymph node dissections are rarely justified and routine surgical staging of regional (para-aortic) nodes in patients with localized paratesticular tumours is not considered necessary by the European groups.[6,9]

The value of secondary operations to achieve complete remission should be distinguished from procedures undertaken merely to confirm clinical or radiologic complete response. Secondary operations, and even multiple biopsies for verification of local control, are not indicated if there is no visible tumour clinically, endoscopically, or on CT or MRI scanning. A significant minority of patients thought to be in partial remission after initial chemotherapy in the IRS III study were shown actually to be in complete remission at second-look surgery. Secondary surgery to achieve local control after initial chemotherapy remains an important aspect of treatment but depends on the site of disease. For example, surgery has little or no role in the primary management of orbital RMS and has only a selective place in the local control of head and neck tumours in general. Surgery at this point in treatment should generally be conservative, whatever the site of disease, anticipating that the morbidity of radiotherapy may be more acceptable than radical operations which result in important functional (e.g. total cystectomy) and/or cosmetic (e.g. amputation) consequences. However, in some circumstances the morbidity of radical surgery to achieve local control may be preferred, for example, to avoid pelvic irradiation in very young children.

Chemotherapy Chemotherapy is an essential component of treatment for all children with RMS. Experience since the 1970s has defined the efficacy of a variety of chemotherapeutic agents, the value of multi-agent chemotherapy combinations, and the importance of adjuvant therapy in patients without macroscopic residual disease after initial surgery. It has long been recognized that treatment of large unresectable tumours with chemotherapy could reduce the extent of subsequent surgery or radiation therapy. However, the role of intensified chemotherapy in reducing or avoiding the need for local therapy remains controversial. This has been most consistently explored by the SIOP MMT studies.[7,10] The strategies of the IRS and of the other European (German and Italian) cooperative groups still tend to retain a systematic approach to local therapy regardless of chemotherapy response, except in patients who achieve complete primary tumour resection with initial surgery. Overall, it seems likely that some patients who achieve complete tumour control with chemotherapy can be spared local treatment, but it is important to recognize that local recurrence is the predominant pattern of relapse in non-metastatic disease and clinicians must not disregard the relevance of local therapy for many patients.

Vincristine (V), actinomycin D (A), cyclophosphamide (C) and doxorubicin [Adriamycin® (Adr)] have been the most frequently utilized agents in the treatment of RMS and have been used in various combinations (VA; VAC; VACAdr) in the sequential IRS studies. Doxorubicin is an active agent when used alone, but its role remains controversial and concern about potential cardiotoxicity justifies caution in its use as part of primary treatment. The introduction of newer drugs has not always been accompanied by clear evidence of their benefit as single agents within phase II studies. Such data are available for cisplatin, etoposide, and DTIC, all of which were introduced into IRS III. However, it was not possible to show that cisplatin, with or without etoposide, offered any survival advantage, although the combination of cisplatin with doxorubicin in MMT 84 produced significant response rates in patients who failed to show an adequate response to IVA.[7]

The substitution of cyclophosphamide by ifosfamide in combination with vincristine and actinomycin D (with or without doxorubicin) has been the hallmark of all recent European studies. Ifosfamide appears to convey some advantages over its analogue cyclophosphamide, showing a lack of cross-resistance and a lower myelotoxicity profile, thus permitting the possibility of administering larger doses. The rate of response to ifosfamide-containing regimens appeared favourable in the historical comparison of the SIOP and CWS studies.[11,12] A prospective randomized trial comparing an ifosfamide-based combination (IVA) with a cyclophosphamide-based combination (VAC) was conducted in the IRSG IV study. The doses of cyclophosphamide and ifosfamide in each cycle were respectively $2.2\,g/m^2$ for 1 day and $1.8\,g/m^2/day$ for 5 days (these doses were previously found to produce comparable myelosuppression). No differences in either 3-year survival or failure-free survival rates were seen between different regimens (84 per cent and 75 per cent for VAC compared with 84 per cent and 77 per cent for IVA).[5] Both drugs require concurrent administration of mesna to avoid haemorrhagic cystitis, but ifosfamide carries a risk of renal toxicity not experienced with cyclophosphamide and VAC remains the combination of choice for future North American studies. Nevertheless, the European groups have decided to keep IVA as standard combination because data suggest that there is only a small risk of significant renal toxicity at cumulative ifosfamide doses $< 60\,g/m^2$ and a higher risk of gonadal toxicity with cyclophosphamide.

A collaborative European protocol for patients with metastatic disease introduced carboplatin and epirubicin (Epiadriamycin®) into first-line therapy as part of an intensive six-drug schedule denoted CEVAIE (with ifosfamide, vincristine, actinomycin D, and etoposide) designed to overcome drug resistance. The choice of carboplatin and epirubicin was based on preferential toxicity profiles compared with cisplatin and Adriamycin®. This chemotherapy strategy was also incorporated into MMT 89 for the treatment of high-risk patients with lymph node disease and produced a significant improvement in outcome compared with historical data from similar patients treated in the previous study (MMT 84). Current European protocols are exploring this six-drug combination in a direct randomized comparison with conventional IVA (SIOP Group) or VAIA (German and Italian Groups) for patients with non-metastatic disease. Ifosfamide and doxorubicin given as a phase II 'window' in children with newly diagnosed metastatic RMS showed a response rate (complete remission and partial response) of 63 per cent and should be considered for inclusion in front-line therapy for children with intermediate- or high-risk RMS.[13]

Topotecan was studied in a classic phase II study in 24 relapsed patients with no response and 48 chemotherapy-naive patients in a window study with 46 per cent response rate.[14] Results of treatment with irinotecan are awaited.

High-dose therapies The place of high-dose chemotherapy strategies necessitating autologous bone marrow or peripheral blood stem cell rescue remains unclear. Some experience has been gained in single institutions utilizing a variety of chemotherapy schedules and, predominantly, in patients with relapsed disease. More recently, the European collaborative groups agreed a shared strategy for the treatment of newly diagnosed patients with metastatic disease. This study was initially intended to explore the value of high-dose chemotherapy only amongst patients with incomplete response to initial chemotherapy, but a modification to the study design in 1991 encouraged the use of high-dose melphalan as consolidation therapy for all patients who achieved complete remission after six courses of CEVAIE. Preliminary analysis suggests that there is no survival advantage for those who received consolidation chemotherapy with melphalan compared with those, treated in the earlier phase of the study, who did not.[15]

Radiotherapy Early experience with radiation therapy demonstrating local control in up to 90 per cent of patients included in the IRS studies has confirmed that doses >50 Gy are not usually required when given by conventional (once daily) fractionation. However, there is also evidence that doses <40 Gy may be insufficient, particularly in patients with macroscopic residual disease. The dose used in the SIOP studies is 45 Gy regardless of site or age (although particular efforts are made to avoid irradiation in young children), with a possible boost to 50 or 55 Gy to a reduced field when there is bulky residual macroscopic disease at initiation of therapy. Randomization studies within IRS I–III studies have established that radiotherapy is unnecessary for patients with embryonal histology and tumour completely resected at diagnosis (IRS Clinical Group I). However, analyses from the same studies indicate that radiotherapy does offer an improved failure-free survival in patients with completely resected alveolar RMS.[16] Current guidelines for therapy within the IRS Group vary the prescribed dose from 40 to 55 Gy depending on the site, size, and histology of the tumour, as well as on the age of the child.

Studies from the European groups have attempted to relate the use of radiotherapy to the response to initial chemotherapy. The most radical approach has been used in the SIOP protocols, where patients in IRS Clinical Group III (SIOP pT3b) disease avoided radiotherapy if complete remission had been achieved with initial chemotherapy, with or without second surgery, except for parameningeal RMS. This approach has proved feasible,[17] but the psychologic impact of relapse and the burden of second-line therapy are important and the definition of such favourable patients should be refined.

Treatment must always be given using megavoltage equipment. Electron treatment may be useful for superficial tumours, either as a direct electron field or as a boost to a linear accelerator planned field. Adequate margins must be used (usually 2–3 cm), and treatment for patients with parameningeal disease is normally planned to the initial tumour volume. In tumours at other sites that show a good response to initial chemotherapy, treatment can be planned to the residual volume (plus margins).

Conventional treatment is usually given as a single daily fraction of 1.8 Gy. Interest in hyperfractionated schedules has been explored in both the IRS IV and (to a more limited extent) MMT 89 studies. Overall, the data suggest that no benefit in disease control can be expected from the use of hyperfractionation,[18] and standard conventional fractionation is still used by most cooperative groups.

Early experience in the treatment of parameningeal tumours was discouraging. Local failure rates were high and there was a high incidence of local extension into the adjacent meninges, often with spinal subarachnoid spread and high mortality. Investigation suggested that these patients were receiving inadequate dose and volume of radiation treatment, and the IRS studies were modified to include earlier introduction of radiotherapy, wider fields (extending to whole brain and spine in some cases), increased dose to the site of bulk disease, and the concurrent administration of intrathecal chemotherapy. This resulted in a much improved survival rate. In fact, radiotherapy to the target volume with systemic chemotherapy are successful treatments for the majority of patients with localized parameningeal sarcomas, and guidelines have been liberalized, particularly in relation to the volume of treatment, so that whole-brain treatment is avoided whenever possible. However, all groups agree that patients with parameningeal disease require mandatory radiotherapy regardless of response to chemotherapy. This is especially important as assessment of complete response can be difficult at these sites and surgery rarely offers a valid alternative approach to local control. Intrathecal chemotherapy has never been used routinely in the SIOP studies and there seems to be little justification to do so in the majority of patients who do not demonstrate evidence of CSF or spinal dissemination.

Interstitial radiotherapy (brachytherapy) using intracavitary moulds or implanted wires may be of particular relevance for small tumours at selected sites, notably in the vagina and perineum. Occasionally this technique is utilized at other genitourinary sites, including tumours of the bladder base and prostate, and there is limited experience of its application to head and neck sites.[10]

Outcome

The most recently published IRS Group study (IRS IV) reported the outcome for 883 patients recruited between 1991 and 1997.[5] Overall, 3-year failure-free survival and overall survival were 77 per cent and 86 per cent, respectively, and did not differ from those of similar patients treated in IRS III with a 5-year progression-free survival of 65 per cent. This compares with the 5-year EFS and overall survival of 57 per cent and 71 per cent, respectively, reported in SIOP MMT 89 and of 59 per cent and 69 per cent, respectively, reported in CWS 86.[19] As discussed previously, these studies used significantly different approaches to local treatment, and the larger difference between overall survival and EFS in the SIOP studies reflects a higher relapse rate with successful salvage therapy for some patients.

Table 18.6 gives details of the outcome of treatment according to site in four cooperative group studies. These confirm the prognostic effect of site with an obvious difference between the favourable outcome associated with orbital and genitourinary sites, and the poor results achieved with tumours presenting in the limbs and at 'other' sites.

Late effects of treatment

'Cure at what cost?' is the difficult, yet essential, issue to be addressed when reviewing the outcome of survivors of all forms of cancer in childhood, particularly when survival relates to different philosophies and treatment modalities. The importance of accurate prognostic assessment at diagnosis is as much to ensure that patients with good prognosis are not

Table 18.6. Five-year survival by primary sites according to collaborative group trials

Primary site	IRS III		SIOP-89		CWS-86		ICS-88	
	N	Survival (%)	N	Survival (%)	N	Survival (%)	N	Survival (%)
Orbit	107	95	19	88	36	71	23	74
Head and neck	106	78	17	77	28	51	29	79
Parameningeal	134	74	41	58	55	60	43	74
GU bladder/prostate	104	81	14	79	30	70	26	88
GU non-bladder/prostate	158	89	35	88	38	89	29	97
Extremity	156	74	23	65	25	56	18	56
Other	147	67	37	45	39	58	50	59

GU, genitourinary.

overtreated as to identify those with a poorer prognosis who require a more aggressive approach. Much concern has been focused on the late sequelae of local treatment for RMS, particularly after radiotherapy and the types of aggressive surgery that result in significant functional or cosmetic problems (e.g. orbital exenteration, retroperitoneal lymph node dissection, and total cystectomy). Chemotherapy is also associated with significant sequelae in some patients, and the concept that more intensive chemotherapy may reduce the use of local treatment must be balanced against the additional toxicity that it may cause. The more recent use of ifosfamide has raised concern about long-term renal damage, whereas the continuing use of high doses of alkylating agents and, more recently, etoposide may result in second malignancies. Long-term follow-up and prospective evaluation of all survivors is required in order to document the frequency and functional significance of all possible late effects of therapy.

Non-rhabdomyosarcoma soft tissue sarcoma

The term non- rhabdomyosarcoma soft tissue sarcoma (NRSTS) includes a group of rare tumours with marked clinical, histologic, and biologic heterogeneity. Most histiotypes are more common in adults and occur sporadically in children. However, in some cases, clinical behaviour may be peculiar to a paediatric presentation, justifying a different treatment approach.

Overall, NRSTS show two peaks of incidence, the first in children aged <5 years and the second in early adolescence. The relative frequencies of different histologic subtypes vary with age; for example, fibrosarcoma is common in children aged <2 years and synovial sarcoma and malignant peripheral nerve sheath tumour (MPNST) most commonly affect adolescents.[20] Other NRSTS include extraosseous primitive neuroectodermal tumour (PNET)/extraosseous Ewing sarcoma (EOE), undifferentiated sarcoma (US), vascular tumors (haemangiosarcoma, haemangiopericytoma), epithelioid sarcoma and alveolar soft part sarcoma. More recently, new entities such as intraabdominal desmoplastic small round cell tumour have been added to the NRSTS group. Very rare entities include liposarcoma, malignant fibrous histiocytoma, and leiomyosarcoma. The incidence of NRSTS as registered by the Italian cooperative group is shown in Figure 18.8.

NRSTSs share several clinical characteristics with the more frequent RMSs. They can occur anywhere in the body, usually as a painless growing mass which shows symptoms only when an adjacent organ or structure is invaded. They mostly arise in the extremities, the wall of the trunk, and the retroperitoneum, while head and neck or genitourinary locations are extremely rare. Evidence of regional and distant metastases at diagnosis is less frequent than in RMS, with involvement of regional lymph nodes present in 10 per cent of cases and distant metastases in about 10–12 per cent.

Open biopsy is recommended and sufficient material should be analysed by an expert pathologist to confirm the diagnosis of NRSTS and to grade the tumour appropriately. Molecular biology is of increasing importance as a number of specific translocations have been identified. This can be an important tool to assist the diagnosis of these rare tumours and for research purposes. Detection of fusion gene product is used for the primary diagnosis of Ewing sarcoma and PNET and for the detection of metastatic or residual disease. A list of the more common genetic abnormalities in NRSTS is presented in Table 18.7.

In general, the diagnostic workup and staging systems are the same as those adopted for RMS. The IRS grouping system and the TNM staging system are commonly used. A histologic grading system has been developed for paediatric NRSTSs which identifies three prognostic groups based on histology, amount of necrosis, number of mitoses, and cellular pleomorphism.[21] The prognostic importance of this has not yet been confirmed in large clinical trials.

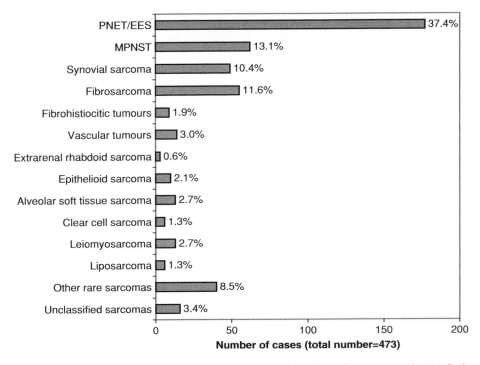

Fig. 18.8 Incidence of different NRSTSs in childhood (data from the Italian Co-operative Studies).

Generally, management of NRSTS has been derived from treatment used for RMS and from adult experience. Increasing data from single institutions and cooperative groups should allow the design of more specific clinical trials for at least some histiotypes in the near future.

Prognostic factors

The search for prognostic variables in such rare tumours presents difficulties. However, some factors are consistently present when analysing data from larger series containing different histiotypes or small series dedicated to a single histiotype.[22–29] These can be summarized as follows.

◆ Disease extension at diagnosis: survival is very poor in children with disseminated disease.
◆ Initial surgery: complete tumour resection gives 70–80 per cent chance of cure in most histiotypes.
◆ Tumour site: influences tumour resection.
◆ Tumour size: lesions >5 cm have an increased risk of local and distant relapse.
◆ Tumour invasiveness (T stage): this is often associated with tumour size.
◆ Histology: different histiotypes have different biologic behaviour and response to treatment.
◆ Grading.
◆ Age: tumours in older children behave more like adult sarcomas and carry a worse prognosis.

It has been suggested that, as in adults, risk factors for local recurrence may be different from those for metastatic relapse, with the latter being more correlated with tumour size, invasive-

Table 18.7. Specific chromosomal abnormalities identified in soft tissue sarcoma

Tumour	Chromosomal abnormalities
Rhabdomyosarcoma	
Alveolar	t(2,13)(q35;q14) or t(1,13)(p36;q14)
Embryonal	LOH chromosome 11p
Fibrosarcoma	
Congenital	t(12;15)(p13;q25)
Adult type	t(2,5) and t(7,22)
Extraosseous PNET/Ewing sarcoma	t(11;22)(q24;q12) or t(21;22)(q22;q12)
Synovial sarcoma	t(X;18)(p11;q11)
Malignant peripheral nerve sheath tumour	Loss or rearrangement of 10p, 11q, 17q and 22q
Alveolar soft part sarcoma	t(X;17)(p11.2;q25)
Clear cell sarcoma	t(12;22)(q13;q12)
	t(9;22)(q22;q12)
Extraskeletal myxoid chondrosarcoma	t(9;17)(q22;q11.2)
Desmoplastic small round cell tumor	t(11;22)(p13;q12)
Myxoid liposarcoma	t(12;16)(q13;p11)
	t(12;22)(q13;q12)
	t(12;22;20)(q13;q12;q11)
Dermatofibrosarcoma protuberans	t(17;22;)(q22;q13)
Leiomyosarcoma	12q rearrangements; loss of 1p, 6q, 11p, 22q

ness, and high histology grading.[22] This may determine the selection of patients for adjuvant chemotherapy after complete surgical resection.

Treatment

A complete tumour resection with wide margins is advocated in adults. Radiotherapy is added if resection margins are close to the tumour and sometimes may be administered preoperatively. Adjuvant chemotherapy is a contentious issue because response rate is quite low and few studies have shown benefit in terms of disease-free and overall survival.

Surgery is also considered the mainstay of NRSTS treatment in children, although a more conservative approach is usually adopted. Limb-sparing procedures and non-compartmental resections are preferred, and therefore the concept of radical surgery in children allows closer surgical margins than are generally acceptable in adults. A complete resection may be the only treatment needed for some histiotypes. If resection is considered unlikely at diagnosis, an incisional biopsy is required for diagnostic purposes (fine-needle biopsy does not usually provide sufficient accuracy) and other treatment modalities need to be considered before referring the child back to the surgeon for a definitive procedure. However, this conservative approach must be balanced against the higher risk of local relapse of NRSTS compared with RMS, and therefore a more aggressive approach to local treatment is generally required.

Radiotherapy is administered when residual disease is present or suspected after resection. Several reports suggest that radiotherapy is effective for maintaining local control only when the residual disease is minimal. In some cases radiotherapy may be considered preoperatively to target the volume better and to make the subsequent tumour resection easier. Doses of at least 40–50 Gy are used but concern about late effects can constrain the use of irradiation, especially in young children. Occasionally, alternative techniques, such as brachytherapy, may be considered.

The benefit of chemotherapy is far from established for NRSTS and represents one of the main therapeutic problems, particularly for the less common entities. Sporadic reports of chemotherapy response exist for several histiotypes, but in general response rates are much lower than those reported in RMS. Some recent data suggest that NRSTS can be divided in three different groups.

- Tumours with proven chemosensitivity: PNET/EOE and US. These tumours respond to treatments adopted for RMS.
- Tumours with possible chemosensitivity: synovial sarcoma, malignant fibrous histiocytoma, liposarcoma, and congenital–infantile fibrosarcoma. Although encouraging chemotherapy responses have been reported, the benefit in terms of improved survival is not well established.
- Tumours with unproven chemosensitivity: juvenile or 'adult type' fibrosarcoma, MPNST, alveolar soft part sarcoma. Responses to chemotherapy have been reported for these entities, and therefore a trial of chemotherapy may be justified when conservative surgical surgery is not considered feasible at diagnosis.

Peripheral neuroectodermal tumours and extraosseous Ewing sarcoma

PNET and Ewing sarcoma are histologically similar and share the same chromosomal translocation, typically t(11;22). Therefore they are grouped in the Ewing family of tumours. Traditionally, paediatric PNET and Ewing sarcoma arising outside bone have been included in soft tissue sarcoma protocols in many countries. However, there is ongoing debate to establish whether or not they should be treated differently from osseous Ewing tumours. Extraosseous PNET/Ewing tumours are considered to be aggressive, but the advent of effective multimodality therapy has improved prognosis and 5-year survival is reported to be ~60 per cent.[23] Unfortunately, survival in patients with metastatic disease at diagnosis remains very poor despite aggressive treatment. Regimens including alkylating agents (ifosfamide or cyclophosphamide) plus actinomycin D and vincristine have been used. Anthracylines are considered important drugs in the treatment of osseous Ewing tumours. However their role has been questioned in soft tissue PNET/Ewing tumours.[23] Aggressive surgery and radiotherapy is recommended for local control.

Fibrosarcoma

Fibrosarcoma represents ~10 per cent of paediatric NRSTSs and is the most common soft tissue sarcoma in infants aged <1 year. Two forms of fibrosarcoma are recognized: congenital–infantile fibrosarcoma that occurs in children aged <2 years, and juvenile or 'adult-type' fibrosarcoma that is more typical of children aged 10–15 years. They are not distinguishable on the basis of histology, as both forms are composed of spindle-shaped fibroblasts which may show different growth patterns (solid, haemangiopericytoma-like, and herringbone), exhibiting variable collagen production and showing no evidence of other differentiation. The clinical characteristics of the tumour, patient age, and cytogenetic differences are considered the main factors in distinguishing the infantile and adult forms. A recurring t(12;15); (p13;q25) translocation has been documented in congenital–infantile fibrosarcoma. Interestingly, the same chromosomal anomaly has been found in congenital mesoblastic nephroma, a usually benign renal tumour occurring in infants. Other translocations [t(2,5) and t(7,22)] have been described in adult-type fibrosarcoma.

Congenital–infantile fibrosarcoma

Typically, this diagnosis is applied only to children aged <2 years although some authors extend this limit up to 4 or 5 years. The tumour is usually located in the distal region of the extremities and presents as a painless rapidly enlarging mass. Despite the rapid growth, evolution may be indolent with a tendency to recur locally without metastatic spread. Spontaneous regression has also been described. Complete tumour resection is the only treatment necessary for most patients, but a trial of chemotherapy is warranted for inoperable tumours. Responses have been reported using regimens including vincristine, dactinomycin, and ifosfamide or cyclophosphamide. Despite a risk of relapse, ~80 per cent of patients with congenital fibrosarcoma are long-term survivors[24] and recently it has been suggested that the presence of translocation (2;5) conveys a better prognosis.[30]

Adult-type fibrosarcoma

In older children fibrosarcoma has clinical features similar to those found in adults. The tumour usually grows slowly and the typical locations are the proximal region of extremities, deep trunk, and cavity sites. Aggressive surgery is advocated to obtain a complete tumour resection. Radiotherapy is used when postsurgical residues are evident or suspected. Response to chemotherapy has been reported, but its role remains uncertain. Unfortunately, local relapse is frequent and this may precede the development of distant metastases. Long-term survival rates of ~50–60 per cent are usually achieved.[24]

Synovial sarcoma

Synovial sarcoma is a malignant undifferentiated mesenchymal tumour resembling normal synovial tissue. It represents 5–10 per cent of all soft tissue tumours in adults and is one of the most common non-rhabdomyosarcoma cancers in the paediatric age range (15–25 per cent),[20] occurring primarily in adolescents. Histologically two major subtypes are described: the monophasic form, characterized by spindle cells, and the more frequent biphasic form, characterized by spindle and epithelial cells organized in glandular structures. Cytogenetic studies have reported the presence of a characteristic translocation t(X;18)(p11;q11) in ~90 per cent of cases. Two fusion transcripts, SYT–SSX1 and SYT–SSX2, are derived from fusion of the SYT and SSX genes localized on chromosomes 18q11 and Xp11, respectively.

Synovial sarcoma usually arises in extremities, and the thigh and knee are the most frequently affected sites. The lungs are by far the most common metastatic site. Prognosis is related to the presence of metastatic lesions, tumour size (>5 cm) and invasiveness, tumour site (distal locations fare better than proximal), and complete resection. Histologic subtype influences outcome, with the biphasic form being more favourable. The type of fusion transcript has also been correlated with survival (patients with SYT–SSX2 tumours do better than those with SYT–SSX1 tumours).

Wide excision of the primary tumour is the mainstay of treatment. The use of radiotherapy and chemotherapy is controversial. Irradiation is usually recommended to improve local control when resection is incomplete. Chemotherapy has been shown to be active in paediatric trials, with response rates of up to 60–70 per cent,[25] and is used in inoperable and disseminated cases. However, the role of chemotherapy after a complete resection is questionable, although survival rates in paediatric series, where chemotherapy has been used systematically, is usually better than in adult series, where chemotherapy is used less frequently and the metastatic relapse rate is higher. A recent multicenter multivariate analysis has shown overall 80 per cent 5-year survival, 88 per cent for patients with tumours grossly resected at diagnosis (IRS Groups I and II) and 75 per cent for patients with localized unresectable tumor (IRS Group III). Adjuvant chemotherapy did not seem to have an impact on survival in patients in IRS Groups I or II, and tumour size appeared to be the most relevant prognostic factor.[25]

Also based on experience in adults, ifosfamide and doxorubicin seem to be the most active drugs and there is a need to test this combination in a randomized international trial.

Malignant peripheral nerve sheath tumour (malignant Schwannoma)

MPNST is strongly associated with neurofibromatosis type I (NF-1): ~20 per cent of patients with MPNST present NF-1 features and up to 15 per cent of children with NF-1 are at risk of developing a MPNST. The NF-1 gene, localized at 17q11.2, is thought to have a role as a tumour suppressor gene, and its inactivation or loss may be involved in the neoplastic transformation of cells. The extremities, retroperitoneum, and trunk are the primary sites most commonly involved, and MPNST tends to be locally aggressive with only few patients showing metastases (mainly in the lungs) at diagnosis.

The most important prognostic factor is the completeness of tumour resection. Radiotherapy, in doses up to 50–60 Gy, is used in cases of microscopic postsurgical residual. The role of chemotherapy is uncertain, although a response (complete or partial) was documented in 30 per cent of a series of 64 patients enrolled by the Italian and German Cooperative groups. In some cases the tumour shrinkage achieved with chemotherapy facilitates its removal, and a trial of chemotherapy (based on ifosfamide and doxorubicin) is warranted in patients with initially unresectable tumour. The 10-year overall survival in this series was 45 per cent, but survival was much worse (5 per cent) in patients with NF-1 in whom the tumour tended to be larger, unresectable, and highly chemoresistant.

Vascular tumours

Vascular neoplasms represent the most common mesenchymal lesion of subcutaneous and deep soft tissue in the paediatric age range. However, ~90 per cent of them are benign and a subset is considered to have limited local aggressiveness. Malignant lesions include angiosarcoma, malignant haemangioendothelioma, and Kaposi's sarcoma. Haemangiopericytoma is also included in this group, although it originates not from the endothelium but from pericytes.

Angiosarcoma is an aggressive tumour with a high propensity to recur locally and to metastatize to local lymph nodes, lung, and liver. It can occur anywhere in the body, but mostly arises in the skin and superficial soft tissue. The head and neck region is the commonest site of origin. Previous radiotherapy, chronic lymphoedema, or environmental toxins (thorotrast, steroids) are all linked to the occurrence of angiosarcoma. Complete tumour resection is important, but this is not generally sufficient to ensure local control. Therefore radiotherapy is recommended in adults. The use of drugs usually administered for soft tissue sarcomas has not improved outcome, and long-term survival is ~30 per cent.[26]

The term haemangioendothelioma includes several different entities. Malignant haemangioendothelioma and epithelioid haemangioendothelioma exhibit an aggressive or borderline malignant potential, respectively. Malignant haemangioendothelioma is considered similar to angiosarcoma. Epithelioid haemangioendothelioma may present as a single lesion of the limbs or with multifocal lesions involving bone, lung, or liver. Surgery is of paramount importance, but no response to chemotherapy has been reported. New approaches are needed for vascular tumours, and the use of paclitaxel in angiosarcoma and interferon-α in haemangioendothelioma have both shown promising results.

Haemangiopericytoma derives from mesenchymal cells with pericytic differentiation. Two distinct clinical entities are described in the paediatric age group: the infantile type, occurring in young infants, and the adult type, occurring in children aged >1 year. Infantile haemangiopericytoma typically occurs in the subcutis and oral cavity. Multifocal lesions may occur and spontaneous regression has been described. Adult-type haemangiopericytoma has a more aggressive behaviour, similar to that seen in adults, with metastatic potential to lung and bone. Late relapses have been described. Wide tumour excision is the treatment of choice. However, both forms of haemangiopericytoma have shown good response to chemotherapy, and this should be implemented in cases where primary resection is not feasible. Radiotherapy is also recommended after incomplete tumour removal in adult-type haemangiopericytoma. Prognosis appears good for infantile-type haemangiopericytoma, with >80 per cent of children surviving at 5 years. The outcome for adult-type haemangiopericytoma in children seems to be better than that in adults, with 5 year EFS rates >60 per cent.[26]

Alveolar soft part sarcoma

Alveolar soft part sarcoma accounts for 1–5 per cent of paediatric NRSTS and occurs more frequently between 15 and 35 years of age. Females outnumber males, especially during the first two decades of life. Histologically, alveolar soft part sarcoma is composed of aggregates of polygonal cells separated by vascular spaces. The degeneration of the central cells produces the alveolar pattern, although the most distinctive feature is the presence of intracytoplasmic periodic acid, diastase-resistant inclusions of unknown nature. There is still considerable uncertainty as to the exact histiogenesis of this tumour.

Alveolar soft part sarcoma usually arises in the extremities, although the head and neck region, including the orbit and tongue, is a more common region in children. Metastatic lesions are present at diagnosis in ~20 per cent of patients; these involve lung, bone, and, less frequently, the central nervous system.

The clinical course is often indolent and patients may survive for several years with evidence of disease. Patients cured of localized lesions may present with metastases after prolonged disease-free intervals, sometimes exceeding 10 years.[27] Complete surgical resection is the strongest prognostic factor and may represent the only treatment for localized disease. The role of adjuvant chemotherapy and radiotherapy is not well defined. Because of the rarity of the tumour and the need for long-term follow-up, it is not clear whether chemotherapy reduces the rate of metastatic relapse. However, chemotherapy responses have been reported, and a trial of chemotherapy seems appropriate when the tumour is not resectable. Radiotherapy may improve the local control when there is postsurgical residual disease.

Overall, the prognosis seems favourable when metastatic lesions are not present at diagnosis. In a recent paediatric series the overall survival was 80 per cent, with 93 per cent disease-free survival for patients with localized disease. Favourable outcome was related to the completeness of tumour resection in most cases.[28] These figures are better than those reported for adults, where alveolar soft part sarcoma seems to have a higher propensity to metastasize.

Desmoplastic small round cell tumour

Since its first description in 1989 by Gerald and Rosai, desmoplastic small round cell tumour (DSRCT) has been increasingly identified but its histiogenesis remains uncertain. It is distinguished from the other small round cell tumours by a characteristic histologic appearance marked by nests of cellular growth within abundant desmoplastic stroma, and a specific polyphenotypic differentiation with coexpression of epithelial, mesenchymal, and neural markers. A recurrent specific chromosomal translocation, t(11,22)(p13;q12), involving the *EWS* and the *WT1* genes has been identified.

The tumour predominantly affects young males, usually in their second decade of life. DSRCT typically presents as a large abdominal mass, often widely disseminated at the time of diagnosis, with extensive spread to the regional lymph nodes, peritoneal seeding, and distant metastases to liver, lung, and bone. Other, less frequent, primary sites are the paratesticular region and the thoracic cavity, sometimes with extensive involvement of the pleura.

DSRCT seems to be chemosensitive, and aggressive multimodality treatment including surgery, radiotherapy, and high-dose chemotherapy based on alkylating drugs has been used. However, early relapses after completing the treatment are common, and the survival is <40 per cent at 30 months.[29]

Future treatment for non-rhabdomyosarcoma soft tissue sarcoma

The experience achieved by the Italian and German Cooperative groups with various histologic types is detailed in Tables 18.8 and 18.9. In most of them surgery is still the best and often the only proven treatment. The role of radiotherapy and chemotherapy is difficult to establish because of the small number of studies published. However, irradiation is widely recommended when there is evidence of residual tumour in the surgical margins. In some cases radiotherapy

Table 18.8. Non-rhabdomyosarcoma soft tissue sarcoma: retrospective analysis of single histotypes from Italian and German group studies

Histiotype	Patient no.	Treatment	Results
Synovial sarcoma[25]	220	82% CT, 60% RT	5-year EFS = 72%; 5-year OS = 80%; CT response rate = 61%
Malignant peripheral nerve sheath tumour	166	80% CT, 40% RT	10-year OS = 45% (5% in NF1); CT response rate = 30%
Fibrosarcoma[24]	25	72% CT, 24% RT	5-year OS 78% infantile type, 51% adult type; CT response 3/8
	52	54% CT, 10% RT	5-year OS 92% infantile type, 60% adult type
Epithelioid sarcoma	44	Not reported	OS = 89% for IRS I, 41% for II–III, 0% for IV; 81% < 5 cm, 33% > 5 cm; CT response 3/8
Leiomyosarcoma[31]	16	56% CT, 19% RT	5-year OS = 73% (size 100% vs 45%)
	54	60% CT, 18% RT	OS 85%, CT response rate 43%
Malignant fibrous histiocytoma	45	55% CT, 33% RT	5-year OS = 89%, 100% in IRS Group I–II; CT response 3/7
Liposarcoma	34	65% CT, 50% RT	5-year OS 100% for IRS I, 67% for II, 22% for III, 33% for IV; 100% <5 cm; CT response 7/13

CT, chemotherapy; RT, radiotherapy; EFS, event-free survival: OS, overall survival.

Table 18.9. Non-rhabdomyosarcoma soft tissue sarcoma: retrospective analysis for single histiotypes from Italian and German group studies

Histiotype	Patient no.	Treatment	Results	Conclusions and comments
Clear cell sarcoma[32]	28	71% CT, 25% RT	5-year OS = 69%; CT response 1/7 Univariate analysis: surgery, size, site	Only surgery for small resected tumour Uncertain role for CT and RT
Angiosarcoma[26]	18	78% CT, 33% RT	5-year OS = 31%; EFS = 21%; CT response 3/9	Poor prognosis, high rate of metastatic relapses Surgery insufficient
Haemangiopericytoma[33]	27	85% CT, 55% RT	Infants: OS = 85%; CT response 5/6 Adult type: OS = 69%; CT response 70%	Infants: myofibroblastic lesions? Adult-type: CT and RT seem effective, size as prognostic factor
Haemangioendothelioma[34]	18	72% CT (four patients received IFN-α)	OS = 83%; EFS 60%; no response to CT 2 PR + 2 SD with IFN-α	Heterogeneous group CT completely ineffective, role for IFN-α
Alveolar soft part sarcoma[28]	19	79% CT, 42% RT	5-year OS = 80%, 92% for localized disease; 100% <5 cm, 31% >5 cm; CT response 2/7	More favourable prognosis than adults Surgery mainstay of therapy Size strongly correlates with outcome
Desmoplastic small round cell tumour[35]	6	All patients received CT	Alive in CR 4/18 (with short follow-up)	Disappointing survival Complete resection + intensive CT ± RT crucial for good prognosis

CT, chemotherapy; RT, radiotherapy; EFS, event-free survival: OS, overall survival; IFN-α, interferon-α; CR, complete remission.

may be considered in the preoperative phase to improve the possibility of obtaining a complete resection.

Chemotherapy responses have been documented in leiomyosarcoma, liposarcoma, epithelioid sarcoma, and sporadically in other histiotypes. However, it is not clear whether this translates into a higher survival rate.

In the past, paediatric non-RMS soft tissue sarcomas have been treated according to strategies developed for RMS, but there is increasing evidence that this should not be the case. The characteristics of many of these tumours seem to be similar to those of the same diagnoses treated by adult oncologists, although survival seems better in children and some entities show differences in biology, clinical behaviour, and sensitivity to chemotherapy (e.g. infantile fibrosarcoma and haemangiopericytoma). There is a need for trials specifically designed for these rare sarcomas. In view of their rarity, wider multinational collaboration will be needed to perform meaningful studies to identify prognostic factors and effective treatments.

References

1. **Rodary C, Flamant F, Donaldson SS** (1989). An attempt to use a common staging system in rhabdomyosarcoma. A report of an international workshop initiated by the International Society of Paediatric Oncology. *Med Pediatr Oncol* 17, 210–15.

2. **Newton WA, Jr., Gehan EA, Webber BL,** *et al.* (1995). Classification of rhabdomyosarcomas and related sarcomas. Pathologic aspects and proposal for a new classification—an Intergroup Rhabdomyosarcoma Study. *Cancer* 76, 1073–1085.

3. **Barr FG** (1997). Molecular genetics and pathogenesis of rhabdomyosarcoma. *J Pediatr Hematol Oncol* 19, 483–91.

4. **Donaldson SS, Draper GJ, Flamant F,** *et al.* (1986). Topography of childhood tumors: pediatric coding system. *Pediatr Hematol Oncol* 3, 249–58.

5. **Crist WM, Anderson JR, Meza JL,** *et al.* (2001). Intergroup rhabdomyosarcoma study—IV: results for patients with nonmetastatic disease. *J Clin Oncol* 19, 3091–102.

6. **Stewart RJ, Martelli H, Oberlin O,** *et al.* (2003) Treatment of children with nonmetastatic paratesticular rhabdomyosarcoma: results of the Malignant Mesenchymal Tumors studies (MMT 84 and MMT 89) of the International Society of Pediatric Oncology. *J Clin Oncol* 21, 793–8.

7. **Flamant F, Rodary C, Rey A,** *et al.* (1998). Treatment of non-metastatic rhabdomyosarcomas in childhood and adolescence. Results of the second study of the International Society of Paediatric Oncology: MMT84. *Eur J Cancer* 34, 1050–62.

8. **Cecchetto G, Guglielmi M, Inserra A,** *et al.* (2001). Primary re-excision: the Italian experience in patients with localized soft-tissue sarcomas. *Pediatr Surg Int* 17, 532–34.

9. **Ferrari A, Bisogno G, Casanova M,** *et al.* (2002). Paratesticular rhabdomyosarcoma: report from the Italian and German cooperative group. *J Clin Oncol* 20, 449–55.

10. **Martelli H, Oberlin O, Rey A** (1999). Conservative treatment for girls with nonmetastatic rhabdomyosarcoma of the genital tract: a report from the Study Committee of the International Society of Pediatric Oncology. *J Clin Oncol* 17, 2117–22.

11. **Stevens M, Flamant F.** (1990) Ifosfamide for children with solid tumours. *Lancet* 335, 1398–1400.

12. **Treuner J, Koscielniak E, Keim M.** (1989). Comparison of the rates of response to ifosfamide and cyclophosphamide in primary unresectable rhabdomyosarcomas. *Cancer Chemother Pharmacol* 24, S48–50.

13. **Sandler E, Lyden E, Ruymann F,** *et al.* (2001). Efficacy of ifosfamide and doxorubicin given as a phase II 'window' in children with newly diagnosed metastatic rhabdomyosarcoma: a report from the Intergroup Rhabdomyosarcoma Study Group. *Med Pediatr Oncol* 37, 442–8.

14. **Pappo AS, Lyden E, Breneman J,** *et al.* (2001). Up-front window trial of topotecan in previously untreated children and adolescents with metastatic rhabdomyosarcoma: an Intergroup Rhabdomyosarcoma study. *J Clin Oncol* 19, 213–19.

15. Carli M, Colombatti R, Oberlin O, *et al.* (1991). High-dose melphalan with autologous stem-cell rescue in metastatic rhabdomyosarcoma. *J Clin Oncol* 17, 2796–803.

16. Wolden SL, Anderson JR, Crist WM, *et al.* (1999). Indications for radiotherapy and chemotherapy after complete resection in rhabdomyosarcoma: a report from the Intergroup Rhabdomyosarcoma Studies I to III. *J Clin Oncol* 17, 3468–75.

17. Oberlin O, Rey A, Anderson J, *et al.* (2001). Treatment of orbital rhabdomyosarcoma: survival and late effects of treatment–results of an international workshop. *J Clin Oncol* 19, 197–204.

18. Donaldson SS, Meza J, Breneman JC, *et al.* (2001). Results from the IRS-IV randomized trial of hyperfractionated radiotherapy in children with rhabdomyosarcoma—a report from the IRSG. *Int J Radiat Oncol Biol Phys* 51, 718–28.

19. Koscielniak E, Harms D, Henze G, *et al.* (1999). Results of treatment for soft tissue sarcoma in childhood and adolescence: a final report of the German Cooperative Soft Tissue Sarcoma Study CWS-86. *J Clin Oncol* 17, 3706–19.

20. Stiller C. (2002). Epidemiology of cancer in adolescents. *Med Pediatr Oncol* 39, 149–55.

21. Parham DM, Webber BL, Jenkins JJ 3rd, *et al.* (1995). Non-rhabdomyosarcomatous soft tissue sarcomas of childhood: formulation of a simplified system for grading. *Mod Pathol* 8, 705–10.

22. Spunt SL, Poquette CA, Hurt YS, *et al.* (1999). Prognostic factors for children and adolescents with surgically resected nonrhabdomyosarcoma soft tissue sarcoma: an analysis of 121 patients treated at St Jude Children's Research Hospital. *J Clin Oncol* 17, 3697–705.

23. Raney RB, Asmar L, Newton WA Jr, *et al.* (1997). Ewing's sarcoma of soft tissues in childhood: a report from the Intergroup Rhabdomyosarcoma Study, 1972 to 1991. *J Clin Oncol* 15, 574–82.

24. Cecchetto G, Carli M, Alaggio R, *et al.* (2001). Fibrosarcoma in pediatric patients: results of the Italian cooperative group studies (1979–1995). *J Surg Oncol* 78, 225–31.

25. Okcu MF, Munsell M, Treuner J, *et al.* (2003). Synovial sarcoma of childhood and adolescence: a multicenter, multivariate analysis of outcome. *J Clin Oncol* 21, 1602–11.

26. Ferrari A, Casanova M, Bisogno G, *et al.* (2002). Malignant vascular tumors in children and adolescents: a report from the Italian and German soft tissue sarcoma cooperative group. *Med Pediatr Oncol* 39, 109–14.

27. Pappo AS, Parham DM, Cain A, *et al.* (1996). Alveolar soft part sarcoma in children and adolescents: clinical features and outcome of 11 patients. *Med Pediatr Oncol* 26, 81–4.

28. Casanova M, Ferrari A, Bisogno G, *et al.* (2000). Alveolar soft part sarcoma in children and adolescents: A report from the Soft-Tissue Sarcoma Italian Cooperative Group. *Ann Oncol* 11, 1445–9.

29. Gerald WL, Ladanyi M, de Alava E, *et al.* (1998). Clinical, pathologic, and molecular spectrum of tumors associated with t(11;22)(p13;q12): desmoplastic small round-cell tumor and its variants. *J Clin Oncol* 16, 3028–36.

30. McCahon E, Sorensen PH, Davis JH, *et al.* (2003). Non-resectable congenital tumors with the ETV6-NTRK3 gene fusion are highly responsive to chemotherapy. *Med Pediatr Oncol* 40, 288–292.

31. Ferrari A, Bisogno G, Casanova M, *et al.* (2001). Childhood leiomyosarcoma: a report from the Soft Tissue Sarcoma Italian Cooperative Group. *Ann Oncol* 12, 1163–8.

32. Ferrari A, Casanova M, Bisogno G, *et al.* Clear cell sarcoma of tendons and aponeuroses in pediatric patients: a report from the Italian and German Soft Tissue Sarcoma Cooperative Group. *Cancer* 94, 3269–76.

33. Ferrari A, Casanova M, Bisogno G, *et al.* (2001) Hemangiopericytoma in pediatric ages: a report from the Italian and German Soft Tissue Sarcoma Cooperative Group. *Cancer* 92, 2692–8.

34. Ferrari A, Casanova M, Meazza C, *et al.* (2001). Vascular tumours in pediatric age. *Ital J Pediatr* 27, 774–8.

35. Bisogno G, Roganovich J, Sotti G, *et al.* Desmoplastic small round tumour in children and adolescents. *Med Pediatr Oncol* 34, 338–42.

Chapter 19

Osteosarcoma

Stefan S. Bielack and Mark L. Bernstein

Epidemiology

Osteosarcoma is the most frequent primary cancer of bone. The approximate annual incidence is 2–3 per million in the general population; it is <1 per million in children aged <five years, 2 per million at age 5–9 years, 7 per million at age 10–14 years, and peaks at 8–11 per million at age 15–19 years. In the period of peak incidence in adolescents aged 15–19 years, it accounts for more than 5 per cent of all cancers. A second smaller age peak in older patients is due to osteosarcomas arising in abnormal bones, such as those affected by Paget's disease or prior irradiation. This chapter describes osteosarcoma in children and adolescents. Tumours of older individuals will not be discussed further.

Osteosarcoma affects males approximately 1.4 times more often than females (Fig. 19.1). The primary tumour is usually located in the metaphysis of a long bone of an extremity, with the distal femur and the proximal tibia being the most frequent sites of involvement, followed by the proximal humerus and proximal fibula. In sum, two-thirds of all paediatric osteosarcomas arise around the knee (Fig. 19.2). Tumours of the axial skeleton or craniofacial bones occur almost exclusively in older patients.

Histology

By definition, osteosarcoma is a mesenchymal malignancy in which the malignant cell population produces osteoid [Fig. 19.3(a)]. The extent of osteoid production can vary considerably. Both abundant production leading to hard and sclerotic tumours and very scanty production are consistent with the diagnosis. Conventional osteosarcoma, a high-grade central malignancy of bone, accounts for 80–90 per cent of all osteosarcomas. Its most frequent subtypes are osteoblastic, chondroblastic, and fibroblastic osteosarcomas. Unusual histologic subtypes, such as sclerosing osteoblastic, osteoblastoma-like, chondromyxoid-fibroma-like, malignant-fibrous-histiocytoma-like and chondroblastoma-like osteosarcomas, as well as giant-cell-rich and epithelioid osteosarcomas, are also included among the conventional osteosarcomas.[1] Conventional, telangiectatic, high-grade surface and small-cell osteosarcomas all have a very similar clinical course and must be treated by multimodal regimens which include chemotherapy. Low-grade central and parosteal osteosarcomas are treated by surgery only. Craniofacial osteosarcomas, apart from those of the skull, metastasize less frequently than conventional osteosarcomas, as do periosteal osteosarcomas, so that there is no general consensus as to whether they should be treated by surgery alone or by surgery plus chemotherapy. Extraskeletal osteosarcomas, usually high-grade malignancies, are rare and are included among the soft tissue sarcomas.

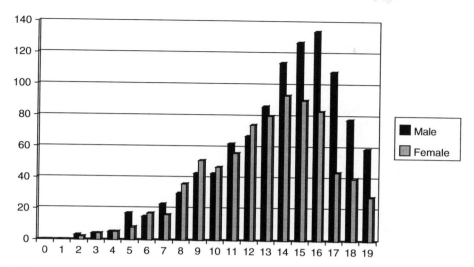

Fig. 19.1 Age and sex distribution of 1791 paediatric patients from the Cooperative Osteosarcoma Study Group (COSS) with primary high-grade central osteosarcoma.

Aetiology

The aetiology of osteosarcoma remains obscure in most patients. Trauma has often been accused, but little evidence exists to support a causal relationship. The predilection of osteosarcoma for the age of the pubertal growth spurt and the sites of maximum growth suggest a correlation with rapid bone growth. There has been a suggestion of a higher incidence in taller individuals, but epidemiologic studies have not been conclusive. A minority of osteosarcomas are caused by radiation exposure. The risk is related to the dose administered. Exposure to alkylating agents may also contribute to osteosarcoma development. Together, radiation therapy, alkylators, and genetic tumour predisposition, as described below, make osteosarcoma one of the most frequent secondary solid malignancies following therapy for childhood cancer. A viral aetiology has been suggested based on evidence that bone sarcomas can be induced in select animals by viruses and by the presence of SV40-like sequences in some human osteosarcomas. However, no convincing evidence has emerged that viruses are a major aetiologic factor in humans.[2]

The incidence of osteosarcoma is increased in several well-defined hereditary disorders associated with germ-line alterations of tumour suppressor genes, but even taken together, these account for only a few per cent of all osteosarcomas. Survivors of hereditary retinoblastoma with germ-line mutations of the retinoblastoma gene *RB1* on chromosome 13q14 carry a risk which is 500–1000 times greater than that of the general population. The Li–Fraumeni cancer family syndrome, in which germ-line mutations in the p53 gene are found, is associated with a 15-fold increase. Among patients with sporadic osteosarcoma, approximately 3 per cent will have germ-line p53 mutations. Although germ-line mutations of p53 and *RB* are rare, these genes are altered in many osteosarcoma tumour samples. Consequently, loss of function of the p53 and *RB* tumour suppressor genes, which regulate cell cycle progression in normal cells, are believed to have an important role in osteosarcoma tumourigenesis. Rothmund–Thomson

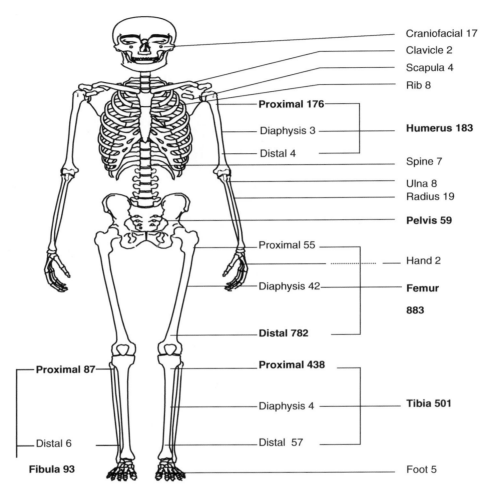

Fig. 19.2 Skeletal distribution of osteosarcoma (based on 1791 primary high-grade central osteosarcomas in paediatric COSS patients).

syndrome and Bloom syndrome, rare conditions caused by mutations in tumour suppressor genes coding for helicases, are also associated with an increase in osteosarcomas, as is Werner syndrome (adult progeria) (see Fletcher *et al.*[1] for reviews of congenital and inherited disorders associated with osteosarcoma development.

Numerous oncogenes are also altered in osteosarcoma tumour cells. These include amplifications of the product of the murine double minute 2 gene, amplification of cyclin-dependent kinase 4 and overexpression of human epidermal growth factor receptor 2. Although it is clear that alterations in tumour suppressor genes and oncogenes are necessary to produce osteosarcomas, it is not clear which of these events occurs first and why or how it occurs. Moreover, it is not clear which, if any, of the alterations is essential for tumour development and therefore might represent a therapeutic target.

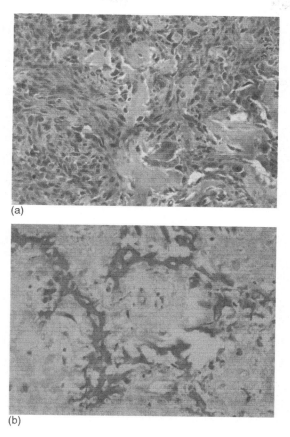

(a)

(b)

Fig. 19.3 Osteoblastic osteosarcoma (a) before and (b) after preoperative chemotherapy, showing a good response to induction chemotherapy. (Courtesy of H. Bürger.)

Signs, symptoms, and natural disease course

Patients with osteosarcoma usually do not feel ill until very late in the course of the disease. They typically seek medical attention because of first intermittent and then continuous pain, which is often erroneously attributed to a recent trauma of the involved region, for instance a sports injury. Tumour-related swelling and loss of function of the adjacent joints usually develop later. In approximately 10 per cent, the first sign of disease is a pathologic fracture. Pain at bony sites other than the primary may represent metastatic involvement. However, metastases are most likely to occur in the lungs, and these produce respiratory symptoms only with extensive involvement. Systemic symptoms, such as fever and weight loss, occur rarely in the absence of very advanced disease.

The differential diagnosis of osteosarcoma includes traumatic lesions, osteomyelitis, benign bone tumours such as exostosis, fibroma, osteoid-osteoma, chondroma, giant cell tumour of bone, bone cysts, and others, as well as other primary malignant lesions of bone such as Ewing sarcoma or lymphoma, and metastases from malignancies such as neuroblastoma or soft tissue sarcoma.

At diagnosis, even the most accurate staging procedures will reveal metastases in no more than 10–20 per cent of patients. Primary metastases are limited to the lungs in 80 per cent of affected individuals. The remainder have bone metastases with or without additional pulmonary involvement. Skip metastases (isolated tumour foci within the same bone as the primary tumour) occur in a minority of patients. Regional lymph node metastases are rare, and other sites are almost never involved at initial diagnosis.[3] If no systemic treatment is given, most patients with seemingly localized disease will go on to develop metachronous metastases within 1–2 years. Lungs and, to a lesser extent, distant bones are again the organs involved. Death is usually due to respiratory failure caused by extensive pulmonary involvement.

Diagnostic evaluation

History and physical examination

The evaluation of suspected osteosarcoma begins with a detailed history, physical examination, and plain radiographs. As stated above, most patients present with a history of pain of the involved region. Physical examination is typically remarkable only for a mass at the primary site. Loss of motion of neighbouring joints, infiltration of the skin, and neurologic deficits may occur, depending on the location and extent of the tumour.

Laboratory studies

There are no known specific laboratory parameters. Increases of alkaline phosphatase or lactic dehydrogenase (LDH) serum levels, which are observed in a considerable number of patients, do not correlate reliably with disease extent but may have negative prognostic significance.

Imaging

The characteristics and extent of the primary tumour must be evaluated by plain radiographs and cross-sectional imaging techniques. On plain radiographs, which are mainly used to describe the bony compartment, osteosarcoma often presents with lytic or sclerotic changes, or both. Ossification in the soft tissue in a radial or 'sunburst' pattern is a typical finding, but neither sensitive nor specific. Periosteal new bone formation with lifting of the cortex leads to the appearance of Codman's triangle [Fig. 19.4(a)]. MRI is the most useful tool to define the intramedullary tumour extent, soft tissue component, and relation of the tumour to vessels and nerves [Fig. 19.4(b)].[4]

The search for metastases must focus on the two organ systems in which >95 per cent of all osteosarcoma metastases arise: the lungs and the skeleton. Plain radiographs [Fig. 19.5(a)] and a CT-scan of the thorax [Fig. 19.5(b)], preferably high-resolution spiral CT, must be performed to exclude pulmonary metastases. Bone metastases are searched for using a [^{99m}Tc]MDP bone scan [Fig. 19.6]. Skip metastases may also be visualized on the bone scan, but MRI of the whole bone is preferable because of its higher sensitivity. There is currently no established role for positron emission tomography (PET), which is inferior to CT for the detection of lung metastases and to bone scintigraphy for the detection of bone metastases. Whole-body MRI may lead to a higher detection rate of bone metastases, but its place in diagnostic evaluation remains to be defined.

Biopsy

While imaging will often result in a high index of suspicion, the diagnosis of osteosarcoma must always be verified histologically. In order to ensure appropriate biopsy techniques and an appropriate evaluation of the material obtained, it is strongly recommended that biopsies should be performed only in specialized centers. Open biopsy may be most suitable to obtain sufficient material for histologic evaluation and ancillary studies. The biopsy specimen should be forwarded to the pathologist without prior fixation.

Staging systems

Previous editions of the TNM staging system were not very well adapted to the necessities of bone sarcomas. Most clinicians, especially tumour surgeons, still prefer the system developed by the Musculoskeletal Tumour Society (MSTS)[5] The MSTS system categorizes localized malignant bone tumours by grade (low grade = stage I or high grade = stage II) and by the local anatomic extent (intracompartmental = A or extracompartmental = B). The compartmental status is determined by whether or not the tumour extends through the cortex. It remains to be seen whether the latest edition of the TNM classification,[6] which allows a more

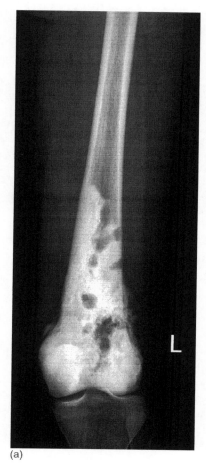

(a)

Fig. 19.4 (a) Conventional radiograph of an osteosarcoma of the distal femur in a 15-year-old girl with extensive intramedullary sclerosis and typical cloudy soft tissue calcifications. (Continued)

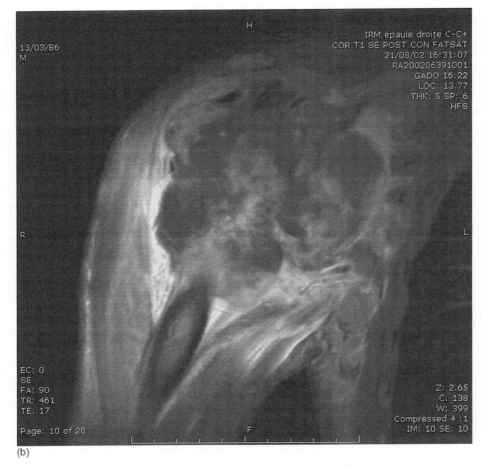

(b)

Fig. 19.4 (Continued) (b) MRI of a large osteosarcoma of the proximal humerus.

accurate description of osteosarcomas than previous versions (Table 19.1), will gain wider acceptance than its predecessors.

Treatment strategy

Many patients with osteosarcoma can be cured (Fig. 19.7). Inappropriate use of diagnostic tools and suboptimal initial therapy can irrevocably compromise a patient's chances. Therefore all patients with osteosarcoma should be treated in specialized experienced centers able to provide access to the full diagnostic and therapeutic spectrum. Treatment within prospective clinical trials is considered standard clinical practice in many countries. An intergroup trial, the European and American Osteosarcoma Study (EURAMOS-1), is currently being performed by several European and North American study groups.

Local treatment of osteosarcoma is surgical. However, most patients have already developed micrometastatic disease by the time their osteosarcoma is detected. Prior to the 1970s, when treatment was exclusively surgical, the outcome was extremely poor. Almost 90 per cent of patients who presented with apparently localized disease developed recurrences and died within 1–2 years of diagnosis. This dismal outlook was dramatically improved when multi-agent chemotherapy was added to surgery. Many trials have since reported disease-free survival rates in the range of 50–70 per cent. Most investigators believed that the favourable results of single-arm studies of surgery plus combination chemotherapy were sufficient to demonstrate the superiority of the combined modality approach over surgery alone. However, a minority questioned the validity of historical comparisons. Therefore the American Multi-Institution

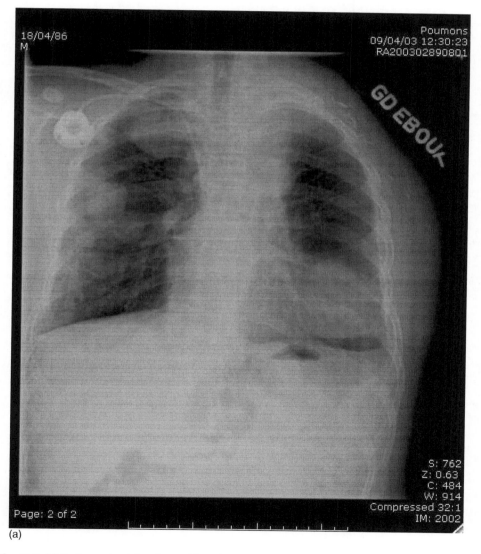

(a)

Fig. 19.5 (a) Radiograph of the chest with multiple pulmonary metastases after forequarter amputation for an osteosarcoma of the proximal humerus. (Continued)

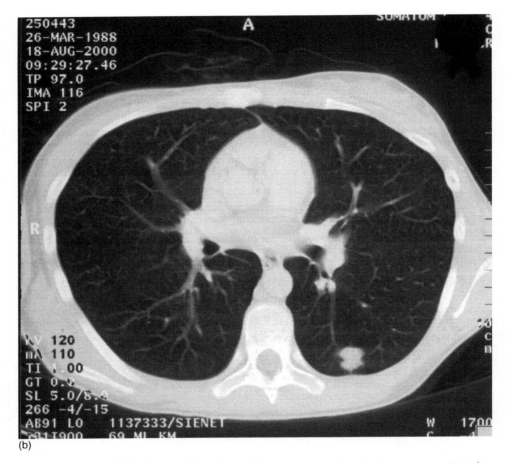

```
250443                              A              SOMATOM
26-MAR-1988                                           C
18-AUG-2000                                         .R
09:29:27.46
TP 97.0
IMA 116
SPI 2
R
kV 120
mA 110
TI : 00
GT 0.0
SL 5.0/8.4
266 -4/-15
AB91 LO     1137333/SIENET          W      1700
T900    69 ML KM                  C
```

(b)

Fig. 19.5 (Continued) (b) CT scan of the chest with pulmonary metastatic osteosarcoma. Note the round metastasis in the dorsal periphery of the left lung.

Osteosarcoma Study (MIOS) randomized patients with localized extremity osteosarcoma between surgery plus adjuvant multi-agent chemotherapy and surgery plus observation. Not surprisingly, this study confirmed the low cure rate (only 11 per cent disease-free survival) for patients who did not receive chemotherapy, while 66 per cent of the patients who received adjuvant chemotherapy were disease-free survivors.[7] Ever since, the multimodal approach has remained the undisputed standard of care.

Effective agents

The majority of current treatment protocols are based on two or more of only four active agents: doxorubicin, cisplatin, high-dose methotrexate, and ifosfamide, although its absolute role has still not been estabished. Even after more than two decades of experience with these agents against osteosarcoma and despite numerous clinical trials, the exact role of each of the agents and the optimal way in which they should be combined and delivered are still being debated, as is the potential benefit of additional drugs.

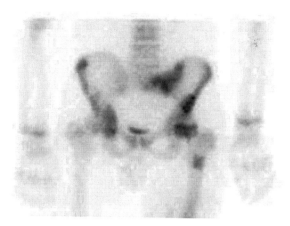

Fig. 19.6 [99m]TC bone scan showing increased uptake in multiple foci in the pelvis (and proximal femur) in a 16-year-old patient with multifocal osteosarcoma

Table 19.1. TNM classification (6th edition) for malignant bone tumours and suggested staging system[1,6]

TNM classification	
Tx	Primary tumour cannot be assessed
T0	No evidence of primary tumour
T1	Tumour ≤8 cm in greatest dimension
T2	Tumour >8 cm in greatest dimension
T3	Discontinuous tumours in the primary bone site
NX	Regional lymph nodes cannot be assessed
N0	No regional lymph node metastasis
N1	Regional lymph node metastasis
MX	Distant metastases cannot be assessed
M0	No distant metastases
M1	Distant metastases
M1a	Lung
M1b	Other distant sites
Staging system	
Stage IA	T1, N0, M0 (low grade)
Stage IB	T2, N0, M0 (low grade)
Stage IIA	T1, N0, M0 (high grade)
Stage IIB	T2, N0, M0 (high grade)
Stage III	T3, N0, M0 (any grade)
Stage IVA	Any T, N0, M1a (any grade)
Stage IVB	Any T, N1, any M (any grade)
	Any T, any N, M1b (any grade)

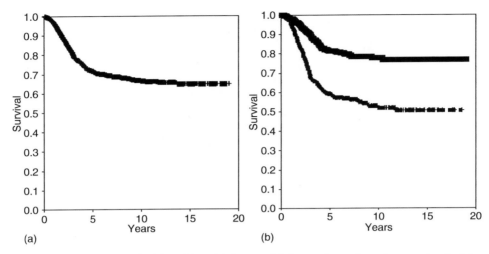

Fig. 19.7 (a) Overall survival with multimodal therapy. (b) Comparison of good responders (solid curve) and poor responders (broken curve). A good response is defined as <10% viable tumour. Results are from 1152 COSS patients aged <20 years with localized extremity osteosarcoma.

Doxorubicin

Doxorubicin was first introduced into osteosarcoma treatment in the 1970s and has remained an integral part ever since. A large meta-analysis of osteosarcoma trials concluded that, of all agents, only the dose intensity of doxorubicin was closely related to efficacy.[8] Given the threat of long-term anthracycline cardiotoxicity, doxorubicin administration to young patients with a fairly high cure rate is troublesome. Some osteosarcoma protocols include measures aimed towards reducing doxorubicin cardiotoxicity. The use of cardioprotectants such as dexrazoxane and the reduction of anthracycline peak levels by continuous doxorubicin infusions feature most prominently. Sequential studies by American and European groups suggest that there is no major loss of efficacy, but no controlled studies evaluating whether cardiotoxicity can be reduced without influencing efficacy against osteosarcoma have been reported.

Methotrexate

Methotrexate, a folate antagonist, blocks the action of dihydrofolate reductase, the enzyme responsible for reducing folate to its active form, tetrahydrofolic acid. In osteosarcoma, methotrexate is given at supralethal doses, usually in the range $8-12 \, \mathrm{g/m^2}$. The severe toxicity which follows high-dose methotrexate administration must be antagonized by the antidote leucovorin (activated folate), thereby bypassing the blocked enzyme. The treatment concept of high-dose methotrexate is based on the assumption that normal cells can be rescued more effectively than tumour cells, which may lack active folate transporters. High-dose methotrexate therapy requires meticulous attention and extensive supportive measures, including hydration, alkalinization of the urine, and leucovorin administration adapted to methotrexate serum levels. Inadequate supportive care will result in severely delayed methotrexate clearance and excessive toxicity, including myelosuppression, increases of serum creatinine or frank renal failure, and severe gastrointestinal side effects. Some patients will experience such toxicity despite adequate supportive care; the risk appears to increase with increasing patient age. The enzyme carboxypeptidase G2, which cleaves methotrexate, may be of benefit in selected patients with renal failure and severely delayed methotrexate clearance, but most cases of delayed methotrexate clearance can be handled with high-dose leucovorin as sole therapy.

No other drug used against osteosarcoma has been associated with as much controversy as high-dose methotrexate. There is no doubt that some osteosarcomas show marked responses to this therapy. The superiority of high over conventional doses was clearly demonstrated in the randomized IOR I trial from Italy.[9] There is still no consensus as to whether individual pharmacokinetic parameters, such as the peak methotrexate serum level, correlate with efficacy. Some investigators believe that the overall efficacy of any osteosarcoma protocol is strongly related to the amount of methotrexate included and the way in which it is administered. In contrast, the European Osteosarcoma Intergroup has claimed that the incorporation of methotrexate into doxorubicin/cisplatin-based protocols may compromise efficacy.[10] The conclusions from their randomized trial EOI 80831 have been questioned, as the overall success rate in both arms was comparatively low, doxorubicin and cisplatin dose intensity was lower in the arm with methotrexate, and the chosen methotrexate dose of $8 \, g/m^2$ was relatively low. Given the relative lack of myelotoxicity and the resulting ability to schedule methotrexate at times when other more myelotoxic agents cannot be administered, most groups continue to incorporate high-dose methotrexate into their osteosarcoma protocols.

Cisplatin

The efficacy of cisplatin against osteosarcomas was demonstrated in early phase II trials. The agent was subsequently incorporated into most multi-agent regimens. Cisplatin therapy requires supportive hyperhydration. Oto- and nephrotoxicity are dose-limiting toxicities. Both can be reduced by administering the drug as a continuous infusion. Intra-arterial cisplatin administration directly into the artery supplying the tumour was investigated in the 1980s, but was later largely abandoned when comparative trials could not demonstrate enhanced anti-tumour effects compared with intravenous administration.[11]

Ifosfamide

Following positive phase II trials, ifosfamide has been part of many osteosarcoma protocols since the mid-1980s. Its efficacy may be related to the dose administered. Supportive measures necessary to prevent the otherwise frequent haemorrhagic uropathy after ifosfamide include hydration and the administration of mesna (Uromitexan). Ifosfamide may also lead to chronic renal tubular toxicity (the Fanconi syndrome) and sterility.

Based on the results of sequential trials, both the Istituto Rizzoli and Cooperative Osteosarcoma Study (COSS) group have reported that the inclusion of ifosfamide into their respective multi agent regimens was associated with improved event-free survival rates. However, a recent randomized trial by the Pediatric Oncology Group (POG) and the Children's Cancer Group (CCG) (intergroup 0133) could not demonstrate that the addition of standard dose ifosfamide to a regimen of high-dose methotrexate, doxorubicin, and cisplatin improved outcome.[12] The results of intergroup 0133 must be interpreted with caution, as a second randomization of liposomal muramyl tripeptide (MTP-PE) may have interfered with the ifosfamide question. Also, the ifosfamide arm contained no preoperative cisplatin.

Other agents

No other agents have come even close to replacing the four standard substances described above. A combination of bleomycin, cyclophosphamide, and actinomycin D (BCD) was used in the early days of chemotherapy, but was later largely abandoned because of questionable efficacy. Carboplatin has some activity against osteosarcoma, but seems to be less active than cisplatin. Etoposide is almost inactive when given as a single agent, but may enhance the effect of carboplatin or ifosfamide. Negative phase II studies have been reported for paclitaxel, docetaxel, and topotecan. Gemcitabine seems to be marginally active, with stable disease having been reported for some patients. High-dose chemotherapy with autologous peripheral blood stem cell transplantation was unsuccessful in the few reported series.

Neoadjuvant chemotherapy

Currently, most institutions use an approach consisting of preoperative chemotherapy (also called neoadjuvant chemotherapy or induction chemotherapy), followed by definitive surgery and postoperative adjuvant chemotherapy. The neoadjuvant concept was first introduced into osteosarcoma therapy ~25 years ago. The theoretical advantages include early treatment of micrometastatic disease and facilitation of the eventual surgical procedure because of tumour shrinkage and decreased vascularity. A theoretical concern is that delayed removal of the bulk tumour could lead to the emergence of chemotherapy resistance. Only one relatively small randomized trial has prospectively compared patients treated by pre- and postoperative chemotherapy with patients treated by primary surgery followed by the same chemotherapy. In this POG trial, treatment results did not differ between the two arms.[13] Similarly, the COSS Group could not detect a survival difference between the two approaches in a large retrospective comparison of 157 patients with primary surgery and 1451 with primary chemotherapy.[14] Given the advantages in facilitating limb salvage procedures and assessing chemotherapy efficacy, the use of induction chemotherapy has become the standard treatment approach. Response of the tumour to induction chemotherapy can be evaluated histologically to assess the effectiveness of therapy [Fig. 19.3(b)]. Most investigators would define a good response as <10 per cent viable tumour.

Prognostic factors

Several prognostic factors have been identified. The largest reported series of 1702 osteosarcoma patients found primary metastases, axial or proximal extremity location, and large tumour size to be of independent negative prognostic value.[14] Survival may be better in fibroblastic and telangiectatic tumours than in osteoblastic and chondroblastic tumours.[15] Other factors associated with an adverse outcome in some series include very young age or older age, high serum levels of alkaline phosphatase or LDH, and the immunohistochemical detection of p-glycoprotein or *HER2–erbB2*. However, the relative risk associated with any presenting factor is lower than that of two treatment-related variables: Incomplete surgery was the most important negative prognostic indicator in the COSS series, followed by a poor histologic response to induction chemotherapy.[14] There is ample evidence that axial, primary metastatic, and even secondary osteosarcomas can be cured if a complete surgical remission of all affected sites can be obtained.

Response and outcome

Response to induction chemotherapy is believed by many to be the most important prognostic factor for resectable osteosarcoma. However, response is not an all-or-nothing effect. Even a very moderate response is associated with a better prognosis than no response at all.[14] Response rates may be higher in fibroblastic and telangiectatic tumours and lower in chondroblastic tumours.[15] Methods used to predict response preoperatively include serial evaluation by angiography, quantitative bone scans, dynamic MRI, or PET. Early reports from the Memorial Sloan–Kettering Cancer Center suggested that the poor prognosis associated with poor response could be improved by altering postoperative chemotherapy.[16] However, the COSS Group's trial COSS-82 failed to detect a benefit of salvage treatment even in poor responders who had received only very low intensity treatment preoperatively and then went on to very intensive doxorubicin/cisplatin salvage therapy.[17] A reanalysis of the Sloan–Kettering results failed to confirm the salvage effect reported earlier.[18] Several other attempts have been made to improve the prognosis of poor responders by altering postoperative chemotherapy, but none of these was a randomized trial in which a salvage approach was compared with unaltered postoperative chemotherapy. The only trial suggesting that salvage chemotherapy might work was the second study by the Rizzoli Institute, Bologna, where ifosfamide/etoposide was added postoperatively for those patients whose osteosarcomas had responded poorly to ifosfamide-free preoperative regimens.[19]

Local therapy

Despite the efficacy of chemotherapy against microscopic disease, it cannot reliably control clinically detectable osteosarcoma. Therefore surgery of the primary tumour and, if present, all metastases remains an integral part of successful therapy. Radiotherapy does not reliably sterilize osteosarcomas and is reserved for inoperable sites or those that can only be operated on with inadequate margins.

Osteosarcoma surgery has three aims: First and foremost, the tumour must be removed completely. Secondly, the patient should be left with good extremity function. Thirdly, surgery should, if possible, result in a cosmetically acceptable appearance. Complete tumour removal is of paramount importance, while functional and cosmetic aspects can only be secondary goals.

Definitive surgery must be planned and performed so that the complete tumour, including the biopsy scar and biopsy track, is removed with an unviolated cuff of normal tissue surrounding it. This corresponds to 'wide' margins as defined by the Musculoskeletal Tumour Society.[5] The MSTS classification distinguishes between radical, wide, marginal, and intralesional resection margins (Table 19.2). Radical and wide margins are considered adequate, while marginal or intralesional margins are associated with an increased risk of local recurrence,[20] which in turn carries a very poor prognosis.

The type of surgery needed to achieve wide margins varies according to the location, size, and regional anatomy of the tumour. *En bloc* resection with limb salvage is possible in many cases, but ablative techniques, such as amputation, will be required in others. The relation of the tumour to nerves and vessels of the popliteal fossa or axilla as well as structures of neighbouring joints must be carefully evaluated before deciding upon the type of surgery.

Table 19.2. Surgical margins in musculoskeletal oncology[5]

Type	Dissection
Intralesional	Within the lesion
Marginal	Through the pseudocapsule or reactive tissue
Wide	Lesion (including biopsy scar), pseudocapsule and/or reactive zone, and an unviolated cuff of normal tissue completely surrounding the mass removed as single block
Radical	Entire anatomic compartment containing the tumour removed as single block

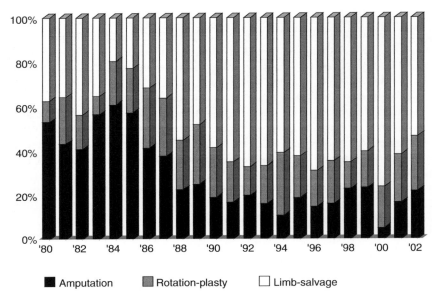

Fig. 19.8 Changing distribution of definitive surgical procedures for extremity osteosarcoma (based on paediatric and adolescent COSS patients, 1980–2000).[14]

Particular care must be taken in tumours with insufficient response to preoperative induction chemotherapy, as this is associated with an excessive local failure rate in the case of inadequate margins.[20] If pathologic evaluation of the resected tumour specimen reveals inadequate (marginal or intralesional) margins, this is usually an indication for revision surgery, even if this implies severe mutilation. Radiotherapy is indicated in cases where even the most aggressive surgical approaches will not result in wide margins, as is often the case in pelvic tumours.

Only a minority of osteosarcomas are located in expendable bones, such as the proximal fibula, where no reconstruction is required. In all other cases, the choice of reconstruction must be based on the bone, nerves, vessels, soft tissues, and skin remaining after wide resection of the tumour. Many patients have not yet reached their final height at the time of tumour surgery, so that the remaining growth expectation must also be included in the decision-making process. Until ~30 years ago, amputation was the only form of bone sarcoma surgery. This has since changed dramatically, and limb-salvage techniques are now used in the majority of cases (Fig. 19.8). Even today, however, amputation may be the most appropriate type of surgery for selected patients with unfavourable tumour characteristics. Advantages of amputation include oncologic safety, a low complication rate, and a low rate of revision surgery. Disadvantages include mutilation, phantom sensations, and functional deficits. The functional outcome is often rather poor after proximal amputations, but below-knee amputations can lead to a good functional outcome.

Rotation-plasty, used for osteosarcomas of the distal femur and occasionally the proximal tibia, is the classic example of a resection–reimplantation procedure. The knee is removed *en bloc* together with the tumour; the only structure left *in situ* is the popliteal nerve bundle. The distal part of the tibia, together with the foot, is then rotated by 180°, the tibia is fused with the femoral stump, and anastomoses are created between the femoral and tibial vessels. The result of this reimplantation is a shortened extremity, in which the rotated foot substitutes for the knee and carries the prosthesis. Advantages of rotation-plasty include oncologic safety even in very large tumours, lack of phantom sensations, and an infrequent need for revision surgery, as well as an extremity function rivalling that of even the most favourable limb-salvage procedures. The highly unusual cosmetic appearance of the rotated foot is the main disadvantage of the procedure.

Today, most osteosarcoma patients are operated on with limb-salvage procedures. Retaining the extremity requires reconstruction of bony and soft tissue defects resulting from tumour resection with wide margins. Because of the predilection of the tumour for the metaphyses of the long bones, this usually implies replacement of one of the major joints. Allografts are used by some surgeons, but modular endoprosthetic systems which can be assembled to fit in the operating room are employed more commonly (Fig. 19.9). Autologous bones, such as a vascularized fibula bridging the defect left by the resection of an osteosarcoma of the femoral diaphysis, can be employed in selected situations. Special expandable endoprostheses are available for growing extremities, but these carry with them a need for multiple revision procedures. Disadvantages of limb salvage include a significant complication risk, to which infections, fractures, and prosthetic wear contribute. Several publications report a local recurrence rate which is approximately three times higher than after amputations or rotation-plasties, pointing to the fact that the resection margins achieved with limb-salvage procedures may sometimes not be as wide as expected.

Treatment of primary metastatic and relapsed disease

Detectable metastases must be removed by surgery if therapy is to be curative. As most metastases develop in the lung, this usually implies thoracotomy. There is evidence that a significant proportion of patients with apparently unilateral lung metastases may, in fact, have bilateral disease. In general, acceptable surgical alternatives include bilateral thoracotomy or median sternotomy. Complete resection of osteosarcoma pulmonary metastases requires palpation of the lung, which is not possible thoracoscopically.

Approximately a quarter of all patients with proven metastatic disease at diagnosis and 40 per cent of those who achieve a complete surgical remission of both the primary and all metastases in the context of an intensive polychemotherapy regimen will go on to become long-term survivors. Patients with solitary primary metastases may have a prognosis similar to those with localized disease.[3]

Osteosarcoma recurrences also usually involve the lung. Bone metastases and local recurrences are much less common, and other sites are rarely affected. Unfortunately, the survival rates after relapse are low, with <20 per cent of affected patients becoming long-term survivors. A short latency period and more than one or two metastases at relapse are associated with an especially poor outcome. Complete surgical removal of all sites of recurrence is the only therapeutic measure with unequivocally proven impact on survival. It may be prudent to irradiate suitable inoperable lesions in order to slow the progression of disease, but it is unlikely that this will lead to permanent cure. In a recent Italian series[21] patients with inoperable osteosarcoma relapse who received chemotherapy survived longer than those who did not. The exact role of adjuvant chemotherapy in the treatment of operable relapsed osteosarcoma is still being debated. So far, success has been limited at best, and there is no accepted standard regimen outside clinical trials.

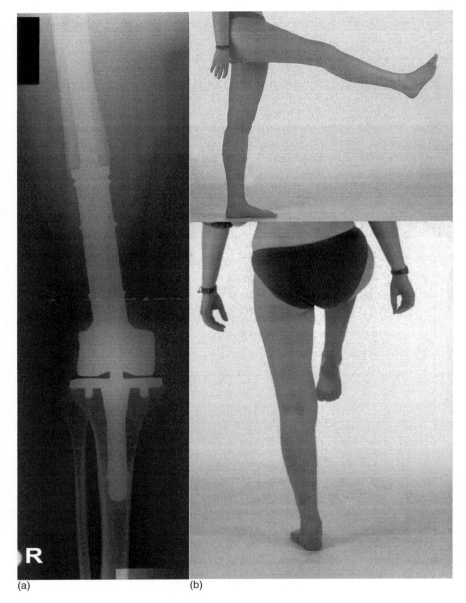

(a)   (b)

Fig. 19.9 Modular endoprosthetic replacement after surgery for a distal femur osteosarcoma: (a) radiograph; (b) extremity function.

Follow-up

Remission status

Suggestions for a follow-up programme are given in Table 19.3. The intervals between clinic visits mirror the declining risk of relapse with time. As there have been no prospective trials addressing follow-up, all suggestions must necessarily remain somewhat arbitrary. However,

Table 19.3. Suggestions for a follow-up schedule after multimodal therapy for osteosarcoma

Time	Tumour-directed	Late effects
Baseline	Chest radiograph and CT Radiograph and CT/MRI of primary site	Echocardiogram, audiogram, liver and kidney function, hepatitis B/C and HIV serology
Years 1 and 2	Chest radiograph every 6–12 weeks Radiograph of primary site every 4 months	Echocardiogram every 1–2 years, audiogram[a], liver[a] and kidney[a] function
Years 3 and 4	Chest radiograph every 2–4 months Radiograph of primary site every 4 months	Echocardiogram every 1–2 years
Years 5–10 Thereafter	Chest radiograph every 6 months[b] A few relapses reported as late as two decades after treatment Discuss with patient whether to continue chest radiograph every 6–12 months	Echocardiogram every 2–4 years[c] Echocardiogram every 2–4 years

Every clinic visit must include detailed history and physical examination. Many institutions will add complete blood counts. Evaluate any site with unexplained pain or swelling. A chest CT scan is optional, but should always be performed if the chest radiograph shows metastasis or is inconclusive. Add consultation with orthopaedic surgery and physical therapy as indicated. Offer fertility testing for males. Additional investigations may be indicated.
[a]Need not be repeated if normal at 1 year.
[b]Some groups recommend continued annual radiographs of the primary site until year 10.
[c]Longer interval if normal function and post-pubertal at diagnosis.

any follow-up for osteosarcoma must include regular assessments of the remission status as well as tests for possible late effects of (successful) treatment. Tumour-directed follow-up should focus on the few organ systems where relapses are likely to occur. Pulmonary metastases, which are part of >80 per cent of recurrences, are potentially curable only as long as they are resectable.[21] They will usually not cause symptoms until they have reached a very large size or penetrate the pleura. In order to detect them at an earlier stage, lung metastases must be searched for by appropriate imaging studies, which include serial radiographs and/or CT scans of the thorax. Local recurrences and bone metastases occur in a much lower percentage of patients and are often first detected because they cause symptoms, most noticeably pain. However, most centers will include sequential radiography of the primary site into the follow-up programme. There is no evidence that serial bone scans are beneficial.

Late effects

Fortunately, many former osteosarcoma patients will go on to lead relatively normal and productive lives. However, it cannot be expected that intensive therapy for an otherwise deadly disease can remain free of late effects. Late complications may be caused by the tumour itself or by the surgery and chemotherapy needed to control it. Functional and cosmetic consequences for the musculoskeletal system depend on the location and extent of the osteosarcoma as well as the type of surgery employed. Amputations, and even more so rotation-plasties, carry the stigma of mutilation, but may lead to functional results which are similar to those after limb-salvage procedures. Ablative surgery is most often definitive, while revision surgery is frequently needed after limb-salvage procedures where periprosthetic infection, loosening, fractures, and prosthetic wear can occur. The use of expandable prostheses in skeletally immature patients is predictably associated with the need for multiple revision procedures.

Anthracycline cardiomyopathy is a feared complication of osteosarcoma therapy in which most protocols include high cumulative doxorubicin doses. Lifelong cardiac follow-up is required. This is usually accomplished by serial echocardiograms. Renal function may be permanently compromised by cisplatin, where changes usually affect glomerular filtration, or ifosfamide, with proximal tubular damage. If end-of-treatment evaluations do not reveal impaired kidney function, it is unlikely to manifest later. The same holds true for hearing loss due to cisplatin. High-frequency loss is frequent, but only a minority of patients will require hearing aids. Protocols incorporating ifosfamide lead to sterility in most males and in some females. Secondary malignancies will develop in $\sim$3 per cent of patients within the first 10 years after treatment. Both the mutagenic side effects of cytostatic treatment and individual predisposition contribute to the development of second cancers.

Perspectives

Osteosarcoma remains a disease that presents challenges to the treating team. It is sensitive to a small number of medications, all of which have significant short- and long-term toxicities. Radiation is of limited effectiveness. Even sensitive tumours are incompletely eliminated by chemotherapy. Therefore surgical resection and reconstruction are necessary, with their attendant morbidity and imposed requirement for intensive rehabilitation. About two-thirds of patients with localized disease at initial diagnosis are cured, whereas only one-third of those with initially metastatic disease achieve cure. Patients whose disease has recurred are difficult to cure, but there is a somewhat better outlook for those with isolated resectable metastases.

New initiatives are required. These include the investigation of newer cytotoxic agents, singly or in combination. An example is the combination of trimetrexate and high-dose methotrexate, designed to circumvent dysfunction of the reduced folate carrier present in many osteosarcoma cells at the time of initial diagnosis. A phase I study to demonstrate tolerability of the combination is being planned at Memorial Sloan–Kettering Cancer Institute (R. Gorlick, personal communication, Spring 2003). Other avenues must be sought as well. An example is the use of trastuzumab in patients who have widely metastatic tumours that express her2 at initial diagnosis, which is currently being studied by the Children's Oncology Group. Another is the use of interferon-α as maintenance therapy after the completion of standard cytotoxic chemotherapy, since it may have both anti-angiogenic and anti-neoplastic activity, as is planned in the upcoming European–North American (EURAMOS) study. Augmentation of the fas, fas ligand death pathway through the use of granulocyte-monocyte colony stimulating factor (GM-CSF) as an inhalation in patients with isolated pulmonary metastatic disease will soon be studied by the Children's Oncology Group, and will be followed by a study of the combination of ifosfamide and inhaled GM-CSF. Investigations of the underlying oncogenic defect, possibly a loss of genomic control, are ongoing. In addition, increasing collaborative efforts with veterinary colleagues, to take advantage of the higher rate of osteosarcoma in large dog species, are underway. Initial studies of the role of bisphosphonates in the therapy of osteosarcoma are planned (C. Khanna and J. Hock, personal communication, Spring 2003). Recent reports suggest that in selected cases external beam radiotherapy, which is not reliably effective against inoperable osteosarcoma, may be augmented by targeted internal radiotherapy with high-dose [^{153}Sm]EDTMP plus blood progenitor cell support. It is hoped that exploration of these novel approaches and the increasing cooperation of European and North American investigators will lead to improved outcome for patients with osteosarcoma.

References

1. **Fletcher CDM, Unni K, Mertens K (eds)** (2002). *WHO Classification of Tumours. Pathology and Genetics of Tumours of Soft Tissue and Bone.* Lyon: IARC Press.

2. **Fuchs B, Pritchard DJ** (2002). Tumor biology: etiology of osteosarcoma. *Clin Orthop* 397, 40–52.

3. **Kager L, Zoubek A, Pötschger U, et al.** (2003). Primary metastatic osteosarcoma: presentation and outcome of 202 patients treated on neoadjuvant Cooperative Osteosarcoma Study Group (COSS) protocols. *J Clin Oncol* 21, 2011–18.

4. **Sanders TG, Parsons TW III** (2001). Radiographic imaging of musculoskeletal neoplasia. *Cancer Control* 8, 221–31.

5. **Enneking WE, Spanier SS, Goodmann MA** (1980). A system for the surgical staging of musculo-skeletal tumors. *Clin Orthop* 153, 106–20.

6. **Sobin LH, Wittekind C** (2002) *UICC TNM Classification of Malignant Tumors* (6th edn) New York: Wiley.

7. **Link MP, Goorin AM, Miser AW, et al.** (1986). The effect of adjuvant chemotherapy on relapse-free survival in patients with osteosarcoma of the extremities. *N Engl J Med* 314, 1600–6.

8. **Smith MA, Ungerleider RS, Horowitz ME, et al.** (1991). Influence of doxorubicin dose intensity on response and outcome for patients with osteogenic sarcoma and Ewing's sarcoma. *J Natl Cancer Inst* 83, 1460–70.

9. **Bacci G, Picci P, Ruggeri P, et al.** (1990). Primary chemotherapy and delayed surgery (neoadjuvant chemotherapy) for osteosarcoma of the extremities. The Istituto Rizzoli experience in 127 patients treated preoperatively with intravenous methotrexate (high vs. moderate doses) and intraarterial cisplatin. *Cancer* 65, 2539–53.

10. **Bramwell VH, Burgers M, Sneath R, et al.** (1992). A comparison of two short intensive adjuvant chemotherapy regimens in operable osteosarcoma of limbs in children and young adults: the first study of the European Osteosarcoma Intergroup. *J Clin Oncol* 10, 1579–91.

11. **Winkler K, Bielack S, Delling G, et al.** (1990). Effect of intraarterial versus intravenous cisplatin in addition to systemic doxorubicin, high dose methotrexate, and ifosfamide on histologic tumor response in osteosarcoma (Study COSS-86). *Cancer* 66, 1703–10.

12. **Meyers PA, Schwartz CL, Bernstein M, et al.** (2001). Addition of ifosfamide and muramyl tripeptide to cisplatin, doxorubicin and high-dose methotrexate improves event-free survival (EFS) in localized osteosarcoma (OS). *Proc Am Soc Clin Oncol* 20,1463 (abstract).

13. **Goorin AM, Schwartzentruber DJ, Devidas M, et al.** (2003). Presurgical chemotherapy compared with immediate surgery and adjuvant chemotherapy for nonmetastatic osteosarcoma: Pediatric Oncology Group Study POG-8651. *J Clin Oncol* 21, 1574–80.

14. **Bielack S, Kempf-Bielack B, Delling G, et al.** (2002). Prognostic factors in high-grade osteosarcoma of the extremities or trunk. An analysis of 1702 patients treated on neoadjuvant Cooperative Osteosar-coma Study Group protocols. *J Clin Oncol* 20, 776–90.

15. **Bacci G, Bertoni F, Longhi A, et al.** (2003). Neoadjuvant chemotherapy for high-grade central osteosarcoma of the extremity. Histologic response to preoperative chemotherapy correlates with histologic subtype of the tumor. *Cancer* 97, 3068–75.

16. **Rosen G, Caparros B, Huvos AG, et al.** (1982). Preoperative chemotherapy for osteogenic sarcoma: selection of postoperative adjuvant chemotherapy based on the response of the primary tumor to preoperative chemotherapy. *Cancer* 49, 1221–39.

17. **Winkler K, Beron G, Delling G, et al.** (1988). Neoadjuvant chemotherapy of osteosarcoma: results of a randomized cooperative trial (COSS-82) with salvage chemotherapy based on histological tumor response. *J Clin Oncol* 6, 329–37.

18. **Meyers PA, Heller G, Healey J, et al.** (1992). Chemotherapy for nonmetastatic osteogenic sarcoma: the Memorial Sloan–Kettering experience. *J Clin Oncol* 10, 5–15.

19. **Bacci G, Ferrari S, Bertoni F,** *et al.* (2000). Long-term outcome for patients with nonmetastatic osteosarcoma of the extremity treated at the Istituto Ortopedico Rizzoli according to the Istituto Ortopedico Rizzoli/Osteosarcoma-2 protocol: an updated report. *J Clin Oncol* 18, 4016–27.

20. **Picci P, Sangiorgi L, Rongraff BT,** *et al.* (1994). The relationship of chemotherapy- induced necrosis and surgical margins to local recurrence in osteosarcoma. *J Clin Oncol* 12, 2699–705.

21. **Ferrari S, Briccoli A, Mercuri M,** *et al.* (2003). Postrelapse survival in osteosarcoma of the extremities: prognostic factors for long-term survival. *J Clin Oncol* 21, 710–15.

Chapter 20

Ewing sarcoma and peripheral primitive neuroectodermal tumour

Michael Paulussen, Heinrich Kovar, and Herbert Jürgens

Introduction

The Ewing family of tumours (EFT) is a clinically heterogeneous group of malignant tumours including Ewing sarcoma (ES), malignant peripheral primitive neuroectodermal tumour (pPNET) and Askin tumour (ES of the thoracic wall, affecting children, adolescents and young adults). EFT most commonly originate in bone but occasionally arise in soft tissue. Lücke in 1866 and Hildebrand in 1890 first described single cases of this tumour, but James Ewing was the first to recognize Ewing sarcoma as a distinct entity. He published reports between 1921 and 1939 on 'diffuse endothelioma' or 'endothelial myeloma', tumours sensitive to radiation and considered to be of endothelial origin.[1] The exact histogenesis remains unknown, although the current view is that EFT originate from an ubiquitous pluripotent stem cell thought to be of neuroectodermal origin. At the genetic level, EFT demonstrate a tumour-specific chromosomal translocation between the long arms of chromosome 22 and, most commonly, chromosome 11 (85 per cent) or chromosome 21 (10 per cent). These aberrations result in a gene fusion which is diagnostic for EFT and which differentiates them from other childhood malignancies with a similar small round cell phenotype. In James Ewing's time, and up to the late 1960s, >90 per cent of patients died of distant metastases within 2 years of diagnosis despite the well known radioresponsiveness of these tumours. This shows that micrometastases are most likely to be present at diagnosis, or develop very early in the course of disease, in the vast majority of patients. Definitive cure of EFT has only been observed since the introduction of chemotherapy and, with current combinations of multi-agent chemotherapy and local therapy, cure rates of >50 per cent can be achieved.

Epidemiology

In Caucasian populations, EFT represent the second most common primary malignant bone tumour in childhood and adolescence and account for 10–15 per cent of all primary malignant bone tumours. Annual incidence rates are approximately 3 per million in children aged <15 years, and 2.4 per million for patients aged 15–24 years. The median age at presentation is 15 years, more than half of cases occurring in the second decade of life, and there is a male predominance (1.5:1) which increases with age (Fig. 20.1). EFT are almost unknown in African and Chinese populations. There is no evidence for genetic predisposition and it seems unlikely that environmental exposure plays a role in pathogenesis.

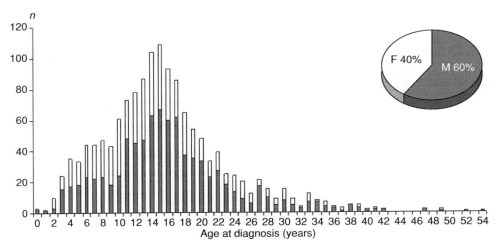

Fig. 20.1 Age and gender. Data based on 1426 patients from the (EI)CESS studies.

Clinical presentation, diagnosis, and staging

Primary sites

The most common sites of the primary lesion are the pelvis, long bones of the extremities, ribs, scapula, and vertebrae (Fig. 20.2). Compared with the skeletal distribution of osteogenic sarcoma, the flat bones of the trunk are more often affected. In long bones, the tumour originates from the diaphysis, either centrally or towards the ends, in contrast with the typical metaphyseal presentation of osteosarcoma.

Signs and symptoms

EFT patients most commonly present with pain. Additional symptoms depend on site and bulk of disease. The pain is often mistakenly related by the patient or health care professional to minor injuries incurred during sport or everyday activity, but it persists for an unusual length of time and is independent of activity (e.g. it occurs at night). A history of increasing persistent pain, followed by swelling of the affected area, can sometimes be misdiagnosed as infection, further delaying the diagnosis. Involvement of the spinal cord or peripheral nerves may produce neurologic symptoms. Bony metastases may be palpable on the skull, ribs, or any superficial bone. Slight to moderate fever is reported in about one-third of patients, and occurs more often in those with metastatic disease at diagnosis.

Laboratory investigations

There are no specific blood or urine tests which identify EFT. Blood tests usually show a moderately elevated erythrocyte sedimentation rate and may reveal some degree of anaemia and leucocytosis. An elevated serum level of lactate dehydrogenase (LDH) correlates with tumour burden and for this reason is of indirect prognostic significance. Urine catecholamine levels are normal.

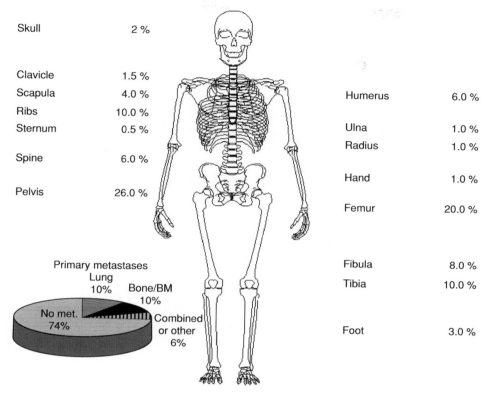

Skull	2 %			
Clavicle	1.5 %			
Scapula	4.0 %	Humerus	6.0 %	
Ribs	10.0 %			
Sternum	0.5 %	Ulna	1.0 %	
		Radius	1.0 %	
Spine	6.0 %			
		Hand	1.0 %	
Pelvis	26.0 %			
		Femur	20.0 %	
		Fibula	8.0 %	
		Tibia	10.0 %	
		Foot	3.0 %	

Primary metastases
Lung 10%
Bone/BM 10%
No met. 74%
Combined or other 6%

Fig. 20.2 Skeletal distribution of Ewing tumours. Percentages based on 1426 patients entered into the consecutive (EI)CESS trials.

Imaging

Plain radiographs, MRI, and CT are required to assess the extent of disease at the primary site, for locoregional extension, and to search for metastases. It is important to define and document tumour size, including its soft tissue components, at diagnosis and to use these measurements to monitor response to chemotherapy, as this is of prognostic significance and helps to plan local therapy. The typical radiograph of a Ewing bone tumour shows a destructive osteolytic lesion of the diaphysis with destruction of the osseous cortex, elevation of the periosteum, and infiltration of surrounding soft tissue. MRI is superior to CT for measuring the extent of the tumour in bone marrow and soft tissue and in defining the relationship between the tumour and its adjacent structures (e.g. blood vessels or nerves). However, a CT scan can identify cortical and bony changes more precisely than MRI. Figure 20.3 shows MRI of a right iliac crest EFT. Chest CT is recommended for detection of pulmonary metastases, and radionuclide bone scanning with technetium-99m is recommended for detection of bone metastases. [18Fluorine]fluorodeoxyglucose positron emission tomography (FDG-PET) has been shown to be of value as another potentially sensitive screening method for detection of metastases in EFT.

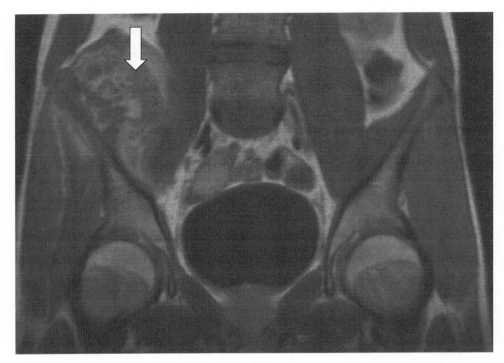

Fig. 20.3 MRI of right iliac crest Ewing tumour.

Biopsy

Open biopsy or needle-core biopsy of the primary tumour is required to confirm the diagnosis. The biopsy track and adjacent tissues must be regarded as contaminated by tumour, and the approach should be planned so that the site can be subsequently included in the local treatment. For this reason, diagnostic procedures should be performed by specialists familiar with this rare disease. About 25 per cent of patients present with detectable metastases at diagnosis (Fig. 20.2), and if there is any doubt, these sites should also be confirmed by biopsy. The biopsy specimen must be sufficient to provide material for standard histology and immunocytochemistry, and fresh/frozen material for molecular biology studies.

Bone marrow involvement

Disseminated tumour cells may not be homogeneously distributed in the bone marrow and thus may escape detection. Therefore it is recommended that marrow samples are obtained from several sites to improve the accuracy of detection. In addition to standard pathologic assessment, micrometastatic disease in the bone marrow can be detected by molecular techniques using reverse transcriptase–polymerase chain reaction (RT–PCR) for tumour-specific *EWS*-fusion transcripts. The prognostic impact of the detection of minimal disease in bone marrow by such techniques is under investigation in clinical trials.

Staging

Staging at diagnosis is based on the the size and extent of the primary tumour and on the presence or absence of lung and/or bone metastases. These factors are of prognostic significance and influence the choice of treatment. A list of staging investigations at diagnosis is given in Table 20.1.

Differential diagnosis

The most important clinical differential diagnosis in EFT is osteomyelitis. The radiologic appearance may be very similar, and occasionally EFT of bone may be secondarily infected. On histologic examination, EFT must be differentiated from other small round-cell tumours, in particular embryonal rhabdomyosarcoma, neuroblastoma (in children aged ≤5 years), small-cell osteosarcoma, and non-Hodgkin lymphoma.

Histopathology

Ewing tumours of bone and soft tissue have a similar appearance and are composed of firm grey-white soft tissue with a glistening moist appearance on sectioning. Macroscopically, the intraosseous component of the tumour is usually of firm consistency, while the extraosseous component tends to be of less firm texture with areas of haemorrhage and cystic degeneration secondary to tumour necrosis. EFT are always high-grade malignancies and when routinely stained with haematoxylin and eosin show microscopically monomorphic small blue round primitive cells, with round nuclei and scanty cytoplasm with variable amounts of glycogen deposition which stain periodic acid–Schiff (PAS) positive (Fig. 20.4). pPNET cells differ from other EFT on electron microscopy by their expression of distinct features of neural differentiation with prominent neurite-like cell processes containing neurosecretory granules and neurofilaments; rosettes and Homer–Wright pseudorosettes are also occasionally identified. However, EFT cannot be differentiated from other PAS-positive small blue round cell tumours on morphologic features alone and the diagnosis must be assisted by immunocytochemistry. The identification of monoclonal and polyclonal antibodies for various differentiation markers provides supportive evidence for the diagnosis of EFT. CD99 (Mic-2 antigen) expression is positive in >95 per cent cases but is not unique to EFT. EFTs show varying degrees of neural differentiation and can be subdivided into typical undifferentiated, atypical differentiated ES, and fully differentiated pPNET by their increasing expression of neural markers such as S-100

Table 20.1. Staging investigations at diagnosis

Investigation	Primary tumour site	Staging for metastases
Radiograph in two planes, whole bone with adjacent joints	Mandatory	At suspicious sites
MRI and/or CT, affected bone(s) and adjacent joints	Mandatory	At suspicious sites
Biopsy, histology, molecular biology	Mandatory	At suspicious sites
Chest radiograph and CT		Mandatory
Bilateral bone marrow aspirates and trephine biopsies		Mandatory
Whole-body technetium bone scan	Mandatory	Mandatory
FDG-PET	Indicated, if available	Indicated, if available

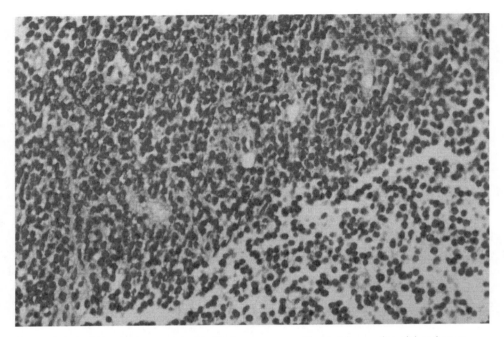

Fig. 20.4 Typical histologic appearance of Ewing sarcoma with round or oval nuclei and poor delineation of cytoplasma of cells.

protein, neuron-specific enolase (NSE), and synaptophysin. Other useful markers include vimentin, desmin, smooth muscle actin, and CD45 (leucocyte common antigen) which help to differentiate between small round cell tumours of myogenic, fibrogenic, and haematopoietic origin.

Molecular biology

Genetic definition of the Ewing sarcoma family of tumours

Historically, ES and pPNET have been considered distinct tumour entities along a gradient of limited neuroglial differentiation. However, after the identification of a tumour-specific chromosomal translocation t(11;22)(q24;q12) and its molecular equivalent, the *EWS–FLI-1* gene fusion in both ES and pPNET, the case was made for a genetically based union. The presence of this gene rearrangement enables unambiguous diagnosis in ~85 per cent of ES and pPNET. In the majority of the remaining cases, variant translocations of the *EWS* gene can be identifed. Today ES, pPNET, and an increasing number of extraskeletal small round cell tumours carrying this genetic marker or one of its similarly structured variants are referred to as the Ewing family of tumours (EFT). This unification implies a common pathogenetic origin and accounts for similar morphology and, at least in part, immunohistochemistry (i.e. high CD99 expression). Patients with EFT are treated according to the same clinical protocols and, despite earlier reports of different clinical outcomes in ES and pPNET, similar treatment results are achieved for ES and pPNET with current multimodal treatment strategies. However, the exact tissue of origin for EFT is still not known. The almost complete absence of unequivocal differentiation markers and the sporadic occurrence of biphenotypic tumours with an *EWS–FLI-1* gene rearrangement imply a primitive pluripotent neuroectodermal or mesenchymal stem cell. At present, however, it cannot be concluded with certainty that ES, pPNET, and all other tumours carrying one of the EFT-specific gene rearrangements originate from the same tissue.

The *EWS–ETS* gene fusion

The molecular key to the disease is the rearrangement of the Ewing sarcoma gene *EWS* on chromosome 22q12 with the *FLI-1* gene on chromosome 11q24.[2] *EWS* encodes an ubiquitously expressed RNA binding protein that appears to be involved in transcription and processing of messenger RNA. *FLI-1* codes for a protein with a carboxy terminal DNA binding domain that is characteristic of members of the *ETS* transcription factor family. As a consequence of the gene fusion, the *EWS* RNA binding domain is replaced by the *FLI-1*-derived *ETS* DNA binding domain, resulting in a novel transcription factor with a strong *in vitro* transactivation potential (Fig. 20.5). Alternative *EWS* gene fusions to other members of the *ETS* gene family (predominantly *ERG*) can be observed in about 10–15 per cent of EFTs (Table 20.2). While *EWS*, as well as its close relatives [*TLS* (*FUS*) and *RPB56* (*hTAF$_{II}$68*)], and *ERG* genes have been found to be involved in several chromosomal translocations in other solid tumours and acute leukemias, the specific combination of *EWS* with an *ETS* gene is restricted to, and therefore diagnostic of, EFT. The *EWS* and *FLI-1* genes comprise 17 and 9 exons, respectively. Breakpoints occur between *EWS* exons 7 and 12 and *FLI-1* exons 4 and 9. The most frequent gene fusions in EFT result in a type 1 chimeric RNA (fusion of *EWS* exon 7 to *FLI-1* exon 6) in about 50 per cent of

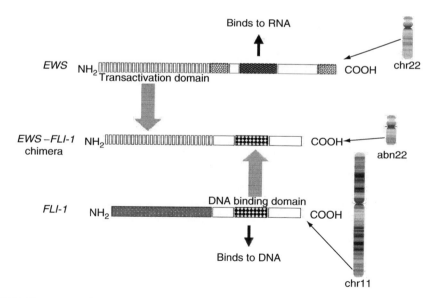

Fig. 20.5 Chromosomal translocation t(11;22)(q24;q12) in EFT. The chromosomal translocation t(11;22)(q24;q12) leads to the generation of a DNA binding fusion protein in EFT. The gene *EWS* for the RNA binding protein is located on chromosome 22 (chr22) in region q12, and the gene *FLI-1* for the DNA binding transcription factor is localized on chromosome 11 (chr11) at q24. The *EWS–FLI-1* chimeric protein is expressed from the abnormal chromosome 22 (abn22), while the reciprocal translocation product on chromosome 11 does not give rise to a gene product in EFT.

Table 20.2. *EWS–ETS* gene rearrangements in EFT

Gene fusion	Cytogenetic equivalent	Observed frequency (%)
EWS–FLI-1	t(11;22)(q24;q12)	85
EWS–ERG	t(21;22)(q22;q12)	10
EWS–ETV1	t(7;22)(p22;q12)	<1
EWS–E1AF	t(17;22)(q12;q12)	<1
EWS–FEV	t(2;21;22)	1

cases or a type 2 product (fusion of EWS exon 7 to *FLI-1* exon 5) in about 27 per cent of cases. In a significant proportion of EFT the specific chromosomal translocation would lead to an out-of-frame gene fusion resulting in a truncated non-functional protein. However, in these cases, alternative splicing restores the correct reading frame for protein synthesis, indicating that there is selective pressure in EFT for the expression of a functional *EWS–ETS* protein.[3] *EWS–FLI-1* antagonists suppress EFT cell growth. Introduction of *EWS–FLI-1* into immortalized murine fibroblasts leads to *in vitro* transformation, and *EWS–FLI-1* transformed cells are tumorigenic in nude mice, with the tumour cells displaying a small round cell phenotype resembling that of EFT.[4] In contrast, oncogenic fusions of EWS to non-*ETS* transcription factors induce a distinct morphology suggesting that the transcription factor moiety of the chimeric gene product determines the tumour phenotype. Most recent studies have demonstrated that *EWS–FLI-1* is capable of suppressing differentiation in pluripotent mesenchymal cells, possibly explaining the largely undifferentiated phenotype of EFT cells. Together, these observations indicate that *EWS–ETS* gene fusion is essential for EFT pathogenesis.

Paradoxically, introduction of *EWS–FLI-1* is toxic to most primary cell types. Impairment of the p53 pathway by either mutation of *p53* or loss of the *INK4A* gene, which play a key role in the regulation of apoptosis in response to cellular stress, including that conferred by several oncogenes, rescues *EWS–FLI-1*-expressing primary cells from programmed cell death. Interestingly, *p53* mutations are rare (<10 per cent) in primary EFT and *INK4A* deletions occur in only ∼25 per cent of cases.[5] However, if present, these alterations appear to be associated with an adverse prognosis. It remains to be established whether other types of secondary mutations rescue EFT cells from *EWS–ETS*-induced cell death or if the EFT progenitor cell is generally tolerant to the chimeric oncogene.

The transforming ability of the EFT-specific oncoprotein requires the presence of at least the *EWS* amino terminus and the *ETS* DNA binding domain, which together confer high transcriptional activity to the fusion gene product. Therefore it is assumed that the oncogenic function of *EWS–ETS* proteins is mediated by deregulation of *ETS* responsive genes. Almost equal numbers of up- and downregulated genes have been observed in response to ectopic *EWS–FLI-1* expression. Several candidate genes downstream of *EWS–FLI-1* have been identified, encoding cell cycle regulatory genes (cyclins D1, p57^{KIP2}, p21), growth factors (PDGF-C), receptors (TGFbRII, EGR), transcriptional regulatory proteins (c-Myc, Id2, c-Fos), molecules involved in intra- and extracellular signalling (EAT2, MNFG), and proteins with a presumed role in the metastatic process (stromelysin, tenascin C). Recently, induction of the cell surface sialoglycoprotein CD99 (MIC2), the immunologic hallmark of EFT, has been found to be induced by transgenic *EWS–FLI-1* in immortalized human fibroblasts.[6] The pattern of *EWS–FLI-1* associated gene expression appears to depend on the cellular context, and it is unclear whether most of the genes identified so far are directly or indirectly affected by *EWS–FLI-1* and what role they might play in EFT pathogenesis. Furthermore, the different *EWS–ETS* gene fusions present in EFT differ with respect to the sets of genes induced/repressed in transgenic murine fibroblasts with only slight overlap. Even different *EWS–FLI-1* fusion types (i.e. type 1 and type 2) differ in the strength of their activating function. How far this variability translates into different clinical behaviour remains a matter of debate. For the group of patients with localized disease, retrospective studies indicated a better event-free survival of patients with tumours expressing type 1 *EWS–FLI-1* when compared with all other *EWS–FLI-1* fusion types. This finding is currently under prospective evaluation as part of the Euro-EWING 99 study. In contrast, no difference in clinical behaviour has been observed between *EWS–FLI-1-* and *EWS–ERG*-containing EFT.

In addition to its transcriptional regulatory activity, *EWS–FLI-1* is likely to be involved in distinct processes that do not depend on a functional DNA binding domain. Because of its interaction with several RNA processing proteins and its documented influence on splice site selection in an *in vitro* model, it may be speculated that alternative splicing might be involved in the oncogenic activity of *EWS–FLI-1*. So far, no targets for this hypothetical *EWS–FLI-1* activity have been identified in EFT.

The strong interest in downstream targets of the primary genetic aberration in EFT derives from the hope of identifing tumour-specific targets for biologically tailored EFT therapy. CD99 (MIC2), which always parallels *EWS–ETS* expression in EFT, and for which engagement by some specific antibodies was found to induce cell death, may provide an example in this respect. However, as this antigen is expressed at variable levels in many tissues, its therapeutic potential may be limited.

Additional chromosomal aberrations

Although t(11;22) or one of its variants may be the only cytogenetically detectable chromosomal anomaly in some EFT, additional recurrent genetic aberrations are frequent. Among them, trisomy 8 and/or 12 are observed in 44 per cent and 29 per cent of cases, respectively. Structural changes commonly affect chromosomes 1 and 16, most frequently leading to a gain of 1q and a loss of 16q and the formation of a derivative chromosome der(1;16). The molecular consequences of these aberrations are not known. Deletion of the chromosomal region 9p21 (the *INK4A* gene), which is lost in ∼25 per cent of EFT, remains cytogenetically invisible in most cases.

Molecular diagnostics

Because of its consistent presence in the disease, *EWS–ETS* gene fusions serve as an unambiguous diagnostic marker for EFT cells. The classical cytogenetic demonstration of t(11;22)(q24;q12) has largely been replaced by fluorescence *in situ* hybridization (FISH) using probes flanking the *EWS* breakpoint region on chromosome 22. Even complex chromosomal rearrangements and rare *EWS* translocations with other *ETS* partner genes can be revealed using this method. However, the most frequently used method of detecting the fusion gene is RT–PCR. This diagnostic approach requires immediate snap-freezing of the biopsy since it relies on extraction of good-quality RNA. The strength of the method lies in its high sensitivity which enables identification of single tumour cells among 10^5–10^6 normal cells. Therefore it is used to evaluate the prognostic significance of minimally disseminated EFT cells in bone marrow, peripheral blood, and stem cell collections for autologous transplantation. Retrospective studies reveal bone marrow involvement in a majority of patients with metastatic disease and in about one-third of patients with localized disease. Preliminary data imply adverse prognosis when the bone marrow tests RT–PCR positive at the time of diagnosis,[7] although these results await confirmation in prospective studies such as Euro-EWING 99.

RT–PCR relies on gene expression. However, nothing is known about the activity of the *EWS–ETS* fusion gene in resting EFT cells. Therefore, at present, it is possible that dormant EFT cells may not be detectable by RT–PCR. Furthermore, as tumour cells may not be evenly distributed in the bone marrow, they may also escape detection. Hence it is necessary to sample the bone marrow from several sites.

Extraskeletal Ewing sarcoma

Extraskeletal ES is uncommon. The major differential diagnosis includes ES of bone with extensive soft tissue extension and an inapparent intraosseous component. The predominant site of initial presentation is the trunk. As distinct from ES of bone, there is no predominance in boys, but the same rules apply for the investigation and systemic treatment of extraskeletal ES as for ES of bone. However, as there appears to be a higher risk of lymphatic spread, local therapy, especially radiation, must be planned according to the same principles as applied to soft tissue malignancies like rhabdomyosarcoma. It can be differentiated from rhabdomyosarcoma, neuroblastoma, and lymphoma by histocytochemistry, and in addition, like all EFT, extraskeletal ES shows the typical chromosomal translocation t(11;22).

Treatment

Until the late 1960s, despite the well-known radioresponsiveness of these localized tumours, >90 per cent of patients died of metastases within 2 years of diagnosis. Since the introduction of multimodal treatment regimens including combination chemotherapy, surgery (where possible), and radiotherapy, cure rates of between 50–65 per cent have been achieved. The high incidence of systemic relapse in localized EFT, despite local and systemic treatment, suggests that disseminated occult tumour cells (micrometastases), possibly present at the time of diagnosis or which develop very early in the course of disease, escape detection and may not be eradicated by current treatment approaches. Improved treatment is the subject of all ongoing clinical trials and, whenever possible, patients with EFT should participate and be treated in a center participating in such studies.

Local therapy

EFT is a systemic disease; nevertheless there is no cure without local control. Local therapy following an induction phase with chemotherapy is now regarded as standard procedure. Radiotherapy is no longer the local treatment of first choice, as surgery, when feasible, has been shown to produce a survival advantage in several studies. Data from the European CESS and EICESS studies indicate that selection bias, owing to the better outcome for small peripheral lesions for which surgery was more feasible, cannot be the only explanation for the difference in local control.

Surgery

Increasing awareness of the risk of local recurrence following radiotherapy has encouraged the use of surgery or surgery with radiotherapy, with chemotherapy as optimal therapy. EFT of bone is rarely limited to the bony compartment and the presence of a soft tissue component

Table 20.3. Enneking classification of surgical intervention

Intralesional resection	The tumour is opened during surgery, the surgical field is contaminated, and there is microscopic or macroscopic residual disease
Marginal resection	The tumour is removed *en bloc*. However, the line of resection runs through the pseudocapsule of the tumour. Microscopic residual disease is likely
Wide resection	The tumour and its pseudocapsule are removed *en bloc* surrounded by healthy tissue within the tumour-bearing compartment
Radical resection	The whole tumour-bearing compartment is removed *en bloc* (e.g. above-knee amputation in tibial tumours)

is common, classifying most tumours as highly malignant extracompartmental tumours. The biopsy track must always be included in the surgical resection. In order to allow comparison of surgical interventions, all surgical procedures should be classified, for example according to the Enneking criteria: intralesional, marginal, wide, or radical resection (Table 20.3). Response of the tumour to initial chemotherapy is classified histologically based on the percentage of viable tumour cells remaining in the resected tumour (Salzer–Kuntschik grades 1–6). In cases of marginal or intralesional resection, or where there is evidence of poor histologic response to initial chemotherapy ($\geq$10 per cent viable tumour cells), surgery should be combined with postoperative radiotherapy. According to experience from several clinical study groups [e.g. the (EI)CESS studies], surgical margins and response to initial therapy correlate with outcome in terms of local control rate and risk of distant metastases (Fig. 20.6). Hence good response to initial chemotherapy and tumour-free margins must be achieved whenever possible.

Situations in which surgical resections are preferable to radiation therapy include lesion in expendable bone, pathologic fracture, distal extremity, bulky primary tumour, and poor response to initial chemotherapy. In every case, a team approach is essential for the evaluation of these patients before local therapy. The treatment plan must be individualized depending upon the location and size of the tumour and the anatomical structures in the vicinity of the tumour which might be affected by the type of treatment selected.

In recent years, surgical options have broadened to include the development of modern modular endoprosthesis systems, autograft techniques such as replacement of tibial bone by contralateral fibula, and modified amputation techniques such as rotation-plasty which have improved the mobility of the patient.

Radiotherapy

The radiosensitivity of ES was recognized by James Ewing in 1921 and radiotherapy has always played a major role in obtaining local control. Preoperative radiotherapy is indicated when there is tumour progression during chemotherapy, in an emergency such as spinal cord compression, or when incomplete surgical resectability is anticipated. Postoperative radiotherapy is indicated by incomplete resection of the tumour or where poor histologic response of the tumour to chemotherapy is determined.

Traditionally, whole-bone irradiation was advised because the tumour was thought to arise in the bone marrow, putting the whole marrow cavity at risk. The advent of improved imaging with MRI, which accurately demonstrates the extent of marrow involvement, and effective chemotherapy has questioned this approach. In a randomized study performed by POG and completed in 1989, it was shown that the results of radiotherapy to initial tumour volume

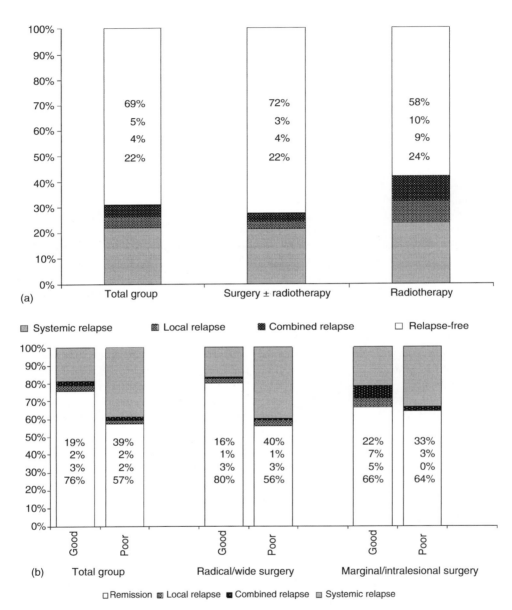

Fig. 20.6 (a) Local therapy and site of failure. (b) Site of failure in surgically treated (with or without radiotherapy) Ewing sarcoma patients according to surgical margins and response.

with a 2-cm safety margin are as good as those obtained after whole-bone irradiation. The compartment dose for radiotherapy of inoperable tumours is 44.8 Gy with a tumour boost to at least 54.4 Gy, but it can vary depending on site of tumour and age of the patient. The standard target volume dose for preoperative radiotherapy is 54.4 Gy. The dose for post-operative radiotherapy depends on histologic assessment of the resected tumour margins and the tumour response to chemotherapy, and varies from 44.8 to 54.4 Gy. Irradiation of the whole anatomical compartment is not required if adequate safety margins around the initial volume of tumour (usually 2–5 cm) can be assured. Areas of scars after biopsy or tumour resection must be included in the radiation fields. To avoid constrictive fibrosis, an adequate strip of skin and subcutaneous tissue should be left when irradiating limb sites and the epiphyseal plates should be spared if possible, particularly in growing children.

Chemotherapy

EFT have been shown to be particularly responsive to alkylating agents such as ifosfamide and cyclophosphamide, to the anthracycline doxorubicin (Adriamycin), and to other agents such as vincristine, actinomycin D, and the topoisomerase II inhibitor etoposide . A combination of agents with complementary mechanisms of action have improved disease-free survival rates. The Intergroup Ewing Sarcoma (IESS) studies showed the superiority of a four-drug regimen with vincristine (V), actinomycin D (A), cyclophosphamide (C), and doxorubicin (D) over a three-drug regimen with vincristine, actinomycin D, and cyclophosphamide (VAC) in terms of disease-free survival (60 versus 24 per cent) and effectiveness of local control (96 versus 86 per cent). Rosen et al.[8] from the Memorial Sloan–Kettering Cancer Center (MSKCC) reported an advantage of using these drugs in combination rather than sequentially. It is important to recognize that a considerable number of patients in earlier series received cumulative doxorubicin doses of over $700\,mg/m^2$ before its use was restricted to a maximum of $400 - 500\,mg/m$ because of the risk of doxorubicin-related cardiomyopathy. The MSKCC and IESS experience led to the wide use of similar four-drug regimens in most therapeutic trials. Thereafter, the treatment of EFT was extended to incorporate ifosfamide (I) (CESS 86) and etoposide (E). In the European EICESS-92 study, patients with localized high-risk disease (tumour volume >200ml) receiving VIDA did not seem to benefit from the addition of etoposide, whereas in the randomized POG–CCG Ewing trial (VACD versus VACD-iE) patients treated with VACD-iE appeared to have a more favourable outcome. Results of selected reported trials[8–23] in localized EFT are summarized in Table 20.4.

The incorporation of granulocyte colony-stimulating factor (GCSF) into treatment regimens allowed for dose intensification by either increasing the dose per cycle or shortening the interval of time between treatment. The IESS-II study compared high-dose intermittent chemotherapy with moderate-dose continuous chemotherapy, resulting in a significant benefit from the more intensive regimen [68 versus 48 per cent disease-free survival at 5 years (Table 20.4)]. The second POG–CCG randomized study explored dose intensification by delivering chemotherapy over either 30 or 48 weeks, although the results so far have shown no difference in outcome between the standard and the dose-intensified arms. The COG are currently exploring dose intensification by decreasing the intervals between cycles (interval compression) while maintaining the same dose per cycle with the use of GCSF.

In patients with metastatic disease, who have a very poor prognosis, treatment intensification has been applied with the use of high-dose chemotherapy and autologous stem cell support. A variety of agents have been used, such as busulphan, melphalan, cyclophosphamide, thiotepa, etoposide, and carboplatin. The addition of total body irradiation does not seem to offer any further benefit, but significantly contributes to toxicity. Analyses from the European EBMT registry have indicated that combinations including busulphan are more effective than other conditioning regimens.

Currently, large phase II–III studies are being conducted in several groups (e.g. in the USA, Scandinavia, and Italy) and within a joint European study group [GPOH, UKCCSG, SFOP,

Table 20.4. Treatment of localized Ewing tumours: results of selected clinical studies

Study	Reference	Treatment	No. of patients	5-year DFS	P-value[a]	Interpretation
Intergroup Ewing Sarcoma Studies						
IESS-I (1973–1978)	9	VAC	342	24%	VAC vs VAC+WLI: 0.001	Value of D
		VAC + WLI		44%	VAC vs VACD: 0.001	Benefit of WLI?
		VACD		60%	VAC+WLI vs VACD: 0.05	
IESS-II (1978–1982)	10	VACD-HD	214	68%	0.03	Value of aggressive cytoreduction
		VACD-MD		48%		
First POG–CCG (1988–1993)	11	VACD	NA	54%	0.005	Value of combination IE
		VACD + IE		69%		
Second POG–CCG (1995–1998)	12	VCD +IE (48 weeks)	492	75% (3 yr)	0.57	No benefit of dose-time compression
		VCD +IE (30 weeks)		76% (3 yr)		
Memorial Sloan-Kettering Cancer Center						
T2 (1970–1978)	8	VACD (adjuvant)	20	75%		After local therapy only, cumulative dose of D up to 600 mg/m^2
P6 (1990–1995)	13	HD-CVD + IE	36	77% (2 yr)		C dose escalation, 4.2 g/m^{2}course
St Jude Children's Research Hospital						
ES-79 (1978–1986)	14	VACD	52	<8 cm 82% (3 yr)		Tumour size as prognostic factor
				≥8 cm 64% (3 yr)		
ES-87 (1987–1991)	15	Therapeutic window with IE	26	Clinical responses in 96%		IE combination effective
EW-92 (1992–1996)	16	VCDIE × 3	34	78% (3 yr)		Tumour size (<8 cm or ≥8 cm) loses prognostic relevance with more intensive treatment
		VCD/IE intensification				
Rizzoli Orthopaedic Institute, Bologna, Italy						
REN-3 (1991–1997)	17	VDC + VIA + IE	157	71%		Surgery in 78% of patients

Table 20.4. (continued) Treatment of localized Ewing tumours: results of selected clinical studies

Study	Reference	Treatment	No. of patients	5-year DFS	P-value[a]	Interpretation
SFOP, France						
EW-88 (1988–1991)	18	VD + VD/VA	141	58%		Histologic response better predictor of outcome than tumour volume
UK Children's Cancer Study Group–Medical Research Council						
ET-1 (1978–1986)	19	VACD	120	41% Extr. 52% Axial 38% Pelvic 13%		Tumour site most important prognostic factor
ET-2 (1987–1993)	20	VAID	201	62% Extr. 73% Axial 55% Pelvic 41%		Importance of administration of high-dose alkylating agents (I)
CESS						
CESS-81 (1981–1985)	25	VACD	93	<100 ml 80% (3 yr) ≥100 ml 31% (3 yr) Viable tumour <10%, 79% (3 yr) >10%, 31% (3 yr)		Tumour volume (<100 ml or ≥100 ml) and histologic response are prognostic factors
CESS-86 (1986–1991)	21	<100 ml (SR): VACD ≥ 100 ml (HR): VAID	301 301	52% (10 yr) 51 % (10 yr)		Intensive treatment with I for high-risk patients. Tumour volume (<200 ml or ≥200 ml) and histologic response as prognostic factors
EICESS (CESS+UKCCSG)						
EICESS-92 (1992–1999)	22	SR: VAID/VACD HR: VAID/EVAID	470	72%/59% 51%/61%	0.5834 0.2913	Tumour volume (<200 ml or ≥200 ml) and histologic response as prognostic factors. Addition of E no major benefit

DFS, disease-free survival; NA, not available; V, vincristine; A, actinomycin D; D, doxorubicin; E, etoposide, I, ifosfamide; WLI, whole-lung irradiation; HD, high dose; MD, moderate dose; SR, standard risk; HR, high risk.
[a]P-values are given only for trials comparing randomized treatment arms.

SIAK, and EORTC–STBSG, forming the European Ewing Tumour Working Initiative of National Groups (Euro-EWING)]. The Euro-EWING 99 study was initiated in late 1999 and serves as an example of a current treatment regimen. All patients receive induction with six courses of vincristine, ifosfamide, doxorubicin, and etoposide (VIDE), followed by consolidation therapy stratified and randomized according to established prognostic factors. Three risk groups are based on initial tumour volume (<200 ml or ≥200 ml), presence and site of metastatic disease at diagnosis, and histologic response to induction therapy. For standard-risk cases with good histologic response to VIDE (<10 per cent viable tumour cells in the surgical specimen), vincristine, actinomycin, and ifosfamide (VAI) consolidation is randomized versus vincristine, actinomycin, and cyclophosphamide (VAC). In high-risk patients with poor histologic response to VIDE (≥10 per cent viable tumour cells in the surgical specimen), VAI is randomized against a high-dose regimen of busulphan and melphalan with autologous stem cell support. In high-risk patients with initial lung metastases, VAI plus lung irradiation is compared with high-dose busulphan and melphalan. The main endpoints of this study are to determine event-free survival and toxicity and to evaluate the role of high-dose therapy in the treatment of patients with high-risk disease. In addition, the predictive value of the detection, by RT–PCR, of minimal metastatic or residual disease in the bone marrow is being investigated for its prognostic significance. Figure 20.7 shows the Euro-EWING 99 treatment strategy (http://euro-ewing.uni-muenster.de).

Metastatic disease

Approximately 15 per cent to 35 per cent of EFT patients present at diagnosis with detectable metastases in the lung and/or in bone and/or in bone marrow. The presence of metastatic disease at diagnosis is a major adverse prognostic factor. The EICESS studies showed that patients with isolated lung metastases may have a better prognosis than those with extra-pulmonary metastases; however, the survival of all has been disappointing (Fig. 20.8). If

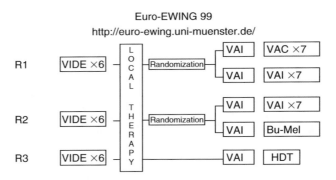

Fig. 20.7 Outline of Euro-EWING 99 treatment protocol. Euro-EWING 99 is a cooperative trial involving GPOH, UKCCSG, SFOP, SIAK, and EORTC. R1, risk group 1 (localized, good histologic response); R2, risk group 2 (localized, poor histologic response, all patients with metastases limited to lungs/pleura); R3, risk group 3 (extrapulmonary metastases); VIDE, vincristine, ifosfamide, doxorubicin, and etoposide; VAI, vincristine, actinomycin D, and ifosfamide; VAC, vincristine, actinomycin D, and cyclophosphamide; Bu-Mel, high-dose busulfan–melphalan therapy with stem cell rescue ; HDT, Bu-Mel or other experimental high-dose therapy.

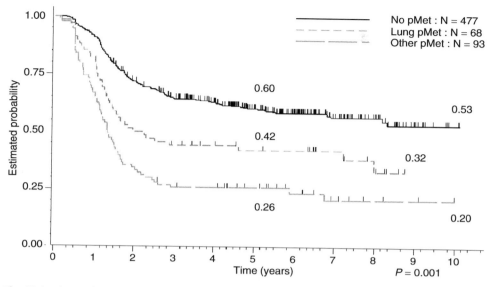

Fig. 20.8 Disease-free survival according to metastatic state.

pulmonary disease is present, patients also receive bilateral pulmonary irradiation at a dose of 14–20 Gy. Patients with solitary or circumscribed bony lesions can receive irradiation to those sites at doses of 40 to 50 Gy, in addition to radiation to the primary site. However, survival rates for patients with multiple bony metastases and/or bone marrow disease are reported to be <10 per cent at 2 years and the discouraging results of treatment for metastatic disease have led to the more aggressive approach with the use of high dose chemotherapy and autologous stem cell reinfusion.

The survival of patients who develop metastatic disease either on or off therapy is poor and second remissions are usually short lived.

Prognostic factors

The classical factors related to poor prognosis include presence of metastases, older age, large tumours, and primary site in the trunk and pelvis (Table 20.5). The specific prognostic factors which concurrently influence treatment regimens include initial volume of the primary tumour (>200 ml), the presence of pulmonary and/or extrapulmonary metastases at diagnosis, the presence of tumour cells in the surgical margins, and poor histologic response of the tumour to induction chemotherapy. The predictive value of other factors such as the degree of neural differentiation (ES versus pPNET), the amount of bone marrow disease detected by RT–PCR, and the type of fusion transcript remains under investigation. So far, studies have shown that EFTs with marked neuroectodermal differentiation such as pPNET do not have a worse prognosis than the typical undifferentiated ES. Among putative molecular determinants of prognosis, loss of the INK4A gene and mutation of p53 have been described as independently associated with poor outcome. The possible influence of the specific EWS–FLI-1 gene fusion type on the prognosis of patients with localized disease is currently under prospective evaluation in Euro-EWING 99. The most clear-cut treatment-related prognostic indicator is tumour

Table 20.5. Prognostic factors in Ewing tumours in order of relevance (poor < good prognosis)

Metastases	Visible at diagnosis < undetectable
	Bone/bone marow < lungs / pleura only
Histologic respose	Poor < good
Tumour size	Tumour extension above 8 cm < less than 8 cm
	Tumour volume above 200 ml < above 100 ml < below 100 ml
Tumour site	Central < proximal < distal
Local therapy	Radiotherapy alone < surgery ± radiotherapy
Age	Over 15 years < under 15 years
Laboratory	Elevated serum LDH < normal serum LDH

LDH, lactate dehydrogenase.

response to chemotherapy. Poor histologic response is defined as the persistence of viable tumour cells within the surgical specimen after presurgical chemotherapy and is a very strong predictor of poor outcome. Finally, early relapse (within 2 years of initial diagnosis) was another predictor of adverse outcome in a recent analysis of two large European trials.

Future prospects

Since EFT are fundamentally systemic diseases, the addition of multi-agent chemotherapy to local control with radiation and/or surgery has improved the disease-free survival rate from only 10 per cent with local therapy alone to ~50–70 per cent. Careful analyses of patterns of failure and the tailoring of the treatment approach to prognostic subgroups of patients appears to be the task for the future in an effort to overcome tumour resistance. Initial chemotherapy following biopsy-confirmed diagnosis prior to local therapy leads to impressive tumour shrinkage in >90 per cent of patients. The optimal combination of agents and the length of initial treatment is still under evaluation, as is the use of high-dose therapy regimens with stem cell rescue for high-risk patients and poor responders to conventional therapy.

High-throughput microarray-based gene expression profiling studies comparing series of different types of small blue round cell tumours have identified a unique gene expression pattern associated with EFT.[24] Thus, in the future, it should be possible to assign a small blue round cell tumour to a specific diagnosis based on its overall gene expression profile. It can also be expected that gene expression studies on large EFT cohorts will lead to the discrimination of prognostically distinct groups to allow better treatment stratification.

In terms of biologically based therapy, hopes have recently focused on the use of tyrosine kinase receptor inhibitors [imatinib mesylate/STI-571 (Gleevec®)]. Among potential targets of this drug are the stem cell factor receptor c-*kit* and PDGF-Rb which are expressed by 30 per cent and 90 per cent of primary EFT, respectively. So far, however, *in vitro* studies and early clinical results suggest only limited therapeutic activity of imatinib mesylate on EFTs.[25] Nevertheless, biologic modifiers with potential antitumour effect may emerge to play an important role in the future treatment of EFT.

Conclusions

The prognosis for EFT patients is determined primarily by tumour dissemination and tumour burden as well as by response to treatment. Tumour burden can only be limited by early diagnosis, but response is subject to the impact of better therapies: These include the design of more effective chemotherapy combinations, increased drug intensity with improved supportive care, and surgical removal of all tumour. In addition, more precise determination of prognostic factors should result in opportunities to improve stratification of treatment intensity, offering the opportunity to limit the risk of late effects from treatment in patients with favourable disease. Because of the rarity of these tumours, treatment should always be performed in centers experienced in EFT treatment and within the framework of controlled clinical trials. In particular, experimental approaches should be restricted to clinical trial settings.

Acknowledgements

This work was supported by Deutsche Krebshilfe and EU-Biomed grants. We thank Christine Jürgens for carefully reading the manuscript.

References

1. Ewing J (1921). Diffuse endothelioma of bone. *Proc N Y Pathol Soc* **21**, 17–24

2. Delattre O, Zucman J, Plougastel B, *et al.* (1992). Gene fusion with an *ETS* DNA-binding domain caused by chromosome translocation in human tumours. *Nature* **359**, 162–5.

3. Zucman-Rossi J, Legoix P, Victor JM, Lopez B, Thomas G (1998). Chromosome translocation based on illegitimate recombination in human tumors. *Proc Natl Acad Sci USA* **95**, 11786–91.

4. Thompson AD, Teitell MA, Arvand A, Denny CT (1999). Divergent Ewing sarcoma *EWS/ETS* fusions confer a common tumorigenic phenotype on NIH3T3 cells. *Oncogene* **18**, 5506–13.

5. Kovar H, Jug G, Aryee DN, *et al.* (1997). Among genes involved in the RB dependent cell cycle regulatory cascade, the p16 tumor suppressor gene is frequently lost in the Ewing family of tumors. *Oncogene* **15**, 2225–32.

6. Lessnick SL, Dacwag CS, Golub TR (2002). The Ewing sarcoma oncoprotein *EWS/FLI* induces a p53-dependent growth arrest in primary human fibroblasts. *Cancer Cell* **1**, 393–401.

7. Schleiermacher G, Peter M, Oberlin O, *et al.* (2003). Increased risk of systemic relapses associated with bone marrow micrometastasis and circulating tumor cells in localised Ewing tumor. *J Clin Oncol* **21**, 85–91.

8. Rosen G, Caparros B, Mosende C, *et al.* (1978). Curability of Ewing sarcoma and considerations for future therapeutic trials. *Cancer* **41**, 888–899.

9. Nesbit ME Jr., Gehan EA, Burgert EO Jr., *et al.* (1990). Multimodal therapy for the management of primary, nonmetastatic Ewing sarcoma of bone: a long-term follow-up of the First Intergroup study. *J Clin Oncol* **8**, 1664–74.

10. Burgert EO Jr., Nesbit ME, Garnsey LA, *et al.* (1990). Multimodal therapy for the management of nonpelvic, localized Ewing sarcoma of bone: intergroup study IESS-II. *J Clin Oncol* **8**, 1514–24.

11. Grier HE, Krailo MD, Tarbell NJ, *et al.* (2003). Addition of ifosfamide and etoposide to standard chemotherapy for Ewing sarcoma and primitive neuroectodermal tumor of bone. *N Engl J Med* **348**, 694–701.

12. Granowetter L, Womer R, Devidas M, *et al.* (2001). Comparison of dose intensified and standard dose chemotherapy for the treatment of non-metastatic Ewing sarcoma (ES) and primitive neuroectodermal tumor (PNET) of bone and soft tissue: A Pediatric Oncology Group–Children's Cancer Group phase III trial. *Med Pediatr Oncol* **37**, 172 (abstr).

13. Kushner BH, Meyers PA, Gerald WL, *et al.* (1995). Very-high-dose short-term chemotherapy for poor-risk peripheral primitive neuroectodermal tumors, including Ewing sarcoma, in children and young adults. *J Clin Oncol* **13**, 2796–804.

14. Hayes FA, Thompson EI, Meyer WH, *et al.* (1989). Therapy for localized Ewing sarcoma of bone. *J Clin Oncol* 7, 208–13.

15. Meyer WH, Kun L, Marina N, *et al.* (1992). Ifosfamide plus etoposide in newly diagnosed Ewing sarcoma of bone. *J Clin Oncol* 10, 1737–42.

16. Marina NM, Pappo AS, Parham DM, *et al.* (1999). Chemotherapy dose-intensification for pediatric patients with Ewing family of tumors and desmoplastic small round-cell tumors: a feasibility study at St Jude Children's Research Hospital. *J Clin Oncol* 17, 180–90.

17. Bacci G, Mercuri M, Longhi A, *et al.* (2002). Neoadjuvant chemotherapy for Ewing tumour of bone: recent experience at the Rizzoli Orthopaedic Institute. *Eur J Cancer* 38, 2243–51.

18. Oberlin O, Deley MC, Bui BN, *et al.* (2001). Prognostic factors in localized Ewing tumours and peripheral neuroectodermal tumours: the third study of the French Society of Paediatric Oncology (EW88 study). *Br J Cancer* 85,1646–54.

19. Craft AW, Cotterill SJ, Bullimore JA, Pearson D (1997). Long-term results from the first UKCCSG Ewing Tumour Study (ET-1). United Kingdom Children's Cancer Study Group (UKCCSG) and the Medical Research Council Bone Sarcoma Working Party. *Eur J Cancer* 33,1061–9.

20. Craft A, Cotterill S, Malcolm A, *et al.* (1998). Ifosfamide-containing chemotherapy in Ewing sarcoma: the Second United Kingdom Children's Cancer Study Group and the Medical Research Council Ewing Tumor Study. *J Clin Oncol* 16, 3628–33.

21. Jürgens H, Exner U Gadner H, *et al.* (1988). Multidisciplinary treatment of Ewing primary sarcoma of bone: a 6-year experience of a European Cooperative Trial. *Cancer* 61, 23–32.

22. Paulussen M, Ahrens S, Dunst J, *et al.* (2001). Localized Ewing tumor of bone: final results of the cooperative Ewing sarcoma study CESS 86. *J Clin Oncol* 19,1818–29.

23. Paulussen M, Craft AW, Lewis I, *et al.* (2002). Ewing tumor of bone—updated report of the European Intergroup Cooperative Ewing Sarcoma Study EICESS 92. *Proc Am Soc Clin Oncol* 21, 393a (abstr).

24. Khan J, Wei JS, Ringner M, *et al.* (2001). Classification and diagnostic prediction of cancers using gene expression profiling and artificial neural networks. *Nat Med* 7, 673–9.

25. Scotlandi K, Manara MC, Strammiello R, *et al.* (2003). c-*kit* receptor expression in Ewing sarcoma: lack of prognostic value but therapeutic targeting opportunities in appropriate conditions. *J Clin Oncol* 21, 1952–60.

Chapter 21

Nephroblastoma

Beatriz de Camargo and Kathryn Pritchard-Jones

Nephroblastoma (Wilms tumour) is the most common renal tumour in children comprising 90 per cent of kidney cancer in this age group. The survival of Wilms tumour patients has improved to 90 per cent in localized disease and >70 per cent for metastatic disease. Challenges remain in identification of histologic and molecular risk factors for stratification of treatment intensity to allow safe reduction in therapy and avoidance of late sequelae for the majority while leading to increased biologic insights and new therapies for the minority of high-risk tumours.

Epidemiology and genetics

Wilms tumour was originally proposed as an index tumour of childhood which could serve to gauge quality of case ascertainment on the grounds that it was thought to have almost constant incidence throughout the world. However, it is now clear that there is international variation. The annual incidence of Wilms tumour has been found to average 7 per million children aged >15 years. A lower incidence has been noted in Asian countries such as Japan, India, and Singapore, as well as in Asian children living in more developed countries. In contrast, a higher incidence is found in Scandinavia, Nigeria, and Brazil. The highest documented rates are among the non-White population of Great Delaware Valley, USA (13.7 per million), the Black population of Los Angeles (11.8) and the SEER Black population (11.1). The incidence rates within Europe range from ~6.5 per million in Spain and Slovakia to >10 per million in Northern European countries.[1] The highest rates are experienced by children aged <5 years, the incidence declines to ~5–6 per million in children aged 5–9 years and approximately 1 per million in those aged 10–14 years. The frequency appears to be equal in males and females. There is some evidence of a difference in age distribution between sexes. Data from the National Wilms Tumour Study Group (NWTS) and the Brazilian Wilms Tumor Study Group suggest that median age at diagnosis is slightly older for girls than boys.[2,3]

Wilms tumour arises in three different clinical situations. First, the majority occur in children with no unusual physical features or family history and are considered 'sporadic'. It can occur in association with several congenital anomalies, especially aniridia, hemihypertrophy, and genitourinary anomalies (cryptorchidism, hypospadias, horseshoe kidney), and with specific syndromes such as the Beckwith–Wiedeman, Denys–Drash and WAGR (Wilms tumour, aniridia, genitourinary abnormalities, mental retardation) syndromes.[4] The third setting in which Wilms tumour arises is within certain families. These findings have helped to identify children at increased risk of Wilms tumour and allowed formulation of recommendations for screening programmes (see later).

In 1972, Knudson and Strong[5] applied the two-step mutational model that had so successfully described the development of retinoblastoma to Wilms tumour. The Wilms tumour suppressor gene *WT1* (at chromosome 11p13) was the second tumour suppressor gene to be cloned. This followed the observation that WAGR syndrome is associated with interstitial deletions of chromosome 11p13 and that tumour tissue at this same locus often displays loss of heterozygosity at this same chromosomal region. The *WT1* gene provides a fascinating example of the close relationship between normal embryonic kidney development and predisposition to cancer. *WT1* plays an essential role in genitourinary development, with different phenotypes associated with different mutations. Complete loss of one *WT1* allele, as in the WAGR syndrome, gives rise to a less severe genitourinary malformation than is seen in Denys–Drash syndrome, where intragenic mutations are associated with early-onset nephritic syndrome and frequent pseudohermaphroditism. Both syndromes are associated with a substantial risk of Wilms tumour of ~ 50 per cent. However, unlike the retinoblastoma model, the *WT1* gene is somatically mutated in only ~20 per cent of Wilms tumours and linkage to the *WT1* locus has been excluded in most familial cases.

Several genes are now known to be involved in predisposition to Wilms tumour and/or in the somatic events occurring in sporadic tumours. The Beckwith–Wiedemann overgrowth syndrome is caused by mutation or deregulation of several genes that regulate somatic growth and are clustered in a locus more distal to the *WT1* gene on chromosome 11 at 11p15.5. These genes (*IGF2, p57KIP2, H19, KVLQT1*) are all subjected to imprinting during normal embryogenesis, which means that the expression from each allele depends on its parental origin. Beckwith–Wiedemann syndrome is associated with either mutation or deregulated imprinting of one or more of these genes, some of which are also affected in sporadic Wilms tumours.

A family history of Wilms tumour occurs in 1–2 per cent of all cases. Typical pedigrees are small, with only two or three affected relatives and without predisposition to other tumour types. Genetic linkage studies in two unusually large pedigrees have localized one gene for familial Wilms tumour, *FWT1*, to chromosome 17q. Another locus has been suggested at 19q and a recent evaluation of all available pedigrees in the UK has confirmed that there is genetic heterogeneity for *FWT* genes with at least four families clearly unlinked to any currently identified Wilms tumour locus.[6] Until these genes are identified, it is difficult to predict what, if any, involvement they would have in sporadic Wilms tumour, at both the constitutional and somatic levels. However, the penetrance of *FWT1* at least appears to be low, of the order of 15–30 per cent. Therefore it is possible that a substantial proportion of apparently sporadic cases of Wilms tumour carry a constitutional mutation in a low-penetrance familial Wilms tumour gene. Very few familial cases are due to *WT1* mutation. The incidence of constitutional *WT1* mutation in apparently sporadic cases is a little higher. In a study of 201 cases of Wilms tumours selected from the NWTS cases, eight constitutional *WT1* mutations were found and these were virtually confined to boys with cryptorchidism as well as Wilms tumour (7/28 patients).[7] A separate study from Germany showed that somatic *WT1* mutation was common in Wilms tumours showing stromal predominant histology (13/26) and, remarkably, nearly all of these (10/13) had a constitutional *WT1* mutation.[8]

Finally, allele loss studies in sporadic Wilms tumours suggest a role of other tumour-suppressed genes at 16q, 1p, and 22q that may be involved in progression to more aggressive tumours. Mutation of the p53 gene is associated with the anaplastic subtype.[9]

The cause of genetic events described is unknown, but several case–control studies of Wilms tumour have identified environmental exposures that may contribute to its development. These include prenatal irradiation, penthrane anaesthesia during birth, household pesticides, parental occupation to pesticides prior to birth, and maternal use of dipyrone.[10,11]

Diagnosis

Clinical presentation

The most common initial manifestation of Wilms tumour is the presence of an asymptomatic abdominal mass. Other associated signs and symptoms include malaise, abdominal pain, gross or microscopic haematuria, fever, anorexia, and hypertension. Abdominal pain may be the result of local distension, spontaneous intralesional haemorrhage, or tumour rupture. The incidence of hypertension is variable because of lack of adequate documentation, but has been reported in 30–63 per cent of children. The aetiology is an increase in circulating renin or a renin-like substance either secreted by the tumour itself or secondary to impaired renal circulation from compression by the tumour mass. Paraneoplastic manifestations associated with Wilms tumour include acquired von Willebrand disease, tumour-induced glomerulonephritis, and erythropoietin and hyaluronidase secretion.

Imaging studies

Imaging studies should be limited to identifying intra- or extrarenal tumour, the presence of a normal functioning contralateral kidney, tumour thrombus in renal vein, inferior vena cava, and heart, and the presence of pulmonary or liver metastases. It is rare for Wilms tumour to metastasize to brain or bone, but imaging of these sites should be performed when other renal tumours (malignant rhabdoid tumour or clear cell sarcoma of kidney, respectively) are identified on histology. Ultrasound, CT scan, and MRI all have their particular advantages. Ultrasound has the specific advantage of assessment of blood vessels for flow and tumour thrombus, and can achieve most of the purposes defined above. CT is superior at evaluating intra- and extrarenal involvement and in demonstrating small lesions within the kidney and liver and the presence of anomalies such as horseshoe kidneys. MRI may possess the advantages of both, but the lesser availability, increased cost, and requirement for sedation probably outweigh the advantages. With current treatment regimens, it appears that chest radiography is sufficient to detect clinically significant pulmonary metastases (see the section on staging for further discussion).

Differential diagnosis

The differential diagnosis on imaging includes other abdominal neoplasms such as neuroblastoma and hepatoblastoma. For a primary intrarenal tumour, the differential includes malignant rhabdoid tumour (MRTK), clear cell sarcoma, hypernephroma (renal cell carcinoma), congenital mesoblastic nephroma (CMN), and benign processes involving the kidney. The likelihood that a primary intrarenal tumour will be a non-Wilms tumour increases with age <6 months (where CMN, MRTK, and renal dysplasia predominate) or >7 years (where other malignancies start to increase).

Biopsy

Immediate biopsy is not always recommended when a tumour has the typical imaging and clinical features of Wilms tumour. The UK Children's Cancer Study Group (UKCCSG) has recently analysed the role of biopsy and shown that 12 per cent of renal tumours with typical features on imaging studies proved to be non-Wilms on pre-chemotherapy biopsy; however, only 1.5 per cent were benign tumours. The morbidity associated with biopsy is small.[12]

Staging

Tumour stage is one of the most important criteria for determining therapy in Wilms tumour, and its accurate determination requires meticulous attention to detail. Staging is based primarily on the anatomical extent of disease, determined after histologic examination of the nephrectomy specimen, as well as surgical factors such as tumour spillage or rupture before or during surgery and completeness of excision.

The staging systems used by two major cooperative groups are somewhat different and reflect that the NWTS system is based on staging of a previously untreated tumour, while the International Society of Paediatric Oncology (SIOP) classification is based on nephrectomy following preoperative chemotherapy (Table 21.1). Staging of a tumour with extension along the renal vein into the inferior vena cava can be problematic. Provided that the tumour can be removed completely *en bloc* from within the inferior vena cava, it remains a stage II. However, if the tumour has to be removed piecemeal, with the likelihood of microscopic residue, or remains adherent to the vessel wall, it should be considered stage III. Cases where only fibrosis is found in the resected vessel wall can usually be considered stage II, but such cases need careful consideration, especially in relation to their prior therapy. For the SIOP staging system after preoperative chemotherapy, the presence of necrotic tumour or chemotherapy-induced change in the renal sinus and/or within the perirenal fat should not be regarded as a reason for upstaging a tumour provided that it is completely excised and does not reach the resection margins (i.e. from stage I to II). However, if evidence of necrotic tumour is found in a lymph node or at the resection margins, the tumour is assigned as stage III because of the possibility that some viable tumour is left behind in an adjacent lymph node or beyond the resection margins.

Assignment of stage IV due to lung metastases has always been based on a chest radiography assessment in all previous international trials. Therefore any move to incorporate detection of 'micrometastases' seen only on CT scan requires careful consideration. Thorax CT will detect pulmonary nodules of size <10 mm that would not generally be apparent on chest radiography (note that a larger nodule apparent on CT but not visualized on chest radiography solely due its

Table 21.1. Clinical pathologic staging

Stage	
I	Tumour limited to the kidney and completely excised[a]
II	Tumour extending beyond the kidney but completely excised Invasion of renal sinus and/or extra renal vessels and/or perirenal fat
III	Invasion beyond capsule Any abdominal lymph nodes[b] Tumour rupture[c] Peritoneal tumour implants Incomplete excision
IV	Haematogenous metastases (lung, liver, bone, brain, lymph nodes outside abdominal pelvic region)
V	Bilateral renal tumours at diagnosis

[a]In the most recent NWTS 5 trial, the definition of stage I was further refined to exclude those tumours showing involvement of blood vessels in the renal sinus.
[b]Previous SIOP studies had a stage II N+ category that is now included in stage III as there are no clear data to suggest that hilar LN metastases confer a better prognosis than para-aortic nodes and it is often difficult to make this anatomical distinction on the pathology specimen.
[c]The NWTS allows minor tumour spillage confined to the flank to remain within the stage II category, whereas in SIOP this is stage III.

position should be considered a metastasis). These nodules may represent either micrometastases or benign lesions. A retrospective review of 141 children treated in the UKW2 trial who had a normal chest radiograph and had a thorax CT performed (but were treated according to the results of their chest radiograph) revealed that 22 per cent had one or more small nodules visible on CT scan only. The median size of these nodules was 5 mm (range 2–8 mm) and all disappeared following chemotherapy. There was no significant difference in pulmonary relapse rate between children with normal thorax CT and those with nodules, with the exception of children treated for stage I tumours with vincristine monotherapy.[13] A similar study from the NWTS also suggests that, provided that presumed 'micrometastases' are exposed to at least two-drug chemotherapy, this is probably adequate therapy. However, neither study incorporates sufficient numbers to reach a definitive conclusion on this important point and prospective studies are needed.

Assignment of the correct tumour stage requires close cooperation between the surgeon and pathologist to ensure that the nephrectomy specimen is delivered intact for proper assessment of any capsular infiltration and completeness of resection margins as well as proper orientation of any additionally resected tissues.

Pathology

Nephroblastoma covers a large spectrum of special variants that differ in their morphologic features and in their prognosis and natural history. Typically, Wilms tumour presents as a solitary spherical unicentric mass, sharply demarcated from the adjacent renal parenchyma. Multicentric lesions and bilateral tumours are not infrequent. Calcification is rare, but may be detected radiographically in 10 per cent of cases, particularly after haemorrhage in the tumour. Most tumours exhibit a so-called 'triphasic' appearance, including blastemal, stromal, and epithelial cell types. However, it is important to recognize that many specimens express only two of these cell types and that monomorphous specimens are not rare. It is important to note that the histologic appearance of a tumour depends on its prior therapy, with different classification schemes used for immediate nephrectomy than for tumours exposed to preoperative chemotherapy (Table 21.2).

Although 'blastemal predominance' is recognized in chemotherapy naïve tumours, this is not the same entity as the 'blastemal type' defined in the new SIOP classification, where survival of large amounts of blastema following pre-operative chemotherapy is believed to confer an adverse outcome with current therapies.

The NWTS classifies tumours into 'favourable' and 'unfavourable' subtypes. Although the latter used to encompass MRTK and CCSK, these have been recognized as distinct biologic entities for many years now. However, any classification scheme of renal tumours of childhood usually retains MRTK and CCSK in a 'high-risk' category, while placing other entities such as congenital mesoblastic nephroma or cystic partially differentiated nephroblastoma in a 'low-risk' category.

A review of the histologic patterns seen in the NWTS-4 showed that tumours composed predominantly of epithelial cell types were usually low stage (81.3 per cent stage I) and presented at a younger age (median 17 months), while predominantly blastemal tumours were much more aggressive (76.3 per cent stage II–IV) and presented at an older age (median 57 months).[14] Similarly, tumours displaying large amounts of stromal elements, particularly those showing differentiation towards skeletal muscle, are known to have a good outcome despite showing little shrinkage in response to chemotherapy. A review of cases treated in a

Table 21.2. The Revised SIOP Working Classification of Renal Tumours of Childhood (2001)[16]

A. Pretreated cases:

I. Low-risk tumours
Mesoblastic nephroma
Cystic partially differentiated nephroblastoma
Completely necrotic nephroblastoma

II. Intermediate-risk tumours
Nephroblastoma: epithelial type
Nephroblastoma: stromal type
Nephroblastoma: mixed type
Nephroblastoma: regressive type
Nephroblastoma: focal anaplasia

III. High-risk tumours
Nephroblastoma: blastemal type
Nephroblastoma: diffuse type
Clear-cell sarcoma of the kidney
Rhabdoid tumour of the kidney

IV. Other tumours or lesions

B. Primary nephrectomy cases:

I. Low-risk tumours
Mesoblastic nephroma
Cystic partially nephroblastoma

II. Intermediate-risk tumours
Non-anaplastic nephroblastoma and its variant
Nephroblastoma: focal anaplasia

III. High-risk tumours
Nephroblastoma: diffuse anaplasia
Clear-cell sarcoma of the kidney
Rhabdoid tumour of the kidney

German study (GPOH) according to SIOP protocols dealt with a group of unilateral localized Wilms tumours which were treated with a standardized preoperative chemotherapy and a small group of immediately operated Wilms tumours. An important difference between the two groups was in distribution of histologic subtypes. The percentage of tumours showing blastemal predominance decreased significantly from 39.4 to 9.3 per cent.[15] This latter group, with blastema resistant to chemotherapy, was more likely to relapse irrespective of stage. The SIOP Working Classification of Renal Tumours of Childhood has recently been revised to incorporate the different clinical behaviours of the various histologic subtypes defined (Table 21.3).[16] Completely necrotic nephroblastoma shows an excellent prognosis and will be included in the low-risk category.[17] However, this subtype tends to be overdiagnosed by local pathologists compared with the review pathologist.

Anaplastic Wilms tumour is a morphologically defined entity containing cells with very large hyperchromatic nuclei associated with multipolar mitotic figures. These changes can be focal or diffuse and occur in about 5 per cent of tumours. Anaplasia is deemed 'unfavourable' or 'high-risk' by both classification schemes. Recently, the definition of focal anaplasia has been limited to tumours showing a single focus of anaplastic features representing <10 per cent of

Table 21.3. Histologic risk groups in Wilms tumour

SIOP		NWTS	
Low-risk	Completely necrotic Cystic partially differentiated Nephroblastoma	Favourable histology	All non anaplastic histologies Focal anaplasia
Intermediate-risk	Nephroblastoma Epithelial type Stromal type Mixed type Regressive type Focal anaplasia		
High-risk	Nephroblastoma Blastemal type Diffuse anaplasia	Unfavourable histology	Diffuse anaplasia

the tumour, and these tumours are now considered to behave in the same way as the 'intermediate-risk' or 'favourable histology' groups.[18] Preoperative chemotherapy does not obliterate or produce anaplasia, but it makes it more obvious because non-anaplastic areas are probably destroyed by chemotherapy while anaplastic foci remain unchanged. Anaplasia is thought to represent a more resistant rather than a more aggressive cell type. The age distribution of anaplastic tumours is distinctive, with a median age of 61 months. Anaplasia is almost never seen in children aged <2 years.

Nephrogenic rests have been considered as precursor lesions of Wilms tumour for several decades. They may become hyperplastic or neoplastic and form multicentric or bilateral renal lesions. Nephrogenic rests have been reported in 25–40 per cent of kidneys harboring Wilms tumour and in almost 100 per cent of bilateral Wilms tumour. Two types of rest have been recognized: perilobar rests (PLNRs) and intralobar rests (ILNRs). PLNRs are more common in patients with hemi-hypertrophy and Beckwith–Wiedeman syndrome, whereas ILNRs are associated with WAGR and Denys–Drash syndromes and with an earlier age of onset of Wilms tumour. Based on their morphology and clinical associations, ILNRs are thought to result from a defect early in nephrogenesis and PLNRs from a slightly later insult to the embryonic kidney.[19]

Clear cell sarcoma and rhabdoid tumour are now considered to be biologic entities distinct from Wilms tumour. Clear cell sarcoma of the kidney (CCSK), the bone metastasizing renal tumour of childhood, is a primitive mesenchymal neoplasm which comprises 4 per cent of renal tumours in children. Bone and brain metastases develop in 23 per cent and 15 per cent, respectively, and may be the first site of recurrence. The need to perform a skeletal survey, or a radionuclide bone scan, and a brain CT at time of diagnosis has been emphasized. The addition of adriamycin to vincristine and actinomycin D has improved survival from 25 to 71.9 per cent (NWTS-3). Rhabdoid tumour is considered to be one of the most malignant tumours of childhood, comprising 2 per cent of childhood renal cancer, and is characterized by a uniform cellular infiltrate with abundant eosinophilic cytoplasm, initially interpreted as rhabdomyoblastic or sarcomatous but which may be of neural crest origin. Most are diagnosed in the first year of life and are characterized by early widespread metastases and a poor response to therapy, with a survival of 25 per cent according to NWTS data. The finding of a common molecular defect, deletion of the SNF–INI1 gene on 22q, in rhabdoid tumours from both renal and extrarenal sites, including the associated brain tumours, shows that these constitute a biologic family of tumours regardless of their anatomical site.

Treatment

Two major clinical trial groups have investigated treatment in Wilms tumour: the International Society of Paediatric Oncology (SIOP) formed in 1970 in Europe, and the National Wilms Tumour Study Group (NWTS) launched in 1969 in North America. Other cooperative groups such as UKCCSG in the UK, GCBTTW in Brazil, and GPOH in Germany have contributed to refining treatment. Overall survival is now approaching 90 per cent for children with Wilms tumour in many countries around the world. Hence the main objective of most trials is to treat patients according to well-defined risk groups in an attempt to achieve the highest cure rates, while decreasing the frequency and intensity of acute and late toxicity and minimizing the cost of therapy. There remain subgroups of Wilms tumour with considerable room for improvement in survival rates.

Combined modality strategies using surgery, radiotherapy, and chemotherapy are the key to success in treating Wilms tumour. Similar outcomes by stage are now reported by all the clinical trial groups (Table 21.4) Therefore the ongoing challenge is to identify better prognostic markers for stratification of therapy, intensifying treatment for patients with poor prognosis, while reducing interventions for those at standard risk. Extent of disease (stage) and tumour histology defined as favourable and unfavourable (NWTS) or low, intermediate, and high risk (SIOP), remain the two most significant prognostic variables for tailoring treatment. Treatment consists of chemotherapy with one to three or more drugs together with surgical excision of the affected kidney. Radiotherapy is used only if there is residual or spilled tumour in the abdomen or metastases.

Preoperative strategies

The benefit of preoperative strategies to facilitate complete surgical removal is well known. The NWTS recommends this approach for a few select groups of patients including those with bilateral renal tumours, tumour extension into the inferior vena cava above the hepatic veins, and tumours found to be inoperable at surgical exploration. The major concern is the potential for loss of important staging information. The approach of SIOP studies is to 'downstage' the disease with preoperative chemotherapy and to avoid radiotherapy in most of the patients. In the SIOP preoperative chemotherapy approach, tumours are downstaged so that only 15 per cent of patients have stage III disease and 50 per cent have stage I. Both approaches have similar cure rates and the advantages and disadvantages of each are constantly discussed. The UKCCSG has recently completed a randomized trial comparing the two approaches in terms of their

Table 21.4. Relapse-free survival with favourable histology

Trial	Survival (%)			
	Stage I	Stage II	Stage III	Stage IV
UK2 (2 years)	87	82	82	70
NWTS (5 years)	92	83	87	75
SIOP-93-01 (2 years)	89.6	89	75.8	68.6

*Note that stage is defined at time of nephrectomy and is therefore not directly comparable. In SIOP-93-01 tumour stage after preoperative chemotherapy. In UK and NWTS trials no pre-operative chemotherapy was used.

impact on stage distribution and overall burden of treatment. One advantage of the preoperative chemotherapy approach is its potential to allow the *in vivo* response to treatment to be used as an individual prognostic parameter for risk-adapted postoperative treatment.

Chemotherapy

Nephroblastoma was the first paediatric malignant solid tumour found to be responsive to systemic chemotherapy using actinomycin D. Others agents such as vincristine, adriamycin, cyclophosphamide, ifosfamide, etoposide, and carboplatin have all been identified as effective in Wilms tumour. Cooperative groups have performed randomized trials to evaluate the necessity of single- or multi-agent chemotherapy in the treatment of Wilms tumour. Lessons learned from cooperative study groups (NWTS, SIOP, UKCCSG, BWTSG) include the following.[20–24]

1. Preoperative chemotherapy is equivalent to radiotherapy in reducing surgical morbidity and tumour stage (SIOP 1 and SIOP 5 trials).
2. Four weeks of preoperative chemotherapy with two drugs is as effective as 8 weeks in producing a more favourable stage distribution for localized tumours (SIOP 9 trial).
3. Limited courses of two drugs (dactinomycin, vincristine) or even a single agent (vincristine) are sufficient for patients with stage I tumours after immediate surgery (NWTS, UKCCSG). Patients with stage I tumours after preoperative chemotherapy with two drugs require only a short postoperative course of the same treatment (SIOP 6 and SIOP 93–01). The blastemal type after preoperative chemotherapy is now considered high risk in the current SIOP WT 2001 trial, where stage I high-risk tumours receive postoperative treatment with three drugs (dactinomycin, vincristine, Adriamycin).
4. A single-dose schedule of dactinomycin is as effective as the standard 5-day divided-dose regimen and is less myelosuppressive as well as reducing the number of hospital attendances for children and their parents (NWTS, BWTSG).[20,21,24] The NWTS reported an unusual hepatotoxicity and reduced the single dose from 60 to 45 μg/kg.[25]
5. For stage II tumours, two drugs are sufficient with excellent cure rates. The addition of adriamycin and radiotherapy did not increase survival in patients treated with immediate surgery (NWTS3). Radiotherapy is not necessary for stage II tumours after preoperative chemotherapy.[20]
6. The need for adriamycin in treatment of stage III tumours is controversial. Previous studies including small numbers suggested that adriamycin was of benefit for disease-free but not overall survival (NWTS3). In view of increasing concerns about long-term cardio toxicity in Wilms tumour survivors, the current SIOP WT 2001 trial is readdressing this question but excluding the newly defined 'high-risk' histology tumours from the randomization between two (vincristine, dactinomycin) and three (vincristine, dactinomycin + adriamycin) drugs postoperatively.
7. Radiotherapy is presumed to be necessary for stage III tumours, although no randomized trials addressing this question have yet been attempted. There is anecdotal evidence that radiotherapy may be avoidable in some younger children.
8. The addition of adriamycin to vincristine and dactinomycin improved survival in stage IV patients (NWTS 2). The question of lung irradiation is discussed in the section on radiotherapy.

Patients with diffuse anaplastic tumours still have a poorer prognosis and there is a need to identify new drugs or schedules with activity. Tumours with focal anaplasia are now treated with less therapy than previously. The prognosis of patients with clear cell sarcoma has improved significantly with the addition of adriamycin. Whether cyclophosphamide should be added is still unanswered. The prognosis for rhabdoid tumours remains dismal.

Surgery

Surgical staging and tumour resection remain a major component of therapy. A large trans-abdominal transperitoneal incision is recommended for adequate exposure. Complete excision without spillage and adequate exploration of the abdominal cavity should be done. Lymph node sampling should be performed even if the lymph nodes appear normal, but radical lymph node dissection is unnecessary. This sampling is important because 11 per cent of lymph nodes believed to be negative for disease by the surgeon will harbour metastatic disease.[26] The obligatory exploration of the contralateral kidney is controversial given the accuracy of modern imaging techniques. Several recent studies have found a very high rate of accuracy of modern imaging in detecting small contralateral lesions.[27] The renal vein and vena cava should be carefully palpated to exclude tumour thrombus. If present, an attempt should be made to remove the thrombus *en bloc* with the tumour. A thrombus extending to the infrahepatic vena cava should be removed through a vena cavotomy.

Radiotherapy

Wilms tumour is a particularly radiosensitive cancer. The addition of postnephrectomy radiotherapy increased the survival of Wilms tumour patients to ~50 per cent. Clinical trials (NWTS and SIOP) have studied the interrelationship of chemotherapy and radiotherapy, and have been able to reduce the indications for radiotherapy and the doses used without apparent deleterious effect on the survival rates. The NWTS now recommends 10 Gy for flank irradiation compared with 14.4 Gy used in SIOP studies. Whole-abdominal irradiation is usually still recommended for diffuse tumour rupture, although its benefit over flank irradiation has been questioned. It is also possible that abdominal radiotherapy can be safely avoided in younger children even when they have stage III tumours.[28]

Current treatment recommendations for the use of radiation as part of the multimodality regimen are as follows.

◆ Stage III: positive lymph nodes and/or diffuse peritoneal spillage.
◆ Stage II–IV: diffuse anaplastic tumours.
◆ Stage IV: sites of metastatic disease (usually lungs).

It should be noted that SIOP studies limit lung irradiation to the ~25 per cent of stage IV patients who do not achieve a complete remission of lung metastases following preoperative chemotherapy and metastatectomy; NWTS retains low-dose lung irradiation for all children with pulmonary metastases visible on chest radiography at diagnosis.

Prognostic factors

Many prognostic factors have been identified, although they may change as treatment becomes more effective. Older age at diagnosis has been identified as an adverse factor in many studies. Conversely, age <2 years appears to identify an exceptionally good prognosis, especially for those with smaller tumours. Extent of disease at diagnosis (stage) and tumour histology remain the two most significant prognostic variables. Although stage IV disease still clearly identifies a group with poor outcome, the prognostic significance of stage in localized tumours has reduced because of the risk-adapted therapy they receive. The most important tumour histologic feature is diffuse anaplasia (see above). Preoperative chemotherapy provides an opportunity to test *in vivo* the chemosensitivity of individual tumours. The new SIOP classification is based on the observation that survival or differentiation of distinct cell types is associated with different clinical outcomes. Tumours in which a substantial proportion of blastema survives preoperative chemotherapy have a poorer outcome than other subtypes.[15] Conversely, tumours in which epithelial or stromal components predominate after preoperative chemotherapy appear to have a very favourable outcome. They are not yet selected for treatment reduction, but this question is being addressed in the SIOP WT 2001 trial. Complete necrosis following preoperative chemotherapy has an excellent outcome.[17]

Molecular prognostic factors are being identified and will be incorporated into treatment strategies in the near future. Loss of heterozygosity (LOH) of markers at chromosome 16q and 1p was associated with a significantly poorer relapse-free survival and overall survival in a retrospective study of 232 children registered on NWTS-3–4.[29] Other retrospective studies have confirmed the adverse prognostic prediction for tumours with LOH on 16q.[30] The NWTS-5 trial was set up to test prospectively the hypothesis that LOH at specific chromosomal loci can identify tumours with a worse outcome. The only other established adverse molecular factor is mutation of the p53 gene which occurs in the majority of anaplastic tumours and may explain their worse prognosis. Involvement of the *WT1* gene, or indeed other genes at 11p15, does not appear to be associated with adverse outcome. The association of many other molecular alterations with clinical outcome is currently under investigation, including gain or over-expression of genes on 1q, telomerase activity, etc.

Another question being considered by the renal tumours committee of the Children's Oncology Group (which has taken over the role of the NWTS) is whether the absence of adverse clinical and molecular prognostic factors can be used to identify a group of stage I tumours curable by nephrectomy only.

Late effects

All treatment modalities are associated with toxic effects, some of which occur early, while others occur months or years later. Long-term deleterious effects of radiation in Wilms tumours patients have been reported in the musculoskeletal system, the gastrointestinal tract, the urinary tract, the endocrine system, and the lungs. In long-term follow-up studies of survivors of Wilms tumour, scoliosis and musculoskeletal abnormalities have been found more frequently in irradiated patients, particularly those treated with orthovoltage radiotherapy. With modern megavoltage techniques and the significant dose reductions now used, late orthopaedic effects are expected to be less frequent. Reduction in stature following megavoltage radiation therapy of the spine is dose and age dependent, and is usually clinically insignificant. Adverse pregnancy outcomes have been reported in Wilms tumour survivors treated with abdominal radiation, with increased rates of perinatal mortality, low birth weight, and congenital malformation.[31] Exposure to doxorubicin and thoracic and left-flank irradiation are risk factors for cardiac toxicity.[32]

Recurrence of Wilms tumour

Overall relapse rates for all patients with Wilms tumour registered on NWTS and SIOP studies is ~17–24 per cent. The majority of relapses occur within 2 years of diagnosis, although with the continued reductions in therapy occurring in most studies, it is possible that this pattern may change in the future. Despite the excellent prognosis at first diagnosis of Wilms tumour, long-term survival is ~30 per cent for most patients with recurrent disease. Prognosis following relapse depends on initial stage, site of relapse, interval from initial diagnosis, and previous therapy. The most favourable prognostic group comprises children treated for low-stage tumours with no more than two drugs and without radiotherapy, who experience isolated pulmonary relapse >6–12 months after diagnosis. All other patients have a poor outcome and a high risk of treatment failure. This has led to the investigation of the role of ifosfamide, etoposide, and platinum compounds as single agents or in combination. These studies have demonstrated response rates >40 per cent. However, the results are transitory and the outcome has continued to be poor. The use of ICE (ifosfamide, carboplatin, etoposide) has shown an overall response rate (partial plus complete) of 82 per cent and a 3-year event-free survival and overall survival of 63.6 $\pm$ 14.5 per cent.[33] High-dose chemotherapy followed by autologous stem cell rescue has been used for the treatment of patients with high-risk recurrent Wilms tumour, and preliminary results are encouraging. Pein *et al.*[34] recently reported on 29 patients with high-risk recurrent Wilms tumour who received treatment with high-dose chemotherapy followed by autologous stem cell rescue. Despite significant treatment related toxicity, the disease-free survival and overall survival at 3 years were 50 $\pm$ 17 per cent and 60 $\pm$ 18 per cent, respectively, an improvement compared with the historical controls.[34] An international randomized trial is being designed to assess the value of consolidation with high dose chemotherapy after intensive re-induction.

Bilateral tumours

Between 5 and 10 per cent of Wilms tumour patients have bilateral renal lesions at diagnosis, usually of low stage individually. Multidisciplinary advances in surgery, chemotherapy, and radiotherapy have markedly improved the expected outcome for these children. The median age at diagnosis is lower than that of patients with unilateral disease and the incidence of congenital anomalies is higher. However, the heterogeneity of conditions associated with bilateral Wilms tumour, as well as the bimodal peak on the age-at-onset distribution curve, suggests more than one causative factor. The management of bilateral Wilms tumour has changed with time, especially with regard to the surgical procedure. Bilateral renal salvage procedures are technically possible and effective in controlling tumours without adversely affecting renal function or survival. Radical excision of the tumour should never be performed at the initial operation. Preoperative chemotherapy is always recommended to reduce the tumour burden and to permit bilateral renal preservation procedures, if feasible. Functional assessment of both kidneys should always be undertaken prior to any planned conservative procedure. Delayed second- or even third-look surgery to attempt tumour resection with maximum preservation of functioning renal tissue may be of benefit. The primary objective of bilateral conservative surgery is to decrease the incidence of renal failure. However, there is a fine balance between preserving nephrons and achieving adequate excision to avoid relapse, as the treatment of recurrent disease has far more deleterious consequences for renal function. Bilateral Wilms tumour patients should be treated individually. Partial nephrectomy, tumour enucleation, radiotherapy, and chemotherapy should be adapted according to response, highest stage, and highest-risk histology. Overall survival rates exceed 80 per cent at 4 years and complete nephrectomy is avoided in ~60–70 per cent of the children.[35,36]

Bilateral Wilms tumour is frequently associated with nephrogenic rests, which are presumed to have the potential for malignant conversion. The role of chemotherapy in influencing this progression is unclear. However, it is currently suggested that prolonged treatment with vincristine and dactinomycin for up to 1 year may be of benefit.

Screening

Certain congenital malformation syndromes carry a high risk of Wilms tumour, of the order of 30–50 per cent. With the discovery of the underlying genetic defects, in some cases subgroups can be defined for screening. For example, in sporadic aniridia, high-resolution karyotyping using probes for the contiguous *PAX6*, *calmodulin* and *WT1* genes on 11p13 can distinguish those children whose aniridia is due to mutation confined to *PAX6* and therefore do not require screening from those with a more extensive deletion involving the *WT1* gene. Similarly, children with early-onset nephrotic syndrome involving diffuse mesangial sclerosis, even without ambiguous genitalia, are likely to harbour a constitutional *WT1* mutation and hence carry an elevated risk of Wilms tumour. In Beckwith–Wiedemann syndrome, it appears that the children with uniparental disomy for 11p15.5 or imprinting abnormalities of the *IGF2* and *H19* genes are at higher tumour risk than those with other types of causative genetic lesion, such as imprinting abnormalities of *LIT1* or point mutations in the p57 gene. A higher tumour risk may also be related to clinical features including the presence of hemi-hypertrophy or nephromegaly during the first year of life. Where the risk of Wilms tumour is of the order of 10–30 per cent, it is generally held that some sort of screening programme is justified. It has not been possible to perform randomized studies in this setting. However, retrospective analyses of the tumour stage at diagnosis in relation to the mode of discovery suggest that if regular ultrasound screening is to be used, it should be performed at intervals of no more than 3–4 months. It is possible to teach parents to perform regular abdominal palpation, particularly at bathtime, but there is no evidence as to whether this is equivalent to ultrasound screening. The risk of Wilms tumour in children with hemi-hypertrophy without other stigmata of Beckwith–Wiedemann syndrome or isolated overgrowth of a single limb is not easily defined, but it does appear to be at a much lower level that raises questions about the justification of an interventional imaging screening programme. Children whose Wilms tumour predisposition results from mutation in the *WT1* gene have a much earlier age of onset of Wilms tumour than those with Beckwith–Wiedemann syndrome (median age at diagnosis 16 months versus 39 months).[37] It is now also emerging that children whose tumorous kidney contains either multifocal tumours or nephrogenic rests are at increased risk of late development of metachronous Wilms tumour. As a safe policy, it is now recommended that all children with these features are screened for a prolonged period of time, at intervals of 3 months until the age of 7 years. These recommendations may become more lenient as the evidence base becomes firmer.

Long-term follow-up

Children who survive relapse free for >3 years after diagnosis of their Wilms tumour are unlikely to suffer a recurrence. Treatment received by the majority means they are at very low risk of developing second cancers related to their treatment. Therefore the main aim of long-term follow up is to monitor renal function. The current UKCCSG recommendations for any child having a nephrectomy are that blood pressure should be checked annually and serum creatinine measured every 5 years. An early morning urine sample should be tested annually for protein-to-creatinine ratio. The risk of renal dysfunction continues into adult life, and it is important that such information is imparted to their adult physicians or general practitioners. Analysis of the molecular genetics of Wilms tumour has provided and continues to provide a fascinating insight into the relationship between developmental abnormalities and embryonal cancers. Identification of genes involved in such processes and their impact on tumour biology may ultimately allow the safe selection of subgroups of children with Wilms tumour requiring only minimal therapy and to modify front-line therapy for those groups with a poorer prognosis. The avoidance of anthracyclines and radiotherapy for an increasing majority would be a major step forward in the successful treatment of this tumour type. The new SIOP WT 2001 trial addresses this issue.

References

1. Stiller CA, Parkin DM (1990). International variations in the incidence of childhood renal tumours. *Br J Cancer* **62**, 1026–30.

2. Breslow N, Olshan A, Beckwith JB, Green DM (1993). Epidemiology of Wilms tumor. *Med Pediatr Oncol* **21**, 172–81.

3. Franco EL, de Camargo B, Saba L, Marques LA (1991). Epidemiological and clinical correlations with genetic characteristics of Wilms' tumor: results of the Brazilian Wilms' tumor Study Group. *Int J Cancer* **48**, 641–6.

4. Clericuzio CL (1993). Clinical phenotypes and Wilms tumor. *Med Pediatr Oncol* **21**, 182–7.

5. Knudson A, Strong L (1972). Mutation and cancer, a model for Wilms tumour of the kidney. *J Natl Cancer Inst* **48**, 313–24.

6. Rapley EA, Barfoot R, Bonaiti-Pellie C, *et al.* (2000) Evidence for susceptibility genes to familial Wilms tumour in addition to *WT1*, *FWT1* and *FWT2*. *Br J Cancer* **83**, 177–83.

7. Diller L, Ghahremani M, Morgan J, *et al.* (1998). Constitutional WT1 mutations in Wilms' tumor patients. *J Clin Oncol* **16**, 3634–40.

8. Shumacher V, Schneider S, Figg A, *et al.* (1997). Correlation of germ-line mutations and two-hit inactivation *WT1* gene with Wilms' tumor of stromal-predominant histology. *Proc Natl Acad Sci USA* **94**, 3972–7.

9. Bardeesy N, Falkoff D, Petruzzi M-J, *et al.* (1994). Anaplastic Wilms' tumour, a subtype displaying poor prognosis, harbours p53 gene mutations. *Nat Genet* **7**, 91–7.

10. Olshan AF, Breslow NE, Falletta JM, *et al.* (1993). Risk factors for Wilms tumor. *Cancer* **72**, 938–44.

11. Sharpe CR, Franco EL, de Camargo B, *et al.* (1995). Parental exposures to pesticides and risk of Wilms tumor in Brazil. *Am J Epidemiol* **141**, 210–17.

12. Vujanic GM, Kelsey A, Mitchell C, Shannon RS, Gornall P (2003). The role of biopsy in the diagnosis of renal tumors of childhood, results of the UKCCSG Wilms tumor study 3. *Med Pediatr Oncol* **40**, 18–22.

13. Owens CM, Veys PA, Pritchard J, Levitt G, Imeson J, Dicks-Mireaux C (2002). Role of chest computed tomography at diagnosis in the management of Wilms' tumor: a study by the United Kingdom Children's Cancer Study Group. *J Clin Oncol* **20**, 2768–73.

14. Beckwith JB, Zuppan CE, Browning NG, Moksness J, Breslow NE (1996). Histological analysis of aggressiveness and responsiveness in Wilms' tumor. *Med Pediatr Oncol* **27**, 422–8.

15. Weirich A, Leuschner I, Harms D, *et al.* (2001) Clinical impact of histologic subtypes in localized non-anaplastic nephroblastoma treated according to the trial and study SIOP-9/GPOH. *Ann Oncol* **12**, 311–19.

16. Vujanic GM, Sandstedt B, Harms D, *et al.* (2002). Revised International Society of Paediatric Oncology (SIOP) Working Classification of Renal Tumors of Childhood. *Med Pediatr Oncol* **38**, 79–82.

17. Boccon-Gibod L, Rey A, Sandstedt B, *et al.* (2000). Complete necrosis induced by preoperative chemotherapy in Wilms tumor as an indicator of low risk, report of the International Society of Paediatric Oncology (SIOP) Nephroblastoma Trial and Study 9. *Med Pediatr Oncol* 34, 183–90.

18. Faria P, Beckwith JB, Mishra K, *et al.* (1996). Focal versus diffuse anaplasia in Wilms tumor—new definitions with prognostic significance. A report from the National Wilms Tumor Study Group. *Am J Surg Pathol* 20, 909–20.

19. Beckwith JB (1998). Nephrogenic rests and the pathogenesis of Wilms tumor: developmental and clinical considerations. *Am J Med Genet* 79, 268–73.

20. Green DM, Breslow N, Beckwith JB, *et al.* (1998).Comparison between single-dose and divided-dose administration of dactinomycin and doxorubicin for patients with Wilms' tumor: a report from the National Wilms' Tumor Study Group. *J Clin Oncol* 16, 237–45.

21. Green DM, Breslow NE, Beckwith JB, *et al.* (1998). Effect of duration of treatment on treatment outcome and cost of treatment for Wilms' tumor: a report from the National Wilms' Tumor Study Group. *J Clin Oncol* 16, 3744–51.

22. Tournade MF, Com-Nougue C, Voûte PA, *et al.* (1993). Results of the Sixth International Society of Pediatric Oncology Wilms Tumor Trial and Study: a risk-adapted therapy approach in Wilms tumor. *J Clin Oncol* 11, 1014–23.

23. Mitchell C, Jones PM, Kelsey A, *et al.* (2000). The treatment of Wilms' tumour: results of the United Kingdom Children's Cancer Study Group (UKCCSG) second Wilms' tumour study. *Br J Cancer* 83, 602–8.

24. De Camargo B, Franco EL for the Brazilian Wilms Tumor Study Group (1994). A randomized clinical trial of single-dose versus fractionated-dose fractionated dactinomycin in the treatment of Wilms tumor. Results after extended follow up. *Cancer* 73, 3081–6.

25. Green DM, Norkool P, Breslow NE, Finklestein JZ, D'Angio GJ (1990). Severe toxicity after treatment with vincristine and dactinomycin using single-dose or divided-dose schedules: a report from the National Wilms Tumor Study. *J Clin Oncol* 8, 1525–30.

26. Othersen HB Jr, DeLorimer A, Hrabovsky E, Kelalis P, Breslow N, D'Angio GJ (1990). Surgical evaluation of lymph node metastases in Wilms' tumor. *J Pediatr Surg* 25, 330–1.

27. Kessler O, Franco I, Jayabose S, Redá E, Levitt S, Brock W (1996). Is contralateral exploration of the kidney necessary in patients with Wilms tumor. *J Urol* 156, 693–5.

28. Pachnis A, Pritchard J, Gaze M, Levitt G, Michalski A (1998). Radiotherapy omitted in the treatment of selected children under 3 years of age with stage III favorable histology Wilms tumor. *Med Pediatr Oncol* 31, 150–2.

29. Grundy PE, Telzerow PE, Breslow N, Mokness J, Huff V, Paterson MC (1994). Loss of heterozygosity for chromosome 16q and 1p in Wilms tumor predicts an adverse outcome. *Cancer Res* 94, 2331–3.

30. Grundy RG, Pritchard J, Scambler P, Cowell JK (1998). Loss of heterozygosity on chromosome 16 in sporadic Wilms' tumour. *Br J Cancer* 78, 1181–7.

31. Green DM, Peabody EM, Nan B, Peterson S, Kalapurakal JA, Breslow N (2002). Pregnancy outcome after treatment for Wilms tumor: a report from the National Wilms Tumor Study Group. *J Clin Oncol* 20, 2506–13.

32. Green DM, Grigoriev Y, Nan B, *et al.* (2001). Congestive heart failure after treatment for Wilms tumor: a report from the National Wilms Tumor Study Group. *J Clin Oncol* 19, 1926–34.

33. Abu-Ghosh AM, Krailo MD, Goldman SC, *et al.* (2002). Ifosfamide, carboplatin and etoposide in children with poor-risk relapsed Wilms tumor: a Childrens Cancer Group Report. *Ann Oncol* 13, 460–9.

34. Pein F, Michon J, Valteau-Couanet D, *et al.* (1998). High-dose melphalan, etoposide, and carboplatin followed by autologous stem-cell rescue in pediatric high-risk recurrent Wilms' tumor: a French Society of Pediatric Oncology study. *J Clin Oncol* 16, 3295–301.

35. **Cooper CS, Jaffe WI, Huff DS, *et al.*** (2000). The role of renal salvage procedures for bilateral Wilms tumor: a 15-year-review. *J Urol* **163**, 265–8.
36. **Horwitz JR, Ritchey ML, Mokness J, *et al.*** (1996). Renal salvage procedures in patients with synchronous bilateral Wilms tumor: a report from the National Wilms Tumor Study Group. *J Pediatr Surg* **31**, 1020–5.
37. **Beckwith JB** (1998) Nephrogenic rests and the pathogenesis of Wilms' tumour: development and clinical considerations. *Am J Med Genet* **79**, 268–73.

Chapter 22

Neuroblastoma

Huib N. Caron and A.D.J. Pearson

Introduction

Neuroblastoma, ganglioneuroblastoma, and ganglioneuroma are embryonal tumours of the sympathetic nervous system derived from the primitive neural crest.

Neuroblastoma has the greatest diversity in clinical behaviour of all childhood solid tumours, with some tumours regressing spontaneously, some being chemo-curable, and others being resistant to intensive chemotherapy. Metastatic neuroblastoma in children aged >1 year is associated with a poor prognosis. Although there is initial response to chemotherapy, relapse with drug-resistant disease occurs in the majority of children.

More is known about the molecular pathology and genetics of neuroblastoma than probably any other adult or childhood malignancy. This knowledge is already guiding therapy so that children can receive individualized treatment, thereby minimizing toxicity in patients with good prognosis and allowing intensive and novel therapy to be delivered only to those children in whom conventional treatment is unsuccessful. A therapeutic classification is at present being developed which is based on patient characteristics and molecular tumour features, such as N-*myc* gene amplification. This classification will be progressively developed.

Epidemiology

The annual incidence of neuroblastoma is 10.5 per million children aged <15 years.[1] There appears to be no significant geographical variation in the incidence between North America and Europe, and similarly there are no differences between races. Neuroblastoma occurs slightly more frequently in males than females (ratio 1.2:1). The peak age of incidence is between 0 and 4 years, with a median age of 23 months. Forty per cent of patients clinically presenting with neuroblastoma are aged <1 year, and <5 per cent are over the age of 10 years. Cases of familial neuroblastoma have been reported.[2]

There are a number of features of neuroblastoma which suggested that screening might have been of value in reducing mortality from the malignancy by detecting poor prognosis disease at an earlier stage. Infants presenting under the age of 1 year tend to have localized good prognosis disease, with favourable molecular features. In contrast, children who are diagnosed over the age of 1 year have a significantly worse outcome, and usually have metastatic disease with genetic features indicative of an aggressive course. Screening for neuroblastoma was pioneered by Japanese investigators who demonstrated that asymptomatic tumours could be detected in infants by measurement of urinary catecholamine metabolites. Although the outlook for the children with the detected tumours was excellent, these studies were not population based and did not demonstrate a resultant reduction in neuroblastoma mortality rates. However, in regions where there were screening programmes, the incidence doubled to 20.1 per million children[3] and the tumours detected all possessed favourable biologic characteristics.[4] Both the Quebec Neuroblastoma Screening Project and the German Neuro-blastoma Screening Study were designed to answer definitively the question as to whether screening a large cohort of infants for neuroblastoma at the ages of 3 weeks, 6 months, and 12 months could reduce the population-based incidence of advanced disease and mortality. Both of these studies demonstrate that screening for neuroblastoma in children aged ≤1 year identifies tumours with a good prognosis and molecular pathology, doubles the incidence, and fails to detect the poor prognosis disease which presents clinically at an older age.[5,6]

Embryology, pathology, and genetics

Embryology

The neural crest is the embryonic structure which gives rise to the sympathetic nervous system. In the third gestational week, the neural plate is formed in the ectodermal germlayer. At the time of the fusion of the neural ridges into the neural tube, the neural crest is formed dorsally to the neural tube. Neural crest cells develop into a large number of mature cell types and structures. They form not only the sympathetic peripheral nervous system, but also part of the facial skeleton, the thymus, the parathyroids, the enteric nervous system, and skin melanocytes. Segmentation and migration are characteristic phenomena in neural crest development. The primitive neural crest cells migrate to a position lateral to the neural tube, forming (segmented) primitive ganglia on each side of it. From these, primitive ganglia neuroblasts migrate along the dorsal pathway to form melanocytes in the skin and dorsal root sympathetic neurons. Neuro-blasts migrating along a ventrolateral pathway will eventually form the side chain (ventrolateral to the spine), the paraganglia (ventral to the spine), the visceral sympathetic ganglia (abdom-inal organs), and the adrenal medulla. The adrenal medulla is formed by neuroblasts which invade the primitive adrenal cortex and differentiate into chromaffin cells. The mature sympathetic nervous system consists of a neuronal part (dorsal root ganglia and side chain) and a hormonal part (paraganglia and adrenal medulla). Both parts produce catecholamines, as neurotransmitters and hormones, respectively. In the first years of life, the majority of systemic catecholamine is produced in the abdominal paraganglia. The adrenal medulla contains very few chromaffin cells at birth and enlarges and matures during the early years of life. It is thought that neuroblastoma develops in immature neuroblasts, ganglioneuroma in more differentiated sympathetic cells (ganglion cells), and pheochromocytoma in differenti-ated hormone-producing cells (chromaffin cells).

Pathology

Histologically, neuroblastomas are very heterogeneous and are composed of two predominant cell types: the neuroblast/ganglion cell and the Schwann cell. Schwann cells are responsible for the stromal element of the tumour. As the neuroblast is an embryonal cell, it can differentiate and mature into a ganglion cell. Evidence suggests that Schwann cells in neuroblastomas are reactive cells arising from non-neoplastic tissues and are recruited into the tumour.[7] The typical histologic appearance of an undifferentiated neuroblastoma is 'a small round blue cell tumour' [Fig. 22.1(a)]. The cells are of uniform size and contain dense hyperchromatic nuclei and scant cytoplasm. Homer–Wright pseudorosettes, from neuroblasts and neuritic processes, are frequently present. Ultimately, a neuroblastoma may differentiate into a mature gang-lioneuroma, which is at the other end of the spectrum and has three components: mature ganglion cells, Schwann cells, and neurophils [Fig. 22.1(b)]. Some neuroblastomas, particularly

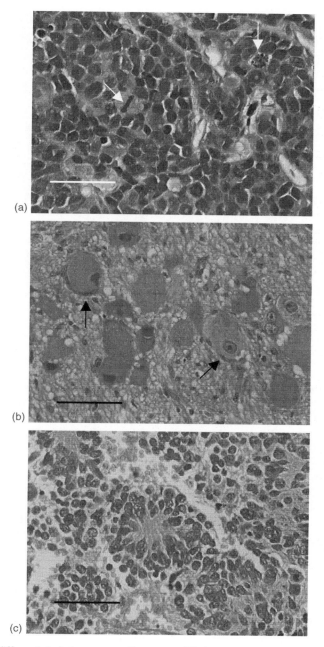

Fig. 22.1 (a) Undifferentiated stroma-poor N-*myc*-amplified neuroblastoma. Haematoxylin and eosin (H & E) stain showing hyperchromatic nuclei without neurophils and a high nuclear-to-cytoplasmic ratio. Mitotic and apoptotic cells are indicated by arrows. (b) Schwannian stroma-rich mature ganglioneuroma with fully mature individual ganglion cells surrounded by satellite cells (arrows). (c) Poorly differentiated stroma-poor neuroblastoma showing Homer–Wright pseudorosettes (rings of neuroblastoma surrounding central core of neurophils).   (Continued)

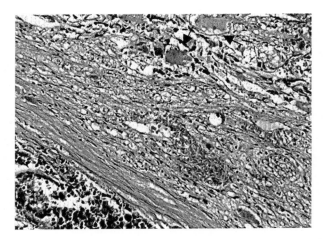

Fig. 22.1 (Continued) (d) Nodular ganglioneuroblastoma. A thickened fibrovascular septum separates the poorly differentiated stroma-poor neuroblastoma (bottom left) from the stroma-rich ganglioneuromatous component (top right). Ganglion cells are indicated by arrows. Scale bars, 50 mM. (Courtesy of Dr D. Tweddle.)

those that are undergoing regression, have a degree of calcification. In the past, a number of histopathologic classification systems of neuroblastoma have been proposed by Shimada and Joshi. The Shimada system is age linked, and the tumours are classified according to the amount of Schwann cell stroma (poor or rich) and the number of cells in mitosis or karyorrhexis. Recently, an International Neuroblastoma Pathology Classification (INPC) has been introduced.[8]

All these classifications are only applicable to tumours before therapy. In the INPC, the four morphologic features which form the basis for the classification are:

- the degree of differentiation of the neuroblasts
- the presence or absence of Schwann cell stroma
- the presence or absence of neuroblastic nodules arising in a mature Schwann cell-stroma-rich tumour
- an index of tumour cell aggressiveness, indicated by the mitotic karyorrhexis index (MKI).

The following tumours can be defined from these features: undifferentiated [Fig. 22.1(a)], poorly differentiated [Fig. 22.1(c)], or differentiating neuroblastoma; intermixed or nodular ganglioneuroblastoma [Fig. 22.1(d)]; ganglioneuroma [Fig. 22.1(b)]. Distinction between the two types of ganglioneuroblastomas is of major importance. Intermixed ganglioneuroblastomas are good prognosis tumours where there is progressive differentiation, with only small nests of neuroblasts. However, there are usually macroscopic, often haemorrhagic, nodules of neuroblasts with the nodular variant [Fig. 22.1(d)], and the associated prognosis is worse.

Genetics

Genetic predisposition

There are very few reported pedigrees of familial neuroblastoma.[2] In those families, the median age at diagnosis is 9 months compared with 2–3 years in sporadic cases. An increased incidence of multiple primary tumours is also apparent. Together, these data suggest that a genetic predisposition for neuroblastoma development exists in these families. Neuroblastoma familial gene loci have been linked to chromosomes 16p and 4p by cytogenetic studies and linkage analyses.[9,10]

Genetic aberrations in neuroblastoma

Broadly speaking, neuroblastoma can be divided into those with a near-diploid nuclear DNA content (~45 per cent) and near-triploid tumours (~55 per cent). Near-triploid neuroblastomas are characterized by whole-chromosome gains and losses without structural genetic aberrations. Clinically, near-triploid tumours are more often localized and show a favourable outcome. Near-diploid neuroblastomas are characterized by the presence of genetic aberrations such as N-*myc* amplification, 17q gain, and chromosomal losses.

N-*myc* oncogene The N-*myc* oncogene is present in an increased copy number in 25–35 per cent of neuroblastomas . N-*myc* amplification is found in 30–40 per cent of stage III and IV neuroblastomas and in only 5 per cent of localized or stage IVs neuroblastomas. N-*myc* amplified neuroblastomas are characterized by highly aggressive behaviour with an unfavourable clinical outcome.[11] Loss of chromosome lp is almost invariable in N-*myc* amplified neuroblastomas.

Chromosome 17q gain Gain of the entire chromosome 17 or gain of parts of chromosomal arm 17q occur in >60 per cent of neuroblastoma. The partial 17q gain most often results from unbalanced translocation of 17q21–25 material to another chromosome (e.g. chromosome 1). Partial gain of 17q identifies unfavourable neuroblastoma.[12] Obvious candidate genes on 17q are the NM23 and survivin genes.

Tumour suppressor genes Loss of tumour suppressor regions is reported in neuroblastomas for chromosome 1 p (30–40 per cent), 4p (20 per cent), 11q (25 per cent), and 14q (25 per cent). Chromosome lp loss occurs more frequently in older children with stage III and IV neuroblastoma and is correlated with increased serum ferritin and serum lactate dehydrogenase (LDH). In almost all samples with N-*myc* amplification, concomitant 1p loss is demonstrated, but loss of chromosome 1p also occurs in N-*myc* single-copy cases. A multivariate prognostic factor analysis showed that 1p loss was the strongest predictor of outcome of all the clinical and genetic factors tested, including N-*myc* amplification.[13] Chromosome 1p loss added considerable prognostic information to the strongest clinical factors. Other studies also report a negative prognostic impact for 1p loss.[14,15]

Caspase 8 inactivation It has been shown that the most frequent mechanism by which neuroblastoma tumour cells evade apoptosis is inactivation of the caspase 8 gene. Loss of the chromosomal region containing the caspase 8 gene and/or hypermethylation of the caspase 8 promoter region lead to a loss of mRNA and protein expression.[16]

Clinical presentation

The clinical manifestations of neuroblastoma are very varied, depending on the site of the primary tumour and whether there is metastatic disease. The classical presentation at age 3–4 years is a pale irritable child with a limp and periorbital ecchymoses, whilst an infant may present with a grossly enlarged liver with subcutaneous nodules (Fig. 22.2). The symptoms of neuroblastoma can be attributed to the primary tumour, metastases, or a paraneoplastic

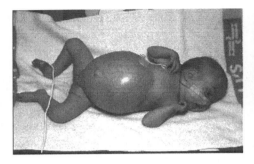
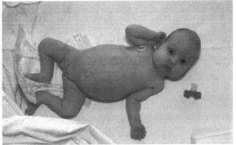
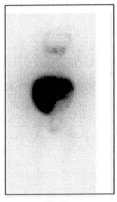
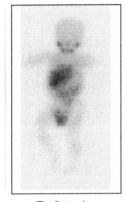

$T = 0$ $T = 2$ weeks

Fig. 22.2 Infant with stage IVs neuroblastoma and spontaneous regression. Primary tumour in adrenal gland and diffuse liver metastasis. (a) The child and ^{123}I-MIBG scan at diagnosis ($T = 0$). (b) the same child after spontaneous regression without any therapy ($T = 2$ weeks).

phenomenon. The clinical presentation of neuroblastoma has changed over the last decade in developed countries, and the disease is now often detected when the child has fewer symptoms.

Primary tumour

Neuroblastoma primary tumours can arise at any location coinciding with normal sympathetic nervous system structures, such as the adrenals, the sympathetic chain, or abdominal para-ganglia. About 25 per cent of primaries are found in the neck or thorax, 70 per cent in the abdomen, and 5 per cent in the pelvis.

A hard fixed abdominal mass causing only mild abdominal discomfort is a frequent presentation. Hypertension can result from compression of the renal vessels by the tumour. Gastrointestinal symptoms are rare, except from pelvic tumours which may cause constipation and difficulties with micturition.

Primaries in the cervical region may manifest only as a mass which is mistaken for cervical lymph nodes. Horner's syndrome with unilateral ptosis, constricted pupil, and absence of sweating may occur with either cervical or thoracic lesions. Although a thoracic primary can cause signs of mediastinal pressure with cough and superior mediastinal obstruction, these are most commonly detected coincidentally on a chest radiograph carried out for other reasons.

Thoracic, abdominal, and pelvic tumours can extend into the neural foramina and compress nerve roots and the spinal cord, resulting in radicular pain, paraplegia, and bowel and bladder symptoms.

Metastatic disease

The most common metastatic sites are bone, lymph nodes, and bone marrow; less common sites are skin, liver, lung and central nervous system. Metastases to the bone are often the presenting symptom, and manifest as painful lesions which produce an irritable unwell child. Frequently, a limp, which is difficult to diagnose, is the predominant feature either at initial presentation or at relapse. Bone marrow involvement generally presents with anaemia and, later, thrombocytopenia. The blood film may show a leuco-erythroblastic picture. Lymph-adenopathy is not usually generalized or massive. Retro-orbital and orbital metastases produce a characteristic appearance of proptosis and periorbital ecchymoses. An infant with stage IVs neuroblastoma can present with significant respiratory distress from a massively enlarged liver, as well as having non-tender blue-tinged subcutaneous nodules (Fig. 22.2).

Paraneoplastic symptoms

Rarely, in 4 per cent of patients, opsoclonus–myoclonus can be a presentation of neuroblastoma. This syndrome comprises myoclonic irregular jerking and random eye movements, often associated with cerebellar ataxia. The symptoms generally tend to occur with good prognosis tumours and mostly resolve with regression of the disease.[17] However, affected children often have significant long-term neuropsychometric damage.[18]

An intractable secretory diarrhoea, probably mediated by vasoactive intestinal polypeptide (VIP), can cause hypokalaemic dehydration (Kerner–Morrison syndrome). Like opsoclonus–myoclonus, this entity usually occurs with ganglioneuromas or ganglioneuroblastomas.[19]

Unlike the presentation in pheochromocytoma, hypertension, tachycardia, and episodes of sweating are less common in neuroblastoma.

Diagnosis and staging

Diagnostic criteria

The diagnostic criteria for neuroblastoma have been clearly defined by the International Neuroblastoma Staging System (INSS) working party.[20] Neuroblastoma can be diagnosed by either a tissue biopsy showing a histologic appearance of neuroblastoma, or the presence of a non-haemopoietic tumour in the bone marrow, together with raised urinary catecholamines. In the bone marrow, neuroblastoma often has the appearance of pseudorosettes with increased reticulin and fibrous tissue. The presence of neuroectodermal antigens on the surface of the malignant cells, detected by monoclonal antibodies, further confirms the diagnosis.

Staging system

There is now an international consensus that the International Neuroblastoma Staging System (INSS) should be used exclusively.

Details are shown in Table 22.1. It is essentially a postsurgical staging system with major dependence on the assessment of resectability and surgical examination of lymph-node

Table 22.1. ISSN International Staging System for Neuroblastoma[a]

Stage I	Localized tumour with complete gross excision, with or without microscopic residual disease; representative ipsilateral and contralateral lymph nodes negative for tumour microscopically (nodes attached to and removed with the primary tumour may be positive)
Stage IIa	Localized tumour with incomplete gross excision; representative ipsilateral and non-adherent lymph nodes negative for tumour microscopically
Stage IIb	Localized tumour with complete or incomplete gross excision with ipsilateral non-adherent lymph nodes positive for tumour; enlarged contralateral lymph nodes must be negative microscopically
Stage III	Unresectable unilateral tumour infiltrating across the midline[b] with or without regional lymph node involvement, or localized unilateral tumour with contralateral regional lymph node involvement, or midline tumour with bilateral extension by infiltration (unresectable) or by lymph node involvement
Stage IV	Any primary tumour with dissemination to distant lymph nodes, bone, bone marrow, liver skin and/or other organs (except as defined in stage 4s)
Stage IVs	Localized primary tumour (as defined for stage I, IIa, or IIb) with dissemination limited to skin, liver and/or bone marrow[c] (limited to infants <1 year).

[a]Multifocal primary tumours (e.g. adrenal primary tumours) should be staged according to the greatest extent of the disease, as defined above, and followed by subscript M (e.g. stage III_M)
[b]The midline is defined as the vertebral column. Tumours originating on one side and 'crossing the midline' must infiltrate to or beyond the opposite side of the vertebral column.
[c]Marrow involvement of stage IVs should be minimal, i.e. <10% of total nucleated cells identified as malignant on bone marrow biopsy or marrow aspirates. More extensive marrow involvement will be considered to be stage IV. The MIBG scan (if done) should be negative in marrow.
Reproduced from G.M. Brodeur et al. (1993) J Clin Oncol **11**, 1466–77.

involvement. The central feature of stage III disease is invasion across the midline by the tumour, with often a main blood vessel being encased. A number of investigations are required to delineate the extent of spread of the disease, and these have been defined by the INSS (Table 22.2).

Radiodiagnostics

Either CT or MRI can delineate the extent of the primary tumour and associated lymph node masses, as well as other metastatic disease. Within the abdomen, detection of liver metastases can be carried out by CT scanning, whilst the extent of lymph node involvement and the margins of the primary tumour can be visualized equally well by either technique. Abdominal ultrasound can replace CT or MRI when carried out by an experienced paediatric radiologist. MRI is the optimal technique to demonstrate intraspinal extension through neural foramina.

MIBG scanning

MIBG (*meta*-iodobenzylguanidine) is taken up preferentially by cells of the sympathetic nervous system involved in catecholamine synthesis. Therefore if the compound is radiola-belled it can localize primary and metastatic neuroblastomas (Fig. 22.2) with a sensitivity of >90 per cent and a specificity of >98 per cent. To prevent uptake of radioactive iodine in the thyroid, the organ is specifically blocked by Lugol's iodine before administration of the isotope.

Less than 5 per cent of neuroblastomas do not take up MIBG; if there is no positivity in the primary tumour, metastases cannot be detected. It is widely recognized that MIBG is the most

Table 22.2. Assessment of extent of disease

Tumour site	Recommended tests
Primary tumour	CT and/or MR1 scan[a] with 3D measurements; MIBG scan, if available[b]
Metastatic sites[b]	Bilateral posterior iliac crest marrow aspirates and trephine (core) bone
Bone marrow	Marrow biopsies required to exclude marrow involvement. A single positive site documents marrow involvement. Core biopsies must contain at least 1 cm of marrow (excluding cartilage) to be considered adequate
Bone	MIBG scan; ^{99}Tc scan required if MIBG scan negative or unavailable, and plain radiographs of positive lesions are recommended
Lymph nodes	Clinical examination (palpable nodes), confirmed histologically. CT scan for non-palpable nodes (3D measurements)
Abdomen/liver	CT and/or MRI scan[a] with 3D measurements
Chest	Anteroposterior and lateral chest radiographs. CT/MRI necessary if chest radiograph positive or if abdominal mass/nodes extend into chest

[a]Ultrasound considered suboptimal for accurate 3D measurements.
[b]The MIBG scan is applicable to all sites of disease.
Reproduced from G.M. Brodeur et al. (1993) J Clin Oncol **11**, 1466–77.

sensitive technique and surpasses [^{99m}Tc]diphosphonate scintigraphy of bones or skeletal survey. However, if there is no uptake of MIBG into the primary tumour, it is recommended that a ^{99m}Tc bone scan is carried out.

Tumour markers

There are a large number of urinary catecholamines, which can be elevated in the urine in patients with neuroblastoma. The most frequently measured metabolites of the catecholamines are vanilglycolic acid (VGA), also known as vanillylmandelic acid (VMA), vanilacetic acid (VAA), also known as homovanillic acid (HVA), vanilglycol (VG), catecholacetic acid (CAA), and vanillactic acid (VLA). In addition, concentrations of the catecholamine dopamine may be assessed. Approximately 90–95 per cent of all patients with neuroblastoma will have increased urinary secretion of these metabolites. Measurement of the ratio of the urinary concentration of the catecholamine metabolite to creatinine in a urine sample gives the most reliable results. The serum concentrations of LDH, ferritin, and neuron-specific enolase are useful prognostic markers.[21] Apart from the urinary concentration of catecholamines, there is no value in monitoring patients during therapy.

Bone marrow examination

Metastatic disease to the bone marrow is one of the most common occurrences in poor prognosis neuroblastoma. Studies in the past have documented that metastatic disease may be present in the bone marrow, but it may not be easy to detect by examination of a bone marrow aspirate. Therefore the international consensus, as specified by the INSS, is that all patients should have histologic examinations of bone marrow aspirate and trephine carried out from two different sites. In this way, the likelihood of detecting 'patchy' bone marrow involvement is increased. Bone marrow aspirate examinations can be assessed using conventional microscopy and, if there is involvement, multiple clumps of a non-haemopoietic malignancy are usually observed. The non-haemopoietic cells tend to cluster and form pseudorosettes. International guidelines suggest that for a bone marrow histologic examination to be adequate, at least 1 cm of haemopoietic tissue should be examined.

Immunocytochemistry of bone marrow aspirates using monoclonal antibodies directed at neuroctodermal antigens can be used to detect neuroblastoma. However, its value in either detecting 'occult disease' at presentation or monitoring disease during therapy has not been confirmed

Treatment strategies

Current therapy

Individualization of therapy according to molecular pathologic features

Amplification of the N-*myc* gene is the most extensively studied marker of all the molecular pathologic prognostic features. At present, therapy for stage III neuroblastoma is determined by N-*myc* gene copy number. Surgery and a short course of chemotherapy are now being recommended for stage III patients with tumours with a single copy of N-*myc*, with survival rates of 85 per cent without intensive chemotherapy, radiation, or myeloablative therapy (MAT). Tumours with N-*myc* amplification progress rapidly and are associated with a 5-year survival of only 20 per cent. In view of this, the consensus is that these tumours should be treated as high-risk disease, in the same way as stage IV neuroblastomas in children aged >1 year.

The consensus is that patients with N-*myc* amplified stage II disease, who have a 50 per cent survival,[22] should also have high-risk therapy. Because of the rarity of stage I N-*myc* amplified tumours, no clear evidence is available and at present an observational policy following surgery is appropriate.

Amplification of N-*myc* also identifies infants with metastatic neuroblastoma (stage IV and IVs) who have a very poor prognosis. These patients should be treated with an intensive chemotherapy regimen and MAT.

No molecular features consistently and reliably identify those patients aged >1 year with metastatic disease who have a worse prognosis, and the prognostic value of N-*myc* amplification is not present in this group. It is expected that other molecular features will soon be confirmed to be of equal value to N-*myc*.

International Neuroblastoma Risk Groups

At present, patient age, tumour stage, N-*myc* amplification, and metastatic pattern in infants are used to determine therapeutic/risk groups. Unfortunately there is not complete international agreement about risk groups, although consensus is greatest for high-risk disease, i.e. stage IV disease at age >1 year and N-*myc* amplification in infants and in stage II and III disease. Efforts are now ongoing to define better risk groups and obtain international consensus.

It is appreciated that age is a continuous variable and that some 'infant' disease will occur in patients aged >12 months, and that some aggressive disease will occur in infants without N-*myc* amplification. Some groups employ pathologic features to define risk groups, whilst others do not. Currently, no group utilizes 1p loss, 17q gain or 11q loss as genetic features to identify different risk groups. Although hyperdiploidy has been suggested to be a good prognostic feature in infants,[23] this has not been incorporated in the International Risk Group Classification. The importance of metastases to bone, lung and central nervous system in infants requires clarification.

Finally, at present the surgeon's decision regarding resectability drives staging and therapy decisions for localized disease, and this must be standardized.

Localized tumours

The most important information with any localized tumour is whether it is resectable without any significant morbidity and if there is N-*myc* amplification.

Stage I and II tumours

The present consensus is that stage I and II tumours should be resected with the major aim being to prevent acute or long-term sequelae. Even if there is residual disease, no chemotherapy or radiation treatment should be given.[22,24] Currently, the Localized Neuroblastoma European Study Group (LNESG) recommends treating recurrent localized tumours by further resection only and it is possible that a recurrent tumour may eventually regress spontaneously. Although allelic deletion of chromosome 1p, 17q loss, and a raised serum LDH concentration have been suggested to be of prognostic importance, to date this has not been verified.

Stage III tumours

In the past, infants with stage III tumours have received postoperative chemotherapy. This has been associated with acute and long-term sequelae from chemotherapy, and there may be significant surgical morbidity and, indeed, mortality. Furthermore, in some reports more deaths result from the effects of therapy than from disease.[25] It is now recommended that careful observation with measurement of urinary catecholamine concentrations and radiologic imaging only is required after surgery. A residual persisting mass associated with some elevation of urinary catecholamines may be a mature ganglioneuroma. Only a definite increase in tumour size should be taken as evidence of progression.

The current approach for stage III disease in patients aged >1 year is to determine whether the tumour is unresectable by imaging and its N-*myc* gene copy number. If resection with very minimal morbidity is not practical, then biopsy is undertaken. If the neuroblastoma does not show amplification of N-*myc*, six courses of chemotherapy are given with, for example, carboplatin and etoposide, alternating with cyclophosphamide, doxorubicin, and vincristine. Surgical resection of the primary tumour is then attempted, again with the emphasis on minimal morbidity, followed by two further courses of chemotherapy. No treatment is given for any residual disease and no radiotherapy, MAT, or 13-*cis*-retinoic acid is administered. The best results for stage III neuroblastoma in patients aged >1 year without amplification of N-*myc* are those of Rubie *et al.*[26] using the above approach. Those stage III tumours with N-*myc* amplification are treated as high-risk disease and receive the same therapy as for stage IV disease in children aged >1 year.

Stage IV tumours in children aged >1 year

The therapeutic approach adopted by most cooperative groups for stage IV disease in children aged >1 year is to administer initial chemotherapy, followed by surgical resection of the primary tumour and consolidation with MAT with haemopoietic stem-cell support, usually utilizing peripheral blood stem cells.[27,28] This is followed by radiation therapy to the site of the primary tumour and differentiation therapy with 13-*cis*-retinoic acid. Randomized trials have established survival benefits of MAT, initially with high-dose melphalan alone[29] and, more recently, with a more complex regimen.[28] The benefits of 6 months of intermittent oral 13-*cis*-retinoic acid have also been established in a randomized study.[28] No randomized trial has investigated the advantages of radiotherapy at the site of the primary tumour in stage IV disease. However, comparison of local relapse rates between North America (where radiotherapy is given) and Europe (where it is not) suggest a benefit. Unfortunately, no randomized comparison has been made of more complex multi-agent MAT regimens compared with high-dose melphalan alone. However, historical comparisons and the European Bone Marrow Transplant Registry data suggest that more complex regimens are of more value. European retrospective analyses indicate that busulphan and melphalan give the best survival results.[30] In contrast, a comparison of North American MAT regimens suggest that carboplatin, etoposide, and melphalan (CEM) yield high event-free survival (EFS) rates (65 per cent). With this background, SIOP Europe Neuroblastoma is comparing, in a randomized study, busulphan and melphalan with CEM as the MAT regimen. There is no convincing evidence to suggest that allogeneic bone marrow is superior to autologous bone marrow,[31] or that there is a benefit in purging the marrow.

Various permutations of the active cytotoxic drugs have been used in induction chemotherapy. However, a platinum compound (either cisplatin or carboplatin), etoposide, and cyclophosphamide are most commonly used.[32] Whether there is a benefit in the inclusion of doxorubicin is unknown. No regimen has been shown to be conclusively better; however, higher doses of agents given in intensive schedules appear to result in better long-term survival. Evidence suggests that increasing dose intensity improves EFS.[33,34] Some of the most widely used induction regimens are Kushner, NB 87 and COJEC.[32,34,35] It is very difficult to compare the efficacy of different induction regimens, as conventional response criteria at the end of induction do not appear to be good surrogates for long-term survival. Only randomized studies comparing different induction regimens will produce appropriate and reliable information.

Infants with stage IVs and IV neuroblastoma

The realization of the major discriminatory effect of N-*myc* amplification in infants, including those with stage IVs disease, has led to a dramatically different approach for those tumours with N-*myc* amplification. Patients with tumours with amplification, including stage IVs, receive intensive chemotherapy, attempted total surgical resection of the primary tumour, radiation therapy at the site of the primary tumour, and MAT.

It has been appreciated since the early 1970s that the majority of infants with stage IVs neuroblastoma require no therapy as their disease regresses spontaneously (Fig. 22.2).[36] Only life- and organ-threatening symptoms, such as respiratory failure due to a rapidly enlarging liver, are indications for treatment. Chemotherapy with carboplatin and etoposide is most effective for these patients. It is essential that the smallest amount of therapy is administered, and frequently only one course is needed to induce regression. The primary tumour should not be resected. Eighty-five per cent of children will be cured with this approach.

The recent appreciation that more neuroblastomas in infants will regress spontaneously has led to the strategy of widening the indications for observation for some infants with stage IV disease. Chemotherapy is only used if there are life- or organ-threatening symptoms. In the current SIOP Europe Neuroblastoma trial, the only infants without life-threatening symptoms to be treated with four courses of chemotherapy are those with metastases to the bone, lung, or central nervous system.

Tumours causing spinal cord compression

Spinal cord compression can occur with stage II, III, and IV tumours. In addition to stage-specific therapy, consideration must be given to the intraspinal disease. With the advent of MRI, asymptomatic extension into the spinal cord is being increasingly detected.

The appropriate therapy depends upon neurologic symptoms and signs, the amount of disease within the spinal canal, and the histology. Decisions regarding therapy should be taken jointly between neurosurgeons, radiation oncologists, and paediatric oncologists.

If there are no neurologic symptoms, provided that no more than 50 per cent of the spinal canal is occupied with tumour, stage-specific therapy should be given and careful clinical and neurologic review undertaken. If >50 per cent of the spinal canal is filled with tumour, dexamethasone should be administered and continued until there is documented regression.

If there is total paraplegia, laminectomy is the preferred approach as modern techniques should reduce long-term surgical sequelae. For other degrees of neurologic symptoms, chemotherapy together with dexamethasone should be considered first. Very careful observation is required and dexamethasone should only be discontinued when there is objective neuroradiologic evidence of response.

Histology of the tumour is also important, as spinal cord compression caused by ganglioneuroblastomas will be less likely to be relieved by chemotherapy or radiotherapy, and laminectomy should be considered more readily.

Recurrent neuroblastoma

Further resection with chemotherapy is required for stage I and II disease. Recurrent stage III disease without N-*myc* amplification warrants further therapy as for high-risk disease. Unfortunately, with recurrent high-risk disease that has received appropriate modern therapy, i.e. MAT, long-term cure is not a realistic possibility and palliative therapy is most appropriate.

MIBG as an anti-cancer agent

The epinephrine analogue MIBG is actively taken up and stored in >90 per cent of neuroblastoma tumours. Incorporation of the ^{131}I radioisotope in MIBG makes it possible to use this for targeted radiotherapy. Currently, [131I]MIBG is used in three groups of neuroblastoma patients:

- those with unresectable localized tumours
- for initial treatment of unresectable stage III and stage IV patients
- in patients with recurrence.

In heavily pretreated recurrent neuroblastoma patients, a single [131I]MIBG treatment results in an objective response rate of >60 per cent. Adequate pain relief can be achieved in >80 per cent of patients. Little or no acute toxicity is seen, and the major side effect is thrombocytopenia.[37] [131I]MIBG treatment has been used to render unresectable mainly abdominal or pelvic neuroblastoma tumours operable, or even to circumvent surgery.

Efforts are underway to use [131I]MIBG as the only initial anticancer agent in unresectable stage III and IV patients. The administration of multiple courses of [131I]MIBG in 43 consecutive patients resulted in an objective response rate of 42 per cent. Following initial MIBG treatment, surgical resection of the primary tumour, intensive combination chemotherapy, and myeloablative therapy were given for stage IV cases.[38]

Treatment results

Stage I and II

An excellent EFS and overall survival is expected for these patients following surgery alone, with >90 per cent survival for stage I and 85 per cent for stage II disease. Stage II tumours with N-*myc* amplification have survival rates of 50 per cent and are now treated as high risk.

Stage III

Overall, 65 per cent of all patients with stage III tumours are long-term survivors. N-*myc* amplification identifies a group with only a 20 per cent probability of EFS, whilst 85 per cent of those with favourable histology without N-*myc* amplification survive.

Stage IV in children aged >1 year

Children aged >1 year with stage IV neuroblastoma have a poor prognosis. In the majority, the malignancy is initially chemosensitive, and then drug-resistant disease recurs. With a regimen employing intensive chemotherapy, surgery, MAT, local radiotherapy, and 13-*cis*-retinoic acid, a survival of 45 per cent can be expected.

Stage IV and IVs in infants aged <1 year

Eighty-five per cent of infants without N-*myc* amplification will be long-term survivors. Some infants die because of large tumour masses and a minority progress to overt aggressive stage IV disease. In the past only 25 per cent of infants with N-*myc* amplification survived. Very preliminary results now suggest an improved survival following intensive therapy.

Novel developments

Antibody therapy

Both murine and chimeric humanized antibodies against the tumour-associated antigen GD2 have been tested in preclinical model systems and in clinical trials in neuroblastoma patients. Phase II trials combining anti-GD2 antibodies and granulocyte–macrophage colony-stimulating factor (GMCSF) for high-risk neuroblastoma patients with residual or progressive bone marrow disease showed a promising bone marrow clearance rate of ~50 per cent.[39] Currently, anti-GD2 antibody treatment, with or without GMCSF and interleukin 2, for minimal residual disease is being prospectively tested in randomized trials by SIOP Europe Neuroblastoma and the Children's Oncology Group (COG).

Detection of minimal residual disease

Several molecular targets for detection of minimal residual disease have been developed. All of them are based on the detection of gene products in general by real-time PCR. The best studied targets are tyrosine hydroxylase, GD2, and GD2 synthase. Substantial evidence for the increased sensitivity of these molecular methods for the detection of neuroblastoma cells compared with conventional cytology has accumulated.[40] The clinical relevance is the subject of ongoing prospective trials.

References

1. **Stiller CA, Parkin DM** (1992). International variations in the incidence of neuroblastoma. *Int J Cancer* 52, 538–43.
2. **Kushner BH, Gilbert F, Helson L** (1986). Familial neuroblastoma: case reports, literature review, and etiologic considerations. *Cancer* 57, 1887.
3. **Yamamoto K, Hayashi Y, Handada R, et al.** (1995). Mass screening and age-specific incidence of neuroblastoma in Saitama Prefecture, Japan. *J Clin Oncol* 13, 2033–8.
4. **Kaneko Y, Kanda N, Maseki N, et al.** (1990). Current urinary mass screening for catecholamine metabolites at 6 months of age may be detecting only a small portion of high-risk neuroblastomas: a chromosome and N-*myc* amplification study. *J Clin Oncol* 8, 2005–13.

5. **Woods WG, Gao RN, Shuster JJ,** *et al.* (2002). Screening of infants and mortality due to neuroblastoma. *N Engl J Med* **346**, 1041–6.

6. **Schilling FH, Spix C, Berthold F,** *et al.* (2002). Neuroblastoma screening at one year of age. *N Engl J Med* **346**, 1047–53.

7. **Ambros IM, Zellner A, Roald B,** *et al.* (1996). Role of ploidy, chromosome 1p, and Schwann cells in the maturation of neuroblastoma. *N Engl J Med* **334**, 1505–11.

8. **Shimada H, Ambros IM, Dehner LP,** *et al.* (1999). The International Neuroblastoma Pathology Classification (the Shimada system). *Cancer* **86**, 364–72.

9. **Maris JM, Weiss MJ, Mosse Y,** *et al.* (2002) Evidence for a hereditary neuroblastoma predisposition locus at chromosome 16p12–13 *Cancer Res* **62**, 6651–8.

10. **Perri P, Longo L, Cusano R,** *et al.* (2002). Weak linkage at 4p16 to predisposition for human neuroblastoma. *Oncogene* **21**, 8356–60.

11. **Seeger RC, Brodeur M, Sather H,** *et al.* (1985). Association of multiple copies of the N-myc oncogene with rapid progression of neuroblastomas. *N Engl J Med* **313**, 1111–16.

12. **Bown N, Cotterill S, Lastowska M,** *et al.* (1999) Gain of chromosome arm 17q and adverse outcome in patients with neuroblastoma. *N Engl J Med* **340**, 1954–61.

13. **Caron H., Van Sluis P, De Kraker J.,** *et al.* (1996). Allelic loss of chromosome 1p as a predictor of unfavourable outcome in patients with neuroblastoma. *N Engl J Med* **334**, 225–30.

14. **Fong CT, White PS, Peterson K,** *et al.* (1992). Loss of heterozygosity for chromosome 1 or 14 defines subsets of advanced neuroblastomas. *Cancer Res* **69**, 1780–85.

15. **Gehring T, Berthold F, Edler L,** *et al.* (1995).Chromosome 1p loss is not a reliable prognostic marker in neuroblastoma. *Cancer Res* **55**, 5366–9.

16. **Teitz T, Wei T, Valentine MB,** *et al.* (2000). Caspase 8 is deleted or silenced preferentially in childhood neuroblastomas with amplification of MYCN. *Nat Med* **6**, 529–39.

17. **Altman AJ, Baehneev RL** (1976). Favourable prognosis for survival in children with coincident opsomyoclonus and neuroblastoma. *Cancer* **37**, 846.

18. **Rudnick E, Khakoo Y, Antunes NL,** *et al.* (2001) Opsoclonus–myoclonus–ataxia syndrome in neuroblastoma: clinical outcome and antineuronal antibodies-a report from the Children's Cancer Group Study. *Med Paediatr Oncol* **136**, 612–22.

19. **Kaplan S, Holbrook C, McDaniel HG,** *et al.* (1980). Vasoactive intestinal peptide secreting tumors of childhood. *Am J Dis Child* **134**, 21.

20. **Brodeur GM, Pritchard J, Berthold F,** *et al.* (1993). Revisions of international criteria for neuroblastoma diagnosis, staging and response to treatment. *J Clin Oncol* **11**,1466–77.

21. **Silber JH, Evans AE, Friedman M** (1991). Models to predict outcome from childhood neuroblastoma: the role of serum ferritin and tumor histology. *Cancer Res* **51**, 1426–33.

22. **DeBernardi B, Conte M, Mancini A.,** *et al.* (1995). Localized resectable neuroblastoma: results of the second study of the Italian Cooperative Group for Neuroblastoma. *J Clin Oncol* **13**, 884–93.

23. **Look AT, Flayes FA, Schuster JJ,** *et al.* (1991). Clinical relevance of tumour cell ploidy and N-*myc* gene amplification in childhood neuroblastoma. *J Clin Oncol* **9**, 581–91.

24. **Kushner BH, Cheung N-KV, LaQuaglia MP,** *et al.* (1996). Survival from locally invasive or widespread neuroblastoma without cytotoxic therapy. *J Clin Oncol* **14**, 373–81.

25. **Berthold F, Hero B, Breu H,** *et al.* (1996).The recurrence patterns of stages I, II and III neuroblastoma: experience with 77 relapsing patients. *Ann Oncol* **7**, 183–7.

26. **Rubie H, Michon J, Plantaz D,** *et al.* (1998). Unresectable localized neuroblastoma: improved survival after primary chemotherapy including carboplatin–etoposide. Neuroblastoma Study Group of the Société Française d'Oncologie Pediatrique (SFOP). *Br J Cancer* **77**, 2310–17.

27. **Philip T, Bernard JL, Zucker JM, et al.** (1987). High dose chemoradiotherapy with bone marrow transplantation as consolidation treatment in neuroblastoma: an unselected group of stage 4 patients over 1 year of age. *J Clin Oncol* 5, 266–71.

28. **Matthay KK, Villablanca JG, Seeger RC, et al.** (1999). Treatment of high-risk neuroblastoma with intensive chemotherapy, radiotherapy, autologous bone marrow transplantation, and 13-*cis*-retinoic acid. Children's Cancer Group. *N Engl J Med* 341, 1165–73.

29. **Pinkerton CR, Pritchard J, de Kraker J.** (1987). ENSG 1. Randomized study of high dose melphalan in neuroblastoma. In: Dicke KA, Spitzer G, Japannath S (eds) *Autologous Bone Marrow Transplantation.* Austin, TX: University of Texas Press, 401–6.

30. **Hartmann O, Valteau CD, Vassal G, et al.** (1999) Prognostic factors in metastatic neuroblastoma in patients over 1 year of age treated with high-dose chemotherapy and stem cell transplantation: a multivariate analysis in 218 patients treated in a single institution. *Bone Marrow Transplant* 23, 789–95.

31. **Matthay KK, Seeger RC, Reynolds CP, et al.** (1994). Allogeneic versus autologous purged bone marrow transplantation for neuroblastoma: a report from the Children's Cancer Group. *J Clin Oncol* 12, 2382–6.

32. **Kushner BH, LaQuaglia MP, Bonilla MA, et al.** (1994). Highly effective induction therapy for stage 4 neuroblastoma in children over 1 year of age. *J Clin Oncol* 12, 2607–13.

33. **Cheung NV, Heller G** (1991). Chemotherapy dose intensity correlates strongly with response, median survival, and median progression-free survival in metastatic neuroblastoma. *J Clin Oncol* 9, 1050–8.

34. **Pearson ADJ, Craft AW, Pinkerton CR, et al.** (1992). High dose rapid schedule chemotherapy for disseminated neuroblastoma. *Eur J Cancer* 28A 1654–9.

35. **Coze C, Hartmann O, Michon J, et al.** (1997). NB87 induction protocol for stage 4 neuroblastoma in children over 1 year of age: a report from the French Society of Paediatric Oncology. *J Clin Oncol* 15, 3433–40.

36. **DeBernardi B, Pianca C, Boni L, et al.** (1992). Disseminated neuroblastoma (stage IV and IV-S) in the first year of life. Outcome related to age and stage. Italian Cooperative Group on Neuroblastoma. *Cancer* 70, 1625–33.

37. **Troncone L, Rufini V** (1997). ^{131}I-MIBG therapy of neural crest tumours (review). *Anticancer Res* 17, 1823–31.

38. **De Kraker J, Hoefnagel CA, Caron H, et al.** (1995). First line targeted radiotherapy, a new concept in the treatment of advanced stage neuroblastoma. *Eur J Cancer* 31A, 600–2.

39. **Kushner BH, Kramer K, Cheung NK** (2001). Phase II trial of the anti-G (D2) monoclonal antibody 3F8 and granulocyte–macrophage colony-stimulating factor for neuroblastoma. *J Clin Oncol* 19, 4189–94.

40. **Burchill SA, Lewis IJ, Abrams KR, et al.** (2001) Circulating neuroblastoma cells detected by reverse transcriptase polymerase chain reaction for tyrosine hydroxylase mRNA are an independent poor prognostic indicator in stage 4 neuroblastoma in children over 1 year. *J Clin Oncol* 19, 1795–1801.

Chapter 23

Germ cell tumours in children and adolescents

Ulrich Göbel, Gabriele Calaminus, and Dominik T. Schneider

Introduction

Germ cell tumours (GCTs) constitute a highly heterogeneous group of tumours that vary significantly with respect to clinical presentation, histology, and biology. In adolescents and adults, they most commonly develop within the gonads. In young men, testicular GCTs represent the most frequent solid tumour. In contrast, childhood GCTs predominantly arise at extragonadal midline sites such as the sacrococcygeal region, the central nervous system (CNS), and the anterior mediastinum. This heterogeneous clinical presentation requires a multimodal treatment that includes the paediatric oncologist in cooperation with appropriate surgical disciplines (paediatric surgeon, urologist, gynaecologist, thoracic surgeon, and neuro-surgeon) and the radiotherapist.

During the past two decades, a dramatic improvement in the prognosis of malignant GCTs has been achieved in both the adult and paediatric populations. This progress can be attributed to national and international cooperative studies that utilize cisplatin-based chemotherapy as part of a multimodal therapeutic approach. The first paediatric trials revealed the particular clinical and biologic features of childhood GCT. Moreover, the early observations have allowed therapy to be tailored more specifically to the paediatric setting and stratification of chemo-therapy according to defined risk groups to be introduced.

In this chapter, we shall review the rapid developments of recent years, and describe what should be considered as state-of-the-art therapy for paediatric GCT.

Epidemiology

GCTs can become clinically apparent in all age groups, ranging from the fetal period to adulthood. Among children aged <15 years, GCTs account for ~3–4 per cent of cancers. Thus the annual incidence can be estimated as approximately 0.5 per 100 000 children aged <15 years. However, it should be taken into account that teratomas may be under-reported to cancer registries, resulting in an underestimation of the incidence rate.

The clinical data reported to the German trials for testicular and non-testicular GCTs show a distinct distribution pattern with regard to site and tumour histology[1]. During childhood, most GCTs present at non-gonadal sites close to the body axis, such as the sacrococcygeal region, the mediastinum, or the pineal gland. Figures 23.1 and 23.2 show that, in general, two incidence peaks can be distinguished. The first peak includes teratomas (in neonates) and yolk sac tumours (during infancy and early childhood). These predominantly arise in the sacrococcygeal

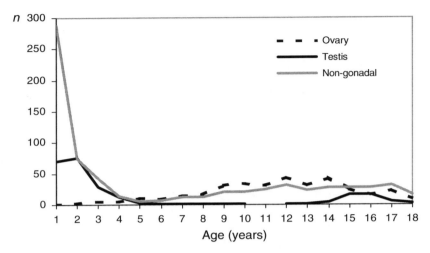

Fig 23.1 Age distribution with respect to primary tumour site in 1307 children and adolescents with germ cell tumours registered in the MAKEI protocols. Reproduced from D.T. Schneider et al. [1]

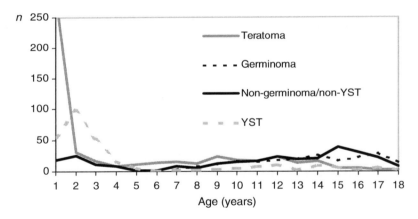

Fig 23.2 Age distribution with respect to histology in 1307 children and adolescents with germ cell tumours registered in the MAKEI protocols. YST, yolk sac tumour. Reproduced from D.T. Schneider et al. [1]

region and testis, and less frequently in the mediastinum or retroperitoneum. During adolescence there is another peak of incidence which is due to gonadal, mediastinal, and CNS tumours. Histologically, these tumours resemble germinoma (also known as seminoma or dysgerminoma) or non-seminomas including embryonal carcinoma, choriocarcinoma, and yolk sac tumour. Spermatocytic seminomas are not observed in adolescents and young adults. In conclusion, the age–characteristic distribution of GCTs has a significant impact on differential diagnostic considerations and should guide therapeutic decisions.

Table 23.1. Histologic classification of germ cell tumours (WHO)

	Synonyms
1. Seminoma (SE)	Dysgerminoma (DYS) (ovary), germinoma (GE) (brain)
2. Yolk sac tumour (YST)	Endodermal sinus tumour
3. Embryonal carcinoma (EC)	–
4. Choriocarcinoma (CHC)	–
5. Teratoma (TER)	
5.1. Mature	–
5.1.1. Solid	–
5.1.2. Cystic	Dermoid cyst
5.2. Immature (IT)	–
5.3. With malignant transformation	–
5.4. Monodermal	–
6. Tumours with mixed histology (MGCT)	–
7. Spermatocytic seminoma (SS)	–
8. Polyembryoma (POLY)	–

Histologic classification of germ cell tumours

GCTs are characterized by a profound heterogeneity in histologic differentiation. They are classified according to the World Health Organization (WHO) classification of testicular, ovarian, and intracranial tumours (Table 23.1). In our experience, these classifications constitute a more precise morphologic description than the traditional British classification as they permit recognition of all histologic components of mixed malignant GCT. As intratumour heterogeneity may be subtle, the initial diagnostic workup should include evaluation by a pathologist experienced in GCT histology in order to achieve a standardized and reliable histopathologic diagnosis and grading (Tables 23.1 and 23.2).

According to the holistic concept of Teilum, GCTs arise from totipotent primordial germ cells which are capable of embryonic and extraembryonic differentiation (Fig. 23.3). Yolk sac tumours and choriocarcinoma follow an extra-embryonic differentiation pattern and are

Table 23.2. Biological characteristics of histologic germ cell tumour subentities

	Histological grading	Tumour marker		Sensitivity to	
		AFP	β–HCG	CT	RT
Seminoma/germinoma	Malignant	–	(+)	+++	≥24 Gy
Embryonal carcinoma	Malignant	–	–	+++	≥45 Gy
Yolk sac tumour	Malignant	+++	–	+++	≥45 Gy
Choriocarcinoma	Malignant	–	+++	+++	≥45 Gy
Teratoma, mature/immature	Benign/potentially malignant	–/(+)	–	?	?

AFP, α-fetoprotein; β–HCG, human chorionic gonadotrophin; CT, chemotherapy; RT, radiotherapy.

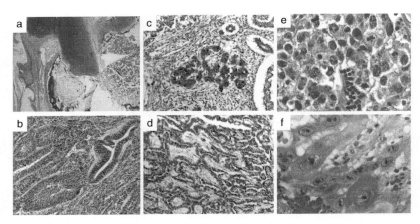

Fig. 23.3 Characteristic histologic morphology of paediatric germ cell tumours. (a) Mature sacrococcygeal teratoma displaying bone, cartilage, bone marrow, fibrous tissue, glial tissue and squamous epithelium (H&E, 10×). (b) Immature sacrococcygeal teratoma with immature neurotubuli (H&E, 10×). (c) Immature sacrococcygeal teratoma with microfoci of yolk sac tumour (AFP immunohistochemistry, 10×). (d) Mediastinal yolk sac tumour with reticular and papillary growth pattern (H&E, 10×). (e) Pineal germinoma with clear cytoplasm and rounded nuclei with prominent nucleoli; scattered nests of lymphocytes (H&E, 40×). (f) Mediastinal choriocarcinoma with syncytiotrophoblastic giant cells (H&E, 40×).

characterized by significant secretion of α_1-fetoprotein (AFP) or human choriogonadotropin (HCG or β-HCG), respectively (Table 23.3). Embryonal carcinomas represent tumours of immature totipotent cells. Teratomas display embryonic differentiation and may mimic organ structures of all germ layers. In teratoma, the histologic grade of immaturity is defined by the extent of immature (predominantly neuroepithelial) elements (Table 23.2).[2] The histologic grading of immaturity correlates with the risk of locoregional relapse, particularly after incomplete resection, and therefore is essential for risk assessment of pure teratomas.[3] Finally, germinomatous tumours [seminoma (testis), dysgerminoma (ovary), germinoma (brain)] display morphologic features of undifferentiated germinal epithelium. In contrast with testicular GCTs of adult patients, paediatric GCTs do not develop from carcinoma *in situ*.

In most patients, the response to the different therapeutic modalities can be predicted from the histologic appearance and the tumour marker profile (Table 23.3). About 25 per cent of all paediatric GCTs present as tumours with more than one histologic type. In this situation therapy and prognosis depend on the component with the highest malignancy.[4]

Table 23.3. Histologic grading of teratomas (Gonzalez-Crussi et al.[2])

Mature teratoma (grade 0)	All tissue components appear well differentiated
Immature teratoma	Some components consist of incompletely differentiated tissue
Grade 1	Occasional foci ≤10% of the sampled surface
Grade 2	10%–50% of the sampled surface
Grade 3	>50% of the sampled surface consist of undifferentiated tissue

Biology

Molecular studies of the imprinting status substantiate the hypothesis that non-gonadal GCTs develop from germ cells that have mislocated during their embryonic development.[5] While no consistent correlation between cytogenetic aberration and primary tumour site has been observed, it is apparent that histology (teratoma versus malignant GCT) and age (prepubertal versus postpubertal) both significantly correlate with distinct genetic profiles.[6] More than 80 per cent of malignant testicular GCTs of young males display a distinct and specific chromosomal aberration, the isochromosome 12p.[7] The remaining isochromosome-12p-negative tumours frequently show amplification of 12p (homogeneously staining regions or tandem repeats), and candidate genes have recently been identified in this region. These aberrations have been observed in both testicular and ovarian tumours, and in mediastinal GCTs. In mediastinal GCTs, there is a considerable association with constitutional Klinefelter syndrome, which constitutes a major risk factor for the early development of malignant mediastinal GCTs.

Ovarian GCTs show a significant association with constitutional aberrations of the sex chromosomes, i.e. lack of the second X chromosome (Ullrich–Turner syndrome) or presence of the Y chromosome at the microscopic or submicroscopic level. In such patients, ovarian dysgerminomas may develop within gonadoblastomas, which may therefore be considered a premalignant stage. Furthermore, these tumours may sometimes be associated with abnormal development of the external and internal genitalia (e.g. streak gonads in Swyer syndrome) and testicular feminization. In characteristic cases, these 'ovaries' histologically resemble testes. A prophylactic removal of the second ovary is mandatory in these patients because of the significant risk of contralateral tumours and the obvious lack of physiologic reproductive function.

In contrast with adult patients, isochromosome 12p has rarely been found in malignant GCT in children aged <10 years. On the other hand, aberrations at chromosomes 1, 6, and 20 and the sex chromosomes have frequently been found. Studies of childhood yolk sac tumours have revealed frequent loss of heterozygosity at the distal part of the short arm of chromosome 1 and the long arm of chromosome 6 in a region that includes the *IGF-2* receptor gene.

Finally, virtually all pure teratomas are cytogenetically normal. However, cystic teratoma of the ovary may present with isodisomic karyotype, consistent with its origin from postmeiotic germ cells.

Diagnosis

In general, GCTs tend to occur as indolent masses and clinical symptoms are mostly related to local tumour growth. For instance, mediastinal GCTs may cause airway obstruction or superior vena cava syndrome, while pelvic GCTs may lead to obstipation. A defined programme of clinical, radiographic, and laboratory investigations has to be followed in a timely fashion in order to address the central strategic questions as to whether a biopsy must be obtained for diagnostic purposes, and whether a primary tumour resection or preoperative chemotherapy followed by delayed resection is preferable.

Tumour markers

Depending on their histologic differentiation, GCT tend to secrete the tumour markers AFP and/or HCG/β-HCG (Table 23.3). These facilitate clinical diagnosis in tumours that present at typical sites.[8] However, it must be taken into account that serum AFP levels may be greatly elevated in neonates and infants.[9] It is important to note that, in contrast with other reports, this series of normal neonates and infants has demonstrated that in a significant percentage of healthy children, AFP does not decline to the normal range of adult patients before the end of the second year of life.[9] Therefore, in the first 2 years of life, only AFP levels significantly above the age-related normal value can be regarded as diagnostic for a secreting GCT.

In general, the tumour marker profile is highly specific for the histologic differentiation of the tumour (Table 23.3).[8] However, there may be secretion of β chains of HCG in seminoma/germinoma (<50 IU/l), which is often related to syncytiotrophoblast-like giant cells. Some patients with immature teratoma show a moderate elevation of the AFP level (<100 μg/l), sometimes associated with histologically detectable small yolk sac tumour foci within the teratoma. On the other hand, microscopic yolk sac tumour foci (Fig. 23.3) may also be present and not result in clinically apparent elevation of AFP. In CNS GCT, tumour markers may frequently be elevated at different levels in CSF and serum. Their values can be within normal range in CSF and elevated in serum or vice versa. Therefore measurement in both compartments is mandatory at diagnosis. About 20 per cent of germinoma may secrete placenta-like alkaline phosphatase (PLAP), which can be used as an additional diagnostic tool if elevated.

Diagnostic imaging

Appropriate radiographic procedures must be performed according to tumour site and potential routes of tumour dissemination. In most patients with extracranial tumours, the initial radiographic assessment of the tumour will be made by ultrasound. During ultrasound, the tumour should be measured in three dimensions, and the abdomen and the lymph nodes should also be screened for metastases. The next step is to perform CT or preferably MRI scans of the tumour.

In pelvic tumours, imaging includes the upper abdomen in order to detect lymphatic spread to the nodes at the renal veins or liver metastases. Sacrococcygeal tumours must be evaluated with MRI including sagittal images to exclude spread into the sacral and spinal canal.

In CNS GCTs MRI examinations should include axial, sagittal, and coronal images of the whole brain and the complete spine, and these must be supplemented by CSF cytology in order to detect CSF metastases. There is a consensus that if a bifocal CNS tumour is diagnosed radiologically (pineal and suprasellar region), the radiologic features together with negative markers in CSF/serum and negative CSF cytology are sufficient for diagnosis of a germinoma.

Skeletal metastases have been observed in ~10 per cent of patients; however, their occurrence has not adversely affected prognosis. Metastases to the CNS, which may be found in ~4 per cent of young males with malignant testicular GCTs are extremely rare (<1 per cent) during childhood. Therefore MRI scans of the CNS are not considered mandatory in extracranial GCTs.

Laboratory studies (pretreatment)

In addition to the tumour markers AFP and β-HCG, serum lactate dehydrogenase (LDH) has proved to be a prognostic marker in adult patients with GCTs. In germinomas, PLAP can be measured in the serum and may then serve as a marker of treatment response during follow-up. In addition to the routine blood tests before chemotherapy, special attention should be paid to renal function (creatinine clearance, urine electrolytes), as several cytotoxic agents such as platinum-compounds and ifosfamide may interfere with this. Finally, a cytogenetic analysis of blood lymphocytes is recommended in female patients with malignant ovarian GCTs and male patients with mediastinal GCTs in order to exclude constitutional aberrations such as Ullrich–Turner or Klinefelter syndromes.

Therapy

Surgery

If the initial radiographic assessment demonstrates infiltration into adjacent organs and/or metastases, initial (up-front) chemotherapy followed by delayed tumour resection is recommended, as preoperative chemotherapy will facilitate complete resection at delayed surgery.[10] Tumour marker measurement in combination with imaging permits a clinical diagnosis at most sites, except the liver and the retroperitoneum.[8] In equivocal cases (i.e. non-diagnostic markers, hepatic or upper retroperitoneal tumours), a diagnostic biopsy is recommended, which should include obtaining fresh tumour tissue for genetic and biologic studies.

If the radiographic assessment indicates a localized tumour without metastatic spread, the treatment of choice is primary tumour resection, except in the CNS as this region carries specific risks of surgical morbidity. In general, there is no role for debulking surgery in paediatric GCT. Surgery must always aim for a microscopically complete resection, as incomplete resection carries the risk of recurrence, even with adjuvant chemotherapy.[10] The criteria of complete resection are the resection of the tumour with capsule and adjacent organs *en bloc*. If this is not achieved, tumour resection has to be regarded as incomplete and an increased risk of recurrence must be considered.

In patients with tumour residues after initial tumour resection, second-look surgery is essential to achieve secondary complete resection. This is also the case in malignant non-germinomatous CNS GCTs. Second-look surgery may at least partially overcome the otherwise unfavourable prognostic impact of incomplete resection.[10] Finally, surgery of metastases is not indicated unless they show insufficient response to chemotherapy.[10,11]

Surgical techniques:

Rescorla[12] has recently reviewed surgical techniques in paediatric GCTs.

Testis

The resection of testicular tumours is performed by unilateral orchidectomy after high inguinal incision. Trans-scrotal biopsy is obsolete and such a procedure will be considered an indication for adjuvant chemotherapy, even in otherwise stage I tumours. Retroperitoneal lymph node dissection is not advocated because of the increased risk of retrograde ejaculation and the overall favourable response to adjuvant chemotherapy in childhood GCTs.

Ovary

The resection of ovarian tumours should be performed after midline laparatomy. Because of the risk of bilateral tumours, a biopsy of the contralateral ovary should be performed in cases of macroscopically suspicious appearance. Intraperitoneal fluid or ascites must be examined cytologically to exclude malignant ascites.

Coccyx

Coccygeal tumours frequently present as large tumours with intrapelvic and sometimes extra-pelvic components. Therefore a dorsal approach is used in most patients. Infiltrated skin areas should be removed *en bloc* with the tumour. Postoperatively, bowel and bladder function recover in the vast majority of patients. The coccyx should be resected *en bloc* to avoid tumour rupture. The so-called hourglass formation of coccygeal tumours refers to a huge tumour partially sited in the bony pelvis incorporating the coccygeal region. In these tumours, an additional ventral approach is useful to achieve a complete *en bloc* resection.

Central nervous system

As most CNS GCTs are located centrally, surgery is often difficult and prone to complications. In addition, it is almost impossible to achieve a complete resection of an intracranial tumour.[13] Therefore radiotherapy has become an integral part of the treatment of intracranial GCTs. As a consequence, surgical interventions should now be reserved for diagnostic biopsies in non-secreting tumours or for tumours with significant residues after chemotherapy and/or radiotherapy. Only neonatal teratomas of the CNS should be considered an exception from this recommendation, as tumour resection constitutes the only meaningful therapeutic approach for these patients who often present with large tumours and hydrocephalus.

The surgical approach to the other extragonadal sites such as the mediastinum or retroperitoneum must be planned according to the presenting situation.

Cisplatin-based chemotherapy

Until 1980, the prognosis of children with malignant GCTs was poor, and outcome was determined by the parameters of age, site, histology, and stage. The modern era of GCT chemotherapy began in the mid-1970s with the identification of the efficacy of cisplatin in testicular GCTs. In 1977, Einhorn and Donohue[14] reported a complete response rate of 85 per cent in patients with metastatic testicular GCTs treated with a combination of cisplatin, vinblastine, and bleomycin (PVB) and tumour resection. Most importantly, in contrast with a previously reported regimen using only vinblastine and bleomycin, the overall good response was also translated into durable remissions.

Nevertheless, relapses or refractory cancers, although rare, established the need for second-line therapies. Etoposide soon emerged as an active drug with a single-agent efficacy superior to vinblastine. Moreover, etoposide shows a more favourable acute toxicity profile with less neuromuscular toxicity. On the other hand, the use of etoposide may be associated with therapy-related leukaemias in ~1–2 per cent of patients.

In addition, the efficacy of ifosfamide in cisplatin-refractory GCTs has been documented. The combination of cisplatin with etoposide and ifosfamide for recurrent testicular GCTs results in a 30 per cent durable remission rate and can now be considered standard treatment for relapse. These observations initiated studies that included etoposide and/or ifosfamide in the first-line treatment of GCTs.

The combination of cisplatin, etoposide and bleomycin (BEP) is now considered standard chemotherapy for GCTs in adult patients. In most patients, a total of three cycles is considered appropriate. The inclusion of ifosfamide in first-line treatment (PEI) did not result in significantly improved outcome but was associated with higher bone marrow and renal toxicity compared with BEP.

In relapsing and refractory GCTs, the therapeutic value of high-dose chemotherapy with autologous stem cell transplantation has been investigated. These analyses have shown only limited efficacy in prognostically unfavourable tumours such as cisplatin-resistant mediastinal GCTs with high β-HCG or multiple relapses. Nevertheless, introduction of high-dose chemotherapy into first-line treatment of high-risk tumours may be beneficial in some patients. Finally, 'modern' drugs, such as paclitaxel and gemcitabine, are currently under investigation.

Development of cooperative protocols for paediatric GCTs

Encouraged by the data discussed above, prospective protocols for gonadal and non-gonadal GCTs in children and adolescents were initiated. The first published trial was conducted by the US Children's Cancer Group (CCG) and included 54 children with malignant non-seminomatous GCT. Patients underwent initial tumour resection followed by VAC + PVB chemotherapy over a 2-year period, second-look resection 4 months after diagnosis, and irradiation if there was residual tumour[15]. Fifteen of 20 evaluable patients with ovarian non-seminomatous GCTs, including a substantial proportion of high-stage tumours, achieved continuous clinical remission. The prognosis of children with non-gonadal GCTs was worse but still encouraging compared with all other previous studies.

The analysis of the following CCG protocol included 93 children and showed that patients with ovarian GCTs had a better prognosis [4-year event-free survival (EFS) of 63 per cent] than children with non-gonadal GCTs (4-year EFS of 42 per cent).[16] This difference was mainly attributed to a higher rate of incomplete tumour resections in non-gonadal tumours.

In the US Intergroup protocol, a watch-and-wait policy was followed in stage I testicular GCTs. Intermediate-risk patients (testicular stage II, ovarian, and non-gonadal stage I–II) received four cycles of cisplatin, etoposide, and bleomycin (reduced to one infusion per cycle compared with three infusions in corresponding adult regimens). Furthermore, the therapeutic impact of cisplatin dose intensification at 200 mg/m^2/cycle was evaluated in high-risk patients (stage III–IV). The analysis of both gonadal and non-gonadal GCTs revealed that higher doses of cisplatin may result in higher response and complete remission rates ($\sim$9 per cent benefit), but with significantly higher renal and auditory toxicity. Notably, two-thirds of patients in the high-dose cisplatin arm required hearing aids after completion of treatment. More recent investigations of this study group aimed to evaluate amifostine protection during cisplatin therapy at escalated doses; however, no significant benefit with regard to ototoxicity has been demonstrated, and amifostine therapy was associated with significant electrolyte imbalances, particularly hypocalcaemia (data presented at the ASCO Conference, 2003).

The analysis of different chemotherapy regimens administered in the British UKCCSG GC I and GC II protocols also demonstrated the high therapeutic efficacy of platinum-based regimens such as BEP or JEB (carboplatin 600 mg/m^2/cycle, etoposide, and bleomycin), which resulted in a 5-year EFS of 57 per cent and 87 per cent, respectively, in non-gonadal GCTs.[17] The recent analysis of the UKCCSG GC II study emphasizes the high efficacy of the JEB regimen, with a 5-year EFS of 88 per cent and a favourable toxicity profile.[18]

The French study group reported 35 children with ovarian and non-gonadal advanced stage GCTs who were treated with a VAC + PB regimen.[19] The French cooperative protocol TGM 85 used a similar chemotherapeutic approach, and in the next TGM 90 protocol cisplatin was replaced by carboplatin (400 mg/m^2/cycle).[20] The results were less favourable with this regimen than with the British JEB regimen. This difference was mainly attributed to the lower single and cumulative doses of carboplatin. In the recent French protocol, alternating combinations of cisplatin with etoposide or ifosfamide are administered, resulting in a superior response rate compared to the previous carboplatin based strategy.

In both the French TGM 90 and the British GC II studies, the analysis of prognostic factors revealed the prognostic impact of high AFP serum levels at diagnosis, a finding that could not be confirmed in other studies using cisplatin-based regimens[10,21] or in the ongoing French protocol.

From 1982 onwards, the German protocols for testicular (MAHO) and non-testicular (MAKEI) GCTs included cisplatin- and etoposide-based chemotherapy regimens integrated into a multimodal approach that also recommended delayed tumour resection after preoperative or neoadjuvant chemotherapy. As early reports indicated an increased risk of bleomycin-associated pulmonary toxicity in children (particularly infants) compared with adults, the German MAKEI protocol recommended the sequential administration of bleomycin and cisplatin. Furthermore, from 1989 onwards, the bleomycin dose was reduced in children aged <2 years and withheld in infants. As a result of the excellent EFS of >80 per cent achieved with the first MAKEI and MAHO protocols, the cumulative chemotherapy was reduced stepwise from a maximum of eight to six cycles, and currently to four or five cycles. This reduction of cumulative chemotherapy did not affect outcome.[10] In addition, a risk stratification of chemotherapy according to age, site, histology, stage, and completeness of resection has been introduced: The favourable outcome for infants with malignant GCTs from whom bleomycin was withheld because of their age, indicated the higher chemosensitivity of malignant GCTs in this age group and encouraged the reduction of chemotherapy to a two-agent regimen with cisplatin and etoposide in some low-risk patients. Moreover, according to the current MAKEI 96 protocol, an expectant watch-and-wait strategy is recommended for patients with completely resected low-stage tumours. This approach makes it possible to avoid chemotherapy in ~75 per cent of patients with stage Ia malignant GCTs. However, patients who relapse during the surveillance require a more intensive regimen with four cycles of three-agent chemotherapy, and therefore therapy is intensified in these patients. In locally advanced and/or metastatic tumours a neoadjuvant approach appears beneficial as it facilitates complete tumour resection and thereby reduces the need for second-look surgery.

In summary, the PEI, BEP, CarboPEI, and JEB regimens (Table 23.4) have synergistic cytotoxic activity and can be considered as standard regimens of comparable efficacy. These regimens are used in the paediatric GCT protocols currently open.

Side effects of chemotherapy

Pulmonary toxicity of bleomycin, which had also been reported as a problem in combination with impaired kidney function or enhanced by anaesthesia, led to the introduction of a regimen without this drug. However, the current US Intergroup Study has demonstrated that a reduction of bleomycin from three to one infusions per cycle does not affect outcome. In this study, no deaths due to pulmonary toxicity have been observed. On the other hand, the highly efficient combination of cisplatin, etoposide, and ifosfamide (PEI) is associated with a higher degree of myelosuppression and carries the risk of tubular nephropathy, particularly in small children. In our experience with this regimen, we observed clinically apparent hearing impairment in 5 per cent of patients. In contrast, two-thirds of patients treated with high-dose cisplatin (200 mg/m^2 per cycle) require hearing aids. Although the auditory toxicity and the renal toxicity of carboplatin regimens are smaller, carboplatin at effective doses (600 mg/m^2/ cycle) causes substantial myelotoxicity.[18] The risk of therapy-related secondary leukaemia is dependent on the therapeutic modalities used, with an estimated cumulative risk of 1.0 per cent (3/442 patients) (Kaplan–Meier method at 10-year follow-up) for children treated with surgery and chemotherapy only and 4.2 per cent (3/174 patients) for children treated with combined radio- and chemotherapy.

Therapeutic strategies of current protocols for malignant germ cell tumours

In general, current paediatric GCT protocols apply different strategies. Some protocols define cumulative chemotherapy according to the response to treatment (e.g. one standard chemotherapy regimen to a total of two cycles after achieving complete remission[17,18]). In other

Table 23.4. Standard chemotherapy regimens in paediatric GCT

PEI (MAKEI 96, SIOP-CNS-GCT 96, MAHO 98, SFOP)

Cisplatin[a]	20 mg/m²	Over 1 h	Day 1, 2, 3, 4, 5
Etoposide	100 mg/m²	Over 3 h	Day 1, 2, 3
Ifosfamide[b]	1500 mg/m²	Over 20 h	Day 1, 2, 3, 4, 5
Two to four cycles			

PVB (MAHO 98)

Cisplatin[a]	20 mg/m²	Over 1 h	Day 4, 5, 6, 7, 8
Vinblastine	3 mg/m² or 0.15 mg/kg	IV bolus	Day 1, 2
Bleomycin[c]	15 mg/m²	Over 24 h	Day 1, 2, 3
Three cycles			

BEP (MAHO 98)

Bleomycin[c]	15 mg/m²	Over 24 h	Day 1, 2, 3
Etoposide	80 mg/m²	Over 3 h	Day 1, 2, 3
Cisplatin[a]	20 mg/m²	Over 1 h	Day 4, 5, 6, 7, 8
Three cycles			

BEP (US Childrens Oncology Group)

Bleomycin	15 mg/m²	Over 24 h	Day 1
Etoposide	100 mg/m²	Over 3 h	Day 1, 2, 3, 4, 5
Cisplatin[a]	20 mg/m²	Over 1 h	Day 1, 2, 3, 4, 5
Four cycles			

High-dose BEP (US Children's Oncology Group)

Bleomycin	15 mg/m²	Over 24 h	Day 1
Etoposide	100 mg/m²	Over 3 h	Day 1, 2, 3, 4, 5
Cisplatin[a]	40 mg/m²	Over 1 h	Day 1, 2, 3, 4, 5
Four cycles			

JEB (UKCCSG GCII)

Carboplatin	600 mg/m²	Over 1 h	Day 2
Etoposide	120 mg/m²	Over 1 h	Day 1, 2, 3
Bleomycin[c]	15 mg/m²	Over 15 min	Day 3
Five cycles, or two cycles after complete remission			

CarboPEI (SIOP-CNS-GCT 96)

Carboplatin	600 mg/m²	Over 1 h	Day 1
Etoposide	100 mg/m²	Over 3 h	Day 1, 2, 3, 22, 23, 24
Ifosfamide[b]	1800 mg/m²	Over 3 h	Day 22, 23, 24, 25, 26
Two cycles			

[a] Plus mannitol-forced diuresis.
[b] Plus mesna uroprotection.
[c] Omitted in children aged <1 year; 7.5 mg/m² in children aged <2 years.

protocols, therapy is stratified according to initial diagnostic parameters, and is only intensified if there is insufficient response to treatment. In the following sections, we summarize the international SIOP-CNS-GCT 96 protocol and the common strategies for the risk-stratified treatment of extracranial GCTs.

SIOP-CNS-GCT 96 protocol for malignant intracranial GCTs

Therapy for malignant intracranial GCTs is stratified according to histologic differentiation (i.e. germinoma versus secreting GCT) and initial dissemination.[22,23] The ongoing SIOP-CNS-GCT protocol aims to evaluate and standardize diagnostic procedures, which include measurement of markers in serum/CSF, CSF cytology, and MRI of head and spine in all patients. Two different therapeutic options in intracranial germinoma are being evaluated with regard to both their therapeutic impact and their specific acute and long-term toxicity. For secreting intracranial tumours and embryonal carcinoma, the effect of a combined treatment with PEI (Table 23.4) and radiotherapy adapted to dissemination is examined.[22]

In pure intracranial germinoma, which accounts for 50 per cent of all intracranial GCTs which do not secrete significant amounts of HCG/β-HCG, histologic verification of the tumour is mandatory. According to the current SIOP-CNS-GCT 96 protocol, patients with germinoma and localized disease can be treated either with craniospinal irradiation with 24 Gy and a tumour boost of 16 Gy or with a multimodal treatment including two cycles of chemotherapy [CarboPEI (Table 23.4)] followed by focal irradiation (40 Gy). In metastatic disease craniospinal irradiation and boost to tumour and metastatic sites is still the treatment of choice. The higher local dose to the primary tumour also aims for the control of potential small foci of non-germinomatous histology such as syncytiotrophoblastic cells that may have been missed by biopsy. To date, data concerning the effect of chemotherapy and localized RT reveal that this approach carries a higher risk of ventricular relapses (Cefalo, data presented at the SIOP Conference, 1995; Alapetite, data presented at the SIOP Conference, 2002). Therefore additional ventricular treatment is implemented in new protocols for localized CNS germinoma. As GCT may arise adjacent to sensitive structures such as the optic chiasma, it is recommended that a paediatric radiotherapist should be consulted about optimal treatment techniques. It has been demonstrated that a 5-year EFS of 91 per cent and 5-year survival of 94 per cent can be achieved with radiotherapy only,[24] but because of the higher risk of ventricular failures, the 5-year EFS of patients treated with combined therapy is ~85 per cent and survival is 92 per cent. Another important risk factor is incomplete staging in germinoma, particularly with regard to marker evaluation in serum/CSF. More than 50 per cent of relapsing patients show secretion of markers which had not been measured at the initial diagnosis of a germinoma (Calaminus, data presented at the SIOP Conference, 2003). The secreting intracranial GCTs show a poorer prognosis than germinomas. In these patients, four cycles of cisplatin-based chemotherapy [PEI (Table 23.4)] are given, followed by delayed tumour resection and radiotherapy. The radiotherapy is stratified according to initial stage. Non-metastatic tumours receive focal irradiation (54 Gy), whereas patients with intracranial or spinal metastases or tumour cells in the CSF receive craniospinal irradiation (30 Gy plus a tumour boost of 24 Gy). Data from Balmaceda reveal[24] that chemotherapy alone is able to cure only 30% of the patients with malignant CNS GCT.

The summary of several cooperative protocols and the preliminary data of the SIOP-CNS-GCT 96 protocol suggest that long-term remission can be obtained in about two-thirds of patients. In the SIOP-CNS-GCT 96 protocol, AFP > 1000 μg/l at diagnosis and residual disease at the end of treatment have been defined as clinical risk factors and will be used for definition of risk groups in the forthcoming SIOP-CNS-GCT II protocol.

Risk-stratified treatment of extracranial germ cell tumours

Both gonadal and extragonadal GCTs are treated according to a similar therapeutic concept. Only in small non-metastatic tumours, in which radiographic evaluation shows no evidence of invasive growth beyond the organ of origin, is a primary resection recommended. In patients with bulky, invasive, or metastatic tumours, preoperative chemotherapy followed by a delayed tumour resection is preferred to avoid the risk of incomplete resection. The fall of the tumour markers according to their serum half-lives indicates a favourable response to chemotherapy.[7,8]

Adjuvant treatment

In current protocols, patients with completely resected testicular stage Ia teratoma or yolk sac tumour are treated according to a watch-and-wait strategy which includes frequent (weekly) controls of the relevant tumour marker AFP. Disease progression can be detected either as failure to normalize AFP according to its half-life or as lymph node metastases at the renal veins. With this treatment approach, chemotherapy can be omitted in >70 per cent of patients. If progression occurs, all patients can be salvaged by conventional chemotherapy. Therefore chemotherapy is reserved for those patients who show disease progression and for patients with malignant testicular tumours that are stage Ib or higher.

Ovarian tumours are treated according to the same strategy. Stage I tumours are followed expectantly and higher-stage tumours receive adjuvant chemotherapy. In the current German MAKEI protocol, completely resected stage II tumours receive two to three cycles of a two-agent regimen [PE (Table 23.4)]. After incomplete resection a three-agent combination is applied [PEI (Table 23.4)]. In other protocols, all stage II–IV patients receive a minimum of four cycles of three-agent chemotherapy (e.g. JEB or BEP). Ovarian dysgerminomas are treated according to the same strategy. Irradiation is omitted to preserve fertility.

Teratoma

Teratoma represent a distinct histologic entity which shows a significant diversity in the clinical course depending on the histologic grade of immaturity.[2,3] Mature teratoma are considered benign, whereas immature teratomas may show clinical features of malignancy. The risk of recurrence can be estimated from the parameters of primary site of the tumour, histologic grade of immaturity, and completeness of tumour resection.[3] The role of adjuvant chemotherapy has not yet been established. However, recent reports have shown that chemotherapy may not be indicated after complete tumour resection, even in the presence of small foci of yolk sac tumour.[3,26] Incompletely resected tumours have a 10 per cent risk of relapse in mature teratomas and a 20 per cent risk in immature teratomas, with increasing risk with respect to the grade of immaturity irrespective of adjuvant chemotherapy.[3] Histologically, half the recurrent tumours may display yolk sac tumour. However, after adjuvant chemotherapy no malignant histology has been observed at relapse, although chemotherapy did not reduce the overall risk of recurrence.

Follow-up

A complete clinical remission is defined as normalization of the tumour markers to within the age-related normal range and the absence of suspicious residual structures, even in patients with normalized tumour markers, as these structures may represent remaining mature teratoma. If any of these criteria are not fulfilled, a diagnostic re-evaluation and change or intensification of treatment, if necessary, is urgently indicated. Most relapses occur within the first 2 years after diagnosis. However, in some patients, late recurrences have been observed up to 5 years after diagnosis of malignant ovarian GCT or intracranial germinoma. Therefore the initial follow-up examinations after completion of chemotherapy must be performed at short intervals, with frequent (i.e. weekly) measurements of the tumour markers AFP and β-HCG early during follow-up. In watch-and-wait patients, the fall in AFP values is evaluated with regard to its serum half-life of approximately 6–7 days. The interpretation of AFP may be difficult, especially in infants aged <2 years, because of the physiologically elevated serum levels. In this context, it has proved helpful to compare the fall in AFP in neonates and infants.[9]

A delayed decline or a secondary rise in AFP levels strongly indicates incomplete tumour resection or a recurrence of yolk sac tumour.

In addition, follow-up examinations include repeated imaging of the primary site of tumour. If there is residual abnormality after chemotherapy of an extracranial GCT, resection is indicated since mature teratoma may have remained and carry the risk of tumour progression. Positron emission tomography has not proved useful in this situation, as often it cannot distinguish between mature teratoma and residual necrosis or scars. Nevertheless, in cases where complete resection after chemotherapy remains difficult or impossible, this new imaging procedure may add important information concerning the remaining metabolic/proliferative activity of the residue.

In intracranial tumours, endocrinologic tests at diagnosis and during follow-up are mandatory, since tumours of the suprasellar region in particular may be associated with endocrinologic symptoms such as diabetes insipidus or panhypopituitrism. A detailed neurologic and if possible neuropsychologic evaluation, with investigation of visuomotor function and cognitive abilities, should be carried out. This information may lead to more structured and individually adapted rehabilitation and reintegration.[27] In children treated with cisplatin-containing polychemotherapy (especially with ifosfamide), renal function must be monitored carefully for tubular nephropathy, and audiometry should be performed at diagnosis and before every course of platinum-based treatment.

In children, prolonged phosphaturia may lead to renal rickets with consequent growth retardation, while adolescents are at risk of renal osteomalacia. These long-term sequelae can be avoided by phosphate supplementation. Further attention should be drawn to the risk of therapy-related secondary leukaemia that depends on treatment intensity and type.

Relapse treatment

Cisplatin-based regimens (preferably PEI) have been successfully used in patients with recurrent or refractory tumours who have previously been treated with a non-platinum or non-carboplatin therapy.[20] Therefore we prefer a cisplatin-containing regimen in patients with relapsed tumours, if the organ toxicities related to the previous treatment allow further cisplatin therapy. On the other hand, patients suffering from severe cisplatin-related toxicity can be treated with a combination of carboplatin and high-dose etoposide (400–600 mg/m^2 on 3 days). Otherwise, there is no international consensus on strategies for treatment of recurrent GCTs. However, in Germany, the following standardized strategy is used for patients with recurrent extracranial malignant GCTs.

In our experience, >90 per cent of relapses occur at the primary site of the tumour. For example, in our series of 104 sacrococcygeal yolk sac tumours only two patients had distant recurrence, whereas 17 patients had local relapse and three patients had combined local and distant relapse.[11] Therefore relapse chemotherapy should be accompanied by intensive local therapy, preferably complete resection of the recurrent tumour after reduction by preoperative chemotherapy. We have been able to demonstrate that patients with local recurrences and poor response to conventional chemotherapy may profit from locoregional hyperthermia combined with platinum-based chemotherapy. This approach significantly enhanced local tumour control.[11,28] However, analysis of treatment of relapsed sacrococcygeal GCTs emphasized the need to use hyperthermia early, as it showed no beneficial effect in late relapses. This probably resulted from cisplatin resistance or delayed chemotherapy due to the myelotoxicity of previous treatment.[11] Finally, high-dose local irradiation at doses >45 Gy has shown some beneficial effect after incomplete resection of the recurrent tumour, whereas irradiation at lower doses was ineffective.[11] In our experience, high-dose chemotherapy with stem cell support, as applied in adult patients, has resulted in long-term remissions only in those patients in whom a clinically complete remission could be achieved prior to high dose chemotherapy.[11] Therefore we regard high-dose chemotherapy as indicated for consolidation treatment only.

In conclusion, failure of local tumour control at the primary site of tumour represents the main problem in most patients. Further significant advances in relapsing GCT will probably be based on additional improvement in local therapy.

The chance of achieving a second remission for malignant CNS GCTs, especially of non-germinomatous histology, which fail after first line treatment is small. Reports from the French SFOP series and observation within the SIOP-CNS-GCT 96 protocol reveal that, although tumours do respond to chemotherapy again, a continuous second remission could only be achieved in cases with complete biologic remission, removal of any residual tumour, and successful application of high-dose treatment with additional irradiation.

Future perspectives

A multimodal approach that utilizes cisplatin/etoposide chemotherapy as well as tumour resection is highly effective for the treatment of paediatric GCTs. In the light of the high cure rates achieved by current protocols, research must now focus on new aims. First, treatment must be further intensified in those patients with cisplatin-refractory or poorly responding tumours. Locoregional hyperthermia constitutes a promising therapeutic concept in extracranial tumours as cisplatin is a very good thermosensitizer. Thus hyperthermia may overcome cisplatin resistance.[28] However, the clinical data show that hyperthermia should be used early. Ideally it should be integrated into first-line treatment of poorly responding tumours.[11]

On the other hand, patients should be identified who are only at a low risk of relapse, and in whom adjuvant chemotherapy can either be withheld or significantly reduced, thus minimizing the impact on short- and long-term quality of life and treatment toxicity. In this context, molecular genetic studies may also reveal important information that may be utilized for risk stratification. In conclusion, in the future clinical and molecular biologic information may help to distinguish low-risk from high-risk patients accurately, thereby facilitating a multimodal approach to the individual patient. International cooperation is vital not only to achieve a standardized diagnosis and treatment for this rare disease, especially for unfavourable sites such as the CNS, but also to detect risk factors, to define risk groups, and to obtain results in a shorter period of time. Another important requirement is to focus on rehabilitation, reintegration and quality of life of the cured patients to determine their quality of survival and, if impaired, to consider these results in future treatment planning.

References

1. **Schneider DT, Calaminus G, Koch S.** et al. (2004). Epidemiological analysis of 1442 children and adolescents registered in the German germ cell tumor protocols. *Pediatr Blood Cancer* 42, 169–75.
2. **Gonzalez-Crussi F, Winkler RF, Mirkin DL** (1978). Sacrococcygeal teratomas in infants and children: relationship of histology and prognosis in 40 cases. *Arch Pathol Lab Med* 102, 420–5.
3. **Göbel U, Calaminus G, Engert J, Kaatsch P,** et al. (1998) Teratomas in infancy and childhood. *Med Pediatr Oncol* 31, 8–15.

4. Göbel U, Schneider DT, Calaminus G, *et al* (2000). Germ-cell tumors in childhood and adolescence. *Ann Oncol* 11, 263–71.

5. Schneider DT, Schuster AE, Fritsch MK, *et al.* (2001). Multipoint imprinting analysis indicates a common precursor cell for gonadal and nongonadal pediatric germ cell tumors. *Cancer Res* 61, 7268–7276.

6. Perlman EJ, Hu J, Ho D, *et al.* (2000). Genetic analysis of childhood endodermal sinus tumors by comparative genomic hybridization. *J Pediatr Hematol Oncol* 22, 100–5.

7. Looijenga LH, Oosterhuis JW (2002). Pathobiology of testicular germ cell tumors: views and news. *Anal Quant Cytol Histol* 24, 263–79.

8. Schneider DT, Calaminus G, Göbel U (2001). Diagnostic value of alpha$_1$-fetoprotein and human chorionic gonadotropic hormone in infancy and childhood. *Pediatr Hematol Oncol* 18, 11–26.

9. Blohm ME, Vesterling-Hörner D, Calaminus G, *et al.* (1998). Alpha 1-fetoprotein (AFP) reference values in infants up to 2 years of age. *Pediatr Hematol Oncol* 15, 135–42.

10. Göbel U, Schneider DT, Calaminus G, *et al.* (2001). Multimodal treatment of malignant sacrococcygeal germ cell tumors: a prospective analysis of 66 patients of the German cooperative protocols MAKEI 83/86 and 89. *J Clin Oncol* 19, 1943–50.

11. Schneider DT, Wessalowski R, Calaminus G, *et al.* (2001). Treatment of recurrent malignant sacrococcygeal germ cell tumors: analysis of 22 patients registered in the German protocols MAKEI 83/86, 89, and 96. *J Clin Oncol* 19, 1951–60.

12. Rescorla F (1999). Pediatric germ cell tumors. *Semin Surg Oncol* 16, 144–58.

13. Nicholson JC, Punt J, Hale J, *et al.* (2002). Neurosurgical management of paediatric germ cell tumours of the central nervous system–a multi-disciplinary team approach for the new millennium. *Br J Neurosurg* 16, 93–5.

14. Einhorn LH, Donohue JP (1977). Chemotherapy for disseminated testicular cancer. *Urol Clin North Am* 4, 407–26.

15. Ablin AR (1981). Malignant germ cell tumors in children. *Front Radiat Ther Oncol* 16, 141–9.

16. Ablin AR, Krailo MD, Ramsay NK, *et al.* (1991). Results of treatment of malignant germ cell tumors in 93 children: a report from the Childrens Cancer Study Group. *J Clin Oncol* 9, 1782–92.

17. Mann JR, Raafat F, Robinson K, *et al.* (1998). UKCCSG's germ cell tumour (GCT) studies: improving outcome for children with malignant extracranial non-gonadal tumours—carboplatin, etoposide, and bleomycin are effective and less toxic than previous regimens. United Kingdom Children's Cancer Study Group. *Med Pediatr Oncol* 30, 217–27.

18. Mann JR, Raafat F, Robinson K, *et al.* (2000). The United Kingdom Children's Cancer Study Group's Second Germ Cell Tumor Study: Carboplatin, etoposide, and bleomycin are effective treatment for children with malignant extracranial germ cell tumors, with acceptable toxicity. *J Clin Oncol* 18, 3809–18.

19. Flamant F, Schwartz L, Delons E, *et al.* (1984). Nonseminomatous malignant germ cell tumors in children. Multidrug therapy in Stages III and IV. *Cancer* 54, 1687–91.

20. Baranzelli MC, Kramar A, Bouffet E, *et al.* (1999). Prognostic factors in children with localized malignant nonseminomatous germ cell tumors. *J Clin Oncol* 17, 1212–19.

21. Calaminus G, Schneider DT, Bökkerink JP, *et al.* (2003). Prognostic value of tumor size, metastases, extension into bone, and increased tumor marker in children with malignant sacrococcygeal germ cell tumors: a prospective evaluation of 71 patients treated in the German cooperative protocols Maligne Keimzelltumoren (MAKEI) 83/86 and MAKEI 89. *J Clin Oncol* 21, 781–6.

22. Calaminus G, Garre ML, Kortmann RD, *et al.* (1998). CNS germ cell tumors in children. Results of the German MAKEI 89 protocols and SIOP-CNS-GCT 93P/96 study. In: Jones DP, Appleyard I, Joffe JK, Harnden P (eds) *Germ Cell Tumours IV.* London: Springer, 247–54.

23. **Calaminus G, Bamberg M, Baranzelli M, et al.** (1994). Intracranial germ cell tumors: a comprehensive update of the European data. *Neuropediatrics* 25, 26–32.

24. **Bamberg M, Kortmann RD, Calaminus G, et al.** (1999). Radiation therapy for intracranial germinoma: results of the German cooperative prospective trials MAKEI 83/86/89. *J Clin Oncol* 17, 2585–92.

25. **Balmaceda C, Heller G, Rosenblum M, et al.** (1996). Chemotherapy without irradiation—a novel approach for newly diagnosed CNS germ cell tumors: results of an international cooperative trial. The First International Central Nervous System Germ Cell Tumor Study. *J Clin Oncol* 14, 2908–15.

26. **Marina NM, Cushing B, Giller R, et al.** (1999). Complete surgical excision is effective treatment for children with immature teratomas with or without malignant elements: a Pediatric Oncology Group/Children's Cancer Group Intergroup Study. *J Clin Oncol* 17, 2137.

27. **Sutton LN, Radcliffe J, Goldwein JW, et al.** (1999). Quality of life of adult survivors of germinomas treated with craniospinal irradiation. *Neurosurgery* 45, 1292–7.

28. **Wessalowski R, Kruck H, Pape H, et al.** (1998). Hyperthermia for the treatment of patients with malignant germ cell tumors: a phase I/II study in ten children and adolescents with recurrent or refractory tumors. *Cancer* 82, 793–800.

Chapter 24

Hepatic tumours

Hitoshi Ikeda, Tadashi Matsunaga,
and Yoshiaki Tsuchida

Introduction

Two-thirds of hepatic neoplasms are malignant (55–65 per cent), and ~90 per cent of the malignant tumours are epithelial tumours, i.e. hepatoblastoma or hepatocellular carcinoma. Benign vascular tumours and malignant mesenchymal tumours account for the rest. The ratio of hepatoblastoma to hepatocellular carcinoma is approximately 1.8:1 in Western countries, but in Japan the incidence of hepatoblastoma is five to six times higher than that of hepatocellular carcinoma.

Hepatoblastoma

Hepatoblastoma is the most common malignant hepatic tumour in children in all parts of the world, except in areas where hepatocellular carcinoma is more common because of endemic hepatitis B infection, accounting for ~1–2 per cent of all malignant tumours in children. The incidence of hepatoblastoma in children aged <15 years is <1 per 1 000 000 in North America. In Japan, the incidence appears to be higher than in Western countries, and the ratio of males to females is 1.2:1. Although hepatoblastoma can be seen at any age <15 years, more than 80 per cent of the tumours are seen in children aged ≤3 years and 45 per cent of the patients are diagnosed during the first year of life.

Genetics and biology

Although most cases are sporadic, hepatoblastoma may occur in association with a variety of congenital anomalies and familial conditions. Beckwith–Wiedemann syndrome and hemihypertrophy carry an increased risk of hepatoblastoma, as well as of Wilms tumour, rhabdomyosarcoma, and adrenocortical tumours. Abnormalities on the short arm of chromosome 11 have been shown in both Beckwith–Wiedemann syndrome and hepatoblastoma, and loss of heterozygosity of 11p15 has frequently been observed. A tumour suppressor gene or a growth factor gene located in the 11p15.5 region may be responsible for the development of the tumour but has not yet been identified.[1] Hepatoblastoma is also a specific malignant tumour in children from families with familial adenomatous polyposis, but inactivation of the adenomatous polyposis coli (APC) gene, which is a putatively mutated tumour suppressor gene in familial adenomatous polyposis, is rare in hepatoblastoma. The relationship between hepatoblastoma and APC may be different from that in colorectal cancer, and an alternative pathogenesis involving β-catenin is apparent. APC controls the degradation of β-catenin, and mutated APC causes the accumulation of β-catenin which acts as an oncoprotein. A high frequency of β-catenin gene mutations (48–65 per cent) has been documented in hepatoblastomas.[2]

Some reports suggest possible connections between environmental exposures and hepato-blastoma, including parental occupational exposure to metals, petroleum products, and paints or pigments. There also appears to be a significant association between hepatoblastoma and low birth weight.[3] Epidemiologic studies have suggested that the lower the birth weight, the higher the risk of hepatoblastoma, but specific perinatal environmental factors responsible for tumour development have not been identified.

Cytogenetic studies have shown that trisomy of chromosomes 2 and 20 is frequently observed in hepatoblastoma, and there is evidence that gains of 2q24, 8q. and 20 are predictive of poor prognosis.[4] DNA content analyses have shown that patients with diploid tumour have a better prognosis than those with aneuploid tumour, and a low proliferation index is another favourable prognostic factor.

Pathology

Hepatoblastoma is usually solitary, but 20 per cent of tumours extend multifocally or infiltrate diffusely into the liver. Macroscopically, the cut surface has a lobulated appearance due to fibrous septae, and multiple variegated nodules with haemorrhage and necrosis are surrounded by a pseudocapsule. The adjacent liver is not cirrhotic. Microscopically, there are two principal subtypes: pure epithelial hepatoblastoma is distinguished from mixed hepatoblastoma which contains mesenchymal tissue in addition to epithelial elements (Table 24.1).[5] The epithelial components exhibit a range of differentiation represented by fetal, embryonal, and anaplastic cells. Well-differentiated 'fetal' cells are smaller than normal hepatocytes and have a low nucleocytoplasmic ratio, minimal nuclear pleomorphism, and small nucleoli. Mitoses are infrequent. The cells are arranged in slender cords, usually two cell layers thick, which often contain canaliculi with or without bile. Sinusoids and vessels resembling central veins are present. Foci of extramedullary haematopoiesis are common (Fig. 24.1). Poorly differentiated 'embryonal' cells have a higher nucleocytoplasmic ratio and mitoses are seen more frequently than in fetal areas. The embryonal cells grow in sheets, assuming a tubular configuration, or rosettes which recapitulate some features of the embryonic liver (Fig. 24.2). Anaplastic (small-cell undifferentiated) type hepatoblastoma consists of sheets of cells resembling those of neuroblastoma which have scanty cytoplasm and a high mitotic rate. The cells are small, undifferentiated, round to oval or spindle-shaped, and monotypic. The term 'macrotrabecular' is used to indicate foci of tumour cells which are repetitively arranged in trabeculae, ≥ 10 cells thick. The tumour cells may be fetal or embryonal in appearance, or indistinguishable from the cells of adult hepatocellular carcinoma. Immature mesenchymal components in mixed hepa-toblastoma include osteoid, chondroid, or, rarely, rhabdomyoblastic tissues, in addition to blood vessels or haematopoietic tissues which are an integral part of the tumour. The epithelial differentiation occasionally yields squamous pearls or mucus-secreting glands. Neuronal dif-ferentiation is rarely seen in hepatoblastoma.

Table 24.1. Histological classification of hepatoblastoma

Pure epithelial hepatoblastoma
Fetal
Embryonal
Anaplastic (small-cell undifferentiated)
Macrotrabecular
Mixed hepatoblastoma (with mesenchymal tissue)

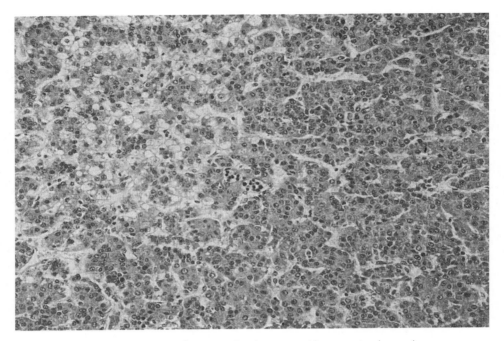

Fig. 24.1 Fetal hepatoblastoma. Cells are smaller than normal hepatocytes, have a low nucleocytoplasmic ratio, and are arranged in slender cords. A cluster of haematopoietic cells can be seen.

The nature of the epithelial components of hepatoblastoma appears to be associated with outcome. The pure fetal type is prognostically favourable when completely resected, but anaplastic (small-cell undifferentiated) histology has an unfavourable effect on outcome even in patients with complete resection.[6] It is not yet conclusive that the presence of macrotrabecular foci predicts a poor prognosis. The prognostic importance of mesenchymal components has not been determined.

Diagnosis

Since a child with advanced disease occasionally presents with anorexia, weight loss, or anaemia, the general condition of the patient should be carefully examined and the necessary supportive care provided.

α-Fetoprotein (AFP) is a glycoprotein synthesized in the yolk sac and the liver at an early stage of fetal life. The production of AFP stops at birth and the serum AFP concentration decreases exponentially from a mean of approximately 50 000 ng/ml to <20 ng/ml at 6–8 months of age. The serum AFP concentration is raised above the upper limit of the normal range for the patient's age in >98 per cent of patients with hepatoblastoma. Although the AFP concentration is relatively higher in hepatoblastomas with embryonal histology than in tumours with fetal histology, this is not prognostically significant or diagnostically discriminatory. Fractionation of AFP by lectin-affinity immunoelectrophoresis can differentiate hepatic malignant tumours from yolk sac tumours and benign hepatic disease, such as hepatitis or cirrhosis.[7] AFP derived from hepatoblastoma or hepatocellular carcinoma includes a subfrac-

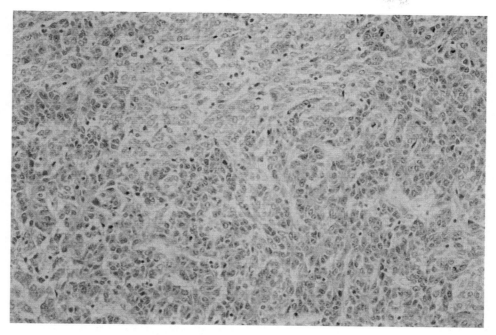

Fig. 24.2 Embryonal hepatoblastoma. Cells grow in sheets, assuming a tubular configuration or rosettes which recapitulate some features of the embryonic liver.

tion which binds to *Lens culinaris* haemagglutinin (LCH), but AFP from a benign hepatic disease does not react with LCH. The presence of a greater amount (>25 per cent) of AFP fraction which is not reactive to concanavalin A (Con A) differentiates AFP derived from a yolk sac tumour from that of hepatic origin (Fig. 24.3). Since serum AFP concentrations are expected to decline exponentially after complete tumour resection and remain within normal limits unless recurrence occurs, the measurement of AFP is very useful in monitoring treatment response, as well as in making a diagnosis.

Isosexual precocious puberty may develop in patients with hepatoblastoma secreting human chorionic gonadotropin (β-HCG). Virilization in male children, with testicular and penile enlargement and growth of pubic hair, has been reported.

Mild normochromic normocytic anaemia is usual and thrombocytosis may be seen in some patients. Interleukin 6, which appears to be produced in stromal cells in response to local secretion of cytokines from tumour cells, has been shown to mediate thrombocytosis and other acute reactions including fever. Routine workup occasionally demonstrates hypercholesterol-aemia or osteoporosis. The latter may be complicated by pathologic fracture.

Pretreatment imaging studies include plain radiography, ultrasonography, and CT or MRI. Plain films of the abdomen occasionally demonstrate the presence of calcification. On ultra-sonography, the echogenicity of the tumour is minimally increased and is usually non-homogeneous. Hypoechoic or anechoic areas, which reflect necrosis or haemorrhage within the tumour, may be seen. The unenhanced CT demonstrates the tumour with decreased attenuation with respect to the surrounding liver parenchyma, which is emphasized with intravenous contrast infusion. T1-weighted images of MRI show decreased signal intensity of

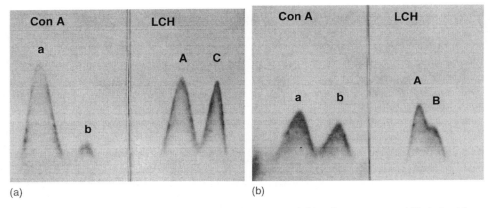

Fig. 24.3 AFP subfraction profiles in (a) hepatoblastoma and (b) yolk sac tumour. AFP derived from hepatoblastoma includes a subfraction which binds to LCH. The presence of a greater amount (>25%) of fraction non-reactive to ConA differentiates AFP derived from a yolk sac tumour from AFP of hepatic origin. a, reactive; b, non-reactive; A, strongly reactive; B, weakly reactive; C, non-reactive.

the tumour, but T2-weighted images show increased signal intensity. In addition to the qualitative evaluation, the surgical resectability of the tumour should be determined from the diagnostic radiology. Tumours involving both lobes of the liver or vascular structures such as the portal veins or the inferior vena cava are usually unresectable. The presence or absence of portal and para-aortic lymphadenopathy and lung metastases are evaluated by either CT or MRI. With modern MRI techniques, adequate information can usually be obtained for surgery, although surgeons may prefer to have an angiogram performed to define the relationship of the tumour to major hepatic vessels. There is occasionally an opportunity for hepatic angiography to be combined with tumour embolization or intra-arterial infusion chemotherapy.

Bone scan should be done to investigate metastatic spread. Bone marrow examination is unnecessary as metastatic disease to this site is extremely unlikely.

Staging

There is no universally accepted system of staging in hepatoblastoma. In the staging system used by the Children's Oncology Group (previously the Children's Cancer Group and the Paediatric Oncology Group) in the USA, stage I tumour is defined as a tumour resected completely at initial laparotomy, stage II as a tumour with microscopic residue, and stage III as a tumour with gross residual tumour. Children with distant metastases have stage IV disease. The same staging system was used in the German Cooperative Paediatric Liver Tumour Study HB-89. The staging system used in the Epithelial Liver Tumour Study Group of the International Society of Paediatric Oncology (SIOPEL) is called PRETEXT (Pretreatment Extent of Disease System) and classifies the tumour by identifying the number of adjoining free section(s) of liver.

PRETEXT is a significant predictor of overall survival in patients with hepatoblastoma,[8] and staging laparotomy is unnecessary as the stage can be determined from the results of imaging studies. The Japanese staging system depends on the number of liver segments involved, the extent of local invasion, the regional lymph node involvement, and the presence of distant metastases. However, the PRETEXT system has been widely used in Japan from the beginning of the Japanese Study Group for Paediatric Liver Tumour (JPLT) 2 protocol.

Surgical treatment

Complete surgical resection is ultimately necessary for cure of hepatoblastoma, but <50 per cent of tumours are resectable at the time of diagnosis. Tumours involving both lobes of the liver or invading the porta hepatis are usually unresectable, and preoperative chemotherapy is required to render them resectable at delayed surgery.[9] In fact, there is evidence that the rate of incomplete resection is lower after primary chemotherapy than in patients with primary tumour resection.[10] However, as there is a significant error rate in the clinical and imaging diagnosis of hepatoblastoma, histologic diagnosis prior to chemotherapy is necessary. A wedge biopsy of the tumour through a small laparotomy incision is preferred to fine-needle aspiration biopsy, and a specimen large enough to provide material not only for diagnosis but also for the investigation of biologic characteristics should be obtained.

The tumour is deemed resectable if it is localized in one or two segments of the liver. Complete resection is achieved by performing a segmentectomy or a standard lobectomy. Left or right trisegmentectomy may be done when the tumour occupies three segments of the liver. The abdomen is entered through a large transverse incision above the umbilicus. The liver is mobilized by dividing the ligaments which attach it to the abdominal wall and the diaphragm to facilitate access to the hepatic veins and the inferior vena cava. Sudden circulatory deterioration may occur if the inferior vena cava is angulated by an excess displacement of the liver. Dissection begins in the porta hepatis, and the branches of the hepatic artery, portal vein, and bile duct are isolated and divided according to the part of the liver to be excised. The hepatic vein should be carefully identified, ligated, and divided, because haemorrhage from an injured hepatic vein is difficult to control and may be fatal in some cases. After ligation of the hepatic vessels, an ischaemic colour change on the surface of the liver demarcates the lobe to be resected. An adequate margin is required, although a narrower margin between the tumour and the dissection line is acceptable in some fetal-type hepatoblastomas. The raw surface of the remaining liver is checked for bleeding and bile leakage, and covered with fibrin glue if necessary. Postoperative chemotherapy should be withheld for 1–2 weeks.

Pulmonary recurrence, which is probably the late appearance of metastatic deposits present at the time of diagnosis or initial operation, may develop within 12 months of diagnosis, rarely later. Intensive chemotherapy should be given before resection of the pulmonary metastases, but they can also be treated by an aggressive surgical approach as long as the number and location of metastatic nodules is precisely identified by radiologic evaluation (Fig. 24.4). Resection of lung metastases can be curative if there is local control of the primary tumour. Patients may survive disease free after several thoracotomies.

Liver transplantation is a promising method of treatment for unresectable hepatoblastomas (see below).[11]

Chemotherapy and clinical trials

The prognosis for children affected by hepatoblastoma has been significantly improved with the introduction of cisplatin (CDDP) into therapeutic trials and, as a consequence, the 3-year overall survival rate has improved from ~30 per cent to 60–70 per cent. The principal chemotherapy regimens used in clinical trials for hepatoblastoma are summarized in Table 24.2.

The SIOPEL Group has been conducting studies of preoperative chemotherapy consisting of cisplatin and doxorubicin. In the SIOPEL-1 study (January 1990–February 1994), patients were treated with continuous 24-h i.v. infusion of cisplatin $80\,mg/m^2$ followed by doxorubicin $60\,mg/m^2$ over 48 h (PLADO) after biopsy and assessment of PRETEXT.[12] Patients were

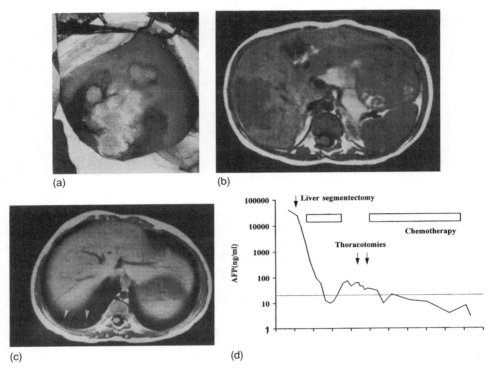

(a)   (b)

(c)   (d)

Fig. 24.4 Hepatoblastoma originating in the right lobe of the liver: (a) gross appearance of the tumour; (b) T1-weighted MRI images showed decreased signal intensity of the tumour; (c) MRI was useful in evaluating the number and location of metastatic nodules (arrowed) ranging from 3 to 5 mm in diameter; (d) serum AFP levels became normal after nine courses of chemotherapy with cisplatin and THP-adriamycin, and the resection of pulmonary metastases.

reassessed after four courses of chemotherapy, at which point the primary tumour was resected where possible. Postoperatively, treatment was completed with two more courses of chemotherapy. A total of 154 patients were registered and 138 patients received preoperative chemotherapy. A partial response with tumour shrinkage and serial decrease in the serum levels of AFP was observed in 113 patients (82 per cent); 115 patients had delayed surgery and 106 patients (including six with liver transplants) had complete resection of the primary tumour. The event-free survival and the overall survival at 5 years were 66 per cent and 75 per cent, respectively. In the latest SIOPEL-3 study, an attempt is being made to avoid exposure to doxorubicin in patients with favourable disease (PRETEXT I–III tumours) who are randomized to receive either PLADO or cisplatin alone. Patients with PRETEXT IV and/or extra-hepatic disease receive intensified treatment with alternating administration of cisplatin and doxorubicin–carboplatin (Super PLADO).

In the USA, the Paediatric Oncology Group (POG) ran a study in the late 1980s to evaluate the survival rate in children with grossly resected hepatoblastoma treated with cisplatin, vincristine, and fluorouracil, and to assess the response and survival rates in children with initially unresectable tumours treated with the same combination. Concurrently, the Children's Cancer Group (CCG) undertook a study to test the feasibility of administering doxorubicin

Table 24.2. Chemotherapy regimens in clinical trials for hepatoblastoma

---

1. International Society of Paediatric Oncology, Epithelial Liver Tumour Study (SIOPEL) 3

PRETEXT I–III

PLADO: cisplatin 80 mg/m^2 over 24 h on day 1 and doxorubicin 60 mg/m^2 over 48 h on days 2 and 3

OR

Cisplatin 80 mg/m^2 alone

PRETEXT IV and/or extra-hepatic disease

Alternating cycle of cisplatin and DOX–carboplatin (Super PLADO): cisplatin 80 mg/m^2 over 24 h, doxorubicin 60 mg/m^2 over 48 h, carboplatin 500 mg/m^2 1 h infusion

2. CCG–POG Intergroup

Stage I (unfavourable histology) and stages II–IV

Regimen A: cisplatin 90 mg/m^2 over 6 h on day 1, and vincristine 1.5 mg/m^2 and 5-fluorouracil 600 mg/m^2 on day 2

OR

Regimen B: cisplatin 90 mg/m^2 over 6 h on day 1, and doxorubicin 80 mg/m^2 over 96 h on days 1–4

Stage I (favourable histology)

Regimen C: bolus i.v. doxorubicin 20 mg/m^2/day on days 1–3

3. German Cooperative Paediatric Liver Tumour Study HB-94

First-line chemotherapy

IFO–CDDP–DOXO: ifosfamide 0.5 g/m^2 bolus on day 1 and 3.0 g/m^2 over 72 h on days 1–3, cisplatin 20 mg/m^2/day on days 4–8, and doxorubicin 60 mg/m^2 over 48 h on days 9 and 10

Second-line chemotherapy

VP16–CARBO: VP16 400 mg/m^2 over 96 h on days 1–4 and carboplatin 800 mg/m^2 over 96 h on days 1–4)

4. Japanese Study Group for Paediatric Liver Tumour (JPLT) 2

First-line chemotherapy

CITA: cisplatin 80 mg/m^2 over 24 h on day 1 and THP–Adriamycin 30 mg/m^2/day by 1 h infusion on days 2 and 3)

OR

CATA-L [trans-arterial chemoembolization (TACE)]: slow transarterial injection of carboplatin 200 mg/m^2 and THP–Adriamycin 30 mg/m^2+ lipiodol

Second-line chemotherapy

ITEC: ifosfamide 3.0 g/m^2/day by 2 h infusion on days 1 and 2, THP–Adriamycin 30 mg/m^2/day by 1 h infusion on days 4 and 5, etoposide 100 mg/m^2/day by 1 h infusion on days 1–5 and carboplatin 400 mg/m^2 over 24 h on day 3)

(by continuous infusion) and cisplatin to patients with unresectable or incompletely resected hepatoblastoma. After these trials, the CCG and POG together conducted a randomized comparison of the two regimens: cisplatin, vincristine and fluorouracil (regimen A), and cisplatin and continuous infusion of doxorubicin (regimen B).[13] A total of 182 patients were enrolled in the study (August 1989–December 1992), and 173 patients, excluding a subset of good prognosis patients (stage I pure fetal histology with minimal mitotic activity), were randomized to receive either regimen after initial surgery. Although toxicities were more frequent with regimen B, there was no statistically significant difference in the 5-year event-free survival (57 per cent and 69 per cent for patients on regimens A and B, respectively).

The German Cooperative Paediatric Liver Tumour Study HB-89 was started in 1989.[14] In this study, patients with a tumour restricted to one lobe of the liver underwent primary resection.

Larger tumours involving both lobes and those with metastases were biopsied and initially treated with a combination chemotherapy of ifosfamide, cisplatin, and doxorubicin (IFO–CDDP–DOXO) and were resected at second-look surgery. The long-term disease-free survival of all patients was 75 per cent. In the HB-94 study (January 1994–December 1998), the efficacy of chemotherapy consisting of IFO–CDDP–DOXO and/or etoposide and carboplatin (VP16–CARBO) was assessed.[15] A total of 69 patients were treated, 53 of whom (77 per cent) remained alive. Primary chemotherapy with IFO–CDDP–DOXO was given to 48 patients, of whom 41 achieved partial remission. Eighteen patients with advanced or recurrent hepatoblastoma were treated with VP16–CARBO, and a response to the regimen was observed in 12 of them.

The Japanese Study Group for Paediatric Liver Tumour Protocol 1 (JPLT-1) ran from March 1991 to December 1999.[16] The chemotherapeutic regimen used for tumours involving over three hepatic sections and/or with metastasis was similar to PLADO, but doxorubicin was replaced by tetrahydropyranyl–Adriamycin (THP–Adriamycin) in an attempt to reduce cardiac toxicity. Half doses were administered to patients with tumours involving one or two hepatic sections. The event-free survival rate at 6 years was 66.0 per cent, and the overall survival rates at 3 and 6 years were 77.8 per cent and 73.4 per cent, respectively. In patients with tumours involving more than three hepatic sections, intravenous chemotherapy was compared with intra-arterial chemotherapy and, although there was a trend to favour intravenous therapy, the difference in outcome was not statistically significant. In the JPLT-2 study, treatment is started with CDDP plus THP–Adriamycin (CITA) or a transarterial chemoembolization (TACE) regimen (Table 24.2). An alternative chemotherapy combination, including ifosfamide, THP–Adriamycin, etoposide, and carboplatin (ITEC) is administered for poorly responding tumours.

Experimental treatment

Despite the aggressive chemotherapeutic regimens described above, ~30 per cent of unresectable tumours remain resistant to treatment and an alternative treatment has to be sought. Options including ligation of the hepatic artery or tumour embolization with materials such as Gelfoam, in combination with chemotherapy, may be effective in decreasing tumour volume and increasing surgical resectability. Immunotargeted chemotherapy with an anti-AFP monoclonal antibody conjugated with Adriamycin or cisplatin has been explored but is still no more than an experimental option.

Liver transplantation may be required as a final approach in the treatment of refractory or unresectable hepatoblastomas. Although only a limited number of patients have undergone the procedure, the results have been encouraging.[11]

Hepatocellular carcinoma

Hepatocellular carcinoma accounts for 10–30 per cent of primary malignant hepatic tumours in Western countries and Japan, but is more prevalent and outnumbers hepatoblastoma in areas where hepatitis B virus (HBV) infection is endemic. For example, in Taiwan, 80 per cent of primary malignant hepatic tumours in children are hepatocellular carcinoma. The tumour usually occurs in children aged >5 years. Male predominance is more prominent than in hepatoblastoma.

HBV infection is causally associated with the development of hepatocellular carcinoma. In Taiwan, nearly 100 per cent of children with hepatocellular carcinoma are seropositive for hepatitis B surface antigen. Maternal transmission is the most important route of infection, but the incidence of childhood hepatocellular carcinoma has declined since the introduction in Taiwan of HBV vaccination for neonates of mothers carrying hepatitis B e antigen.[17] The extremely short incubation period from HBV infection to the genesis of hepatocellular carcinoma in children as compared with that in adults suggests that there may another, so far unrecognized, mechanism which accelerates the carcinogenesis of childhood hepatocellular carcinoma. Hepatitis C viral infection has been recognized to cause hepatocellular carcinoma in adults, but the relationship is not yet fully understood in children.

The tumour is also recognized to be associated with a number of underlying chronic liver diseases, including tyrosinaemia, biliary atresia, idiopathic neonatal hepatitis, and α_1-antitrypsin deficiency. Children with the chronic form of hereditary tyrosinaemia develop cirrhosis and eventually hepatocellular carcinoma. The incidence of the tumour exceeds 35 per cent if the children survive >2 years. Patients with biliary atresia who survive >3 years after portal-jejunostomy are at high risk for the tumour. Patients with α_1-antitrypsin deficiency are also at high risk, but the tumour usually develops in adult life. Glucose-6-phosphatase deficiency (type 1 glycogen storage disease), Fanconi's anaemia, and Wilson's disease are among other associated disorders. Long-term parenteral nutrition and resultant biliary cirrhosis are also underlying causes of hepatocellular carcinoma.

Pathology

The gross and microscopic features of hepatocellular carcinoma in children are similar to those seen in adults, except for the lower incidence of underlying cirrhosis. Pre-existing cirrhosis is present in 5–40 per cent of children, whereas 50–85 per cent of adult hepatocellular carcinomas occur in cirrhotic liver. The tumour occurs as multiple nodules or a diffusely infiltrating mass involving both lobes of the liver. According to the SIOPEL-1 study, 39 per cent of tumours were associated with cirrhosis and >50 per cent of patients had multifocal tumours. The disease was advanced at diagnosis in most cases; 31 per cent had metastases, and 39 per cent had extrahepatic tumour extension or vascular invasion.

The cut surface is often bile stained, and haemorrhage and necrosis within the tumour are seen more often than in hepatoblastoma. Pseudoencapsulation is less conspicuous. The tumour cells are larger than normal hepatocytes. Histologic features distinguishing hepatocellular carcinoma from hepatoblastoma include broad trabeculae, nuclear pleomorphism, nucleolar prominence, and the presence of tumour giant cells. Extramedullary haematopoiesis is not seen in hepatocellular carcinoma.

Diagnosis

Abdominal pain and a palpable mass are the most common initial manifestations, and hepatosplenomegaly is the sign most frequently observed in hepatocellular carcinoma. Fever, weight loss, and jaundice are occasionally observed. Shock due to tumour rupture and intra-abdominal bleeding may be the initial manifestation. Anaemia and mild hyperbilirubinaemia are the principal laboratory abnormalities, and the serum AFP concentration is high in 50–80 per cent of patients. Serologic evaluation for the possible presence of HBV infection is essential.

The radiologic features of hepatocellular carcinoma are similar to those of hepatoblastoma (Fig. 24.5), and differentiation between the two may be difficult. Occasionally, however, the growth patterns of the tumours may be useful in differentiating between these diagnoses; tumours with smaller satellite lesions, those invading the portal vein, or those with distant metastases are more often hepatocellular carcinomas. Metastatic spread is to the lungs, regional lymph nodes, and, rarely, bone.

Treatment

Complete resection is the basis of successful treatment in hepatocellular carcinoma as in hepatoblastoma, but it is often prevented by advanced disease. Primary unresectability and the presence of metastasis are factors indicating unfavourable prognosis,[18] and although intensive chemotherapy regimens of several cooperative study protocols have been used, the results so far have generally been unsatisfactory.

In the German Cooperative Paediatric Liver Tumour Study HB-89, in which unresectable or incompletely resected tumours were treated with a combination of ifosfamide, cisplatin, and Adriamycin, only three of 10 patients were free from the tumour. Data from the SIOPEL-1 study showed that only eight of 40 patients treated with cisplatin and doxorubicin were alive without disease at a median follow-up of 75 months.[18] The CCG and the POG conducted a randomized comparison of treatment with cisplatin, vincristine, and fluorouracil or cisplatin, and with continuous infusion of doxorubicin.[19] There was no difference between the two regimens in terms of outcome, and the 5-year event free survival rates (88 per cent, 8 per cent,

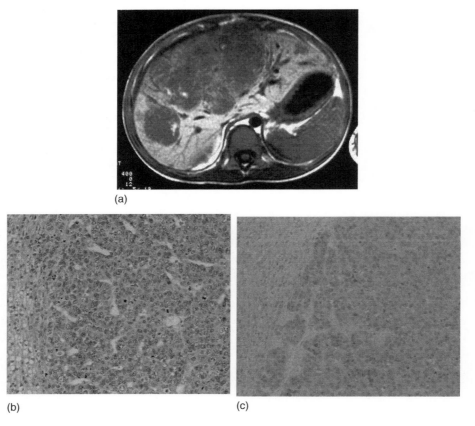

(a)

(b)   (c)

Fig. 24.5 Unresectable hepatocellular carcinoma refractory to multiagent chemotherapy is shown. (a) MRI showed a huge heterogeneous tumour extending to both lobes of the liver. The tumour had a lower signal intensity than the surrounding liver tissue on T1-weighted MRI images. Histologically, tumour cells were growing in (b) a macrotrabecular pattern (haemotoxylin and eosin stain) and (c) were positive for β-catenin (immunostaining).

and 0 per cent for patients with stage I, III, and IV disease, respectively) confirmed the importance of surgical resection.

Total hepatectomy and liver transplantation may be an effective treatment for hepatocellular carcinoma. In one series, a 5-year disease-free survival of 63 per cent was obtained in 19 patients with hepatocellular carcinoma who underwent transplantation.[11]

Fibrolamellar carcinoma (fibrolamellar variant of hepatocellular carcinoma)

Fibrolamellar carcinoma, a distinctive variant of hepatocellular carcinoma, occurs in the non-cirrhotic livers of older children and young adults without sex preference. The tumour is not associated with underlying liver disease, viral infection, or metabolic abnormality. The serum AFP is not high in the majority of patients, but a specific abnormality of the vitamin B_{12} binding protein has been documented and the level of unsaturated vitamin B_{12} binding protein is significantly high in fibrolamellar carcinoma and rises with disease progression. The imaging characteristics are generally similar to those of classical hepatocellular carcinoma. The gross appearance of the tumour generally consists of a single well-circumscribed pseudo-encapsulated mass rather than the diffusely infiltrating mass usually seen in heptocellular carcinoma. Microscopically, fibrolamellar carcinoma is characterized by large plump polygonal cells encompassed by fibrous bands (lamellar fibrosis). The cytoplasm is granular and deeply eosinophilic, and ultrastructurally shows abundant mitochondria.

Fibrolamellar carcinoma differs from the ordinary form of hepatocellular carcinoma in its clinical presentation and biologic behaviour, as well as in histologic features. It is characterized by a longer duration of symptoms prior to diagnosis and increased chance of resectability. Importantly, prolonged disease-free survival is seen compared with that usual for hepatocellular carcinoma if the tumour is completely resected, although it is suggested that the prognostic difference between the tumour types may be insignificant after adjustment for disease stage.

Undifferentiated (embryonal) sarcoma of the liver

Undifferentiated (embryonal) sarcoma of the liver is a highly aggressive tumour most often presenting in late childhood as an abdominal mass, pain, or fever. There is no sex preponderance. Serum AFP is within the normal range. Pathologically, the gross findings are relatively consistent and show cystic areas and gelatinous tissues with extensive necrosis and haemorrhage. Demarcation from the surrounding liver appears sharp, but there may be microscopic infiltration and permeation to the veins. Histologically, the tumour shows a proliferation of spindle cells, with occasional polygonal or round cells loosely or densely arranged in a myxomatous background. Bizarre and multinucleated giant cells and periodic acid–Schiff positive hyaline globules of various sizes are frequently observed. Entrapped bile ducts, together with non-neoplastic hepatocytes, are observed at the periphery of the tumour. Positive immunostaining for histiocytic markers (α_1-antitrypsin, α_1-antichymotrypsin), muscle markers (desmin, muscle-specific actin), and vimentin is fairly consistent. Supported by these pathologic findings, it is suggested that the tumour is of mesenchymal origin, presumably from a very primitive precursor cell.

Radiologic evaluation by ultrasonography and CT typically reveals a large intrahepatic mass with a wide range of solid and cystic components which correlate with areas of haemorrhage, necrosis, and cystic degeneration. Complete excision and adjuvant multi-agent chemotherapy appear to be essential in achieving long-term survival. There is limited information about optimal adjuvant treatment because of the lack of large-scale clinical studies.

Other liver tumours

Other primary malignant mesenchymal tumours of the liver include rhabdomyosarcoma, leiomyosarcoma, angiosarcoma, fibrosarcoma, yolk sac tumour, and rhabdoid tumour. Embryonal rhabdomyosarcomas are rare malignant tumours of the biliary tract, and may be found anywhere from the ampulla of Vater to the liver itself. Tumours with evidence of striated muscle differentiation are diagnosed as rhabdomyosarcoma, but a histologic distinction between undifferentiated sarcoma and rhabdomyosarcoma can sometimes be difficult. Rhabdomyosarcomas are usually seen in patients <4 years of age and tend to present with obstructive jaundice. The tumour often grows as a botryoid gelatinous mass occluding the lumen of bile ducts.[5] Histologically, the tumour cells lie in a loose myxoid stroma beneath the epithelium of the bile ducts and exhibit the typical features of embryonal rhabdomyosarcoma. Although surgery is critical for establishing an accurate diagnosis and determining the extent of regional disease, aggressive surgery is not usually warranted for biliary tract rhabdomyosarcoma. Primary gross total resection is rarely possible; nevertheless the outcome of treatment with chemotherapy, with or without radiation therapy, is good.[20]

Yolk sac tumour and choriocarcinoma, although extremely rare, may arise *de novo* in the liver, and a variety of paediatric solid tumours including neuroblastoma, Wilms tumour, rhabdomyosarcoma, and yolk sac tumour can metastasize to the liver (details are discussed in the chapters describing these tumours).

References

1. **Hartmann W, Waha A, Koch A, et al.** (2000). p57(KIP2) is not mutated in hepatoblastoma but shows increased transcriptional activity in a comparative analysis of the three imprinted genes p57(KIP2), IGF2, and H19. *Am J Pathol* 157, 1393–1403.

2. **Takayasu H, Horie H, Hiyama E, et al.** (2001). Frequent deletions and mutations of the β-catenin gene are associated with overexpression of cyclin D1 and fibronectin and poorly differentiated histology in childhood hepatoblastoma. *Clin Cancer Res* 7, 901–8.

3. **Ikeda H, Matsuyama S, Tanimura M** (1997). Association between hepatoblastoma and very low birth weight: a trend or a chance? *J Pediatr* 130, 557–60.

4. **Gray SG, Kytölä S, Matsunaga T, Larsson C, Ekström TJ** (2000). Comparative genomic hybridisation reveals population-based genetic alterations in hepatoblastomas. *Br J Cancer* 83, 1020–25.

5. **Stocker JT, Husain AN, Dehner LP, Chandra RS** (2001). Hepatic neoplasms. In: Stocker JT, Dehner LP (eds) *Pediatric pathology*, Vol.2. Philadelphia, PA: Lippincott–Williams & Wilkins, 752–81.

6. **Haas JE, Feusner JH, Finegold MJ** (2001). Small cell undifferentiated histology in hepatoblastoma may be unfavorable. *Cancer* 92, 3130–4.

7. **Tsuchida Y, Honna T, Fukui M, et al.** (1989). The ratio of fucosylation of alpha-fetoprotein in hepatoblastoma. *Cancer* 63, 2174–6.

8. **Brown J, Perilongo G, Shafford E, et al.** (2000). Pretreatment prognostic factors for children with hepatoblastoma: results from the International Society of Paediatric Oncology (SIOP) study SIOPEL 1. *Eur J Cancer* 36, 1418–25.

9. **Schnater JM, Aronson DC, Plaschkes J, et al.** (2002). Surgical view of the treatment of patients with hepatoblastoma: results from the first prospective trial of the International Society of Pediatric Oncology Liver Tumor Study Group (SIOPEL-1). *Cancer* 94, 1111–20.

10. **Fuchs J, Rydzynski J, Hecker H, et al.** (2002). The influence of preoperative chemotherapy and surgical technique in the treatment of hepatoblastoma: a report from the German Cooperative Liver Tumour Studies HB 89 and HB 94. *Eur J Pediatr Surg* **12**, 255–61.

11. **Reyes JD, Carr B, Dvorchik I, et al.** (2000). Liver transplantation and chemotherapy for hepatoblastoma and hepatocellular cancer in childhood and adolescence. *J Pediatr* **136**, 795–804.

12. **Pritchard J, Brown J, Shafford E, et al.** (2000). Cisplatin, doxorubicin, and delayed surgery for childhood hepatoblastoma: a successful approach. Results of the first prospective study of the International Society of Pediatric Oncology. *J Clin Oncol* **18**, 3819–28.

13. **Ortega JA, Douglass EC, Feusner JH, et al.** (2000). Randomized comparison of cisplatin/vincristine/fluorouracil and cisplatin/continuous infusion doxorubicin for treatment of pediatric hepatoblastoma: a report from the Children's Cancer Group and the Pediatric Oncology Group. *J Clin Oncol* **18**, 2665–75.

14. **von Schweinitz D, Byrd DJ, Hecker H, et al.** (1997). Efficiency and toxicity of ifosfamide, cisplatin and doxorubicin in the treatment of childhood hepatoblastoma. *Eur J Cancer* **33**, 1243–9.

15. **Fuchs J, Rydzynski J, von Schweinitz D, et al.** (2002). Pretreatment prognostic factors and treatment results in children with hepatoblastoma: a report from the German Cooperative Pediatric Liver Tumor Study HB 94. *Cancer* **95**, 172–82.

16. **Sasaki F, Matsunaga T, Iwafuchi M, et al.** (2002). Outcome of hepatoblastoma treated with the JPLT-1 (Japanese Study Group for Pediatric Liver Tumor) Protocol-1: a report from the Japanese Study Group for Pediatric Liver Tumor. *J Pediatr Surg* **37**, 851–6.

17. **Chang MH, Shau WY, Chen CJ, et al.** (2000). Hepatitis B vaccination and hepatocellular carcinoma rates in boys and girls. *JAMA* **284**, 3040–2.

18. **Czauderna P, Mackinlay G, Perilongo G, et al.** (2002). Hepatocellular carcinoma in children: results of the first prospective study of the International Society of Pediatric Oncology group. *J Clin Oncol* **20**, 2798–804.

19. **Katzenstein HM, Krailo MD, Malogolowkin MH, et al.** (2002). Hepatocellular carcinoma in children and adolescents: results from the Pediatric Oncology Group and the Children's Cancer Group Intergroup Study. *J Clin Oncol* **20**, 2789–97.

20. **Spunt SL, Lobe TE, Pappo AS, et al.** (2000). Aggressive surgery is unwarranted for biliary tract rhabdomyosarcoma. *J Pedatr Surg* **35**, 309–16.

Chapter 25

Retinoblastoma

Guillermo L Chantada and Enrique Schvartzman

Introduction

Retinoblastoma is a malignant endo-ocular tumour of children arising in the embryonic neural retina. It is the prototypical model for hereditary cancer development. Because of its rarity, most paediatricians and paediatric oncologists see few cases of this neoplasm, and diagnosis and management have traditionally been the reponsibility of ophthalmologists. In fact, ophthalmologists usually establish the diagnosis, decide the local treatment modalities, and monitor the response.

Although estimates vary, retinoblastoma occurs with a frequency of ~1 in 15 000–18 000 live births in developed countries. However, it may be more frequent in less developed areas such as Latin America, Africa, and Asia. In such areas, retinoblastoma is diagnosed late when extraocular dissemination has already occurred, leading to higher morbidity (blindness) and mortality. There seems to be no predisposition for race or sex and no predilection for either eye.

Retinoblastoma can occur in two forms, heritable and non-heritable, and the tumours can be either unilateral or bilateral. All patients with bilateral retinoblastoma have the heritable disease, whereas only 10 per cent of unilateral cases have the heritable form. They tend to be younger and often have multifocal tumours. Non-heritable retinoblastoma is always unilateral and unifocal. Retinoblastoma can occur in a familial or sporadic form, but only 6–10 per cent are familial. The average age of patients at diagnosis is 24 months in unilateral cases and 13 months in bilateral cases.

Genetics

In 1971, Knudson developed a mathematical model to explain the heredity of retinoblastoma.[1] He suggested that 'two hits' should occur at a gene level to develop retinoblastoma. In heritable cases, a first event or 'hit' should be a germinal mutation, i.e. inherited and present in all cells of an affected individual. The second 'hit' occurs at some time during the development of the retinal cells, leading to retinoblastoma. In contrast, in non-heritable cases, both events occur in the retinal cells in an acquired fashion. According to this model, heritable retinoblastoma is inherited in an autosomal dominant fashion with approximately 95 per cent penetrance and high expressivity. However, some families show a different pattern characterized by reduced penetrance and expressivity. Some low-penetrance mutations have recently been characterized. Members of these families often develop only unilateral retinoblastoma or spontaneously regressing tumours called benign retinomas.

In 1985, the retinoblastoma gene (*rb1*) was isolated at chromosome 13q14. It is a large gene, spanning over 200 kb, and it is composed of 27 exons. This gene encodes a protein that plays a key role in the regulation of cell growth in normal cells acting at the checkpoint between G_1 and the entry to S phase. The phosphorylated form of the protein dissociates from the transcription factor E2F, freeing itself to promote progression to the cell cycle. In patients with retinoblastoma, functionally altered *rb1* allows uncontrolled entry into the S phase leading to cell division. Sequences of the papillomavirus, which is known to interact with the *rb1* pathway, have been found mostly in tumour tissue of unilateral patients with retinoblastoma from Mexico, suggesting that this virus may play a role in tumour development and possibly in the increased incidence in this area.[2]

Abnormalities at chromosome 13q14 can be detected by conventional karyotyping studies in only 5 per cent of cases. In the remainder, the mutations should be detected using more sophisticated molecular techniques. The mutations found in these cases vary from family to family, making molecular diagnosis very difficult and time-consuming since there are no sites with a high frequency of mutations within the retinoblastoma gene. Nonsense and frameshift mutations are the most frequent DNA alterations described.[3] The first hit is usually a deletion or translocation at the *rbl* gene, occurring in either the maternal or paternal alelle; the second hit frequently involves the loss of heterozygosity of the remaining alelle, leading to neoplastic transformation.

Molecular diagnosis of retinoblastoma plays a key role in genetic counselling. If a germ-line mutation is identified in a given family, unaffected siblings can be tested and periodical fundoscopic examinations (under general anaesthesia in younger children) can be avoided in those who do not carry the abnormal gene. Prenatal diagnosis is also feasible, and when an abnormal retinoblastoma gene is detected in a fetus from an affected family, earlier delivery can be advised to treat the tumours as soon as possible. A useful card for genetic counselling developed by Abramson is shown in Figure 25.1.

Histology

Retinoblastoma is a tumour of neuroepithelial origin, which can be classified as one of the primitive neuroectodermal tumours of childhood. It consists of small undifferentiated anaplastic cells with scanty cytoplasm and large nuclei that stain deeply with haematoxylin, arising from the nucleated layer of the eye. Calcification occurs in necrotic areas and is a common feature of large tumours. Retinoblastoma cells often express antigens of photoreceptor differentiation and neuron-specific enolase but do not express CD99, glial fibrillary acidic protein, or S-100. Retinoblastoma cells express ganglioside GD2 almost invariably. Classically, two types of retinoblastoma have been described. The most common type is composed of highly undifferentiated retinoblasts; the other consists of more differentiated photoreceptor cells with neuroepithelial rosette formation. These Flexner–Wintersteiner rosettes are characteristic of retinoblastoma but they can be present in other ophthalmic tumours (medulloepithelioma). Less commonly seen in well-differentiated tumours is a 'bouquet-like' arrangement of benign-appearing cells with abundant cytoplasm, small nuclei, and long cytoplasmic processes traversing a fenestrated membrane. Depending on the level within the retina from which the retinoblastoma arises, the tumour may grow either in an endophytic pattern into the vitreous cavity or in an exophytic form into the subretinal space. Because of their friable nature, endophytic tumours can eventually seed the vitreous cavity and simulate a severe endophthalmitis. The active seeds of retinoblastoma can remain viable for long periods and eventually re-implant in the retina, giving rise to new tumours. In addition, seeding may occur following chemotherapy or radiation, since portions of the calcified mass break away and may contain viable tumour cells. When the tumour grows from the retina outwards into the subretinal space (exophytic pattern), it produces a retinal detachment, sometimes with no clear view of the

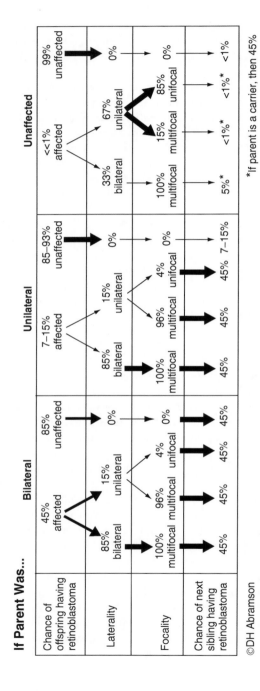

If Parent Was...

	Bilateral	Unilateral	Unaffected
Chance of offspring having retinoblastoma	45% affected / 85% unaffected	7–15% affected / 85–93% unaffected	<<1% affected / 99% unaffected
Laterality	85% bilateral / 15% unilateral → 0%	85% bilateral / 15% unilateral → 0%	33% bilateral / 67% unilateral → 0%
Focality	100% multifocal / 96% multifocal / 4% unifocal → 0%	100% multifocal / 96% multifocal / 4% unifocal → 0%	100% multifocal / 15% multifocal / 85% unifocal → 0%
Chance of next sibling having retinoblastoma	45% / 45% / 45% / 45%	45% / 45% / 45% 7–15%	5%* / <1%* <1%* / <1%* <1%

*If parent is a carrier, then 45%

©DH Abramson

Fig. 25.1 Card for genetic counselling for retinoblastoma.

mass, and can resemble Coats disease or other forms of exudative retinal detachment. Both patterns can occur in the same eye. Neither type is related to prognosis or responsiveness to treatment, but may affect the ease or difficulty in diagnosis evaluation. Another uncommon type of growth pattern, diffuse infiltrating retinoblastoma, is characterized by a flat infiltration of the retina by tumour cells and is usually found in older children. Retinoblastoma can disseminate outside the eye, following the course of the optic nerve and/or the subarachnoid space to the chiasm, the brain, and the meninges. It can also escape from the eyeball through the sclera and invade the orbit and beyond it to the surrounding structures. The tumour cells can also reach the choroid and, from there, they may gain access to the systemic circulation giving rise to haematogenous metastases. Metastatic retinoblastoma usually involves the central nervous system (CNS) either as a solitary mass or multiple lesions, or with leptomeningeal dissemination. It can also invade facial structures such as the pre-auricular lymph nodes and the bones of the skull. It can also give rise to haematogenous metastases involving the bone, bone marrow, and less frequently the liver, lungs, or any other organ.

Presenting signs and symptoms

The presenting signs and symptoms of retinoblastoma vary depending on where in the world a child with retinoblastoma is seen. In developing countries, proptosis and an orbital mass, sometimes with pre-auricular adenopathy indicating extraocular extension, are usually present at diagnosis (Fig. 25.2). In developed countries, parents seek medical care because of leukocoria (Fig. 25.3), strabismus, or, less frequently, for a red painful eye, glaucoma, or poor vision.[4] Less common signs are rubeosis iridis (a reddish coloration of the iris), orbital cellulitis, heterochromia iridis (change in the colour of different parts of the iris), unilateral mydriasis, hyphaema (haemorrhage in the anterior chamber), or nystagmus. Leukocoria, a white reflex known as the cat's eye reflex, is the most common presenting sign of retinoblastoma. The whitish glow seen through the pupil is light momentarily reflected from the tumour. It is only seen when the child looks sideways or if the observer is at an oblique angle to the child's face as he or she looks straight ahead. It can also be noticed by parents or relatives in a flash photograph. Even though leukocoria is a quite specific sign with a narrow differential diagnosis, paediatricians often overlook it. Strabismus, the second most frequent presenting sign of

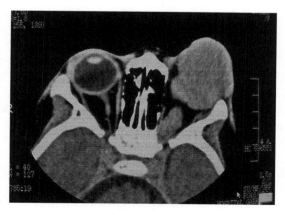

Fig. 25.2 CT scan showing extrascleral extension of retinoblastoma.

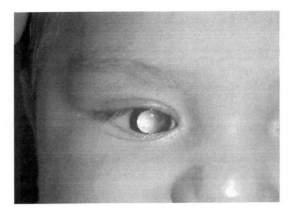

Fig. 25.3 Patient with leucokoria.

retinoblastoma, is a non-specific sign which is present in many normal children, and is also often overlooked. Strabismus occurs when the tumour arises in the macular area, leading to an inability to fixate and subsequent deviation of the involved eye. Therefore a young child with strabismus calls for a dilated examination of the retina under anaesthesia with special attention given to the macula. When retinoblastoma is diagnosed in the first month of life, it is usually detected because of a positive family history.

Poor vision is seldom encountered because most children with retinoblastoma are too young to complain about visual impairment, but it may be the initial manifestation in older children. Another clinical manifestation, although less frequent, is a red painful eye, resembling orbital cellulitis. A syndrome associated with deletion of the long arm of chromosome 13 (the 13q-deletion syndrome) has been reported with the features of microcephaly, hypertelorism, micro-ophthalmos, epicanthal folds, micrognathia, short neck with lateral folds, low-set ears, imperforate anus, hypoplastic or absent thumbs, and psychomotor and mental retardation. Identification of these abnormalities may precede recognition of concomitant retinoblastoma. Such children require karyotype analysis and retinal examination. Another way in which the disease may be diagnosed early is by investigation in infants who have a family history of retinoblastoma.

Diagnosis

The most important step in diagnosis is examination of the eye under anaesthesia through fully dilated pupils, with indirect ophthalmoscopy and scleral indentation by an experienced ophthalmologist. Needle biopsies are not indicated for the diagnosis. Retinoblastoma is one of the few paediatric neoplasms that can be accurately diagnosed without histopathologic confirmation. Ultrasonography can be very helpful in the differential diagnosis of children with leukocoria. Two-dimensional B scan demonstrates the presence of a mass in the posterior segment in cases where the fundus may be obscured by detachment or haemorrhage, and shows a rounded or irregular intraocular mass with numerous highly reflective echoes in the orbit directly behind the tumour.

MRI is the method of choice for evaluating the optic nerve, orbital and CNS involvement, and the presence of an associated pinealoblastoma. This synchronous tumour, an entity that has been termed trilateral retinoblastoma, occurs in 2–3 per cent of bilateral heritable retinoblastoma cases, and it is not considered a metastasis but a separate primary tumour arising from cells of photoreceptor origin in the pineal gland and the suprasellar area. CT scans may be useful to detect intraocular calcifications but are not recommended routinely because they carry the risk of greater exposure to radiation. MRI also helps in differentiating retino-blastoma from Coats disease, a benign condition often confused with retinoblastoma. How-ever, both MRI and CT scans are relatively unreliable for determining extension of the tumour into the sclera, choroid, or optic nerve, and invasion of these structures is only detected by histopathologic examination of the enucleated eye. Intraocular retinoblastoma should be differentiated from Coats disease, *Toxocara* infection, persistent hyperplastic primary vitreous, retrolental fibroplasias, and medulloepithelioma. Differential diagnoses of extraocular retino-blastoma include orbital rhabdomyosarcoma, metastatic neuroblastoma and leukaemia, and lymphoma. Bone marrow examination and biopsy and lumbar puncture for cytologic exam-ination of the cerebrospinal fluid are mandatory when extraocular disease is suspected. Its yield is insignificant in patients with localized intraocular disease. In the presence of symptoms suggestive of metastatic disease (bone pain), a bone scan is indicated.

Follow-up

New tumours can develop up to the age of 7 years in patients with bilateral disease and so these children should be monitored regularly up to that age. Some bilateral cases present as unilateral disease, and tumours in the other eye may develop at follow-up examination up to 44 months of age. When new tumours develop in an eye with retinoblastoma, they seldom involve the macula.

Since tumours can appear in patients aged up to 28 months with a family history, a thorough ophthalmologic examination under anaesthesia should be performed shortly after birth and periodically up to that age in children born to affected parents.

Imaging studies are not routinely performed for the follow-up of patients with intraocular disease, but may be needed for monitoring patients with extraocular extension. The use of head MRI to screen for trilateral retinoblastoma during follow-up in young patients with hereditable retinoblastoma in order to facilitate earlier detection is under evaluation. There is no agree-ment on which imaging schedule (if any) can detect presymptomatic secondary malignancies in patients with heritable retinoblastoma.

Staging

The most widely used grouping system for retinoblastoma was proposed by Reese and Ellsworth (Table 25.1) and has become adopted as the standard for intraocular disease. Here, prognosis refers entirely to preservation of useful vision in the affected eye if radiation therapy is delivered via a lateral portal with photon therapy, and not to long-term survival. There is no widely accepted staging system for patients with extraocular disease.

Treatment

Two aspects of treatment of retinoblastoma must be considered: first, the local therapeutic options to treat intraocular disease and, secondly, systemic therapy for patients with extrao-cular, regional, or metastatic disease.

In developed countries, most patients present with intraocular disease and survival is ~95 per cent. In these cases, treatment planning must consider the potential preservation of useful

Table 25.1. The Reese–Ellsworth staging system for intraocular retinoblastoma

Group I. Very favourable for maintenance of sight
Solitary tumour, smaller than 4 disk diameters in size, at or behind the equator
Multiple tumours, none larger than 4 disk diameters in size, all at or behind the equator

Group II. Favourable for maintenance of sight
Solitary tumour, 4–10 disk diameters in size, at or behind the equator
Multiple tumours, 4–10 disk diameters in size, behind the equator

Group III. Possible for maintenance of sight
Any lesion anterior to the equator
Solitary tumour, larger than 10 disk diameters in size, behind the equator

Group IV. Unfavourable for maintenance of sight
Multiple tumours, some larger than 10 disk diameters in size
Any lesion extending anteriorly to the ora serrata

Group V. Very unfavourable for maintenance of sight
Massive tumours involving more than half the retina
Vitreous seeding

vision, minimizing the long-term sequelae. The size, number, and location of tumours and the status of the remaining eye are taken into account in choosing the best therapy. Even though an increasing number of patients with unilateral retinoblastoma can avoid enucleation in developed nations, eye preservation is uncommon in less privileged areas. Most patients with bilateral retinoblastoma come with advanced intraocular disease, often needing enucleation, in one eye and less advanced disease in the other eye, which can usually be preserved.

In developing countries, retinoblastoma is usually diagnosed after extraocular spread is evident. In these cases, the treatment of retinoblastoma aims to save the patient's life since death from metastatic disease is possible.

Surgery

Enucleation is the simplest and safest therapy for retinoblastoma. Resection of a long portion of optic nerve is mandatory. A prosthetic eyeball is fitted several weeks after the procedure to minimize the cosmetic effects. When enucleation is performed in the first 2 years of life, facial asymmetry develops because of inhibition of orbital growth.

Enucleation is indicated when no useful vision is predicted even if tumours are controlled. Most patients with Reese–Ellsworth stage V tumours require enucleation, especially when no useful vision can be achieved after successful treatment of the tumours. However, if the contralateral eye also has advanced disease, a conservative approach may be undertaken and a few eyes can be retained. Enucleation is mandatory when glaucoma, anterior chamber invasion, or rubeosis iridis are present and when local therapy cannot be evaluated because of a cataract or difficulty in following a patient closely.

Enucleation can be delayed when overt extrascleral extension is evident at diagnosis. Orbital masses usually shrink considerably after a few courses of chemotherapy, allowing enucleation to be performed and therefore avoiding orbital exenteration.[5] There are few, if any, indications for orbital exenteration nowadays. Intraocular surgery, such as vitrectomy, is contraindicated in patients with proven or suspected retinoblastoma since it can increase the risk of orbital relapse.

External-beam radiotherapy

Retinoblastoma is a radiosensitive tumour and external-beam radiotherapy (EBRT) is the most effective local therapy for retinoblastoma. However, long-term side effects limit its use. EBRT is usually delivered using a linear accelerator to a dose of 40–45 Gy covering the whole retina. Infants must be anaesthetized and immobilized during the procedure, and close cooperation between the ophthalmologist and the radiotherapist is essential for planning the fields. Most radiotherapists use a D-shaped lateral field, which minimizes the risk of radiation-induced cataracts. Nevertheless, the anterior retina is underdosed with this technique, and recurrent tumours near the ora serrata are not uncommon.

The success rate of EBRT with this technique depends not only on tumour size, but also on location. Ophthalmoscopic regression patterns following radiotherapy have been characterized. Local control rates range from 58 to 80 per cent. Most recurrences after radiotherapy can be re-treated successfully with cryo- or photocoagulation. Long-term sequelae of radiotherapy are of great concern. Like enucleation, it causes inhibition of growth of the orbital bone, leading to cosmetic disturbances and, more importantly, it has been associated with an increased risk of secondary malignancies.

EBRT is also indicated for overt orbital disease and invasion of the cut end of the optic nerve. In these instances the chiasm should be included in the portal.

Plaque radiotherapy

Radioactive episcleral plaques using ^{60}Co, ^{106}Ru, or ^{125}I are used in the treatment of retinoblastoma. Plaques are inserted in the operating theatre by suturing them outside the sclera. They are removed in a second operation a few days later when the target dose has been administered. Plaque radiotherapy delivers an effective dose to the tumour while preserving the normal surrounding tissues from the adverse effects of radiotherapy. Plaques are usually prescribed for medium-size single tumours that are not amenable to cryo- or photocoagulation, but because of their high success rate, they have been increasingly used as primary therapy after chemoreduction. ^{125}I is the preferred isotope because of radiation safety for both patients and staff.

Cryo- and photocoagulation

Cryo- and photocoagulation are used to treat small (usually <5 mm) accessible tumours. They are widely available and can be repeated several times until local control is achieved. Cryotherapy is usually prescribed to treat anterior tumours and is applied with a small probe placed on the conjunctiva. Photocoagulation is generally used for posterior tumours, and is performed with either an argon laser or a xenon arc. However, photocoagulation should be avoided in tumours near the macula since it may leave a scar causing severe amblyopia. Both modalities cause little or no morbidity or long-term sequelae. The use of thermochemotherapy for posterior pole tumours has been recently described. It is based on the synergistic effect of intravenous carboplatin and hyperthermia administered by a diode laser.[6]

Chemotherapy

In the past, chemotherapy was only used to treat metastatic disease. However, in recent years, most groups have used chemotherapy as primary treatment for intraocular disease not amenable to local therapy in order to decrease tumour size and make the tumours suitable for local therapy.[7,8] This approach, called chemoreduction, may make it possible to avoid either enucleation or EBRT in selected cases. Carboplatin is the agent most frequently used since it has good penetration into the eye. Vincristine and etoposide are also used; however, their penetration into the eye is unknown. Most intraocular tumours usually show dramatic shrinkage after systemic chemotherapy, but consolidation with local treatment appears to be needed in most cases to prevent relapse. Tumour location, patient age, and size of tumour all correlate with responsiveness to chemotherapy. Most patients with Reese–Ellsworth group I–IV tumours respond favourably to chemoreduction, so that enucleation and EBRT are usually avoided. Eye retention ranges from 74 to 100 per cent. Patients with Reese–Ellsworth group V disease, and especially those with vitreous seeds, have proved difficult to treat with this modality. After early encouraging results, it was reported that most require EBRT for effective tumour control and many are ultimately enucleated after chemotherapy and EBRT.[8] Alternative treatment for these high-risk patients includes periocular administration of carboplatin or the association of intravenous cyclosporin with carboplatin in order to circumvent P-glycoprotein-mediated chemoresistance, which has been postulated by some groups as a potential cause of treatment failure.

Even though chemoreduction followed by local treatment has become an established therapy for intraocular retinoblastoma, there are several limitations to this approach. Long-term results and safety are unknown, especially as far as potential induction of secondary malignancies is concerned. The chemotherapy agents used are known to induce secondary leukaemia, especially the epipodophylotoxins used by many groups. The optimal regimen has not yet been determined, and the duration of treatment and the need for local therapy are also still under investigation.

Patients with unilateral disease are frequently best managed by enucleation. However, selected cases may benefit from chemoreduction and local therapy. Finally, treatment with chemoreduction and local treatment is tedious and needs meticulous management which is only available in specialized centers.

The role of adjuvant chemotherapy for patients with putative histopathologic risk factors for relapse is a matter of controversy. Post-enucleation histopathologic staging is essential to define groups with different risk of relapse.[9] The paediatric oncologist faces the dilemma of prescribing adjuvant chemotherapy to all patients with putative risk factors, or of withholding it in controversial cases and treating those who relapse aggressively. Adjuvant chemotherapy does not completely eliminate the possibility of extraocular relapse, and its benefit in groups with low relapse rate is not proven. Because of the low relapse rate of this population, a randomized study comparing adjuvant treatment with observation would require an enormous number of patients. Many authors consider extraocular relapse as a catastrophic event and recommend adjuvant therapy for all patients with histopathologic risk factors.[10] However, in recent years it has been shown that many relapsed patients can be salvaged by intensive therapy.[5,11] Therefore avoiding adjuvant chemotherapy for patients with a low probability of relapse and treating those who relapse aggressively is a reasonable alternative.[12]

There is almost universal agreement that there is no need for adjuvant chemotherapy for patients with intraretinal disease and those with pre-laminar optic nerve invasion.[9,12] The role of chemotherapy in isolated choroidal invasion is controversial. It has been suggested that once the tumour invades the choroid, it may gain access to the systemic circulation, giving rise to haematogenous metastasis and thus justifying adjuvant therapy.[10] However, in our series of 55 patients with isolated choroidal invasion treated only with enucleation, only one had an extraocular relapse.[12] Therefore, according to our data, chemotherapy is not needed in this population. Choroidal invasion may only be relevant when it is combined with post-laminar optic nerve invasion.

Invasion of the optic nerve beyond the lamina cribrosa is a major risk factor for relapse, especially when the cut end is involved. When the cut end is free from tumour, management is controversial. At our center, patients with this condition receive no therapy other than enucleation provided that there is no major choroidal or scleral invasion. In our published series of 21 patients treated with enucleation and no adjuvant therapy, none relapsed.[12] Patients with concomitant major choroidal involvement with or without scleral invasion have a greater risk of relapse, and adjuvant chemotherapy is indicated. Patients with invasion of the cut end of the optic nerve are uniformly considered as having a high risk of relapse. Survival rate has been reported to be as low as 40 per cent. However, with multimodal treatment, including adjuvant chemotherapy and orbital radiotherapy involving the optic chiasm, 11/14 patients survived at our institution.[9] The role of intrathecal chemotherapy in these situations remains to be established. According to our limited experience, patients with microscopic scleral involvement are at high risk for extraocular relapse and should receive adjuvant therapy.[9]

When overt extraocular disease is present, pre-enucleation chemotherapy is warranted.[5] Doz et al.[13] pioneered the use of the combination of carboplatin and etoposide, which became the gold standard. A phase II study showed an overall 60 per cent response rate of extraocular retinoblastoma to idarubicin, which may be the anthracycline of choice.[14] Response to other agents has been studied in single patients or small series. Cisplatin, cyclophosphamide, ifosfamide, vincristine, doxorubicin, topotecan, and thiotepa are frequently used. With a multimodal approach combining chemotherapy, limited surgery, and radiotherapy to the involved areas, a 5-year probability of event-free survival of 84 per cent for patients with overt orbital disease with or without pre-auricular node invasion as their only metastatic site was achieved.[5] However, even though complete remission is usually achieved with conventional chemotherapy in patients with metastatic disease (haematogenous or CNS), it is usually short-lived and ultimate survival is infrequent.[5,9] High-dose chemotherapy followed by autologous stem cell rescue has proven efficacy for the treatment of patients with systemic relapse, but it is of less value in cases of CNS dissemination.[11] Conditioning regimens have usually included the drugs mentioned above at higher dose. There is no effective therapy for these patients, and most centers treat them according to investigational protocols or palliatively. They may need craniospinal radiation to achieve disease control, but the high frequency of neuropsychologic sequelae in young children precludes its use.

The drug combination used for extraocular disease at our center[5] is shown in Table 25.2.

Secondary malignancies

The presence of a germ-line mutation at the retinoblastoma gene confers on affected individuals a lifetime high predisposition for secondary malignancies. Conversely, unilateral retinoblastoma patients without the constitutional mutation are at no risk for developing second tumours. With current therapy, there are more patients with bilateral retinoblastoma dying of secondary malignancies than those who succumb from the retinoblastoma itself. The risk of developing a secondary malignancy exists among these children regardless of the therapy received. However, those patients receiving radiotherapy in the first year of life appear to be at greater risk.[15]

The cumulative risk of second cancers is 1 per cent per year, reaching 51 per cent 50 years after the diagnosis of retinoblastoma. The median latency period is 15 years. Those who survive a secondary malignancy are at increased risk of developing additional malignancies at a rate of about 2 per cent per year.

Table 25.2. Chemotherapy regimens used at the Hospital JP Garrahan,Buenos Aires, Argentina[5]

Patients with post-laminar optic nerve invasion with major choroidal or scleral invasion, cut end invasion, orbital and metastatic disease

Weeks 0,6,12,18: cyclophosphamide 65 mg/kg (day 1), mesna 60 mg/kg (day 1), vincristine 0.05 mg/kg (day 1), idarubicin 10 mg/m^2 (day 1)

Weeks 3,9,15,21: carboplatin 18.7 mg/kg (patients <10 kg) or 560 mg/m^2 (patients >10 kg) (days 1 and 2), etoposide 3.3 mg/kg (patients <10 kg) or 100 mg/m^2 (patients >10 kg) (days 1, 2, 3)

Cut end invasion

Orbital radiotherapy 45 Gy up to the optic chiasm (starting at week 0)

Most secondary cancers seen in patients with bilateral retinoblastoma are sarcomas, usually osteosarcomas of the irradiated orbit. Sarcomas outside the orbit, cutaneous melanoma, thyroid carcinoma, and lung and breast cancer have also been reported. The risk for osteogenic sarcoma is greater at age 10–20 years and brain tumours tend to present later. Secondary malignancies in these patients are usually very aggressive and are frequently fatal. However, they should be treated with curative intent. A high index of suspicion and aggressive treatment have improved results in recent years.

References

1. **Knudson AG** (1971). Mutation and cancer: statistical study of retinoblastoma. *Proc Natl Acad Sci USA* **68**, 820–3.
2. **Orjuela M, Ponce Castaneda V, Ridaura C, et al.** (2000). Presence of human papilloma virus in tumor tissue from children with retinoblastoma: an alternative mechanism for tumor development. *Clin Cancer Res* **6**, 4010–16.
3. **Harbour W** (1998). Overview of RB gene mutations in patients with retinoblastoma. Implications for genetic screening. *Ophthalmology* **105**, 1442–7.
4. **Abramson DH, Frank C, Susman M, Whalen M, Dunkel I, Boyd N** (1998). Presenting signs of retinoblastoma. *J Pediatr* **132**, 505–8.
5. **Chantada G, Fandiño A, Casak S, et al.** (2003). Treatment of overt extraocular retinoblastoma. *Med Pediatr Oncol* **40**, 158–61.
6. **Lumbroso L, Doz F, Urbieta M, et al.** (2002). Chemothermotherapy in the management of retinoblastoma. *Ophthalmology* **109**, 1130–6.
7. **Kingston J, Hungerford J, Madreperla S, Plowman P** (1996). Results of combined chemotherapy and radiotherapy for advanced intraocular retinoblastoma. *Arch Ophthalmol* **114**, 1339–43.
8. **Shields C, Honavar S, Meadows A, et al.** (2002). Chemoreduction plus focal therapy for retinoblastoma: factors predictive of need for treatment with external beam radiotherapy or enucleation. *Am J Ophthalmol* **133**, 657–64.
9. **Schvartzman E, Chantada G, Fandiño A, et al.** (1996). Results of a stage-based protocol for the treatment of retinoblastoma. *J Clin Oncol* **14**, 1532–6.
10. **Honavar G, Singh A, Shields C, et al.** (2002). Post enucleation adjuvant therapy in high risk retinoblastoma. *Arch Ophthalmol* **120**, 923–31.
11. **Dunkel IJ, Aledo A, Kernan NA, et al.** (2000). Successful treatment of metastatic retinoblastoma. *Cancer* **89**, 2117–21.
12. **Chantada GL, Dunkel IJ, de Dávila MT, Abramson DH** (2004). Retinoblastoma patients with high risk ocular pathological features: Who needs adjuvant therapy? *Br. J. Ophthalmol* **88**, 1069–73.

13. **Doz F, Neuenshwander S, Plantaz D, *et al.*** (1995). Etoposide and carboplatin in extraocular retinoblastoma: a study by the Societé Française d'Oncologie Pédiatrique. *J Clin Oncol* **13**, 902–9.

14. **Chantada GL, Fandiño A, Mato G, *et al.*** (1999). A phase II window of idarubicin in children with extraocular retinoblastoma. *J Clin Oncol* **17**, 1847–50.

15. **Moll A, Imhof S, Schouten van Meeteren AY, *et al.*** (2001). Second primary tumors in hereditary retinoblastoma: a register-based study, 1945–1997. *Ophthalmology* **108**, 1109–14.

Chapter 26

Rare tumours

David A. Walker

Introduction

Cancer is a 'moderate-risk' disease of childhood (age 0–14 years), affecting one in 650 children. The tumours included in this chapter are those which are rare among the generality of childhood tumours. They are not rare variants of the common childhood tumour categories and they have been reported to have the capacity to invade and metastasize.

This diverse group of rare tumours is collected together to enhance access to age-specific information on diagnosis, treatment, and outcome. There are often insufficient recent data available to reach a consensus on the best treatment. This lack of information is disabling for the oncologist and a source of anxiety for the child and family when no one seems to be familiar with the condition and its treatment. Many of the tumours are more common in adulthood, and the recommended treatment plans have evolved from adult practice which, if followed without modification, may cause unacceptable morbidity in a developing child.

National groups are focusing on these rare tumours through national tumour registration, development of clinical guidelines, and promotion of a network of clinicians with a special interest. These developments will increasingly provide opportunities for the development and evaluation of new treatment approaches and promote relevant research.

The epithelial cancers (carcinomas) are the single largest group, accounting for 2–3 per cent of all childhood malignant disease in Western populations. For most sites, incidence increases with age throughout childhood and well into adult life. Presumably the childhood cases represent the very beginning of the age–incidence curve, although it is noteworthy that the most common carcinomas of adulthood, those of lung and breast, are exceptionally rare in childhood in all regions of the world. Exceptions to this age–incidence pattern are adrenal carcinoma and nasopharyngeal carcinoma, where there is a bimodal age distribution.

Sex incidence and 5-year survival rates of selected rare malignant tumours are given in Tables 26.1 and 26.2.

Head and neck

Nasopharyngeal carcinoma

Nasopharyngeal carcinomas (NPCs) are the most common epithelial tumour in childhood, accounting for 30 per cent of the nasopharyngeal malignancies in this age group.

Incidence

There is considerable variation in international incidence in childhood. In predominantly White populations, the incidence in childhood is usually no more than 0.4 per million, whereas

Table 26.1. Sex incidence and 5-year survival rate: selected rare malignant tumours from National Registry of Childhood Tumours, UK, 1981–1995

ICD-10 code	Site	Male	Female	5-year survival rate (%)
CO0-06	Mouth	5	7	92
C07-08	Salivary glands	17	18	94
C11	Nasopharynx	32	13	54
C1 5-21,26	Gastrointestinal	12	6	33
CIS-21,26	Malignant carcinoid, gut	3	1	(75)
C25	Pancreas	1	2	(33)
C34	Bronchus, lung	2	1	(33)
C34	Malignant carcinoid, lung	2	0	(100)
C37	Thymus	8	1	(0)
C44	Skin	40	52	99
C56	Ovary	0	19	62
C62	Testis	1	0	(0)
CM	Kidney	13	9	68
C67	Bladder	5	2	100
C73	Thyroid	28	56	98
C74	Adrenal	3	24	38

in the US Black population it is about one per million. In Chinese populations, rates in children are 0.8 per million. The highest incidence is apparently in North Africa; reliable incidence rates are not available, but nasopharyngeal carcinoma could well account for 10 per cent of childhood cancer. There is a bimodal age distribution with an early peak in adolescence and

Table 26.2. Sex incidence and 5-year survival rate: selected rare malignant tumours from National Registry of Childhood Tumours, UK, 1981–1995

ICD-10 classification	Site	Male	Female	5-year survival rate (%)
8720–8780/3	Malignant melanoma	88	110	90
	Skin	78	104	93
	Eye	6	4	(80)
	Central nervous system	4	2	(17)
8971/3	Pancreatoblastoma	3	2	(20)
8972/3	Pulmonary blastoma	0	1	–
9050–9053/3	Malignant mesothelioma	0	2	(50)
9310/3	Malignant ameloblastoma	1	0	(100)
9370/3	Chordoma	4	5	(78)
9590/3	Malignant granular cell tumour	1	2	100

young adulthood in European and American Caucasians but not in Southeast Asians or North Africans. It is more common in males, although this male preponderance is less marked in the younger age groups.

Aetiology

There is evidence for family clustering and an association with specific HLA types. A possible causative role of dietary carcinogen intake has been raised but not proven. Rare cases of NPC complicating invasive juvenile laryngeal papillomatosis have been reported, especially after the use of radiation therapy. An association with the Epstein–Barr virus (EBV) has been clearly established by sero-epidemiologic surveys. Indeed, in Southern China population screening for NPC is performed using EBV serology. The EBV antibody level is used to quantify tumour burden, response to treatment, and screening for relapse. EBV DNA has been shown to be present in premalignant carcinoma *in situ* lesions as well as in active tumour. It has been shown to be clonal and arise from a single EBV-infected cell. The precise role of EBV in oncogenesis remains unclear. Its ubiquitous distribution in populations coupled with wide variations in tumour incidence suggests that genetic and environmental factors interact.

Pathology

The tumours are most commonly undifferentiated carcinomas (WHO type 3) or non-keratinizing carcinomas (WHO type 2). WHO type 2 and 3 NPCs are accompanied by an inflammatory infiltrate of lymphocytes, eosinophils, and plasma cells, which explains the earlier name of lymphoepithelioma. The tumours usually arise in the fossa of Rosenmüller and spread locally to the rest of the pharynx and the base of skull. They metastasize preferentially to cervical lymph nodes, bone, mediastinum, lung, and liver.

Clinical presentation

The most common clinical presentation is with cervical lymphadenopathy (80 per cent); the primary tumour in the nasopharynx is often clinically undetectable. Symptoms related to the primary tumour result from involvement of local structures and include hearing loss, local mass, nasal obstruction, otitis media, epistaxis, cranial nerve palsies, and headache. Disseminated tumour may produce symptoms related to the site of metastasis (<10 per cent). Rarely, a paraneoplastic syndrome in patients with disseminated disease may occur with osteoarthropathy, clubbing, and bone or joint pain. Delays in diagnosis are frequent.

Tumour staging

Tumour evaluation should be directed at the delineation of the extent of the primary tumour, local lymph node involvement, and a search for distant metastases. Nasolaryngoscopy may not reveal a primary tumour, but blind biopsies may be taken. Imaging of the base of skull with plain radiography, CT, or MRI scans (Fig. 26.1) permits definition of tumour size, site, and lymph node involvement as well as local bony or central nervous system invasion which can be confirmed by examination of the cerebrospinal fluid. Evidence of metastatic disease should be sought with radionuclide bone scanning, chest CT, and abdominal ultrasound or MRI. Positron emission tomography may image symptomatic tumour deposits which are not otherwise detectable. Raised serum-IgA antibody to the viral capsid antigen may be of prognostic value and has been used as a tumour marker. The staging system in the 5th edition of the American Joint Cancer Committee (AJCC) is currently used (Table 26.3).

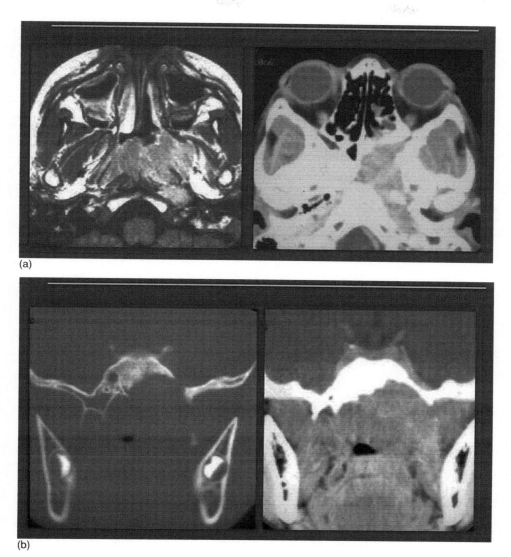

(a)

(b)

Fig. 26.1 CT scans showing (a) axial and (b) sagittal images of a nasopharyngeal carcinoma invading the skull base.

Surgery

The curative role of surgical treatment is limited by the high incidence of early spread of the primary tumour at diagnosis. Surgical efforts are generally limited to biopsy and the treatment of otitis media prior to local radiotherapy. Therefore successful treatment of this tumour depends on the use of radiotherapy and chemotherapy.

Table 26.3. American Joint Cancer Committee (AJCC) staging system for nasopharyngeal carcinoma (5th edition)

T1	Tumour confined to the nasopharynx		
T2	Tumour extends to the soft tissue of oropharynx and/or nasal fossa		
T2a	Without parapharyngeal extension		
T2b	With parapharyngeal extension		
T3	Tumour invades bony structures and/or paranasal sinuses		
T4	Tumour with intracranial extension and/or involvement of cranial nerves, infratemporal fossa, hypopharynx, or orbit		
NO	No regional lymph node metastasis		
N1	Unilateral metastasis in lymph node(s) measuring 6 cm in greatest dimension above the supraclavicular fossa		
N2	Bilateral metastasis in lymph node(s) measuring 6 cm in greatest dimension above the suprclavicular fossa		
N3	Metastasis in lymph node(s)		
N3a	>6 cm in greatest dimension		
N3b	Extension to the supraclavicular fossa		
MO	No distant metastasis		
M1	Distant metastasis		
Stage I	T1	NO	MO
Stage HA	T2a	NO	MO
Stage IIB	T1	N1	MO
	T2a	N1	MO
	T2b	NO-1	MO
Stage III	T1	N2	MO
	T2	N2	MO
	T3	NO-2	MO
Stage IVA	T4	NO-2	MO
Stage IVB	Any T	N3	MO
Stage IVC	Any T	Any N	M1

Chemotherapy

In principle, the high incidence of metastatic relapse favours aggressive systemic therapy early in treatment. The role of chemotherapy in this tumour is now established in children as a result of a number of prospective but non-randomized reports of the use of adjuvant chemotherapy. A recently published randomized study has shown that chemotherapy with 5-fluorouracil, cisplatin, and radiotherapy is superior to radiotherapy alone in adults with advanced disease. Tumour shrinkage with initial chemotherapy has been well documented. Tumours that do not respond to combined chemotherapy and radiotherapy do poorly with other treatments. The recent report of exceptional survival rates using adjuvant interferon also raises the possibility that biologic modifiers may have a role to play in tumour control. The GPOH reported results of multimodality treatment using pre-radiation chemotherapy (methotrexate, 5-fluorouracil, and cisplatin) and radiotherapy to the primary tumour bed (54.9 Gy) and whole neck (45 Gy). Subsequently, all patients were treated with adjuvant interferon-β (105 U/kg, three times a week for 6 months) with a high response rate (91 per cent) and sustained remission.

Radiation

Irradiation of the nasopharynx requires careful planning to encompass the whole tumour volume with adequate margins yet exclude adjacent involved structures. Doses >50Gy have not been shown to be more effective in younger age groups, and so most therapists have avoided the 70-Gy doses advised in the adult population. Irradiation has been used to treat metastatic tumour recurrence with good effect.

Prognosis

The CCSG study from the early 1980s using radiotherapy alone (35–80 Gy) reports overall and relapse-free survival of 51 per cent and 36 per cent, respectively, at 5 years, and 45 per cent and 33 per cent, respectively, at 10 years. Tumour staging predicts outcome; 5-year overall survival for T1–2 and T3–4 tumours are 63–90 per cent and 22–75 per cent, respectively. Survival rates in children and young people (aged <30 years) were better than those in adult patients.

Late effects

In view of the substantial number of survivors, careful consideration must be given to the late effects of therapy. Cervical and temporomandibular joint fibrosis are well-recognized complications which are more common in patients treated with higher doses. Irradiation of the thyroid gland, inner ear, and hypothalamus requires careful monitoring of hearing, growth, and endocrine functions.

Thyroid cancer

Thyroid cancer (TC) has an incidence of 0.2–1.5 per million per year and is considerably more common in girls than boys. Five to ten per cent of all TC occurs in childhood and adolescence.

Pathology

The majority of tumours in the young age group are of the highly differentiated papillary type or the less differentiated follicular and mixed types. Anaplastic tumours are exceptional. Medullary thyroid carcinoma (MTC) accounts for up to 20 per cent of all TCs in childhood, the majority of which are associated with the multiple endocrine neoplasia (MEN) syndrome type 2 in which a high proportion are multifocal and bilateral. TC metastasizes to local lymph nodes, lung, and bone.

Aetiology

Aetiologic factors implicated include a history of exposure to environmental or therapeutic irradiation, genetic predisposition (familial adenomatous polyposis, Cowden's disease) and dietary iodide intake or changes in endocrine status.

Radiation

Ionizing irradiation is strongly implicated in the oncogenesis of TC. Evidence for this comes from clinical reports describing excess risk of TC in those who had previously received therapeutic irradiation. This risk is enhanced in patients with neuroblastoma who had received treatment with *meta*-iodobenzylguanidine (MIBG). The impact of environmental irradiation has been intensively studied since atmospheric testing of nuclear weapons after the Second World War and more recently after the radiation leak at Chernobyl. Incidence rates after the accident were raised by up to 10-fold in heavily contaminated areas and are thought to be related to exposure to radioactive iodine. Younger children, some of whom were irradiated *in utero*, were more vulnerable than adolescents. The tumours have been reported as being more aggressive in their clinical behaviour.

ret proto-oncogene mutations

Oncogenic rearrangements of the *ret* tyrosine kinase receptor have been characterized in patients with both differentiated papillary TC and MTC. Specific somatic rearrangements (*ret–PTC1*, *ret–PTC2*, and *ret–PTC3*) have been identified; all are formed by the fusion of the truncated tyrosine kinase domain of *ret* to the amino terminus of different gene fragments. Their frequency varies according to geographic area, with the highest being in Italy (33–35 per cent) and the lowest in Saudia Arabia (2.5 per cent) and Japan (0–9 per cent). *ret–PTC1* mutation is most common in sporadic cases, whilst *ret/PTC3* is most common in radiation-induced cases in both adults and children. These mutated receptors are now being targeted for new therapies.

Medullary thyroid cancer

MEN type 2 syndromes are associated with MTC development. Previously MEN risk was estimated by the pentagastrin stimulation test in which enhanced calcitonin secretion indicated the existence of the MEN syndrome. Germ-line point mutations of the *ret* proto-oncogene have identified these genes as being causative in MTC. Screening for these mutations in at-risk individuals permits their identification without the use of the pentagastrin stimulation test.

Clinical presentation

Clinical presentation is commonly with thyroid swelling in a euthyroid patient or during surveillance of patients previously irradiated or individuals from kindreds with familial predisposition to TC. The use of family photographs to time the onset of the swelling may be a valuable clue to the differential diagnosis. There may be associated symptoms including hoarseness, dysphagia, dyspnoea, haemoptysis, recurrent laryngeal nerve palsy, or thyrotoxicosis.

Investigation

Scanning of the thyroid with [^{123}I] sodium iodide will differentiate between multinodular goitre and hot and cold nodules. The majority of hot nodules are benign. Cold nodules require further imaging with ultrasound to exclude cysts.

Diagnosis

Fine-needle aspiration biopsy is not recommended in children, in contrast with adult practice. Measurement of serum thyroglobulin (TG) after thyroid-stimulating hormone (TSH) suppression and serum calcitonin will help differentiate between MTCs and TCs. TG is a useful tumour marker. Distant metastases can be demonstrated by ^{131}I uptake studies after resection of the primary tumour and blockade of iodine uptake by the thyroid remnant. Conventional imaging with radiography and CT/MRI scans will demonstrate local spread to the mediastinum and lung.

Surgery

In the papillary/follicular tumours, conservative resection of the primary is recommended with resection restricted to lobectomy and ishiectomy in solitary nodules. Radical neck dissection, with its attendant risks, is generally avoided in children with differentiated tumours. Total thyroidectomy is recommended for MTC in view of the high incidence of multifocal tumours, in individuals affected by MEN type 2A as a prophylactic procedure before the age of 5 years, and in those with MEN type 2B in the first year of life. Complete thyroidectomy is also advocated in patients exposed to significant environmental radiation in order to remove all residual potentially tumour-bearing tissue and in those with papillary tumours occurring at age <10 years because of the reputation of enhanced aggressiveness.

Radiotherapy

Adjuvant therapy with ^{131}I after thyroid ablation is used for treatment of metastatic deposits. Shrinkage of secondary tumours with ^{131}I therapy is easily demonstrated, and repeated doses can be used. Its role in patients without metastases is unknown. The influence of radio-iodine treatment on survival has not been tested in a randomized trial. Its use did not predict for survival in an uncontrolled study of treatment outcome. The long-term side effects of ^{131}I therapy in children are unclear, although post-radiation tissue atrophy in growing tissues and the increased risk of thyroid tumours after external beam thyroid irradiation are well known.

Medical care/chemotherapy

Reduction of thyroid tissue stimulation by thyroxine/tri-iodothyronine suppression of TSH production is used as preoperative preparation. Cytotoxic chemotherapy has not been widely used in these tumours. However, responses to single-agent therapy with etoposide, carboplatin, or cisplatin, and combination therapy with methotrexate and Adriamycin, bleomycin, or vincristine have been reported.

Prognosis

Reports frequently describe thyroid cancer in children as being aggressive with nodal metastases and frequent pulmonary metastases. The indolent nature of the majority of papillary and follicular TCs is associated with a 99 per cent overall 5-year survival (Table 26.1) in UK population-based figures. Series report up to 20 per cent recurrence rates. Deaths due to such tumours have been reported up to 30 years from diagnosis, and the standardized mortality ratio in patients aged <15 years at diagnosis has been calculated as 11.2. Prognostic variables in uncontrolled trials are limited to age at diagnosis, nodal invasion, and degree of tumour differentiation, with more differentiated tumours having a better prognosis. DNA aneuploidy has been associated with increasing age and tumour malignancy, but did not act independently on the prognosis of 125 adult patients. MTCs have a worse prognosis with only 50 per cent survival.

Salivary carcinomas

Salivary gland masses may include benign adenomas, haemangioma, lymphangioma, or malignant tumours such as mucoepidermoid carcinoma, acinic cell carcinoma, adenocarcinoma, soft tissue sarcoma, and leukaemic or lymphomatous infiltrates. Oral carcinoma in childhood may be 10 times as common in Bangladesh as it is in the UK, and some cases may be linked to chewing betel nut and tobacco. In the United States, the incidence among Black children is three times that among White children.

Clinical presentation and investigation

Clinical presentation is with a localized mass with or without facial pain and/or a facial palsy in parotid tumours. Regional lymph nodes may be involved at presentation. Investigation with facial radiography and CT/MRI scanning should be performed to define local tumour extension prior to surgery. A closed or incisional biopsy is not recommended. Staging investigations for distant spread to lung, liver, brain, and bone should be performed in high-grade tumours once the diagnosis has been confirmed histologically.

Pathology

Pleomorphic adenomas are well circumscribed benign solitary lesions; they rarely invade the gland capsule. The most common malignant salivary gland tumour type is the mucoepidermoid carcinoma, followed by acinic cell carcinoma, adenoid cystic carcinoma, and adenocarcinoma. Tumours are graded from I to III according to the level of differentiation.

Treatment

The primary aim of treatment is to achieve complete surgical excision. In the parotid gland, preservation of the facial nerve is highly desirable. Radiotherapy to areas of residual disease may be considered as an alternative to creating a facial palsy, as the cosmetic disfigurement may be less from radiotherapy if considerable facial growth has already occurred. Limited responses to chemotherapy using cisplatin, doxorubicin, 5-fluorouracil, cyclophosphamide, and vinorelbine given alone or in combination have been reported in adult patients. The best response rates reported used a combination of three or four of these drugs. Whether such response rates would be better in children is not reported. It does raise the possibility that chemotherapy might be used in individuals where the facial nerve is involved in order to attempt to make the tumour resectable without sacrificing the nerve.

There is a high incidence of local recurrence in both benign and malignant tumours. Evidence of incomplete resection or disseminated tumour justifies consideration of repeated surgery or radiotherapy if the disease is localized. Chemotherapy should be considered if the disease is disseminated, as this has been shown to produce durable remission and symptomatic relief.

Laryngeal carcinoma

Laryngeal carcinoma is extremely rare in childhood. It occurs most frequently after irradiation of juvenile laryngeal papillomatosis. Presentation is with cough, hoarseness, haemoptysis, stridor, and dysphagia. The tumours present later when located above the vocal cords. Diagnosis is made with microlaryngoscopy. Evidence for distant metastases should be sought with CT/MRI scanning of the chest and bone scanning. Tumours secondary to laryngeal papillomatosis are believed to metastasize rarely.

The rarity of this tumour in childhood has prevented the development of an established treatment approach. Preservation of the larynx is generally a high priority. Laser surgery, partial or total laryngectomy with or without local irradiation, may be employed depending upon the stage of the lesion. Overall survival of 59 per cent has been reported with such an approach. The inhibition of laryngeal growth coupled with the increased risk of secondary laryngeal and thyroid malignancies after irradiation makes the investigation of chemotherapy in these tumours in childhood a high priority. Reports of children being treated with chemotherapy are few, but responses have been noted. A recent review of adult trials of chemotherapy concluded that the use of induction therapy is feasible and delays development of distant metastases, although local and regional control are not improved and overall survival is unchanged. Concomitant chemotherapy and radiotherapy does produce superior survival in adults but remains experimental.

Angiofibroma

This tumour of adolescence occurs almost exclusively in males, suggesting an endocrine aetiology although this is not proven. The tumour is a mixed fibroblastic vascular tumour which is believed to be mesenchymal in origin. It commonly arises in the naso- or oropharynx and invades local surrounding hard and soft tissues; metastases are rare. It has been reported to invade the orbit, maxilla, and hard and soft palate as well intracranially. Clinical presentation is commonly with a unilateral facial swelling, obstructed nares, and recurrent epistaxis. Visualization of the tumour by anterior or posterior rhinoscopy reveals a dark red glistening tumour, warning of its extreme vascularity. Differential diagnosis includes inflammatory polyps, glomus jugulare tumour, capillary haemangioma, and fibromyxoma. Histologic examination is required to confirm this, but **biopsy is not recommended**. Treatment is mainly restricted to surgical resection using conventional or laser techniques. Some tumours are suitable for embolization. Local recurrences can occur. Case reports of tumour regression produced by hormone blockers and chemotherapy (flutamide, Adriamycin and DTIC) may justify trial of these approaches in extensive unresectable or recurrent cases. Stilboestrol and radiation have been used, although short- and long-term side effects in children limit the acceptability of these treatments.

Ameloblastoma (adamantimoma)

In childhood these tumours may be benign or malignant. They most commonly arise in the mandible and maxilla, although they are occasionally reported in the long bones. The facial presentation has been associated with enamel development of the teeth and primordial or dentigerous cysts. Infection, irritation, and nutritional deficiency have been suggested as possible aetiologic factors. Radiographs of the tumour reveal an osteolytic solitary cystic lesion. The treatment of choice is local tumour excision. Local recurrences are more common in the mandible than the maxilla. Radiotherapy has produced tumour responses, and sensitivity to chemotherapy has been reported with a wide variety of conventional agents. Pulmonary metastases have been reported many years after treatment of the primary lesion warranting modality therapy.

Chordoma

This rare tumour is thought to develop from remnants of the notochord and presents as a slow-growing locally invasive lobulated mass. It is more common in boys than girls and can arise anywhere within the axial skeleton, although it is most common in the spheno-occipital and sacrococcygeal regions. It can also occur in vertebral and extra-axial sites such as the facial bones, sinuses, and mediastinum. There is a tendency for chordomas of childhood to be intracranial and more aggressive. Metastatic spread occurs in ~10 per cent of patients as a late event, but is much lower in intracranial tumours. A recent report has identified loss of heterozygosity for the retinoblastoma gene in highly aggressive chordomas.

Clinical presentation is often late, with a prolonged history of symptoms related to tumour invasion or pressure on local structures. Investigation with radiography and CT/MRI scans will define the extent of the tumour. Treatment has been with a combination of local excision and radiotherapy. The restrictions on wide surgical excision imposed by the tumour site lead to a high incidence of local recurrence and a poor prognosis. The use of high radiation doses, close to the limits of normal tissue tolerance, has produced measurable responses and is reported to improve survival compared with surgery alone. More recently, computer-guided radiation techniques including proton beam therapy have been employed to provide highly focused high-dose radiotherapy in unresectable cases, although in skull base tumours this is associated with a significant risk of temporal lobe necrosis. The use of chemotherapy has been reported occasionally, with mixed responses. It is not known whether preoperative shrinkage in sensitive cases may improve surgical resection rate and permit less extensive radiation fields. In our view the risks of extensive surgery and radiation justify a trial of preoperative tumour shrinkage in patients where there is no immediate risk of neurologic deterioration.

Thoracic tumours

Thymoma

Thymoma and thymolipoma account for <10 per cent of all thymic tumours. The incidence of thymoma has decreased in recent years, almost certainly because some cases registered in the past were T-cell lymphoma. The incidence of benign thymolipoma is unknown as they are not ascertained by cancer registries. Thymolipoma is a mixed epithelial and lipomatous tumour which is slow growing and benign. It has characteristic appearances on CT and MR and can reach massive size prior to discovery. Thymoma is an epithelial tumour which can be encapsulated or locally invasive. Metastatic spread is rare.

Clinical presentation

Presentation is often incidental upon chest radiography or with superior vena cava obstruction. Breathlessness, mistaken for asthma, is reported. In adulthood, paraneoplastic syndromes such as myasthenia gravis, pure red cell aplasia, hypo-gammaglobulinaemia, finger clubbing, and new bone formation occur. Reports of EBV in tumour tissue suggest an aetiologic role similar to that in nasopharyngeal carcinoma.

Other causes of thymic masses include lymphoma, carcinoid tumour, and germ cell tumour. As the treatment of choice of thymoma is surgical, diagnostic biopsy is recommended prior to definitive surgery. Histologic grading can separate tumours into well-differentiated (low-grade) tumours and carcinomatous (high-grade) tumours, although this classification is not well validated in children.

Surgery

Surgical/pathologic staging from adult practice is used to dictate therapeutic approaches as follows.

◆ Stage 1 tumours (encapsulated): no adjuvant therapy is recommended.
◆ Tumours with local residual disease involving fat, pleura, or pericardium (stage 2): local radiotherapy.
◆ More extensive local invasion, involving lung, bones, etc. (stage 3): consider both radiotherapy (50–60 Gy) and adjuvant chemotherapy.

Adjuvant chemotherapy

For children, mediastinal radiotherapy is likely to be associated with considerable late morbidity linked to the subsequent growth and development of irradiated structures (e.g. lung, heart, bone marrow, sternum and ribs, and thoracic spine). Such risks must be balanced in individual cases with the response to chemotherapy and surgical staging of the tumour. Regimens using cisplatin, cyclophosphamide, and doxorubicin have been shown to be effective as neo-adjuvant treatment aimed at optimising surgical resection.

Primary lung and pleural tumours

Tumours of the lung and pleura are most commonly secondary to other neoplasms. Their anatomic location dictates the nature of their clinical presentation and helps predict the likely tumour type.

Clinical presentation

In childhood and adolescence, the majority of tumours are peripherally located and present with symptoms or signs of chest-wall involvement such as chest and shoulder pain or Horner syndrome. Centrally located tumours are more likely to present with signs of bronchial obstruction, such as wheeze, recurrent infection, haemoptysis, and superior vena cava obstruction.

Pathology

Rare pulmonary tumour types include adenomas and carcinomas, whilst rare types of pleuropulmonary tumours include pulmonary blastoma, neuroepithelioma (Askin tumour), or malignant mesothelioma.

Investigation

Imaging with chest radiography, CT/MRI scanning, and bone scanning is necessary to delineate the site and extent of the tumour as well as the number of distant metastases.

Pleuro-pulmonary blastoma

Pleuro-pulmonary blastoma (PPB) is a distinct clinicopathologic entity which occurs almost exclusively in childhood. It is an embryonic lung tumour consisting of gland-like structures lined with non-ciliated epithelium and surrounded by mesenchymatous stroma, mimicking the appearances of developing lung. It is found equally in both sexes. Trisomy 2 has been reported as have elevated levels of AFP. Despite failing to find abnormalities of *TP53*, family studies suggest that PPB heralds predisposition to dysplastic or neoplastic disease in 25 per cent of cases. Nearly a third of cases reported have been in association with congenital lung cysts, justifying a surgical approach to their management at diagnosis. The tumours grow aggressively and metastasize early. Primary surgical resection may be complicated by local recurrence. Recent case reports of the use of chemotherapy suggest that responses may be possible, justifying its consideration in tumours which are considered primarily inoperable. A proposed strategy would be to adopt an approach to therapy similar to that used in soft tissue sarcoma of preoperative chemotherapy followed by delayed surgery in order to optimize the chances of complete surgical resection.

Pulmonary adenomas

This term covers a variety of slow-growing tumours with low malignant potential including: carcinoid tumour, mucoepidermoid carcinoma, and cylindroma. They most commonly occur in the main bronchi. Primary treatment of these tumours is by surgical resection.

Lung carcinoma

Such carcinomas are well documented in childhood and are equally represented in both sexes. Histologically, they are most commonly undifferentiated bronchoepidermoid or adenocarcinomas. Lung carcinomas in children are more commonly located peripherally. Their aggressive nature and late presentation may explain the presence of metastases early in their clinical course. Treatment has followed adult guidelines with resection of operable tumours. The use of modern chemotherapy has an established role in the management of adult patients with small-cell lung carcinoma, resulting in a significant prolongation of survival in the majority and cure in a small percentage. Its role in the neo-adjuvant setting is being explored; cisplatin, VP16, gemcitabine, paclitaxel, carboplatin, vinorelbine, and docetaxel all have activity. Novel biologic agents are being investigated with mixed success. Radiotherapy has been used palliatively with some effect.

Breast tumours

The very significant difficulties in assessment and surgical approaches, and the need to support a young patient during diagnosis, treatment, and follow-up, justify referral for assessment of such problems to a paediatric oncology center linked to a collaborating multidisciplinary breast cancer team. Most breast tumours in children are benign. Breast lumps in early adolescence or childhood can be due to premature thelarche, juvenile papillomatosis, fibroadenoma, and, rarely, malignant tumours such as juvenile secretory carcinoma, fibro-, rhabdo-, and liposarcomas, and cystosarcoma phylloides. The benign tumours are more likely to show fluctuations in size and tenderness during the menstrual cycle. Secondary malignant tumours have been reported, as have rare presentations of soft tissue sarcoma and lymphoma. Secondary breast cancers are more common in young women after thoracic wall irradiation. Ultrasound-guided needle biopsy is recommended. Histologic diagnosis is difficult in view of the variable appearance of the developing breast. However, *in situ* studies of oestrogen and progesterone receptors may help to identify hormonally dependent and independent tissues. Areas of secretory carcinoma have been reported within fibroadenoma and juvenile papillomatosis. The rarity of breast tumours in this age group justifies a national/international pathology review process in order to standardize diagnostic criteria before rational treatment programmes can evolve.

Phylloides tumour

Phylloides tumour is a rapidly growing tumour which is most commonly benign, although histology is not always predictive (15 per cent are malignant). Five per cent of all tumours occur during adolescence, and they are not reported in males. Treatment by surgical resection is recommended. In metastatic cases, chemotherapy and radiotherapy have been effective. Long-term follow-up is recommended as there is a sustained risk of recurrence.

Breast carcinoma

Fewer than 0.1 per cent of breast carcinomas occur in children aged <15 years. Malignant tumours are most commonly juvenile secretory carcinomas for which conservative primary surgical resection is recommended, after which long disease-free periods have been observed with occasional late relapses. Their clinical behaviour is one of slow growth with multiple recurrences. Patients with juvenile secretory carcinomas aged <12 years seem to have a better prognosis than older adolescents. Undifferentiated carcinomas have been reported and have a much poorer prognosis, justifying an aggressive multimodality approach to treatment with surgery, chemotherapy, and radiotherapy. The use of radiation has been limited to the treatment of localized unresectable disease.

Malignant mesothelioma

Prognosis

Malignant mesothelioma arises from the mesothelial layer of the pleura, peritoneum, pericardium, and tunica vaginalis. The incidence of mesothelioma is very low in children's tumour registries. Histopathologic classification within these childhood cancer registries is complicated by the lack of a specific internationally recognized disease code coupled with a lack of consensus of histopathologic features. In most childhood cases there is a predominant tubular papillary pattern with solid areas, whilst some tumours show foci of single cells. Immunoreactivity for cytokeratin, epithelial membrane antigen, and vimentin is characteristic. It is not possible to grade these tumours histologically. Peritoneal tumours are often multicystic and have a reduced capacity to metastasize, tending to recur locally.

Biology

Chromosome loss from overlap regions 1p21–p22 and 9p21–p22 have been reported, together with other areas of chromosome loss on 3p, 6q, 14,16,18, and 22. *WT1* tumour suppression gene is expressed in the mesothelial lining during embryologic development. Mutations of *WT1* have been detected in some sporadic mesotheliomas. These observations suggest that there is a multiple step process to tumour development.

Aetiology

In adults, environmental exposure to asbestos (crocidolite) with a latent period of 12–20 years is a well-recognized aetiologic mechanism. It is estimated to account for over half of cases in adults, predominantly in males. In the absence of asbestos exposure, the sex ratio of adult cases is probably close to 1:1. Childhood mesothelioma is fairly equally represented in both sexes. It is not commonly associated with asbestos exposure, although asbestos bodies have been identified in children. A study in the USA failed to identify geographical clustering of childhood cases, although a cluster of cases in the West Midlands, UK, has been identified and remains to be explained. The SV40-contaminated poliomyelitis vaccine has been implicated in the aetiology of mesothelioma, although this was not supported in recent follow-up studies. Of some concern is the number of reports of mesothelioma occurring as a second malignant neoplasm in survivors of childhood as well as adult cancers. The first tumours in the childhood cases were predominantly Hodgkin disease and Wilms tumour.

Clinical presentation

Clinical presentation is most commonly pleural (75–85 per cent), with initial chest pain and subsequent shortness of breath and cough as pleural effusions develop. Peritoneal presentation is with abdominal distension and/or intestinal obstruction. Sixty-five per cent of peritoneal malignant mesotheliomas occur in girls. Multicystic tumours can present with free-floating cystic masses. Congenital presentation has been reported. Detailed imaging of pleural/peritoneal spaces, lung, and bone should be performed with CT/MRI, ultrasound, and scintigraphy scanning. Positron emission tomography has been helpful in monitoring cavitary tumour responses during therapy.

Treatment

Successful treatment is dependent upon complete surgical excision, particularly in the multi-cystic tumour types, although local recurrence is common and repeated resections may be necessary. Systemic chemotherapy has been used; the agents reported to be active include doxorubicin, cisplatin, cyclophosphamide, mitomycin-C, ifosfamide, and vincristine. Intraca-vitary treatment with cisplatin and bleomycin have been used to control recurrent effusions, although this may lead to the development of extensive abdominal adhesions. The use of intracavitary instillations of radioactive gold or phosphorus is being investigated.

Abdomen

Gastric carcinoma

One to two per cent of gastric carcinomas occur in people aged <30 years of age, and 3 per cent of these are in the paediatric age group. They may be associated with immune deficiency states or with features of ataxia telangiectasia. Clinical presentation is often late, with weight loss, iron deficiency anaemia, and anorexia. Barium studies or endoscopy and tumour biopsy will confirm the diagnosis. The tumours are usually unresectable, having a tendency to disseminate early and invade locally. Radiotherapy is of little value in view of the low radiation tolerance of the surrounding structures. Promising results with a variety of chemotherapy regimes have been reported, including VAC and FAM (5-fluorouracil, Adriamycin, and mitomycin) and cisplatin alone and in combination with 5-fluorouracil, Adriamycin and etoposide. Neo-adjuvant chemotherapy is being explored. Intraperitoneal cisplatin has been used in view of the presence of malignant cells in peritoneal washings in up to one-third of patients at surgery. Good anti-emetic therapy is important for the use of chemotherapy in upper gastrointestinal neoplasms if the treatment is to be tolerated. The optimistic reports of chemotherapy in adult patients indicate the need to explore its role as primary treatment of such poor prognosis childhood tumours.

Pancreatic tumours

Benign tumours of the pancreas are either dermoid cysts or cystadenomas. Malignant tumours of the pancreas occur more commonly and are equally distributed between the sexes. There are four main tumour types: pancreatoblastoma, papillary cystic neoplasm (Frantz's neoplasm), islet cell tumours, and adenocarcinoma.

Clinical presentation

Clinically, these tumours present with abdominal pain, an upper abdominal mass, symptoms of disturbed exocrine pancreatic function (diarrhoea, weight loss), duodenal obstruction (vomiting, weight loss), or symptoms related to endocrine products of the tumour such as gastric ulceration, hypoglycaemia, endocrine disturbance, or diarrhoea. Obstructive jaundice is less common in childhood (one-third of patients) than in adults (two-thirds of patients).

Investigation

Locating the mass in the pancreas is best performed by ultrasound, CT/MRI scanning (Fig. 26.2), arteriography, and sometimes endoscopic retrograde cholangiopancreatography

(ERCP). Tumours are most common in the head of the pancreas. Identifying tumours arising from the pancreas as opposed to the liver or other retroperitoneal structures can be difficult. A cytologic diagnosis may be made at ERCP from pancreatic fluid. A variety of tumour markers have been used for diagnosis (carcino-embryonic antigen, AFP, and pancreatic oncofetal antigen). Pancreatic peptides have also been used (Table 26.4).

Pancreatoblastoma

Pancreatoblastoma is the most common malignant neoplasm of the pancreas in early life. The mean age at presentation is 4.5 years; it rarely occurs after 10 years of age. There is a predominance of Asian case reports in the literature.

Pathology

Embryologically there are great similarities between the development of the liver and pancreas from the foregut, and these similarities are mirrored in nature of the embryonic tumours of these organs. Pancreatoblastoma tumours are frequently large and well circumscribed. Microscopically, pancreatoblastoma is a dense epithelial cellular tumour with acinar differentiation and 'squamoid corpuscles'. The tissue is frequently lobulated by fibrous stroma. Cystic change and calcification are described. Immunocytochemically, pancreatoblastoma is positive for α_1-antitrypsin, AFP, and glucose-6-phosphatase. It is a malignant tumour with local invasion, with metastatic disease to local lymph nodes, liver, and lung in up to 35 per cent in one series. It is associated with Beckwith–Wiedemann syndrome and may be associated with elevated levels of serum AFP which might constitute a useful tumour marker.

Treatment

Pancreatoblastoma is potentially a curable malignancy, with survival rates of 50–80 per cent being reported. The higher survival rates are in patients who have had complete resections. The largest series reports an overall 58 per cent survival rate. The similarity to hepatoblastoma and the successes of multimodality approaches to treatment in the SIOPEL studies of that tumour, coupled with the evidence for chemosensitivity in pancreatoblastoma, justify the proposal to adopt a similar multidisciplinary approach; the high-risk strategy of SIOPEL 2 being most suitable. Primary resection should be reserved for localized tumours which are considered easily resectable. Biopsy is followed by a trial of chemotherapy and delayed resection for those deemed initially unresectable.

Table 26.4. Pancreatic endocrine tumours: cell types, ectopic hormones and clinical presentation

Cell type	Hormone secreted	Tumour type	Clinical presentation
A	Glucagon	Glucagonoma	Adult
B	Insulin	Insulinoma	Hypoglycaemia
C	Gastrin	Gastrinoma	Peptic ulceration, Zollinger–Ellison syndrome
D	Somatostatin	Somatostatinoma	Primarily adult
D1	Vasoactive intestinal polypeptide (VIP)	VIPoma	Diarrhoea

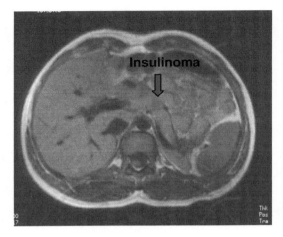

Fig. 26.2 MRI scan showing a pancreatic tumour (insulinoma).

Papillary cystic tumour of pancreas (Frantz's tumour)

Papillary cystic tumour of pancreas (PCTP) has been variously referred to by a heterogeneous collection of terms, and varying degrees of malignant behaviour are described. It is a relatively slowly growing tumour predominantly affecting girls (one-third occur at <16 years of age) and young adult women.

Pathology

PCTP is typically encapsulated and associated with pancreatic inflammation, pseudocyst formation, and calcification. Mitoses are rare, although capsular invasion is common and may extend to the duodenum and hepatic portal vein. Microscopically it consists of solid and papillary components. The solid elements typically form rosettes and degenerate into cysts. The papillary components stain positively for periodic acid–Schiff reagent. Immunocyto-chemically, the tumours stain positively for α_1-antitrypsin and α_1-antichymotrypsin. Studies of oestrogen and progesterone receptors may be justified in some cases as they may provide an option for therapy in difficult cases.

Treatment

Surgical resection for both primary tumour and any metastases is the treatment of choice, justifying extensive surgical procedures to achieve this. Chemotherapy and radiotherapy have been reported to be effective. However, these treatments are generally restricted to those with residual or metastatic disease.

Islet cell tumours

Islet cell tumours are endocrine tumours. They are the least common group of tumours of the pancreas and secrete either insulin or gastrin. They are most commonly solitary and benign. Individuals with MEN type 1 may present with adenomatosis of the pancreas. In the case of insulinomas, a plasma glucose-to-insulin ratio >1, with a normal C peptide, is diagnostic. The tumour may be difficult to localize and is most commonly benign. Gastrinomas are diagnosed by the identification of elevated serum gastrin levels. They are more commonly malignant although they grow slowly. Treatment for these tumours is by surgical resection where the tumour is solitary and resectable. Multiple or metastatic tumours are best treated medically to control exocrine or endocrine symptoms.

Carcinoma of pancreas

As in adults, ductal adenocarcinoma followed by acinar cell carcinoma are the most common types. Cases have been described in patients aged as young as 3 weeks. Surgical resection provides the only hope of cure. Chemotherapy (usually 5-fluorouracil, gemcitabine) produces partial responses, as does radiotherapy. However, survival benefit is yet to be demonstrated. Some authors believe that children may have a better prognosis than adults.

Adrenal cortical carcinoma

Adrenal carcinoma (ACC) accounts for 0.2 per cent of childhood malignancies with an international incidence of 0.5–1 per million. It is more common in girls than boys (1.5:1) and has a bimodal age distribution, with a peak incidence in early childhood and adolescence. In early childhood the ratio of girls to boys is at least 2:1. A 5-year survival of 38 per cent is reported by the CCRG in the childhood age range (Table 26.1).

Aetiology and biology

There is clear evidence of a genetic aetiology for many cases of ACC. It is one of the tumours linked to the family cancer syndrome originally described by Li and Fraumeni. The presence of ACC in such families is rare, but it occurs 100 times more frequently than would be expected by chance. Most families with classic Li–Fraumeni syndrome have a germ-line mutation of *TP53*. As 50 per cent of cases with ACC have germ-line mutations of *TP53*, the diagnosis of ACC in a family is likely to be the first sign of a familial cancer predisposition justifying consideration of referral for genetic counselling. ACC is also associated with two tissue-overgrowth syndromes: hemi-hypertrophy and Beckwith–Wiedemann syndrome. A possible metabolic aetiology is suggested by the association with a previous history of salt-losing congenital adrenal hyperplasia. Finally, an environmental toxic aetiology is suggested by a study of parental toxic exposures in children identified with ACC within the Manchester Children's Tumour Registry and the observation of a threefold increase in population incidence in southern Brazil compared with international incidence. St Jude's Children's Research Hospital has established an international ACC paediatric tumour register.

Clinical presentation

Clinical presentation is with virilization/precocious puberty (90 per cent), abdominal mass (60 per cent), Cushing syndrome (<50 per cent), or a combination of these. Occasionally rapidly growing carcinomas present with abdominal pain, weight loss, fever, and an abdominal mass in the absence of endocrine disturbances.

Pathology

Differentiating histologically between adenoma and carcinoma is difficult as features of malignancy, including frequent mitoses, cellular pleomorphism, and vascular invasion, may be seen in both categories. A modification of the Weiss criteria based upon atypical mitoses, confluent necrosis, and nuclear grade is believed by some to predict clinical outcome. However, tumour size is more widely accepted as a predictor of tumour behaviour; tumours of weight <100–150 g and diameter >5–6 cm or volume >200 ml are more likely to be malignant. In the author's view, this assumption is counter-intuitive. A preferable assumption would be that all tumours have malignant potential if left to grow untreated, which is supported by the adverse prognostic factors of older age at presentation, increased urinary steroid excretion, and delays in diagnosis.

Investigation

Investigations are directed at clarifying the endocrine status by differentiating between Cushing disease, congenital adrenal hyperplasia, and adrenal tumours. Adrenal carcinomas are associated with markedly elevated basal urinary 17 ketosteroid production (>40 mg/24 h), and urinary androgens, plasma levels of cortisol, dihydroepiandrosterone sulphate, and 17-hydroxy progesterone may be raised. ACTH levels are low because of pituitary suppression. It is important to determine the endocrine profile in order to monitor response to treatment. Imaging with abdominal ultrasound and CT/MRI scans will permit definition of tumour size and local and distant spread (Fig. 26.3). Vascular invasion of the inferior vena cava may occur and its demonstration is important prior to surgical removal.

Surgery

Primary surgical removal is the treatment of choice and may be curative for smaller tumours. Patients with residual disease are seldom cured. Staging criteria are given in Table 26.5.

Endocrine management

In tumours characterized by excess hormone production, great care is needed to manage steroid deficiency in the postoperative period. Treatment with mitotane (o, p′-DDD) has been used to control steroid side effects and has been reported to reduce primary and secondary tumour size. Response rates reported are 19–34 per cent in adults and 30 per cent in the most recent study in children. No reports claim curative success with this treatment. In a large adult study it was not shown to improve survival. Mitotane is administered orally (starting dose 0.5 g) and is associated with a range of troublesome symptoms including vomiting,

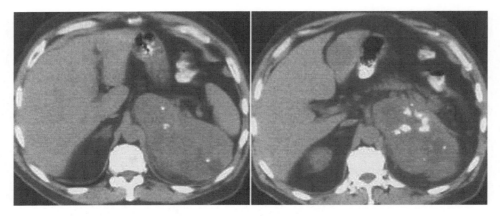

Fig. 26.3 CT scans showing an adrenal tumour with calcification.

Table 26.5. Anatomical staging systems for adrenal carcinoma

Stage 1	Total excision of tumour, volume < 200 cm³
	Absence of metastases and normal hormone levels after surgery
Stage 2	Microscopic residual tumour, tumour volume > 200 cm³
	Absence of metastases yet persistently elevated adrenocortical hormone levels after surgery
Stage 3	Gross residual or inoperable tumour
Stage 4	Distant metastases

diarrhoea, neurologic disturbances, lethargy, dizziness, somnolence, and muscle weakness. Careful monitoring is essential. It is most effective when the serum level >14 mg/l. Concomitant mineralocorticoid and glucocorticoid therapy may need to be intensified during mitotane therapy since deaths from adrenal insufficiency, despite replacement therapy, have been reported.

Chemotherapy

Cytotoxic chemotherapy has generally been restricted to the treatment of relapse. Responses have been reported with combination regimens such as 5-fluorouracil, Adriamycin, and cisplatin, streptozotocin and mitotane, CAP (cyclophosphamide, Adriamycin, and cisplatin), OPEC/OJEC (cisplatin, carboplatin, vincristine, VM26, VP16, and cyclophosphamide), cisplatin and etoposide, and cisplatin and etoposide in combination with mitotane. The precise role of chemotherapy in clinical management, despite this evidence of tumour sensitivity, is not established in the literature. However, the importance of complete resection coupled with demonstrable chemosensitivity would justify a trial of preoperative treatment in large and predictably unresectable tumours.

Radiotherapy

Radiotherapy has been used to eradicate residual disease. However, secondary tumours within the irradiation field have been reported which in the presence of a high risk of genetic cancer predisposition suggests an enhanced sensitivity to radiation-induced second tumours, especially in the breast in girls.

Colon and rectal carcinoma

Epidemiology and pathology

Almost all of the 1 per cent of cases of colorectal malignancy that arise in patients aged <30 years are carcinoma. It is almost unheard of in infancy, and the majority of cases that are reported occur during adolescence where boys are affected twice as commonly as girls. Predisposing factors such as familial adenomatous polyposis, Turcot syndrome, and ulcerative colitis are recognized but accounted for a minority of reported cases in the literature.

Clinical presentation

Clinical presentation is with vague abdominal pain, rectal bleeding, weight loss, altered bowel habit, and abdominal distension. Screening is not possible in the childhood population; delays in diagnosis are frequent and <50 per cent have the diagnosis made prior to operation. The majority of tumours occur in the sigmoid and rectum. Barium enema, colonoscopy, and biopsy are the optimal diagnostic investigations in suspected cases. Histologically, the tumours are most frequently mucus-secreting adenocarcinomas (50 per cent) or are poorly differentiated, hence the high incidence of rapidly disseminated disease. Sixty to eighty per cent present with Duke stage C or D involvement at diagnosis and are often inoperable.

Treatment

As in adult practice, successful treatment of colon cancer depends upon complete surgical resection. Adult studies of systemic chemotherapy have identified that high-dose 5-fluorouracil combined with leucovorin and irinotecan improves survival of more advanced stage patients. Intra-arterial or portal chemotherapy has been used for hepatic metastases but the results are inconclusive. Chemotherapy produces responses in >50 per cent of cases in childhood but they are not sustained. The overall survival is poor, with 5-year survival rates <10 per cent.

Successful treatment of rectal carcinoma in adult practice is again based upon the extent of surgical resection. There is controversy surrounding the optimal method of defining margins of resection. Preoperative radiotherapy can improve resection rates in 35–75 per cent of patients but seems to be less effective after surgery. Most recently, biologic therapies targeting epithelial growth factor receptor and vascular endothelial growth factors are being combined with conventional chemotherapy and are producing improved and sustained responses in refractory patients.

Pelvis

Genital tract and bladder tumours

The majority of genital tract tumours in childhood are rhabdomyosarcomas or germ cell tumours. Carcinomas may occur throughout the genital tract in girls, whilst in boys they have only occasionally been reported in the testis and bladder.

Clear cell adenocarcinoma of the vagina and cervix

An association between intrauterine exposure to diethylstilboestrol (DES) and an increased incidence of clear cell vaginal adenocarcinoma with vaginal adenosis was suspected after two case–control studies. Prospective screening of the at-risk population established an association between intrauterine DES exposure and vaginal and cervical adenosis. However, the risk for having clear cell carcinoma after intrauterine DES exposure was small (0.14–1.4 in 1000) and the evidence for a causative association with clear cell vaginal carcinoma in young women has not been clearly demonstrated. The use of DES during pregnancy was widespread in the USA but only limited in the UK, and its use was discontinued in 1971. Screening has been recommended for exposed children from the age of 14 years or menarche. Clinical presentation may otherwise occur with abnormal vaginal bleeding in the prepubertal and adolescent years.

Investigation and treatment

Presentation is with premenarchal vaginal bleeding. Diagnosis is dependent on abdominal and pelvic ultrasound/MRI and vaginal examination including colposcopy, which may necessitate an anaesthetic. Evidence for metastatic spread should be sought with chest CT and clinical evaluation of lymph nodes, including the supraclavicular region. The tumour is locally invasive and may metastasize to the lungs as well as to local and distant lymph nodes. Local treatment is dictated by the stage of the tumour at presentation. The staging system of the International Federation of Gynecology and Obstetrics (FIGO) is used. Interstitial or transvaginal radiotherapy, which spares the ovaries from ablative irradiation, is reserved for stage I lesions. More extensive disease is treated by radical surgery, followed by vaginal reconstruction, or external irradiation of the entire pelvis. The use of chemotherapy has been reserved for the treatment of recurrent disease. Responses to cyclophosphamide, melphalan, actinomycin D, 5-fluorouracil, and carboplatin have been reported.

Prognosis

Overall survival is ~80 per cent (stage I, 85 per cent; stage II, 70 per cent; stage III, 50 per cent; stage IV, 0 per cent). Older patients (>19 years) do better than younger patients (<15 years), and this difference in survival is attributed to the prevalence of tubulocystic differentiation in the older age group. The extensive surgery or radiotherapy recommended in advanced stages has many long term physical and psychologic side effects which may justify the exploration of early chemotherapy if less radical local treatment could be considered after initial tumour shrinkage.

Tumours of the Fallopian tubes

Malignant tumours of the Fallopian tubes are either pure carcinomas or mixed Müllerian tumours, which are biphasic tumours containing both mesenchymal and carcinomatous elements. Conventional treatment approaches to such tumours depend upon a combination of radical surgery and radiotherapy. Chemotherapy with a wide variety of agents is currently under investigation. Anecdotal reports of responses to chemotherapy with BEP (bleomycin, VP-16, and cisplatin) in mixed Müllerian tumours justify further investigation in an attempt to reduce iatrogenic morbidity and distant failures associated with continued surgery and radio-therapy.

Transitional cell carcinoma of the bladder

Transitional cell carcinoma of the bladder occurs rarely during the first two decades of life. Gross haematuria is the most common presenting symptom. Preoperative imaging frequently detects the tumour, although cytoscopy is necessary to obtain histology. The malignancy is usually low grade and non-invasive, with a low recurrence rate. Transurethral resection or fulguration is the treatment of choice, and the prognosis is favourable. Trials of intravesical chemotherapy and local microwave hyperthermia for recurrence are being reported, with gemcitabine and carboplatin being the investigatory drugs.

Ovarian carcinoma

Adeno- or cystadenocarcinomas of the ovary account for 12–18 per cent of malignant ovarian tumours in children. Their clinical presentation is with acute or chronic lower abdominal pain in the majority, together with abdominal distension and a palpable mass. Pelvic and abdominal ultrasound is important to differentiate between solid and cystic masses. Most, but not all, cystic masses are benign. Careful surgical staging is important, as is tumour monitoring with C125. Management is effectively as for adult disease. Surgery is recommended for solid, palpable, or calcified masses and for those that present with persistent fever to rule out appendix abscess. At surgery, where a tumour is suspected, oophorectomy with or without salpingectomy is recommended. Second-look procedures to monitor response are widely used. Postoperative chemotherapy with combinations of cyclophosphamide, hexamethylamine, cisplatin, and Adriamycin have been used successfully in extensive disease. A recent phase III trial in adults showed a

survival advantage for a paclitaxel–cisplatin regimen, and a randomized comparison of paclitaxel with topotecan showed that topotecan performed favourably with respect to response rates
and time to progression. Dose-intense and high-dose therapy with stem cell rescue have been
tested in recurrent adult cases. Intraperitoneal chemotherapy is also used.

Other tumours

Melanotic primitive neuroectodermal tumour of infancy (MPNET, melanotic progonoma)

This tumour is unusual in that it is made up of two populations of cells derived from the neural
crest, neuroblasts and melanocytes. Ninety-five per cent of the tumours occur in infants aged
<1 year. The sites of presentation include the maxilla (60 per cent), the skull (13 per cent), the
epididymis (9 per cent), the mandible (6 per cent), and the brain (6 per cent), as well as a
variety of other bony and soft tissues. Urinary vanillylmandelic acid (VMA) excretion may be
elevated in a small proportion of tumours. This is of no prognostic significance, but it is useful
as a tumour marker. It has a favourable prognosis, with a low malignant potential (2–7 per
cent) and low (10–15 per cent) local recurrence risk. Indications for adjuvant treatment are
governed by the clinical nature of the tumour at presentation. Mixed responses to chemotherapy agents have been reported.

Malignant melanoma

Malignant melanoma is an aggressive skin tumour derived from melanocytes which are cells
which arise in the neural crest in the fetus.

Epidemiology

In the UK, the annual incidence in childhood is about 1.2 per million with a male-to-female
ratio of 0.8:1. A Swedish population-based study showed that the incidence rates for childhood
malignant melanoma were stable, whilst the incidence rates for adolescents are rising in line
with adult figures. In Australia, crude rates of 5 per million nationally and 10 per million in
Queensland have been recorded. There is a different pattern of disease incidence between those
malignant melanomas arising in childhood (<14 years) and those arising during adolescence.
The malignant melanomas arising in childhood are predominantly associated with skin types
susceptible to damage by ultraviolet radiation, children who have a family history of the
disease, and tumours which present as a complication of a congenital melanocytic naevus.
Families with a strong history of melanoma may demonstrate 'genetic anticipation', where
successive generations have the condition diagnosed earlier than their parents. Whether this is
due to improved surveillance or genuine genetic anticipation is not proven. The increasing
incidence in adults and adolescence is thought to be related to enhanced skin exposure to
sunlight, although the epidemiologic evidence is conflicting. Exposure to phototherapy given
in infancy for hyperbilirubinaemia has not been identified as a risk factor for the development
of malignant melanoma.

Clinical presentation

More than 90 per cent of childhood malignant melanomas are skin tumours. Rarely, ocular and
central nervous system leptomeningeal primaries are also seen. Over half of the skin tumours

are of the superficial spreading type and most other specified cases are nodular. Staging investigations looking for 'in transit' metastases, regional lymph node involvement, and distant metastases in lung, brain, and bones should be carried out. Cerebral metastases occur in ~20 per cent of patients. The presence of brain metastases is associated with a very poor prognosis.

Pathology and prognosis

The histologic diagnosis should only be made by experienced pathologists. A recent EORTC study identified only 60 per cent of centrally referred malignant melanoma as true malignant melanomas. In adults, malignant melanomas are graded by their thickness (Breslow thickness > 3 mm) which correlates with their risk of metastatic spread. The EORTC study identified a thickness >2 mm as predictive of a higher risk of metastatic spread and fatal outcome. Overall 5-year survival rates were greater than 80 per cent (Table 26.2).

Large congenital melanocytic naevi

A study of 289 cases of large congenital melanocytic naevi (LCMN) identified only 38 (13 per cent) which developed primary cutaneous malignant melanomas, all of which arose within LCMNs located at axial sites and none within LCMNs located on peripheral (limb) sites. Two others developed malignant melanoma at uninvolved sites. A striking finding in this study was the absence of malignant melanomas in any of the many thousands of satellite lesions. Removal of LCMN is an area of controversy. Curettage or surgical removal has been performed within the first few weeks of life for cosmetic reasons, and in older children removal has been directed at preventing development of melanoma. There is little evidence that radical surgery of this sort reduces the incidence of metastatic disease.

Surgery

Newly diagnosed patients with malignant melanoma should have wide surgical excision and pathologic assessment of the lesion by an experienced pathologist. There is a place for surgical resection of solitary accessible cerebral metastases.

Drug therapy

No further therapy is recommended for completely resected thin lesions (Breslow thickness <3 mm) in adults. Adjuvant therapy with high-dose interferon given over a year has shown a 10 per cent survival advantage for locally advanced disease (Breslow thickness > 3 mm), regional lymph node involvement, or 'in transit' metastases. Metastatic disease in adulthood is treated with DTIC, and trials are under way to evaluate the use of chemotherapy in combination with biologic therapies such as interferon and interleukin. Such treatments are considerably more toxic than chemotherapy alone. There are no trials open in the UK specifically recruiting children. The nitrosourea analogue fotemustine is licensed for treatment of cerebral metastases in a number of countries, but not in the UK or the USA. Preliminary experience with responses to temozolomide have been reported. Twenty per cent response rates have been reported to both fotemustine and temozolomide, which are well tolerated as they are given orally.

Radiotherapy

The role of radiotherapy in cerebral metastases is controversial as few patients have sensitive disease.

Future developments

A number of conclusions can be drawn from considering these rare tumours.

There is a strong need for an individual case to be managed in the children's multidisciplinary team, supported by specialists from disciplines familiar with technical aspects of specific tumour types, for example breast cancer team, head and neck cancer team, radiotherapists, endocrinologists, urologists, gynaecologists, geneticists, neurosurgeons, maxillofacial surgeons, and upper and lower gastrointestinal teams.

Advances in therapy will be promoted by national cancer registration, central pathologic review, the development of guidelines, trials of novel therapies, and adoption of new techniques from adult practice.

The rarity of these tumours makes them attractive for research in aetiology and biology (adrenal carcinoma, thyroid cancer), new treatments (mesothelioma, pleuropulmonary blastoma), and, where relevant, publicity aimed at prevention (melanoma).

Patient/family information should be developed to reduce the sense of isolation that these families experience when their condition is referred to as 'rare' and they become the focus of medical curiosity.

Acknowledgements

The author would like to acknowledge the invaluable assistance of Dr Charles Stiller of the Children's Cancer Research Group, Oxford, UK, and Dr Richard Grundy of the University of Birmingham.

Bibliography

Walker DA, Grundy R, Stiller C (2002) Rare tumours of childhood. In: Souhami R, Tannock I, Hohenberger P, Horiot JC (eds) *Oxford Textbook of Oncology* (2nd edn). Oxford: Oxford University Press, 2669–91.

Index

THE CONSUL'S DAUGHTER

Caseley is the 21-year-old daughter of Teuder
Bonython, successful shipyard owner and consul
for Mexico. When Teuder falls ill, Caseley takes
responsibility for the shipyard, the consulate, and
her father's health, but in Victorian England, she
must hide her talents in a world dominated by
men. Not conventionally beautiful, Caseley also
resigns herself to a life without love ... until she
encounters a half-Spanish captain, Jago Barata.
Their every encounter sets them at each other's
throats, until Caseley must deliver an important
letter to Spain and the only ship leaving in time
is Jago's...

THE CONSUL'S DAUGHTER

by

Jane Jackson

Magna Large Print Books
Long Preston, North Yorkshire,
BD23 4ND, England.

British Library Cataloguing in Publication Data.

A catalogue record of this book is
available from the British Library

ISBN   978-0-7505-4427-6

First published in Great Britain by Accent Press Ltd 2016

Published in Large Print 2017 by arrangement with Accent Press

Magna Large Print is an imprint of Library Magna Books Ltd.

Printed and bound in Great Britain by
T.J. (International) Ltd., Cornwall, PL28 8RW

Chapter One

'Drunk again?'

Rage flushed Teuder Bonython's pallid complexion. He tugged with shaking fingers at the neck of his white nightshirt. 'He needs a thrashing to knock some sense into him.' He closed his eyes, labouring to breathe, the grooves in his forehead deepening.

Seated on the side of the bed, Caseley leaned forward. 'Are you in pain, Father? Will you have your drops now?'

'Where is he?'

'Ben is putting him to bed.'

He looked up at her. The wretchedness and frustration in his gaze wrenched her heart. 'How many times is that this week? I want the truth.'

'Four, I think.' She looked at his blue-veined hand clenching the sheet. 'He's going through a difficult–'

'Damn it, Ralph is twenty-five years old.' Bitterness and despair twisted his mouth. 'My only son.' He looked at her. His pale eyes, usually so sharp beneath shaggy grey brows, now held bewilderment. 'Why, Caseley? Why is he doing this? To me, to the family?'

'He's unhappy,' she said softly.

A strangled laugh tore itself from her father's throat. 'Good God in Heaven, what's he got to be unhappy about? How much more does he want?'

Not more, less. Caseley said nothing. She reached forward to the bedside table and unscrewed the top from a fluted brown bottle resting on a silver tray. Pouring several drops of amber liquid into a glass she added water from a carafe.

'I don't need that,' Teuder growled. But as she held the glass to his lips he drank obediently. The burst of anger had drained him, and though the purple tinge had faded, beneath the flush on his cheeks his skin was grey.

'You're a good lass,' he muttered. 'You should be tending a husband and children, not burdened with me and the business and your wastrel brother.'

'You're no burden.' Caseley smiled. He had no idea how much the well-meant words hurt.

'If only your mother were here.'

'It wouldn't help Ralph, Father,' she said as gently as she could. 'Try to sleep now. Dr Vigurs is coming tomorrow, and if you don't look better than you do now, he'll keep you in bed for another week.'

'Doctors,' Teuder grunted, his papery eyelids drooping. 'What do they know?' But he didn't protest as she straightened the covers and blew out the candle. She leaned down and kissed his forehead.

'Goodnight.' He grunted again and she limped out. She closed the door quietly. Turning she saw a stocky man in his early thirties carrying an oil lamp coming along the passage.

'How is my brother?'

'Sleeping. He've parted with most of it, begging your pardon, miss. But I brung the bucket back up, just in case.'

She hid her distaste at the all too vivid image Ben's reply conjured. She should be used to it by now. Hadn't she done her share of holding Ralph's head? She understood the desperate battle raging within him, and admired his talent. But she was tired of his self-destructive behaviour.

'He'll have some thick head come morning.'

'Where was he found this time?'

'In the alley behind the Marine Hotel. Henry didn't know how long he'd been there. He wouldn't have seen him at all but for taking out a couple of barrels. He put him in a cab and sent him home.'

'I'll see Mr Voss is paid for his trouble.' Caseley mentally added this to the already long list of tasks for the morning. She opened the kitchen door. 'I expect you'd like something to eat before–' She broke off.

The large scrubbed table was set with a knife and fork, a mug of ale, and a plate of cold beef, pickled onions, and a lump of cheese. A spotless white apron tied over her grey calico dress, mousy hair gathered into a bun, Liza-Jane, thin as a willow and strong as an ox, emerged from the pantry carrying a crusty loaf.

'Evening, miss.' Her brown eyes slid past Caseley and a blush crept up her throat to stain her sharp features. 'I just done a bit of supper for Ben.' Picking up a long knife in a work-roughened hand that trembled slightly she began to slice the bread.

Despite her exhaustion, Caseley had to smile. 'He's earned it, Liza-Jane.'

The maid's colour deepened and in the soft

9

light from the gas-mantle she looked eighteen instead of twenty-eight. What must it be like, to care so much for someone that his mere presence was transforming?

Caseley looked round. 'Where's Rosina?'

'She've gone up bed, miss,' Liza-Jane said. 'Got one of her headaches. I brewed up some mint and marjoram, and when I looked in a few minutes ago she was sleeping.'

Caseley had a strong suspicion that the housekeeper's headache was more diplomatic than real. Until her husband's untimely death, swept overboard from his fishing boat ten years ago, Rosina Renfree had been blessed with a very happy marriage, and she took every opportunity to encourage the growing attachment between Liza-Jane and Ben Tonkin, who had joined the household a year ago as valet, gardener, and handyman.

'Want a cup of something, do you, miss? It won't take a minute.'

Caseley shook her head. 'No, thank you.' She took a lamp from the shelf, lit it, and replaced the glass funnel. 'Ben, I'm grateful.'

'No trouble, miss.'

'Goodnight.' She paused at the door. 'Liza-Jane, make sure the copper is lit first thing, will you? Dr Vigurs is coming and Father's bed linen must be changed. Mrs Clemmow will be here by eight thirty.'

'Right, miss. 'Night.'

Caseley sensed their relief as she closed the kitchen door. As she climbed the stairs once more, the brass lamp cast distorted shadows on wall and ceiling.

10

In her room she set the lamp down on top of her writing cabinet. A tall clothes press filled an alcove. The brass bedstead gleamed above the lilac spread. Behind the door a flower-patterned ewer and basin stood on the marble top of the night table and several white towels were folded over a rail at the side.

She sank into her chair, gazing at the litter of invoices, orders, requests for quotations, and other paperwork generated by a busy and successful shipbuilding and repair yard. The long narrow drawer holding her pens and ink was pulled out, everything exactly as she left it when her father had called, woken by Ralph's drunken shouting.

Caseley rested her head against the chair's high back. What would Miss Hester say seeing her now?

Under the meticulous eye and strict discipline of the Misses Hester and Amelia Wills who ran the School for Young Ladies on Florence Terrace, she had learned to compose and address correspondence for every occasion in beautiful flowing script. She had studied literature, mathematics sufficient to ensure she could balance a household budget, deportment, piano and watercolour painting. Miss Hester deemed her embroidery exquisite.

Though being able to dance was another important accomplishment, she had been excused due to the accident that had left her with a crushed foot and pronounced limp. Her classmates sympathised, but no one wanted to partner her. So while they mastered the complexities of the waltz and mazurka, she studied Spanish.

11

It would have shocked Miss Amelia deeply to know that instead of reading Castilian poetry, her star pupil was gazing at a letter penned in Mexican Spanish requesting information concerning the qualities of different steam pumping engines for use in the Guanajuato silver mines.

Propping her elbows on the paper-strewn writing slope, Caseley buried her face in her hands.

There was a quick tap on the door and Liza-Jane walked in carrying a cup and saucer. 'I know you said you didn't want nothing, but you're looking proper wisht. I've brung you some camomile tea.' Beneath the severe centre parting her forehead puckered in concern. 'All right, are you?'

Caseley looked up, her eyes hot with unshed tears. 'Actually, I was laughing.'

'Bleddy cry if you didn't, eh, miss?'

Caseley lifted one shoulder. 'It wouldn't help though, would it?' She sat up straight. 'Thank you for the tea.'

Liza-Jane placed the cup and saucer by the lamp. 'Drink it while it's hot.'

'Ben's a lucky man. I hope he realises it. And Liza?' The maid turned in the doorway. 'Thank him again for taking care of Ralph. I couldn't have faced it tonight.'

After Liza-Jane had closed the door Caseley picked up the cup and cradled *in* between her palms. Sipping the honey-sweetened liquid she stared into space, disjointed thoughts and images tumbling through her mind.

Ralph's ashen, sweaty face had lolled against Ben's shoulder, as the manservant carried him upstairs.

Her great bull of a father, weakened by illness, was unable to understand his son's rejection of the business that should have been his inheritance. She remembered finding her father hunched over the desk in his office, his face dusky grey and creased with pain.

'Tired, that's all,' he gasped. 'A few days' rest and I'll be fine. You can stand in for me.'

The responsibility terrified her. 'Father, I can't. I don't know enough. Surely Uncle Thomas or Uncle Richard would–?'

'This is *my* business, girl,' he croaked. 'Thomas can only think in figures. While there's no one to beat Richard at finding cargoes for our vessels and those we're agent for, neither of them knows a thing about shipbuilding or repair. You must stand in for me.'

He clutched her hand, his grip painful. 'If word gets out I'm sick, people will take their work elsewhere. Once we lose a vessel to another yard we won't get it back. You've been translating letters and replies long enough to know what's needed. You must act for me, Caseley. It won't be for long. In a week or two and I'll be fine.'

So under the disapproving eye of Dr Vigurs her father had – through her – continued to run his business. But he was not recovering as quickly as either of them had hoped.

Unable to remain in the office after official closing time, partly to avoid speculation about the true state of her father's health, but also because Bar Road linked the docks with the town and at night was crowded with sailors and prostitutes, she had started bringing work home.

A soft knock on the door brought her head up as Liza-Jane looked in.

'I'm going up bed, miss. Doors is all locked and the lights out. Finished your drink, have you?'

Caseley looked down at the still-full cup, now cool. 'Not quite,' she smiled. 'But I will. Goodnight, Liza-Jane.'

''Night, miss.'

Swallowing a mouthful of tea, Caseley set the cup on the saucer and studied the letter from Mexico. But the words would not register.

Obeying an impulse she slipped off her shoes, opened the door, and padded quietly along the passage and up the dark narrow staircase to the small tower that gave the house its name.

The captain who had built the house had added the windowed tower so he could point his telescope over the narrow spit of land at the back of his property to the bay beyond and know which ships were coming into port long before they arrived.

But it was not to the open sea that Caseley looked. Resting her forehead against the cold glass, she gazed out over the inner harbour. Below her, on the far side of the road, the Bar with its warehouses, boatyards, saw pits, and timber pools curved round to the left. They were quiet during the hours of darkness. But daybreak would bring renewed noise and activity.

Above the wharves and quays, the town rose from the river to sprawl over the hillside. A fat pale moon, veiled by scudding cloud, hung low over the village of Flushing on the far side of the harbour, its ghostly light silvering the dark,

14

rolling water.

The rising wind keened and sighed in the rigging of ships moored in the harbour and alongside the quays. It clapped ropes against masts and made the beech trees creak and rustle in the garden next door.

Along the road the door of the Dock and Railway Inn opened. A man staggered out, his arm around a laughing woman. As they stopped in the shadows she turned away and went back to her room.

Chapter Two

Jago Barata eased himself up, leaned against the wooden headboard, lit a thin brown cheroot, and blew a thin plume of fragrant smoke. Cropped short, black curls clung to his forehead and temples. Sweat glistened on his broad shoulders, chest, and flat belly. Against the damp sheets and pillows his caramel skin glowed with animal health and as he raised his arm to tap ash from his cheroot, muscle and sinew flexed, gleaming in the lamplight.

Why was there no news? Alfonso Gaudara, his father's agent in Spain, had promised the writ holding his schooner in the blockaded port of Bilbao would be rescinded. Word of this should have been waiting for him yesterday when he arrived back from South America.

Twice today he had called to see George Fox,

vice-consul for Spain at his office in Arwenack Street. Both times the man had been out and, though apologetic, the clerk had been adamant. There was no message for Captain Barata.

Tomorrow he would go to the telegraph office. Each day the *Cara* lay idle in Bilbao he lost money. He had only a part-share in *Cygnet*. Though she handled well, and he was glad to have use of her, he wanted the *Cara* out of Spain in time for the fruit trade from the Azores starting in December. In the meantime he would use *Cygnet* for whatever deep-water runs he could get.

Unloading at the docks had been completed this evening and the hides he had carried from the Rio Grande were in the warehouse ready for transport to leather factories. He would need to allow a couple more days to rid the ship of the stench and for repairs to the jib boom and two jib sails.

It had been a close call, a collision that should never have happened yet could have been so much worse. That master would not tangle with him again. In the wrong place at the wrong time he had lacked the seamanship to get himself out of the way. Jago had little sympathy for him.

They had made a fast passage, only fourteen days across the Atlantic from the Gulf of Mexico. But it was more than two months since they had touched Cornish shores. His men would welcome a day or two with their families.

He knew the value of a contented crew. At sea since the age of sixteen, he had neither time nor inclination for any but brief casual relationships. He was baffled by his mate's willingness to walk

16

the eight miles from Falmouth to Feock to spend twelve hours with his wife and children then walk back to be on board in time to catch the tide. Yet when turnaround was expected to be even shorter, he supervised the unloading himself so the mate could still make his visit home.

He gained the mate's gratitude and unswerving loyalty, and used the time for paperwork. Knowing he was in his cabin ensured the crew worked hard and fast.

He knew he had a reputation as a hard but fair master with eyes in the back of his head. An ironic smile lifted one corner of his mouth. Despite the old tales about dual ancestry, his had produced no special powers or sorcery. His gifts were simply an instinctive understanding of human nature, and intelligence that required him to curb his impatience with those less mentally agile than himself.

The woman beside him stirred and sighed, drawing her legs together from their abandoned sprawl as she pulled the sheet over her full breasts in a gesture of studied coyness.

'You've forgotten I'm here,' she pouted.

Jago stubbed out the cheroot. 'My dear Louise, how could I forget you, even for a moment.'

The hotel's bedroom window faced out onto Market Street. Porters shouted names and information to the desk clerks. Parties who had enjoyed a good meal and fine wines in the dining room laughed and chatted beneath the portico while awaiting their cabs. In the passage outside the bedroom, guests came and went, pageboys carrying messages knocked on doors.

Then the blast of a horn and the thunder of hooves and iron-rimmed wheels announced the arrival of the late evening mail.

Jago reached for his watch on the night table beside the bed.

Louise stuck her lower lip out even further. 'I suppose you want me to go.'

'Will your husband not wonder where you are?' He asked mildly.

'Him?' She gave a derisive snort. 'He wouldn't notice if I lay naked on the slab between a side of beef and a leg of pork.'

Jago's mouth twitched. 'No man worthy of the name could fail to be moved by your beauty, Louise.'

She tossed her untidy mane and preened. 'You got some lovely way with words. 'Tis true though. He've got three shops, and when he isn't working in one he's visiting the others. Money, money, money, that's all he think of.'

Jago regarded her with faint amusement. 'But surely that was why you married him?'

''Course it was,' Louise agreed readily. 'I got three older sisters. I wanted a nice house, and nice clothes nobody else had worn first. He'd have got good value from me. But I aren't no ornament, just for show, to be took down and dusted off once a month.' Sighing, she lifted Jago's hand to her breast. 'I'm a woman and I do need a man.'

The blend of coyness and invitation in her soft purr stirred him not at all. He freed his hand without haste. 'No, Louise.' As her full mouth grew sulky he added, 'I am concerned for your–' He hesitated over the word *reputation,* aware that,

18

offended by his rejection and her husband's neglect, she could with truth accuse him of having
little concern for it before. Guarding her good
name was her responsibility, not his. But that
would carry little weight with her in this mood.
'For your well-being. What if your husband should
return home and find you not there?'

'He's at a Chamber of Commerce meeting. They
talk for hours in the Council Chamber, then go
and talk some more in the King's Head.' She
raised herself on one elbow, allowing the sheet to
drop as she arched her magnificent breasts towards him. 'C'mon, Jago. Just once more?'

He smothered a pang of irritation. He liked her
earthy honesty. But she never seemed to realise
when enough was enough. He pushed back the
sheet and with one lithe movement rose from the
bed. Taking one of the towels from the washstand
he wrapped it without haste or shyness around
his lean hips.

'Go home, Louise.' He spoke softly, but the
steely edge to his voice had her scrambling quickly
into her clothes.

'See you again soon?'

'I expect so.' He took two notes from his wallet
and picking up the little blue velvet drawstring
purse trimmed with ribbon that matched her
dress, pushed them into the gathered neck.

'You don't have to do that.' Her tone was a
blend of resentment and gratitude.

'I know. But a gift is always welcome, is it not?'

'Come again next week, shall I?' she asked,
twisting her frizzy hennaed hair into an untidy
coil, then pinning her hat on top and tilting it at

19

a rakish angle.

'No. Tonight you bribed a porter to let you in here while I was out. You will not do that again.'

She gazed at him, clutching the little purse, hearing the paper money crackle beneath her fingers. 'But you said you'd see me soon.'

He hadn't said that. '*I* will make any future arrangements.'

'I might decide not to come.' She shook out her skirts.

Jago inclined his head. 'That would be your choice, and I shall accept your decision.'

Louise's shoulders drooped and suddenly she looked much older than her thirty-one years. 'You arrogant bastard.' There was no malice in her tone, just weary acceptance and a hint of admiration. Unlocking the door, she glanced up and down the passage then left without another word, closing it softly it behind her.

Rubbing one hand over his dark beard, Jago's aquiline nostrils flared at his own scent. After opening the sash window he tugged the bell-pull.

When the boy appeared, he ordered hot water. 'I want a bath.'

'*Now,* sir?' the boy asked, startled.

'Now,' Jago growled. The taste of wine was sour in his mouth. 'Bring a pot of coffee as well.' As the door closed he lit another cheroot and propped himself on pillows against the headboard. He had much to think about.

In the big double bed, his striped nightshirt buttoned up to the neck, Thomas Bonython looked up from a large leather-bound ledger and peered over his spectacles.

'What was that, dear?'

Seated at her dressing table his wife glared at him in the gilt-framed mirror as she rubbed cream into her fleshy face. A lace-frilled cap covered her hair and she wore a voluminous peignoir of peach satin with deep flounces of lace at the neck and cuffs.

'I said it's ridiculous, Caseley in Teuder's office trying to look as if she knows what she's doing. At least she hasn't the cheek to use his desk. When I called in yesterday she was working on that little walnut bureau of her mother's in one corner. I told her Teuder should have done the proper thing and appointed you to take over while he was—'

Thomas jerked upright. 'You did *what?*'

'She said *you* could discuss the matter with Teuder when he's better.' Her tone was venomous. 'Just who does she think she is?'

'She's young,' he placated automatically, his thoughts racing. 'She'll be finding the situation difficult.'

Margaret swung round on the tapestry-covered stool. 'That is exactly my point, Thomas. She should not even be there. You are next in age to Teuder. You should have been asked to take over.' She turned back to the crowded dressing table, opened another jar, and began to rub almond-scented cream into the backs of her plump white hands.

'Teuder would have had to raise your salary, or at least increase your share of the profits. We need the money, Thomas. Look at this place.' She gazed

21

with obvious discontent around the over-furnished room. 'Heaven knows what Bess did to those curtains when she had them down in the spring. They have never looked right since. And Charlotte needs at least three new dresses for Christmas.'

'Three?' Thomas bleated.

'In case you hadn't noticed, our daughter is now fourteen years old. She's a young lady and will be a laughing stock among her friends if she has to wear last season's clothes to the parties and dances.'

'Yes, but do they all have to be new?' He hesitated. 'Surely some different trimmings, an alteration here and there.' He waved a vague hand.

His wife's thin mouth tightened in disapproval. 'Regardless of our grievances against certain members of the family, we Bonythons have a position to uphold. If Charlotte appears in last season's dresses she will be snubbed.'

'Come now.' Thomas felt his smile wilt as he tried once more to defuse his wife's wrath. 'I am certain Charlotte's friends would not be so unkind.'

Margaret raised her eyes to the ceiling and sighed. 'How can you be so naive? I'm not talking about her friends. Though I don't doubt some young hussy would delight in sharpening her tongue and her wits at our daughter's expense. People in our position excite jealousy, Thomas. It is the mothers we have to guard our little girl against. And I cannot possibly invite the Trembaths here again until we have the Chesterfield re-covered. I saw Maria Trembath eyeing the worn patch on the seat. Apricot velvet would look nice.'

She stood up and blew out the candles in their gilt holder, then took off her wrapper to reveal a long white flannel nightdress with a pie-frill collar and full sleeves. Climbing between the starched sheets, she settled herself on the two feather pillows and pursed her lips. 'So, what are you going to do about it, Thomas?'

He closed the big leather book and placed it on the bedside table. 'About what, my dear?' Time was running out. The audit was due shortly. If he could persuade Teuder to let him do it himself, he might be able to juggle the figures.

'About Caseley, of course.'

Thomas removed his spectacles and placed them carefully on the polished table alongside the accounts ledger. He had promised himself it would be once only. But now, with so many demands to meet, he could see no other option. They could count him in. He would tell them tomorrow. Excitement stirred, warming his pallid cheeks.

'Nothing, my dear.'

Margaret's head jerked off the pillow as she glared at him. 'Nothing? You mean–'

'I mean,' Thomas's interruption startled his wife into silence. 'I am happy for Caseley to remain exactly where she is. I never liked Teuder looking over my shoulder, always checking up on me. Since his illness Caseley has so much to do at the yard that she leaves all financial matters to me. For the first time I am my own master, and I like it.'

'What about me? People are talking behind our backs about you being passed over. But because Teuder is sick and you don't have to report to him like a – a – schoolboy, you are happy.'

'You don't understand.'

'No, I don't. I thought that with my encouragement you could make something of yourself, show Teuder that he had underestimated you. This would have been the perfect opportunity. You are content with so little, Thomas.'

'Will you listen?' He fought to contain his simmering rage, terrified of what might happen should he let it loose. 'Caseley is clever, but she's young and too much is being asked of her. Teuder's main interest is the yard. That is where he is directing her attention.'

'How does that help you?'

He hesitated. He had been warned to tell *no one*. But they weren't married to Margaret. They had no idea of the pressures a wife like her inflicted on a man. He *had* to tell her. Not everything, just enough, or she would play the martyr for weeks. Besides, it would show her he was as capable as Teuder of handling complicated business deals. Though obviously he could not give too many details. But the extra money would be a boon. She would welcome that. And when Margaret was happy she was more *accommodating*.

'It allows me to run a little private enterprise. Certain items will be brought to me, and all I have to do is ensure they reach the people who want them. For this service I will receive a commission.'

Seeing her expression sharpen he knew he had her. 'How much?'

'That depends on the value of the goods. But the items we have in mind should make the

24

venture well worthwhile.'

'You said *we*. Who–?'

He shook his head. 'No names. I had to promise. I shouldn't even be telling you this much.' He placed a tentative hand over his wife's. 'My only contact is the man who brings me the goods. I arrange transport to their destination. The first consignment arrived yesterday and will be on its way to London on the mail coach tomorrow morning.'

'When will you be paid?' Her expression was avid.

'Within forty-eight hours, provided the buyer receives the package intact.' His voice quivered with suppressed excitement. 'Teuder has done me a favour by bringing Caseley in. Be nice to her, Margaret. We want everything to remain exactly as it is.' His hand crept upward to rest on his wife's large, flannel-covered breast.

She did not move. 'It has been an exhausting day, Thomas. Perhaps by the weekend we may have something to celebrate.' She rolled away, dislodging his hand. 'Turn the lamp out, dear.'

He did as he was told.

Chapter Three

Caseley's dreams were filled with people pursuing her demanding decisions and information she didn't have. Restless, disturbed, she kept waking and listened to the wind rattling the window and causing a door left unfastened in the yard opposite to bang monotonously.

Soon after dawn, unable to remain in a bed that offered neither comfort nor escape, she had got up. Slipping a robe over her nightgown, her hair rippling down her back, she had worked on a reply to the letter from Mexico. She was busy writing at her desk when Liza-Jane brought in hot water.

She dressed in a plain bottle green skirt gathered to fullness at the back waist and a shirt-like bodice the colour of thick cream with a round neck and buttoned cuffs. She brushed her hair until it gleamed like burnished bronze then bundled it into a net secured on her nape with two pins.

Examining her reflection in the ornate mirror she pinched her cheeks to give them some colour. About the shadows under her eyes she could do nothing.

Passing her father's door she heard Ben's voice as he washed and shaved her father.

She ate a boiled egg and a slice of toast, drank the last of her tea, and was dabbing her mouth with her napkin when the door opened.

Unshaven, his hair tousled, with one hand shading his eyes against the sunshine streaming in through the window, Ralph walked carefully to the table and eased himself down onto a chair.

'God, I feel awful.' He supported his head on hands that trembled. His crumpled shirt was unfastened at the neck and wrists and his dark trousers were stained.

'Why do you do it, Ralph?' Caseley asked softly.

'No lectures, Caseley. Not today, especially not

26

now.' He let his hand drop and leaned back. His bloodshot eyes were narrowed against the bright morning and the pain she guessed was hammering at his temples. 'Give me something, Caseley. One of your brews? I can't stand this.'

About to say that he didn't have to, that he wouldn't suffer if he simply left the cork in the bottle, she knew she'd be wasting her breath.

'Please?' He sounded desperate.

'All right.' She stood up. 'I won't be long.'

'I'm not going anywhere.' He sank his head into his hands once more.

She paused in the doorway. 'Could you eat anything?'

He shook his head, clearly regretting the movement as his thin shoulders tensed against renewed pain.

As Caseley entered the kitchen Rosina looked up from the pastry she was making. 'All right, my 'andsome? Want something more?'

'Some lime tea for Ralph. His nerves are in a dreadful state.' She went to one of the large wooden cupboards.

'I bet his stomach don't feel too happy neither. A teaspoon of grated nutmeg on a slice of bread and butter, that's what he need.'

'Maybe later.' Caseley measured a teaspoonful of dried lime flowers into a cup. 'I doubt he'd keep it down right now.' She lifted the heavy kettle from the black-leaded range and poured boiling water onto the flower heads then returned the kettle to the slab with its gleaming brass rail. 'How's your head?'

The housekeeper looked up in surprise. 'My–?'

She lowered her voice. 'I reckon 'tis me time of life.'

Caseley strained the lime infusion into a fresh cup. 'Odd that they usually happen in the evenings.'

'Do they? Well, I never.' Rosina's amazement was beautifully judged. 'Some strange that is.'

Before Caseley could reply, Liza-Jane came in from the scullery carrying a large basket of wet washing.

'I'll just get this put on the line for Mary. Some lovely drying day it is.' She turned to Rosina. 'You was right about Louise Downing.' Her voice held mingled censure and excitement. 'She have got another fancy man.'

'I knew it. Didn't I tell you?' Rosina crowed. 'Is it Jimmy Mitchell? I seen the way he do look at her. 'Tis all Ada Mitchell can do to serve her. But then Ada always look like she's sucking lemons.'

Caseley knew she shouldn't condone gossip. But since her father fell ill she was spending most of each day discussing cargos and destinations with Uncle Richard or ship repairs, labour costs, and wholesale rates for oakum, pitch, Norwegian pine, and English oak with her father. She translated letters relating to his consular work, and relayed his instructions for work at the yard. A little local gossip made a welcome change.

''Tis never right, her carrying on like she do,' Liza-Jane said.

''Tis his own fault.' Rosina sprinkled flour on the pastry board before rolling out a lump of dough. 'If he spent a bit less time with they dead carcasses and a bit more on the live one he's married to, she wouldn't stray. Anyhow, who's the new fancy man? She've kept this one quiet.'

'Because he's foreign,' said Liza-Jane.

Rosina looked up. 'He isn't a Falmouth man?'

Liza-Jane rolled her eyes heavenward. 'He isn't *English*. Leastways, that's what Mary said. Betty Chard told her she seen Louise coming out of the Royal Hotel about ten o'clock last night.'

'That don't mean anything.' Rosina pursed her lips as she pushed the rolling pin to and fro. 'Louise have been seen coming out of stranger places than that at ten of an evening.'

Caseley opened the jar of honey and stirred a spoonful into the lime tea.

'Well, Betty's eldest is a boot boy up the hotel and he says he've seen her in there four or five times in the past six months, and always at the same time as they foreigners.'

Rosina gasped, the pastry forgotten. 'There's more than one?'

Liza-Jane nodded. 'That's what Betty told Mary.'

Rosina snorted. 'Get on, 'tis just guessing. What Betty don't know she do make up. That woman is some terrible gossip.'

Biting her lip to hide her smile, Caseley picked up the cup and saucer and returned to the breakfast room. Ralph was where she had left him, hunched forward, elbows on his knees, face buried in his hands.

She felt a pang of sympathy as she set the cup on the table beside him. 'Drink it while it's hot, Ralph. It will help.'

He turned to look at her. Despite the bloating

29

and the stubble his face appeared young and defenceless. 'I can't go on like this.'

Caseley looked at the long sensitive fingers, now grimy and trembling, at the thin body taut with nervous tension and the pain of yet another hangover, at the stained, dishevelled clothing. 'No,' she agreed quietly. 'You can't.'

'What am I to do, Caseley?'

'You have to talk to him.'

'He won't listen.'

'Ralph, you haven't tried.'

He glared at her. 'Of course I've tried–'

'To tell him what you really want? Have you, Ralph? I've heard you rant about what you *don't* want. You've ridiculed all the ideals he grew up believing in. But I've never once heard you explain quietly and reasonably exactly what your ambitions are. Do you even know?'

'How can you say that?' He was deathly pale. 'I thought you understood. Are you turning against me as well?'

'No, of course I'm not. But you're destroying yourself, drinking like this.'

His expression grew sullen. 'Don't preach, Caseley. I'll deal with this my own way.'

She crouched beside him. 'But you're not dealing with it. You're just running away.'

He leaned back. 'You don't understand at all. My whole life's at stake and all you can do is babble on about the demon drink, like some ... Methodist.' He spat the word.

Caseley stood up, clasping her hands tightly. 'What about *my* life, Ralph? I've listened and I've tried to understand. I know you are suffering.

30

But I can't do anything to change it. Only you can do that, either by talking to Father and settling it once and for all, or by leaving.'

'Leave? Where would I go? What would I live on?' He grew petulant. 'Why should I leave? This is my home. I'm entitled to be here.'

'Yes,' she agreed. 'And as the only son no doubt when Father dies the house will be left to you, along with shares in the yard, which you don't want. You will be a wealthy man, Ralph. You'll be able to drink yourself to death in style.'

Shaken, he stared at her. 'What's the matter with you? You've never spoken to me like this before. You don't understand at all.' He flung the words at her like stones. 'You have no idea what I'm going through.'

'Perhaps you're right, Ralph. But I have tried. God knows I've tried. Drink your tea.' She turned away.

He caught her hand. 'Don't go, Caseley. Don't leave me. I need someone to talk to.'

His hand was cold and clammy. She held it between her own. 'Then talk to Father,' she urged. 'Or to Dr Vigurs. He'll be in later.'

'Vigurs?' Ralph snatched his hand away, his mouth curling bitterly. 'He'll only lecture me about filial duty and Father's health and the inheritance I ought to be grateful for.' He glared at her. 'Anyway, where are you going that's so important?'

'To do your job.'

She went to her room to collect the books and papers she would need for the day's business, placing them in the leather music case she used

31

to carry them to and from the yard office. She would not think about Ralph. If she did, exasperation and rage would make it impossible for her to concentrate and she needed all her wits about her.

Swirling a hip-length cape of chocolate brown worsted around her shoulders against the morning chill, she went in to say goodbye to her father.

'Dr Vigurs will be calling later.' She moved the bed-table containing his breakfast tray.

'I don't care what he says. I'm getting out of this bed tomorrow. A man could die of boredom lying here.'

Sitting in the armchair while she changed his sheets had exhausted him and he'd been glad to return to bed and rest until his breakfast arrived. But mentioning it would only upset him.

'Shall I bring the newspaper up for you? Or a book?'

'Books? What do I want with books?' he snarled. 'I want the sun on my face and the smell of the sea in my nostrils. I want to be back in my yard and see what's going on. Books!' he grunted in disgust.

She knew better than to argue. She poured out his drops and handed him the glass, watching as he stared at the liquid, clearly debating whether or not to swallow it.

'Dr Vigurs will be impressed by your determination, Father,' she said with studied calm. 'Especially if you are tranquil and your blood is not overheated.'

Teuder grunted then gulped the mixture down. 'What time is he coming?'

'Before lunch, I believe. A nap now will conserve your strength and help you order your thoughts.' Caseley was aware of his gaze as she straightened the bedcover.

'What are you doing about that engine for Guanajuato?'

'I have drafted a letter to Fox's foundry requesting them to send details of engines they think would be suitable, plus shipping costs, to Señor Mantero.'

'Why Fox's? Why not–?'

'Because,' she cut in, plumping his pillows, 'Fox's foundry and engineering works have been operating at Perran Wharf for over twenty years. They've sent pumping engines to tin mines, copper mines, and gold mines all over the world.'

She paused to control the rising tension in her voice. 'I simply don't have time to make enquiries of all the other possible companies. Anyway, none of them have the freight and transport facilities that Fox's do.'

Making a huge effort she smiled at her father. 'I drafted a reply to Señor Mantero telling him of the company's reputation for reliability and high quality workmanship, and assuring him he will receive Mr Fox's personal attention in the matter.'

Teuder's tired eyes held a glint of admiration as he looked up at his daughter. 'A neat move, girl. Let Fox's do all the work, eh?'

Caseley tugged the bell-pull. 'Aunt Margaret's visit yesterday put me behind.'

'Margaret? What did she want? Poisonous old biddy.' Teuder scowled. 'Was she snooping?'

'No,' Caseley hated lying. But relating her

aunt's comments would only upset him and she didn't have time for that. 'She wanted to share some good news. Frances Lashbrooke–'

'Good news? It will be a rare day when any good news that woman wants to pass on doesn't have a sting in the tail.'

How well her father knew his sister-in-law. After a quick knock on the door the maid walked in.

'You can take Father's tray, Liza-Jane. He's going to rest now. Will you bring him some beef tea at eleven? The doctor should be here soon after.'

'Yes, miss.' Liza-Jane picked up the tray. Caseley kissed her father's forehead then followed her to the door.

'Try to sleep, Father. I'll come up and see you as soon as I get home.'

He raised one hand a few inches off the coverlet. 'Has *Dora* left the yard yet?'

'Will moved her round to the quay. He's taking her out on the morning tide. The account for her repairs was settled yesterday.'

'Where's she bound?'

'Par, to load china clay for Liverpool. She'll bring back salt.'

Teuder's eyelids were dropping. 'I must see him when he gets back. Tell him...'

'I'll try and catch him before he leaves. Sleep well.'

Teuder roused himself. 'Who's sleeping? I'm just resting my eyes until that damn doctor arrives. Don't forget to tell Will.' His eyes closed.

Shutting the door quietly, Caseley went downstairs to the kitchen. She could hear the splash of water and the creak of the wooden mangle as Mary Clemmow wrung out the sheets.

A moment later Mary's head appeared round the door. Greying hair had worked loose from the bun on her nape and floated in wisps about her flushed face as she wiped her red hands and forearms on a threadbare towel.

'Beg pardon, miss, but we need more blue bag. I got enough for today's sheets, but 'twill all be gone by Monday.'

Caseley nodded. 'I'll make sure it's added to the list, Mrs Clemmow.'

Mary bobbed her head and disappeared. Moments later the mangle resumed its creaking.

The scent of cloves and cinnamon made Caseley's mouth water as Rosina lifted a golden-crusted pie from the oven and set it on the scrubbed table beside two others.

'That's one apple, one apple and blackberry, and one plum. They saffron cakes is ready to go in. Fancy anything else do you, my 'andsome? I'll do a slab of 'eavy cake.'

'Thank you, Rosina. As it's the end of the month, be sure to pay both the butcher's and grocer's accounts. Add blue bag to the list. I've left money with the accounts in the drawer of the side-table in the dining room.' Caseley handed her a small key. Experience had taught her never to leave cash where Ralph might see it.

'Put the receipts and change back in there, shall I?'

Caseley nodded. Liza-Jane came in from the passage carrying dusters and polish. 'The wind have broke that low branch on the apple tree.

35

Dragging on the ground, he is.'

'Ask Ben to saw it off, Liza-Jane. And make sure he brings in plenty of coal.

At last Caseley got away. The wind whipped her skirt against her ankles and pushed her along the pavement edging the dirt road. Dust eddies whirled. Leaves and scraps of paper were snatched up, spun then dropped as the gust blew itself out. Puffs of cloud raced across the hazy sky as gulls screamed and wheeled.

Glancing into the grain warehouse as she passed, Caseley saw men loading sacks of oats and barley onto horse-drawn carts. She could hear the *shush* of the mill wheel turning in the tidal pool as water poured through the sluice.

'Caseley!'

Glancing round she saw a familiar figure close the garden gate of an elegant terraced house. Ever fashionable, Tamsyn was wearing short maroon coat over a pink flounced skirt gathered into a bustle topped by a large maroon bow. Her fair hair had been drawn back into a cluster of ringlets. Perched on the front of her head was a small hat with an upturned brim fastened with two pink roses. Matching ribbons tied in a bow hung down at the back. She always looked as if she had just stepped out of the pages of one of the ladies' fashion magazines.

Caseley felt a pang of envy, but it was small and easily ignored. She had neither the time nor the inclination to spend hours on her toilette. Besides, who would notice?

'Hello, Tamsyn. You're looking well. In fact you look radiant.'

36

'So I should,' Tamsyn laughed. 'That is exactly how I feel.' She gripped Caseley's forearm. 'William and I are to be married before Christmas.'

Caseley laid her hand over her friend's. 'I'm so pleased for you.' She meant every word. Resenting other people's happiness was mean, small-minded, and reminded her of Aunt Margaret.

'You must come to the wedding, Caseley. Papa is holding the reception at the Falmouth Hotel. There is to be an orchestra and dancing–' Her pretty face sobered. 'Oh, I'm sorry. I didn't think.'

'It's fine. Don't worry.'

'I cannot wait to be married. You would not believe how much there is to think about and plan!' Full of bliss, she hurried away towards the town.

Glad for her old schoolfriend, Caseley crossed the road to her father's boatyard, passing beneath the one-word sign over the tall double gates.

Her grandfather had claimed the Bonython name was enough. 'Word of mouth brings us all the business we want. Them that come here know what we do. No point wasting money to have it writ up there.'

In seventy years of building and repairing quay punts and fishing smacks, ketches, and schooners, the sign had never been altered. Nor had Bonython's ever lacked work.

As she passed the blacksmith's shed, the rhythmic clang of hammer on anvil stopped and a cloud of steam billowed out as red-hot metal was plunged into the cooling trough.

'Good morning, Mr Reece, have you seen Will Spargo?'

'Morning, miss.' The brawny smith emerged from his shed. In his huge fist long-handled tongs gripped a bent iron bar dripping water. His scarred and blackened leather apron reached almost to his heavy boots. 'I b'lieve he's down by the slip.'

'Thank you.' Caseley hurried across the yard past a stack of seasoning timber. She breathed in the acrid smell of hot tar coming from the riggers' shed and the sweet scent of fresh sawdust.

Reaching the slip she saw *Dora*, with Will at the helm, already twenty yards off, her sails set as she headed towards the Carrick Roads and the sea beyond.

Caseley sighed. She would jot down a reminder as soon as she reached the office. About to turn away, she saw a two-masted schooner approaching. It was coming in fast – too fast – under a single staysail.

A dark-haired figure stood at the wheel. As she watched he raised one arm then brought it down. A crewman waiting in the bow loosed the staysail sheets. The canvas flapped, spilling the wind, then slid swift and smooth to the deck. The schooner slowed and Caseley saw that the jibboom was broken off level with the bowsprit cap, the guys and bobstay neatly coiled and fastened to the bowsprit.

As the vessel glided alongside, a second seaman and a boy leapt onto the wharf and, whipping ropes around the bollards fore and aft, brought her gently to a stop. The boy let out a delighted whoop and the seaman cuffed him playfully as he jumped back on board.

The man at the wheel smiled, his teeth flashing white in his bearded face. He moved towards the companionway hatch then paused, suddenly still.

The speed of the schooner's approach had held her rooted to the spot, apprehension spiked with curiosity as she noticed the broken spar.

During her recent visits to the yard she had become acquainted with most of Bonython's fleet, except the *Lily*. Loading cod in the tiny harbours around St John's on the Labrador coast, *Lily* had been away for months and was due back in two weeks' time, mid-September.

If the schooner was one of theirs, then who was the man at the helm? The accuracy with which he had judged both the wind and the speed of the hundred-foot vessel proclaimed him a first-class seaman.

But the arrogant tilt of his head and his cool stare stirred unexpected and unwelcome agitation. The yard and everyone in it faded away, leaving just the two of them.

Startled and self-conscious, Caseley turned quickly away, retracing her steps across the yard and out onto the road.

Barely glancing at the overgrown ruins of the Manor, she hurried past the row of four-storey properties with deep windows and pillared porches that housed several of the town's eminent people, including Dr Vigurs.

She would call at his consulting rooms on her way home. She needed to know the truth and her father told her only what suited him.

The breeze whipped the waters of the inner harbour into a sea of white horses. Waves slapped and broke against the sea wall on the other side of the road. Small boats moored to rings in the wall and bollards along the top bobbed like corks on the choppy water.

Gulls flapped and screamed overhead, diving for scraps thrown overboard by fishermen sluicing decks and holds. The clink of caulking irons driving oakum between hull planks rose and fell on the gusting wind. Horses' hooves clopped, cart and carriage wheels rumbled, children squealed and squabbled, hammers clanged in foundries and women packing pilchards in the curing sheds gossiped and shrieked with laughter.

Turning in through the gateway of Bank House she climbed the granite steps. The glossy black door with its polished brass knocker swung open easily on well-oiled hinges. She walked along the tiled hall and up the wide, curving staircase to Bonython's offices on the first floor.

Entering her father's, she removed her cape, her gaze skimming over the glass-fronted bookcases, shelves packed with ledgers, and the small walnut bureau in the corner, its open top covered with neat stacks of papers.

It had been her mother's and usually stood in a corner of the drawing room. She had made Ben bring it down. To see her seated at her father's desk would have offended Uncle Thomas. Working at the small bureau signalled to anyone entering the office that she was simply helping out until her father's return.

Her gaze lingered on the framed letters of consulship approval and appointment. The first signed by Queen Victoria and her Home

Secretary, the second by the President of Mexico, Benito Juarez, and his ambassador in London.

She hung her cape on the coat stand and was tucking escaped curls back into their confining net, when the door opened and Uncle Richard waddled in.

Short and plump, wearing black coat and trousers, her father's youngest half-brother resembled an earnest mole. His stiff collar and cravat made his neck appear very short and it merged into shoulders rounded by years of poring over ledgers.

In his early forties, his fair hair was fast receding despite luxuriant side-whiskers. Concentration had furrowed deep grooves in his forehead. Yet he had only to smile for people to realise he was not the dry old stick they imagined. He was smiling now.

'How is the old curmudgeon this morning?'

Laying her music case on her father's desk, Caseley gave a wry smile. 'Determined to be back in the office tomorrow. Dr Vigurs is seeing him later this morning.'

'Irresistible force meets immovable object.' Richard grinned.

'I'm relieved I won't be there. How is Aunt Helen's cold?'

'Improving, though she has not yet recovered her voice. She did manage to rebuke Oliver this morning for some misdemeanour, but a whispered scolding lacks the desired effect.' As he spoke of his wife Richard's habitually fraught expression softened into warm affection.

Brisk footsteps approached along the passage, the door opened wider, and in strode the man

41

Caseley had seen at the helm of the damaged schooner. Instead of the navy reefer jacket, he was wearing a frock coat of fine dove-grey cloth over dark trousers, and in one hand he carried a tall hat with a narrow brim.

Their eyes met, and the impact was like a clenched fist. She looked down at her case trying to hide her shock.

Chapter Four

'Good morning, Captain Barata. Welcome back.' Richard stepped forward, offering his hand. 'A successful voyage, I trust?'

As the two men shook hands, Caseley released a quiet shaky breath, unable to understand her reaction.

'Profitable, certainly. We finished unloading cargo at the Docks yesterday. I picked up a mooring in the harbour overnight and brought *Cygnet* into the yard this morning. She needs a new jibboom and two new jib sails.' His voice was deep and though his English was perfect, a faint trace of accent would have told Caseley of his ancestry even if his name had not.

'I see.' Richard did not sound surprised. 'Do you wish your contribution to the cost of repairs deducted from your share of the profit?' Richard picked up a thick ledger from the desk and riffled through the pages. 'I believe this is the usual arrangement?'

Caseley glanced at the newcomer. Masters did not pay for repairs unless they were also part-owners. She had shares in *Cygnet,* a twenty-first birthday present from her father. Even so impersonal a connection with this man made her uneasy.

'As you will.' A brief gesture disposed of the matter.

Richard looked up from the entry he was making in the ledger. 'Bad weather in the Atlantic?'

'An incompetent master who got in my way.' The cold indifference in his reply sent a shiver down Caseley's spine. 'Where is Captain Bonython? I wish to speak with him.'

Stiffening at his imperious tone, Caseley moved round behind her father's desk so it became a physical barrier between her and the bearded man. But Richard did not appear in the least put out.

'Of course.' His frown cleared as he set the ledger down on top of another. 'You have been two months away. You will not have heard.'

'Heard what?'

'My brother has succumbed to a mild indisposition aggravated by overwork. As you are aware, Captain, it has been his policy to maintain an interest in every aspect of the business.'

'Indeed,' came the dry agreement.

'So to ensure a speedy return to health, his doctor advocated a short period of rest.'

Caseley could not help admiring her uncle's smooth explanation even as she shrank inside at the yawning chasm between what he believed and the truth of her father's condition. She was

43

startled to see Richard steer the visitor towards her.

'Allow me to present Captain Bonython's daughter.'

When he first entered the room his surprise made her wonder if he recognised her from the yard. But he had not mentioned it. Perhaps a woman in a consular shipping office was reason enough for astonishment.

His expression gave her no clue to his thoughts. But the sharpness of his gaze made her wary.

He started forward, a smile lifting the corners of his mouth.

A smile designed to flatter anyone lacking the perception to see the pirate underneath. Why should she think such things? She knew nothing at all about this man. Yet every instinct was warning her to be wary.

Despite glimpsing her uncle's bewilderment, she remained behind the desk, her fingertips resting lightly on her music case, her chin high.

One dark brow lifted fractionally and she saw a gleam of amusement in his narrowed gaze as he bowed. 'Jago Lantsallos Barata, at your service, Miss Bonython.' His voice was low-pitched and as smooth as dark chocolate.

It was a battle of wills and the force of her reaction overrode polite dishonesty. She cared nothing for his health and she was certainly not pleased to meet him. Remaining silent, she inclined her head briefly.

No longer smiling he turned to Richard. 'Perhaps we could go to your office. There are matters I wish to discuss and I have other appointments.'

He started towards the door, irritation crossing his aquiline features when Richard did not immediately follow.

'I fear you do not understand, Captain Barata.' Richard's smile was uncertain as his gaze darted between them. 'I did not introduce my niece out of social convention.'

'I'm relieved to hear it. Apparently Miss Bonython is not sociable.'

'I do not play games, sir,' Caseley said, stung into speech.

He cast a brief sharp glance in her direction. 'Nor do I, madam. You would do well to remember that.'

'Er – what I meant was,' Richard intervened, clearly bewildered. 'She is here at her father's insistence.'

'For what purpose?'

'Miss Bonython enjoys her father's complete confidence. She is more than capable of conveying even the most complex matters to him.'

Caseley felt a rush of gratitude towards her uncle.

'I see.' Coolly Jago looked her up and down. 'It appears I misunderstood. For a moment I thought – a foolish mistake. So, you are a messenger.'

Caseley looked down to hide her wince. As far as Richard and Thomas were aware, that was precisely the extent of her involvement. Anxious to avoid further friction between her father and his half-brothers, she had tried hard to make it appear that she was simply a courier, that it was her father who answered the questions, solved the problems, and made the decisions.

Concerned for his wife's health and busy with his own side of the business, Richard might well have forgotten how long his half-brother had been away from the office.

He relayed his queries to her and the following morning she gave him answers. It was natural he should assume that Teuder was dealing with matters from his bed.

Only she knew it wasn't so. Weakness and delirium had often made it impossible for her father even to hold a rational conversation.

It was totally beyond him to balance materials, manpower, and available berths against deadlines set by owners and agents who wanted repairs done, yet needed their vessels in ports many miles away to collect cargoes won against fierce competition.

One morning four weeks ago, having taken half the night and dozens of sheets of paper to work out the figures, she had gone to the yard and handed the foreman, Toby Penfold, a list of vessels due in for repair the following week, and a countersigned order for materials.

Then she had walked to the office and handed Richard the list of dates, a sheaf of letters to owners and agents, and a page of figures for Thomas to enter in his invoice and accounts ledgers.

When Richard asked how her father was, Caseley referred to the previous evening's delirious ramblings as 'a slight fever.'

Richard smiled, shaking his head. 'He really is amazing, managing to do all this despite a fever.'

Caseley had opened her mouth to tell him the

46

truth. But he didn't give her the chance.

'Of course, it's the business that keeps him going. It means everything to him. After losing his first wife, then your mother and Philip, it was the yard that kept him sane. A lesser man would have given up, but not Teuder. He put aside his grief and built up one of the busiest shipping agencies and repair yards in Falmouth. There were ups and downs, but he never gave in. Even now he is working from his sickbed. What a man.'

After that, telling him was impossible. That evening she took home more letters needing immediate replies, an enquiry from the Lloyd's agent regarding preliminary inspection of *Fair Maid* for her A1 classification, and a polite refusal by the Embassy to reimburse the expenses incurred in repatriating two injured Mexican seamen.

The letter stated that information had come to light proving that their wounds had been sustained not, as they claimed, when their ship sank in a storm, but during their attempt to commit an act of piracy. By repatriating them in his capacity as Consul, Teuder Bonython had, albeit unwittingly, abetted the escape of two felons. Therefore he would have to bear the cost.

Finding her father weak but lucid, she had fully intended to tell him what she had done. But then she recalled her uncle's praise for his half-brother. If she revealed her deception she might deal him a blow from which he would not recover.

So she read him the correspondence, soothed him over the Embassy decision and, as she was writing his reply to the Lloyd's agent, she announced casually that she had done all he'd asked

47

her to the previous evening and both Richard and Toby were delighted to have the matter settled.

She passed him the copies from her music case, hardly daring to breathe. His forehead was deeply furrowed and she could see the effort it was costing him to check the pages that had taken her hours.

What if she had made some glaring error that would demolish her fabrication like a house of cards? What if he thought, as he must, that *he* was responsible? Would he be able to shrug it off as the effect of his illness? Or would it undermine his confidence and erode his belief in himself? If that happened, Caseley knew he was as good as dead. His body might linger, but his spirit would wither away.

As the strain became unbearable and she was on the point of confessing, he sighed and shook his head.

'I don't remember any of this.'

Moistening dry lips, Caseley took the pages gently. 'You had a spell of fever last evening, Father.'

He gave a tired smile and sank back against the pillows. Caseley replaced the papers in her case, relief leaving her shaky.

'I'll do it, girl,' Teuder grunted. 'I'll keep the vultures away and the yard working just like it always has. Truth to tell, there have been days when I just couldn't think straight. The doubts came then. It was all getting away from me.'

Pride shone in his watery eyes as he pointed an unsteady finger at her case lying on the coverlet. 'But I've been running that yard so long I can do it in my sleep. You keep on bringing the work home. I'll be out of this bed soon and when I get back to my yard and the office, no one will know I was ever away.'

That had been four weeks ago. Four long busy weeks, during which she had repeated the deception daily, gaining in knowledge and experience but terrified of getting it wrong and being found out.

She was used to solitude. Ever since the accident her disability had set her apart from her contemporaries. But never in her life had she felt so achingly lonely.

There was no one in whom she could confide, no one to share her anxiety and the crushing burden of responsibility.

Having promised her father she would not reveal the severity of his illness to Thomas and Richard, nor could she reveal the extent of her deception.

Standing behind her father's desk she linked her hands and dug her right thumbnail into her left palm. The pain helped her to focus, gave her strength.

'Yes, Captain Barata, you will find me an adequate messenger.' She lowered her lashes at a sudden sharpening of his gaze.

'Might I be permitted to visit Captain Bonython at home?' His voice was silky smooth.

'Oh no. That is out of the question.' Richard's apologetic smile softened the rejection. 'Even my brother Thomas and I have been dissuaded from calling.'

'Oh?' Jago Barata's black brows rose.

Caseley knew that on no account could she afford to underestimate this man. Formidably intelligent, he was also predatory. She sensed he was listening not just to her words and the timbre of her voice, but to all she was *not* saying.

She made herself relax. Exhaustion was causing her to over-react. Her imagination was playing tricks. For weeks she had kept the severity of her father's illness, and her part in keeping the business going a secret from Richard, Thomas, and Toby. Jago Barata had been in the office only a few minutes. He couldn't know anything. It wasn't possible.

Yet her reaction to him had been instinctive and violent. He represented danger. As a battle raged inside her she managed a contrite smile.

'Perhaps you think me over-anxious, Captain Barata, but my father is very dear to me.'

'I do not doubt it, Miss Bonython.' She recognised genuine sincerity and felt a little of the tension leave her. 'I trust your protectiveness has served its purpose and your father will shortly be well enough to return. He has been away for several weeks?'

'Yes, but we have every hope–'

'When?' he enquired pleasantly.

'It – it is not easy to–'

'But you must have some idea?' He was relentless.

Desperate to be rid of him and free of his probing she blurted, 'A few days.'

'Really?' Richard beamed with pleasure. 'Caseley, that's wonderful. I didn't realise you had definite news of his return.'

Hotly conscious of Jago Barata's steady, speculative gaze, she could not backtrack. 'I– Father wanted it to be a surprise. He – he intended to come in and simply pick up the reins as if he had never been away.' That much was true.

She smoothed damp palms down her skirt. 'Under the circumstances, Captain Barata, no doubt you would prefer to return later in the week and conduct your business with my father in person.' With all her strength she willed him to leave.

Neither his expression nor his shuttered gaze gave any clue to his thoughts. Eventually he smiled.

'I wish that were possible. But as I mentioned earlier I have other appointments and may not be free at a time convenient to your father. On reflection it suits me better to accept your uncle's recommendation and avail myself of *your* talents – as a messenger.' The pause was brief, but Caseley knew it was deliberate.

He turned to Richard. 'Doubtless there is much requiring your attention, Mr Bonython. I will call in at your office when I have finished here.'

Caseley stiffened. He was dismissing her uncle like a servant. But Richard seemed oblivious, still smiling at the news of Teuder's return.

'Yes, yes, do. I cannot wait to tell Thomas. He will be as delighted as I am.'

'Uncle Richard!' Caseley did not want to be left alone with Jago Barata. He was a threat. But she did not know *why*. She shot a desperate look at her uncle, only to have it intercepted. Realising her nervousness was bound to encourage speculation she reached into her case and pulled

51

out two letters, both unfolded.

'One is for Señor Mantero at Guanajuato, the other for Fox's foundry,' she offered them to her uncle.

'Allow me,' Jago murmured. Taking them from her trembling grasp he passed them over.

Richard nodded. 'I'll see they go in the afternoon post. Sam can take them.'

'I was not aware Bonython's had interests in Mexican silver mines,' Jago said, one hand on the door as Richard disappeared back to his office.

She wanted to tell him to leave it open, but something stopped her. She was afraid for her father and for the tangled web of deceit she had spun to protect him. But the slightest hint of fear would re-ignite the curiosity and scepticism lurking in Jago Barata's slate-grey eyes.

The door closed with a soft click and panic tightened her throat. She swallowed. 'We don't. But as consul my father is frequently asked for information concerning the purchase and shipping of mining equipment.'

'Yes, of course.' One corner of his mouth tilted up. 'Are we not known for our expertise in all aspects of mining? Wherever there is a hole in the ground, a Cornishman will be found at the bottom of it.'

'*You* claim to be Cornish?' The words were out before she could stop them.

One brow lifted. 'My claim is legitimate, I assure you.'

'But your name—' She broke off in confusion, keenly aware it was not simply his name that had convinced her he was of foreign descent. The

Cornish were brilliant engineers, fine seamen, and knew more about mining than any other race on earth. They were hardworking, loyal, and self-contained.

Jago Barata might have any or all of those attributes. But he had something else; a patrician arrogance that was as much a part of him as his limbs. She also sensed ruthlessness and a cold implacability that would make him a terrible enemy. Though she brushed the thought aside as fanciful nonsense, her skin tightened in a shiver.

'Surely you know that Jago is Cornish for James?' He was toying with her like a cat with a mouse. 'My maternal grandfather, Joseph Lantsallos, came from Redruth, and my mother's family bible records ten generations born in that area. But you are right, Miss Bonython, I've other blood in my veins. My father's family came originally from Castile. I see you are fluent in Spanish.'

The statement hit Caseley like a slap. 'How–?'

'The letters. The same hand wrote both, a firm neat hand betraying no sign of weakness. Did it take you long to compose them?'

She saw the trap just in time. 'Captain Barata, I am, as you say, simply a messenger. You mentioned having other appointments. If you would care to tell me what it is you wish my father to know, I will detain you no longer.'

He gripped the back of the visitor's chair angled in front of the desk.

'You are not detaining me, Miss Bonython.' His half-smile mocked, and Caseley felt warmth climb her throat and flood her face. 'I am here because *I* choose to be. Shall we sit? The message I have for

53

your father is not unduly complicated but it does deserve your full attention.'

He moved round the chair. 'No doubt you are about to tell me you can attend perfectly well on your feet. That may well be so. However, courtesy does not permit me to sit while you stand and, despite your apparent aversion to introductions, I cannot believe you are entirely lacking in manners.'

Feeling her face flame, she sat on the edge of her father's chair, her back ramrod straight, her hands tightly folded. She could feel herself trembling with anger.

'Your message, sir?'

He settled himself comfortably, crossing one leg over the other. 'I want the post of senior captain. I also want your father's word that if the writ holding my ship in Bilbao is not rescinded in time, I, and no one else, will skipper *Fair Maid* to the Azores in December for the start of the fruit trade.'

Caseley gazed at him in horror. 'No, you can't,' she whispered, completely forgetting she was supposed to be merely a go-between.

'Why?' he enquired calmly.

'The post is not available. We already *have* a senior captain—'

'Will Spargo,' he broke in. 'He's a good seaman, excellent on coastal trading. But for the Atlantic he is too old.'

'No,' Caseley repeated, her voice rising. 'Will Spargo has sailed Bonython ships all his life. He started as a cook's boy with my grandfather and worked his way up to master. He has earned his rank and the privileg

'Of course he has.

runs make a fair profit

to his family every week

six months.'

'You don't care about

Caseley cried. 'You just wai.

Jago's eyes narrowed. 'Why

there is. I have equalled all cr

broken several. I have sailed   ╷torm,

typhoon, and hurricane without   ╷g a ship or

a cargo.'

It was no boast. He was simply stating facts. But Caseley recalled *Cygnet's* broken jibboom.

'A situation due more to luck than judgement if the vessels you command require repair every time you reach port.' Her heart thumped painfully against her ribs.

'So it *was* you,' he murmured. 'What is wrong with your foot?'

'That is none of your business.' He had been fully occupied bringing *Cygnet* in alongside the wharf and she had been many yards away among the sheds and stockpiles in the yard. Yet he had noticed her limp.

'So, you will convey my requirements to your father.' It was not a request.

Before she could respond he stood up. The sunlight caught his close-cropped curls and they gleamed like polished ebony. It cast bars of shadow across the fine material of his frock coat whose superb cut defined the breadth of his shoulders. Tanned by wind and sun his skin glowed bronze against his white collar. He leaned

...ipped black beard reminded ...ure entitled *Lucifer* in a book of ...es favoured by Miss Amelia.

...fering your father the chance to make ...hon's a major force in international mari-...ne trade. He will want me, do not doubt it.' Caseley stared at him. He smiled. 'So be sure my message is delivered in its entirety. Good day, Miss Bonython. I will see you again. Very soon.'

He gave a mocking bow and strode out.

Chapter Five

A few minutes after Jago Barata left, her uncle Thomas burst in, startling her.

'Is it true? Will Teuder be returning to the office in a few days?'

She had never seen him so fraught. He was usually such a quiet, retiring man. But he must be feeling the strain of her father's absence almost as much as she was.

He had been so helpful, refusing to allow her to carry the heavy ledgers home each evening. Instead he had prepared a weekly balance sheet so her father could see at a glance that all was well. But Teuder had complained bitterly, demanding to see the books. The implied slur on his character and ability had offended Thomas.

Desperate to keep the peace, she had begged her father to accept the sheets. Reluctantly and with much grumbling he had agreed.

'I – I was going to tell you a bit nearer the time,' she stammered. 'We cannot be sure of the *exact* day. It should be soon though.' She had been compelled to tell so many lies, what difference could one more make?

'Then I must get back. Lots to do.' Reaching the door he glanced back. 'Caseley, as soon as you know for certain you must tell me.' He must have seen her surprise at his urgency. 'So we can arrange a small celebration.'

'I don't think he'd want that, Uncle Thomas,' she said quickly.

'No, perhaps you're right. But you will let me know?'

'Yes, of course.'

As he left the offices and turned towards the town centre, Jago reviewed his encounter with Teuder Bonython's daughter. Caseley: an unusual name for a prickly young woman who apparently cared little for appearance, fashion, or men. With a mental shrug he dismissed her, climbed the five steps, and entered the red brick building that housed the offices of GC Fox and Company.

Only she would not be dismissed. There were hollows beneath her high cheekbones, a wide soft mouth above a stubborn chin, and dark lashes she used to veil emerald eyes flecked with bronze. There was no coyness in her manner. She appeared genuinely reluctant to have anything to do with him. He found that intriguing. As was her refusal to offer her hand.

On his sixteenth birthday, as a gift to mark his entry into manhood, his father had arranged for him to lose his virginity to an attractive young widow. His sensual mouth curved at the memory of Genez. From her he had learned consideration and the exquisite rewards of curbing his youthful impatience. He had believed himself deeply in love with her. With kindness and humour she had convinced him he wasn't.

In the eighteen years since he had never lacked female company. His striking appearance, punctilious manners, and a background combining wealth and nobility ensured his name appeared on the guest list of every family of rank and many of those with aspirations. But he had avoided emotional entanglements.

His physical needs slaked, he had devoted his energy to his chosen profession, the sea, frequently returning to his ship sooner than planned simply to escape designing mothers. Faced with his lack of interest in their simpering daughters, more than a few hinted at their own availability, colouring his opinion of women and marriage with cynicism.

He had been celibate for a while before starting his liaison with Louise. She was earthy, generous, and honest, shunning many of the pretensions of others in her position. Physically she satisfied him as no woman had since Genez. But she was seeking more than he was inclined to give.

Opening the door he promptly forgot her.

'My apologies for not being here to receive you in person yesterday, Captain Barata,' George Fox said as they shook hands. 'However, I'm afraid there is still no message.'

'I will send a telegraph from the post office,' Jago took the chair Fox indicated. 'Perhaps you

58

can tell me the latest news from Spain?'

'The newspapers–'

'Say very little. They are more concerned with the proposed pilot service around the Lizard, the lack of passenger revenue on the railway, and strike-breakers bound for collieries in the north where mine owners are refusing to employ union men.' Jago crossed one long leg over the other.

'Mr Fox, my ship is being held under writ in Bilbao. You are Vice-Consul for Spain, and I need to know exactly what's happening out there.'

'Yes, of course.' Fox sat down. 'May I offer you some coffee, or perhaps a glass–'

'Nothing, thank you.'

George Fox shook his head. 'The information we receive is garbled and on occasion contradictory. As you can imagine, communication is difficult and the situation changes daily. But it is a bloody war, captain. The *guerilleros* are behaving with appalling savagery. This is no disciplined army supporting the rights of Don Carlos to the Spanish throne. It is a rabble of murderers using the rebellion to satisfy their lust for blood and money.'

'How far have they reached? The last news I had was that Don Carlos had stormed the port of Bilbao, and his brother Don Alfonso was moving south.'

George Fox nodded. 'Don Alfonso's forces plundered and terrorised their way through Aragon and invaded the heart of Castile.' He paused. 'With the capture of Cuenca they managed to come within eighty miles of Madrid. The citizens resisted for two days, but when Cuenca fell–' His voice quavered and he avoided Jago's gaze. 'The mob, for they are little better, was unbelievably ruthless. They took few prisoners. The streets literally ran with blood.'

While Fox struggled to regain his composure, visibly distressed by the terror and wanton destruction convulsing the country whose interests he represented, for Jago this news was infinitely more painful. Spanish blood ran in his veins. Spain was part of his heritage. But his features remained impassive.

'However, there is some good news,' Fox said. 'The siege of Bilbao has been lifted. General Serrano's army defeated the Carlist forces but it was a hard-won victory and the town was a bloodbath. Rumour has it that Don Carlos fled across the border into France. Some are saying the rebellion is ended. But I have my doubts.'

He struck the desk lightly with the edges of his clenched fists. 'Forty years this vendetta has lasted. Two branches of the same family fighting for the crown, and the republican faction adding to forty years of carnage and misery that would never have started if Ferdinand had not bypassed his brother to hand the throne of Spain to his daughter, Isabel.' He shook his head. 'Forgive me, Captain.'

Waving the apology aside, Jago stood up. 'Your concern does you great credit, sir, and I appreciate it.' He offered his hand and Fox rose to shake it warmly. 'You'll contact me if—'

'I will,' Fox promised.

Needing exercise to dispel his tension, Jago strode along Arwenack Street, heedless of the in-

60

terest aroused by his dark good looks and proud bearing. Working men, recognising authority, tipped their caps. Men of substance and breeding acknowledged with a nod one of their own caste.

Respectable married ladies glanced at him then averted their eyes, smothering pangs of yearning and their guilt at such inappropriate thoughts. Girls stared openly, then clutched at each other to giggle and sigh. Sullen youths with catcalls on their lips changed their minds as cold grey eyes swept over them and they perceived beneath expert tailoring a muscular physique that owed nothing to padding.

The aroma of freshly baked bread and roasting coffee wafting from a refreshment house reminded him that he'd eaten little breakfast, but his stride did not falter.

The street was busy. Women shopped; errand boys darted to and fro across the dusty street. A hansom rolled past, the driver sitting high at the rear, cracking his whip above the horse's ears to quicken its pace. An argument in the boot-mender's doorway had attracted a knot of onlookers.

The sun was high, but the tall buildings on both sides of the street acted as a funnel for the keen-edged easterly wind. The smells of fish and horse dung competed with rotting vegetables, burning wood, and the gas works.

He crossed the square in front of the church, passed the King's Head hotel and, a few yards further on, entered the new and beautifully faced post office building. The first rush had eased and he reached the counter with little delay.

'Good morning, Mrs Cox. My mail, if you please?'

The postmaster's wife had a naturally pale complexion, emphasized by the high-necked black bombazine she usually wore. But she was quite pink as she raised one hand in a reflex gesture to untidy, sandy-grey hair that appeared to be on the point of escaping the bun into which it had been loosely gathered.

''Morning, Cap'n. I heard you was back.'

Jago's mouth twitched. There was very little that escaped Mrs Cox, the post office being a clearing house for both local gossip and news brought in by crews of vessels returning from all over the world.

'Staying at the Royal again are you? Only Mrs Sandow up along Woodlane have got a lovely house to rent if you was interested.' She reached up to one end of a large wooden rack that covered half the wall its shelves partitioned into dozens of small compartments, and took down a wad of letters. As she passed them to him under the ironwork grill she leaned forward, her round face close to the heavy mesh. 'She asked me to find a *gentleman*. She said you can't be too careful these days.'

'And you thought of me?' Jago wondered what Mrs Cox would have thought had she seen him cuckolding the town's leading butcher the previous night. He picked up the letters. 'That was kind of you, Mrs Cox.'

''Tis a sad day if we can't help one another.'

'A worthy sentiment indeed. Is Mr Cox in the office?'

'No, Cap'n. He've gone out to meet the

steamer to collect the mails. It give'n a break. The post office make'n work from seven in the morning till ten at night. If I wasn't here to help I don't know how he'd do it.'

'Please give him my regards, Mrs Cox.' He bent towards the grill. 'And take good care of yourself. For where would your husband, and all of us, be without you?'

'Get on, Cap'n,' she bridled, her cheeks glowing, one plump ink-stained hand touching the cameo brooch at her throat.

Jago left and climbed the stairs to the telegraph office on the first floor. After sending cables to Farando, his agent in Bilbao, and Ramon Gaudara, his father's representative in Madrid, he returned to the hotel for a late lunch.

At his table, from where he could observe without being too easily seen, he ordered sea-bass with a cream and tarragon sauce, and white wine, remembering with wry amusement the boiled salt beef, figgy duff, and stewed tea he had eaten the evening before he docked.

He flicked though his mail, tossing aside envelopes he recognised as containing social invitations. This left two letters. The first was from a local solicitor informing him that the last will and testament of his maternal grandmother, Sarah Ellen Bray, had been proved, probate granted, and if he would call at the office in Market Street when convenient, the keys to the property could be handed over.

He glanced at the date on the embossed paper. 29th July 1874. It had lain at the post office for over a month. He felt a self-mocking smile curve his mouth. He, who had always travelled light, rejecting the ties imposed by personal possessions, was now a man of property.

He thought of Mrs Cox and her well-meaning attempts to prise him loose from the hotel and establish him in a house like a 'proper gentleman', and wondered how long it would take for the news to reach her ears.

The second letter was from his father. His mother was well, but Elena, the companion who had moved with her from Spain to Mexico, had succumbed to a chronic digestive complaint. The *estancia* was showing a higher profit this year and cattle sales were up. The Indians worked well under the new foreman and the unrest that had cost the estate so much in time and money, had settled down.

Then he came to the heart of the letter. 'There has been another disaster at the Pachuca Silver Mine,' Felipe Barata wrote, his bold scrawl flowing across the pages. 'Fifteen killed and more than thirty injured, such waste! Indian labour might be cheap but owners risk dire consequences from both the law and political vigilante groups if they do not observe basic safety rules.

'As for our own mines, investment in new crushing equipment had proved worthwhile and production has increased. However, the quicksilver for the extraction process has not arrived from Spain this month. I have written to Guadara in Madrid and to Juan at the mine, but have received no replies. I ask you, my son, to find out what is happening. While we are still mining some nuggets at Carmelita, the bulk of our silver

64

is extracted from lead and copper ores and we need the quicksilver urgently. I am enquiring for supplies here, but am not hopeful as competition is too fierce.'

Jago completed his meal with a cup of coffee. How recently had his father written to Gaudara? The letter did not say. Maybe the tide *had* turned in the war and stability would soon be restored. But until then communication would pose an insoluble problem. He would have to allow at least twenty-four hours for Ramon to reply to this morning's cable.

Meanwhile, assuming he managed to find some quicksilver, all he could do was co-ordinate shipping arrangements from the nearest free Spanish port. He might have to collect it himself, bring it back to Falmouth, then trans-ship it to be sent on to Mexico. Though as he was already committed to an appointment concerning unloading facilities on the wharves and another at his bank, he could not return to the shipping office until the following day.

Immediately an image of Caseley Bonython formed in his mind, her slender neck and the heavy mass of chestnut hair bundled into its confining net. She looked tired and had been as approachable as a porcupine. He brushed the image aside as he would a fly.

Yet for the rest of the afternoon her memory plagued him. Why, he could not understand. Her clothes were plain and understated to the point of making her invisible. And while her low-pitched voice offered a welcome contrast to the usual female shrillness, her tongue possessed a cutting

65

edge that ill-became a young woman. He grew more irritable as they day wore on.

Somehow Caseley got through the rest of the day. But despite valiant efforts to concentrate on the ledgers and papers in front of her, images of Jago Barata kept intruding. Over and over again she heard his cool voice with its subtle, taunting inflections, pictured the wintry gaze that saw too much and revealed so little.

It was late afternoon when she left the office and walked briskly to Dr Vigurs's consulting rooms.

'He can return to the office? And the yard?' Caseley couldn't hide her surprise. Despite his bluster and determination, her father still seemed weak and far from well. But perhaps he had simply been too long indoors, deprived of the sunshine and fresh air he craved.

Dr Vigurs nodded. His portly figure was draped in formal black frock coat, winged collar, and grey striped trousers. Sitting behind his desk he toyed with his pince-nez. 'An hour a day to begin with, and he must keep his drops with him at all times.'

She would be free. Able to relinquish the responsibilities she had been forced to shoulder. But what would take their place? What in her life required a fraction of the intelligence and energy she had discovered as a result of her father's dependence on her? She pushed the thought away.

There was plenty demanding her attention: neglected friends, domestic duties that had been postponed. She would soon fill her days. And she would not be obliged to be civil to Jago Barata. She need not see him ever again.

But as the doctor's gaze met hers, sudden apprehension squeezed her heart. 'There's something else, isn't there?'

'Caseley, what I have to tell you will not be easy to bear. However, you are strong and I know you will be able to accept it and act accordingly.'

I'm not strong. I don't want to hear. I can't take any more. I'm too tired. But not a word escaped as she sat stiff-backed on the edge of the chair and waited.

'You father is still full of grit and determination, and his spirit is as willing as ever.' He paused.

'But?' she prompted softly, a hollow growing in her stomach.

'But his heart has been damaged beyond repair. He will never be the man he was.'

'Are you saying he will be a permanent invalid?'

'Not exactly,' Robert Vigurs replied carefully.

'I don't understand. You are letting him go back to work.'

The doctor placed his hands flat on the blotter in front of him. 'Given the right conditions your father could live for many months.'

'Months?' she echoed, deeply shaken. 'But I thought– Only *months?* So what are the right conditions? Should he have a special diet? Are there medicines we could buy?'

'The conditions I speak of are not purely physical, they relate to the mind and spirit. But one thing I am sure of. There is nothing more medicine can do for him. Your father's life is in the hands of Providence, and I see little point in demanding he conserve his energy for a future he may not have.'

'That's why you're letting him return to work?' she whispered. 'But the stress could kill him.'

'On the other hand, it might not,' the doctor pointed out. 'And if it does, do you not think he will die a lot happier? He *wants* to go back, Caseley. It serves no purpose to stop him. Indeed it would be cruel.'

Her eyes stung and her throat ached. 'Have you told him?'

'There was no need. He already knows and has accepted it.'

'But–'

'We all die, Caseley. That is the only certainty in this life. You have the hardest task, knowing what you do, to allow him to live his life his way until the end.'

She stood up, swallowing her tears. 'Thank you. I'm glad you told me.'

He came round the desk and took her gloved hand in both his. 'I'm here if you should need me. The drops will ease any pain he may have. As for the rest, there's no way of knowing how long...' He allowed the sentence to hang unfinished in the air.

She nodded, unable to speak. He walked with her to the front door. She had known him all her life. He had brought her and her two brothers into the world. At this moment at least she was not entirely alone.

'It will be a difficult time for you, my dear. Never doubt that your father loves you. But each of us must make the final journey on our own, and your father has already begun his.'

Chapter Six

That night, halfway through his beef with a second glass of claret in front of him, Jago was hailed by a loud voice from the far side of the room.

He looked up to see the mop-headed, reed-thin figure of Luke Dower plunging through the crowded dining room towards him, scattering cheerful apologies as he bumped into chairs and scraped against tables.

'Jago, you old bastard,' he bellowed. 'How's it going, my son? When did you get back?'

'Good evening, Luke,' Jago drawled, raising his glass in salute. Not for an instant was he taken in by the other's expansive smile and bonhomie. 'How are you?'

Luke Dower did his drinking in the waterside inns and public houses. His presence in the best hotel in Falmouth meant a business deal was brewing for which he needed funds. Jago guessed this was no chance meeting.

Luke sat, slammed his glass onto the table, and, with a visibly trembling hand, poured brandy from the bottle he was clutching. 'I'm doing fine. I got a regular run to Portugal, taking out wool and cotton, bringing back wine and lace. Been doing it a few weeks now.'

'I'm glad for you. Last time we met the bank was threatening to foreclose and Trembath–'

'All in the past, my son.' His wide smile revealed

69

stained and broken teeth. 'Old Luke bounced back like he always do. 'Tis looking good.'

Jago finished his beef and pushed the plate away. He sat back, turning the stem of his wine glass.

Luke hitched his chair closer and Jago noted the greasy shine on his forehead, smelled the stale sweat and tobacco smoke that permeated his clothes. Luke's shirt was grubby and there were spots and stains on his coat and trousers.

'I got a deal you–'

'I don't think so.'

'Wait till you hear. You'd be mad to turn this one down.'

'What is it this time?'

Luke tapped the side of his nose. 'My client has a commodity he wants to dispose of in this country. I bring it over and pass it on to a third party.'

'From Portugal?'

Luke nodded. 'Part of the regular run. No diversions, no problems.'

'No customs duty,' Jago's tone was dry.

'Now why should we give the poor buggers all that extra work? They got too much to do already.' Luke grinned.

'So why do you need me?'

Luke stiffened. 'I never said I did.' He gulped a mouthful of brandy, grimacing as the fiery spirit burned its way down. 'I'm offering you a chance to make some easy money. But if you aren't interested, there's plenty who will be.'

Jago moved one shoulder. 'As you like.'

Luke swallowed another mouthful, wiped his mouth with the back of his hand then leaned forward to confide. 'Look, I shouldn't be telling you this. But I've already got one partner. I'm naming no names, but 'tis a well-known family, solid business background. Would a man like that get involved if it wasn't a sound proposition?'

Jago shrugged. 'That depends on *his* reasons.'

'Look, you and me both know you got to invest if you want to make a profit. My outlet is guaranteed. So instead of me acting as an agent and getting a piddling little commission for handling the goods, it makes better sense for me to *buy* then re-sell. That way I can sell to the highest bidder and control the market.'

'So you're looking for capital.'

'Well, I can't go to the bank, can I?' Luke retorted. 'This is the chance of a lifetime. Turn it down and you'll regret–'

'What is the commodity?'

Luke's eyes flickered sideways.

'You can't expect me to invest if I don't know what I'm buying.'

'You're in then?'

'I didn't say that.'

Luke drained his glass, gripping it with both hands. 'Moidores,' he muttered reluctantly.

'Are you mad?'

'Each one of those coins is worth twenty-seven shillings,' Luke was defensive.

'Have you forgotten the penalty for smuggling bullion?' Jago demanded in an undertone. 'Do you know how many men with schemes like yours died of typhus in Bodmin Gaol last year? You've got work, a regular run. Why in God's name are you risking it all?'

71

'I don't get an owner's share,' Luke hissed. 'With freightage of two or three pounds a ton to be divided three ways after paying port expenses, wages, and food, there's bugger-all left.' He glanced round again. A look of cunning crossed his face, quickly masked by a wolfish smile.

Curious, Jago turned his head and saw Thomas Bonython weaving through the crowded tables towards them.

Spotting Jago, he hesitated, then came forward, a worried frown creasing his forehead and dragging the corners of his mouth. After a polite nod to Jago, Thomas turned to Luke.

'I must speak with you.' His whisper was urgent.

Luke lurched to his feet and threw an arm over Thomas's shoulders. 'No need to look so tragic, my old son.' He grasped the brandy bottle by its neck. 'Whatever it is we'll sort it out. Let's find a quiet corner. We'll have a drink, and you can tell me what's on.' He winked at Jago, while Thomas twisted his hands together.

'No, I don't think you understand–'

As Luke pushed him through the crush, Jago watched them go, his gaze thoughtful.

A restless night disturbed by dreams of a chestnut-haired girl with shadows in her eyes drove Jago from his bed in a foul temper before six.

Wearing his navy reefer jacket over a clean white shirt and a red kerchief knotted loosely round his throat, he locked his door and left the hotel, heading for the yard.

The wind had dropped and the morning was crisp and fresh. Through opes and alleys leading down to the quays, warehouses and workshops he saw a forest of masts. The water was calmer, changing colour from indigo to sapphire as gold-washed clouds moved slowly across a pearly sky.

By the time he reached the yard his head had cleared and his temper improved. Despite the early hour the yard was busy. Grey smoke belched from the smithy chimney. Two boys called to one another as they staggered with newly cut planks from the sawpit to the dry timber store. A man tended a crackling fire beneath a steaming-box in which planks were being softened and shaped to fit a curving hull.

As he headed towards *Cygnet*, Jago could see pitch bubbling in buckets over fires built within small brick squares and hear the musical clink of caulking hammers. Before he reached the schooner his nostrils flared at the pungent odour escaping from the companionway hatch, fo'c'sle scuttle and ventilators despite their heavy covering of canvas.

'All right, Cap'n?'

He turned and saw the short, stocky figure of the yard foreman coming towards him. Toby Penfold had skin the colour and texture of old leather and iron-grey fluff fringing his skull. His navy-blue Guernsey was darned in several places, as were his paint-smeared work trousers.

''Morning, Toby. When did you start fumigating?'

'Last night. I put four sulphur candles in the cabin, four in the fo'c'sle, and same again in the hold. I'll open her up in an hour. But you won't want to spend time below till tonight. Better still,

73

leave it till the 'morning. Want something from inside, did you?'

'Nothing that can't wait. I'd rather see those damn bugs killed.'

'The sulphur will do that all right, Cap'n. But give it a week and 'twill be bad as ever. The little buggers nest in they timbers behind the lockers and panelling. There idn no way to reach the eggs, and the sulphur don't touch 'em.' He gave a philosophical shrug.

'How soon can you have *Cygnet* ready for sea again?'

The foreman scratched his head and drew air between his teeth with a slow hiss. 'We should keep her at least two weeks. She's spewing oakum. I got Joe and Henry caulking her now and we'll seal her with pitch.' He shook his head. 'I'd like to replace that there bowsprit with a longer spar and save all the trouble with the jibboom. I know,' he said before Jago could speak, 'you wouldn't have space for extra canvas. But the shroud plates is loose, and 'tis time–'

'Toby.'

The foreman sighed. 'Three days.'

'Thanks,' Jago grinned and Toby shook his head in resignation. 'How far have you got with *Fair Maid?*'

Toby scratched his head again as they crossed the wharf to the dry dock. 'She've had her new felt and metal sheath fitted, and a new mainmast step. Penrose's sent word that her fore, main, and mizzen sails will be ready by Thursday. We already got her squares and topsails and we kept her old foresails and jibs. All her masts, spars,

74

and yards have been scraped and oiled. Standing and running rigging will be fitted by the end of next week.'

The three lofty masts lay in wooden cradles along the dock, the close-grained yellow pine gleaming under its coating of oil. Even without them, *Fair Maid* had the slim lines and pronounced curve at deck level that marked her as a thoroughbred. Her bulwarks were freshly painted and the new varnish on her rail reflected the sun.

As his critical gaze softened in admiration, Jago thought of his own vessel, held for months in the northern Spanish port. What would she look like now? Not wanting to think about the damage she might have sustained during the siege and blockade, he turned to the foreman.

'Has Captain Bonython's illness caused problems in the yard? I didn't know about it until yesterday.'

Pursing his lips Toby leaned back, feet planted wide, resting gnarled knuckles on his hips. 'I can't say it have. We've missed him about the place. But the work's gone on same as always. He's some lucky with Miss Caseley. As for that brother of hers,' Toby turned his head and spat. 'Little twerp should have had his backside leathered years ago. He won't have nothing to do with the yard. He'd sooner be out drinking or painting pictures.'

He glared up at Jago. 'What's it coming to?' After he lost his eldest boy, Mr Teuder was some pleased when Ralph was born. Gived that boy everything, he did. Sent him to school and all.' Toby grunted in disgust. 'Fat lot of good that did.

75

Bone idle, he is, and I'd tell him to his face except he never come near the place. Near broke his father's heart. If it wasn't for Miss Caseley I dunno what would have happened here these past weeks. She's some lovely maid. Clever too. Henry's wife had these sores on her legs. Miss Caseley made some herb stuff for her to put on them and they was all gone in a week. Good as gold, she is. The men think the world of her. But though they haven't noticed, 'tis plain to me.'

Trying to reconcile the foreman's description of a warm-hearted, friendly, smiling girl with the defensive hostile creature he had been introduced to, Jago almost missed what Toby had said.

'Noticed what? What is plain?'

Toby shook his head. ''Tis getting too much for her, and no wonder.'

'Looking after her father? Surely–'

'No,' the foreman scoffed impatiently. 'Running this here yard.'

Jago was suddenly very still. 'Are you suggesting–?'

'No, I aren't.' Toby was curt. 'I'm *telling* you.'

'But Richard Bonython said...' Jago broke off as his initial incredulity gave way to thoughtfulness. 'How do you know?'

'I've worked in this yard since I was a boy. I know the way Mr Teuder do think. The orders I get when Miss Caseley come in of a morning, well, they don't have the stamp of her father.'

'Have there been mistakes?'

Toby shook his head. 'No.' There was a note of surprise in his voice. ''Tis just the feel of it.'

'Have you mentioned this to anyone else?'

''Course I haven't!' Toby was indignant. 'Family business, isn't it? Dunno what I'm telling you for.'

'It will go no further,' Jago promised. 'If you're right, it's my belief she's the only member of the family who knows. I have some personal business to take care of but I'll be back in a day or two. I trust *Cygnet* will be ready?'

As the foreman sucked in a breath, Jago lifted one eyebrow. The foreman threw up his hands.

'I'll do my best, but I can't promise.'

'Your best is all I ask. I may have to go to Spain to pick up a cargo my father needs urgently.'

His thoughts buzzing like a swarm of angry bees, Jago pushed the half-open door wide. Caseley was replacing a file on a high shelf. His gaze swept over her, lingering briefly on the swell of her breast beneath the sprigged muslin blouse. She glanced round, flushing as she recognised him, but the colour quickly drained, leaving her ashen. Her eyes had bruise-like shadows beneath them. Compassion caught him an unexpected blow.

She circled round behind the wide desk, graceful despite her limp, attempting to maintain as much distance as possible between them in the small room. Her back was stiff and she radiated antipathy.

He fought an urge to reach out, tell her she had nothing to fear. Then his habitual cynicism returned, overriding emotion both unexpected and unwelcome.

'Can I help you, Captain Barata?'

Though he had heard her voice over and over

in his mind, its musical quality struck him anew despite her icy manner.

He was equally cool. 'I hope so. Does Bonython's have any vessels due to sail for Spain or Mexico during the coming week?'

'You must speak to my uncle Richard. It is he who coordinates cargoes and transport.' Her chin rose a little higher. 'As I'm sure you are already aware.' She placed some papers in another folder, picked it up and hugged it in an unconscious gesture of self-protection. She waited, clearly expecting him to leave.

He did not move. 'You do not assist him?'

'No, Captain Barata, I do not. I am here solely to help my father, and his work involves the yard and the consulship.'

'So Richard Bonython would arrange cargoes or shipping to Portugal?' His gaze never left her face.

She shook her head. 'That would be most unlikely. Mr Fox is consul for Portugal so their agency handles all commerce with that country.' There was no hesitation, nothing in her voice but mild impatience. Jago realised that whatever connection Thomas Bonython had with Luke Dower, it was not official business for the company. Surely the man had more sense than to get involved in such a dangerous venture, unless...

'Was there anything else?'

Beneath her coolness he heard a thread of anxiety. It had not been there when she answered his questions. Clearly she wanted him gone.

He had used Bonython's agency to find cargoes for his own vessel for the past five years, ever since deciding to make Falmouth his base for lucrative deep-water runs to the Azores for the fruit trade and the Labrador coast for salt fish.

Teuder Bonython had made him master of the *Cygnet* after his own schooner, *Cara,* had been seized when he landed in Spain to load a cargo of salt for St John's. He had bought shares in *Cygnet* as an investment and a gesture of good faith. Never before in his dealings with the company had he sensed the undercurrents and tension that existed now.

'Just one more question,' he said smoothly. 'What news of your father? When will he be back at his desk?'

A spasm of anguish crossed Caseley's face and her grip on the folder tightened. 'Probably to-morrow.'

Jago arched one black brow in surprise. 'Indeed?'

'I mentioned his imminent return when you came by yesterday,' she blurted.

'So you did. Yet I had the impression you did not entirely believe what you were saying.'

He saw her flinch. But she recovered quickly. 'I also told you that I care very much for my father. Perhaps I am over-protective.' Her mouth quivered but she controlled it. 'However, the doctor sees no reason to keep him at home any longer. Now, if you will excuse me, I have a great deal to do.' As she looked down at the crowded desk and gathered papers, he sensed desperation.

'Far more, I think, than most people are aware of. At least, that is Toby Penfold's opinion.'

Her head jerked up, eyes wide, and it was obvious that the foreman had guessed correctly. 'How did you–?'

Realising she had betrayed herself, her entire body sagged. She leaned on her hands, her head dropping forward like a blossom too heavy for its stem. 'Was there a mistake? Did I get something wrong?' Her voice was unsteady and full of dismay.

'No. Toby couldn't fault anything. He only guessed because, to use his own words, it *felt* different.'

She nodded without raising her head, merely acknowledging what he had said.

'Why did you do it?' he demanded. 'What were you trying to prove?'

She raised her head and eyed him with a mixture of bewilderment and disgust. 'I have nothing to *prove*, Captain Barata. My father needed my help.'

Jago felt her disdain like a whiplash on raw flesh. Incensed by her defiance, his voice was a deadly purr. 'Then no doubt he is very proud of you. I must congratulate him on having raised a daughter whose gifts, while certainly less common than those of her peers, are plainly far more useful. Good day, Miss Bonython.' He made a mocking bow and turned to leave.

'No.' The word was wrung from her.

He turned slowly. 'I beg your pardon?'

'Congratulations would be out of place.' She laid the folder on the desk with exaggerated care, squaring the corners. 'I only did what was necessary. There is nothing praiseworthy in that.'

He caught the anxiety in her voice and wondered. 'I cannot agree. Such devotion, such a sense of duty and responsibility cannot go unmarked. I shall make a point–'

'No!' She made a heroic effort to control herself. 'It is not your concern, Captain. Please, I – I beg you, don't...' She fell silent under his scrutiny.

'You *beg* me? And with such passion,' he murmured, comprehension dawning. 'I doubt Caseley Bonython has ever begged for anything in her life. Most women seek compliments like water in a desert, but you–'

'Forgive me, Captain Barata.' She drew herself up, her face taut with dislike. 'I should have known better than to request anything of you. I do not wish the matter spoken of because...' She swallowed. 'Because my father did not know what I was doing.'

'I see. May I ask the reason for this deception?'

Caseley hugged herself as if cold. 'To protect him.'

Jago was sceptical. 'From what?'

She half-turned to gaze out of the window. Several seconds passed and he could see her trying to decide how much to tell him. 'No one knew how ill he was, not even the family. He made me promise ... he was afraid the business would suffer.'

'I assume from what you're saying that there were occasions when your father was not capable.'

Her eyes flashed splinters of ice. 'Rare occasions, Captain, very rare. I saw no reason then, nor do I now, to–'

'Shatter his confidence? I agree entirely, Miss Bonython. No purpose would be served, especially as he is now sufficiently recovered to take control once more.'

'He never relinquished it,' Caseley shot back.

'No?' He enquired softly. As a tide of dusky rose flooded her face her eyes defied him. But he gave her no chance to reply. 'Still, no doubt you will be pleased to withdraw from this unfamiliar world and return to more feminine occupations.'

'I don't follow you, Captain.' Her gaze was stormy, her tone quiet and controlled.

His gesture encompassed the paper-laden desk, the small writing bureau in the corner, the shelves stacked with boxes, files, and ledgers.

'Surely you are out of place here?' It was unusual for a young woman to accept such a burden of responsibility. Even more unusual for her to acquit herself so well that only one person guessed the depth of her involvement.

Was that why she disturbed him in a way no other woman ever had? Though neatly dressed, she seemed totally uninterested in her appearance. A sensual man himself, he recognised passion in her of which she was totally unaware.

She irritated him yet he could not get her out of his mind. She didn't fit into any of the categories to which he usually assigned women. That offended his sense of order.

He heard her soft intake of breath.

'Perhaps ladies of your acquaintance are rarely required to use their brains,' she retorted with acid sweetness. 'However I should have been of little help to my father were my only accomplishments the ability to play the piano and discuss the finer points of fashion.'

'Rest assured it had not occurred to me to credit you with either of those attributes. Good day.' He inclined his head, pausing in the doorway. 'You gave your father my message?'

'Of course.' Her eyes were glacial, but the hurt in their depths made him despise himself. That made him even angrier.

'Then I will return tomorrow so we may agree terms.'

'I shall be occupied elsewhere.'

'Did you not hear me? I said *we*. That means your father, myself, and you.'

Her eyes widened. 'But – I am not– It has nothing to do with me.'

'On the contrary, we both know you are deeply involved.' He pulled the door wider. 'I trust you will not fall victim to a sudden indisposition.' Twin spots of colour staining her cheekbones told him the thought had crossed her mind.

'Until tomorrow, Miss Bonython.' He closed the door quietly behind him.

Chapter Seven

Teuder Bonython leaned back in his chair and nodded. 'This is more like it.' He sighed with deep contentment.

Caseley knew the twin patches of crimson on his cheeks were not a sign of good health but evidence of his damaged heart labouring. His clothes hung loose on his large frame, the bones of his face and skull were clearly defined, and his grey-white hair lay flat and thin. But his smile was broad and his watery eyes twinkled.

'I've missed this place. Open that window a bit more. I want to hear the town.'

She did as he asked. A hansom had picked them up outside the front door and dropped them in the courtyard of Bank House. The stairs had seemed endless, but her steady flow of chatter had covered the slowness of their ascent. Even so, by the time they reached his office, he had been breathing heavily.

Hanging up her cape and his hat and coat she had seen pain flicker across his face, and started towards him, but he had shaken his head.

She busied herself around the office, to allow him a few moments in which to recover, and to hide the dampness on her lashes.

If he could pretend then so must she. It would be all too easy to fuss over him and so reveal her deep concern. But he would hate it, and it would be self-indulgent on her part.

'I still say we should have stopped off at the yard,' he grumbled. 'Dammit, we had to pass the gate. It wouldn't have taken long.'

A knock on the door made Caseley jump. Busy with her father she had managed to avoid thinking about Jago Barata. But now they were in the office, not knowing when he would appear, each footstep in the passage, each knock on the door, stretched her nerves ever tighter.

The door opened and Sam peered round holding a bundle of letters. Caseley hurried forward to take them, fearing the clerk's reaction on seeing the change in his employer. 'Back to normal, eh, miss?'

Caseley managed a smile. 'Back to normal, Sam.'

The clerk withdrew and she placed the letters in front of her father. 'You're needed here, Father,' she said gently. 'I know you'd rather be in the yard. But Toby is following your orders and everything is running smoothly.'

She shivered as fear rasped her nerves. Jago Barata had promised to say nothing about her part in keeping the yard functioning. But could she trust him?

Teuder grunted. 'You open them.' He leaned back in the chair, resting his head. 'Cutting down a tree to build a ship, that's right and proper. A ship has a heart and spirit. But destroying forests to make paper,' he shook his head. 'That's terrible.'

The door opened. Taut as a bowstring, Caseley glanced round then relaxed as Richard bustled in.

'I heard you arrive but I was–' He broke off, his warm smile of welcome fading as he came face to face with his brother for the first time in two months.

'Good morning, Uncle Richard.' Her mouth smiled while her gaze begged. 'We heard voices in your office. I told Father you'd be along as soon as you were free.' She watched her uncle struggle to hide his shock.

'Yes. Yes, indeed. It *is* good to see you once again in your proper place, Teuder.' His sincerity made Caseley's heart swell with gratitude. 'We

85

have missed you, though less than we expected, for Caseley has coped admirably.'

'So I should hope,' Teuder was gruff. 'All she had to do was relay my instructions.'

Caseley lowered her gaze. He didn't intend to hurt. He was simply stating what he believed to be the truth. Dr Vigurs had warned that her father would feel resentful. He had never been ill in his life and equated it with weakness, something to be ashamed of and denied. Compliments on her performance in his absence rubbed salt in his wounded pride.

The door opened again. As Caseley turned, her pulse quickening, Thomas entered. Catching sight of Teuder he stopped.

'My God!'

'No,' Teuder said, droll and impatient. 'Just me. I suppose you've noticed I've lost a bit of weight. Feel all the better for it too. Now we've got that out of the way, I want to know why we're losing Liverpool cargoes to Broad's. Richard, Jimmy Morrison is still our agent up there, isn't he? Find out what he's doing. He's not being paid to let another company steal our bread and butter. Thomas, those balance sheets were pretty enough but I've got a feeling they're not telling me the whole story. I shall do an audit next week and I want the books, *all* the books, up to date and on my desk by Wednesday.'

Seeing both men about to protest, Caseley linked her arms through theirs and drew them out into the passage.

'Try to understand,' she pleaded. 'It's his first day back. He's just settling in.'

'And unsettling everyone else,' Thomas retorted resentfully. 'He doesn't look fit to be out of bed.'

'He's like an old tom cat marking his territory.' Richard's smile was perceptive. He sighed. 'I'd better put a squib under Jimmy Morrison.'

'Stop that whispering,' Teuder roared. 'Caseley, get back in here. There's work to do.'

With an apologetic smile to her uncles, she went back into the office. But as she turned from closing the door her breath caught. Her father was slumped in his chair, eyes closed against the pain that tightened his mouth and scored grooves in his forehead. One hand was pressed to his upper chest. The other clutched the chair arm.

She grabbed the bottle of drops from her case. Biting her lip as she tried to steady her trembling hands she measured out a dose, relieved she had remembered to tell Sam to put a tray with a glass and carafe of fresh water on one corner of the desk. Stirring the mixture she held it to her father's lips.

'This will help.' Her calm voice betrayed no hint of the terror flooding her body. It couldn't be yet. Months, Dr Vigurs had said. *Please not yet.*

Draining the glass he lay back, breathing heavily. Caseley recapped the bottle and moved the tray, watching him.

His breathing eased and he began to relax. His eyelids flickered then opened.

'I'll send Sam for a cab to take you home.' Relief weakened her legs. 'This is your first day back. Best not to overdo it.'

'I'm all right,' Teuder rasped. 'Just give me a

87

minute. I'll be fine.'

'Father, please—'

'Stop your fussing.' What his voice lacked in strength it made up for in irascible determination. 'I'm staying. I didn't ask you to come in today. It was your idea. If there is something you would rather be doing, go and do it. Sam can see me home when I'm ready to leave.'

Caseley turned away. She did not want to stay. But how could she leave him? If he had another attack – if he could not reach the drops – overshadowing it all was the spectre of Jago Barata. If she was not here, if he carried out his threat to tell her father... She had no choice.

She swallowed the ache in her throat. 'There is nowhere else I would rather be, Father. If I seem to fuss it's only because I care. I will try to control it.'

'All right then.' He cleared his throat loudly. 'Let's get this blasted paperwork out of the way.'

Caseley drew the visitor's chair close to the opposite side of the desk and reached for paper and pen. After reading the first two letters and dictating replies, her father pushed the third across to her.

'Here, you read it to me. No sense keeping a dog and barking yourself.'

She saw the drops were taking effect. Now the pain had gone he was becoming drowsy. Settled comfortably in his chair, his fingers linked over his waistcoat and what remained of his paunch, his gaze wandered round the room as she read a request from the owner of a Penzance trading ketch for a new main lower and top mast within ten days.

'Last time I was in Penzance was in '72,' he mused. 'Toby and his son and two nephews came with me in *Ada* to see the Channel Fleet. There was a big sea running but the wind was fair and Toby had every stitch of canvas he could lay hands on up that mast. We were flying.' He smiled at the memory.

'Those ironclads were a sight to behold. Anchored about a mile off the pier head they were. Little steamers were taking parties out for a closer look. *Sultan, Achilles, Agincourt,* and *Black Prince,* names to stir the heart and put fire in a man's belly. We got quite close to *Minotaur.* Twenty-six guns she had, and five iron masts. That ship weighed ten thousand tons if she weighed an ounce. That was a day to remember.' He nodded, lapsing into silence.

Caseley leaned over the desk and moved one of the ledgers across in front of her father. 'Shall I stop by the yard later and ask Toby if he'll be able to accept Mr Tresawle's ketch? They're very busy at the moment.'

Behind her the door opened. The tiny hairs on the back of her neck prickled and her stomach clenched. She knew without looking that Jago Barata had entered the room.

She tried to hide panic she could neither explain nor control. Laying her notepad and pen carefully on the desk she rose and turned, her face carefully expressionless.

'Good morning, Captain.' Her voice was calm and clear despite the sensation of standing on shifting sand.

'Good morning, Miss Bonython.' His coolness matched hers. Then taking her completely by surprise, he caught her right hand and raised it to his mouth, brushing her knuckles with warm lips that sent tiny flames along every nerve.

Her breath stopped in her throat and she snatched her hand back, furious at the scalding blush. Clasping her hands, she rubbed her knuckles, not caring what he thought, desperate to erase the sensation of his mouth.

One black brow arched and his eyes gleamed. Then he walked past her to greet her father, extending his hand across the desk. Teuder leaned forward to grip it with both his.

'Good to see you again, Jago. How did it go?'

Standing to one side, Caseley watched Jago as he gave a brief account of cargoes and ports of call during his two-month absence. Not by the flicker of an eyelash had he betrayed the shock he must have felt at her father's changed appearance. Perhaps after what she had been forced to tell him, he had prepared himself – but for a moment her dislike and mistrust were pushed aside by gratitude.

It didn't last.

'So, that is the past. Let us look to the future. Your daughter told you of my proposition?'

'She did.'

Caseley looked away. She had reminded her father of Will Spargo's years of loyal service and prior claim, urging him not to give way to Jago Barata. He let her finish then demolished every objection.

'You can't afford a soft heart in business, girl. I

90

know Will's value, and I'll see he don't lose by it. But Bonython's can't afford to miss this chance. If I don't make Jago Barata chief captain, Broad's or Fox's will.'

'Let them,' Caseley cried. 'We don't need him.'

'Don't be so bloody daft, girl.' Teuder had been testy. 'You don't give an advantage to your rivals. Has your sense gone begging? Seems to me you've taken against him, though for the life of me I can't think why. How many times have you spoken? Once? Twice?' He had shaken his head in disgust. 'Dear life!'

What could she say that he would understand? He was talking competitors and potential profits. All she had was intuition.

'He's a pirate.'

Clearly startled, her father had nodded, admiration stealing across his tired features. 'Could be you're right. But then so was I. We're the ones who run risks. We push hard. We take what we want, and pay for it,' he added. 'But we get things done and build something that will last long after we've gone.'

It was the first time he had mentioned a future in which he had no part. It had cost her dearly not to react.

'I'd be a fool to turn him down. I have faults a-plenty, but I'm not stupid. He's half Spanish. He speaks the lingo. He can negotiate new contracts and markets that will put Bonython's leagues ahead of our competitors. Not just in Spain, but South America. And we need 'em, make no mistake about that. The railways are taking a good part of our freight, and road hauliers are developing their own transport networks at competitive prices. We have to develop our foreign trade. That's where the future lies.'

'Don't you agree, Miss Bonython?' Cool and ironic, Jago Barata's voice jerked Caseley back to the present.

She looked up at him and the amusement in his grey eyes told her he was well aware her thoughts had been far away.

Her skin burned but she did not shrink from his gaze. 'I'm afraid I wasn't listening, Captain.' His mouth twitched at her candour. 'If you'll excuse me, I will leave you and my father to discuss your business privately. It is not my concern so–'

'Indeed it is,' Jago interrupted.

'I don't understand.'

'Then allow me to explain.' A smile still hovered at the corners of his mouth, but his eyes were as hard as granite. 'I made your father a business proposition. I believe he is about to accept it. However, there is something I wish to add.'

'I'm not looking for further inducement, Jago,' Teuder grunted. 'I reckon we'll both do well out of the arrangement.'

'We will. This is no inducement. I am making a request. No, a demand,' he amended without taking his eyes from Caseley.

She stared back, her breath and heartbeat quickening as apprehension crawled along every nerve.

'Demand, is it?' growled Teuder. 'Go on then.'

Jago rested one lean hip on the edge of the desk. 'My maternal grandmother died some months ago and has left me a property along Greenbank.'

'Nice houses, they are,' Teuder said. 'You planning to sell it?'

'No, I plan to live there. Though it is structurally sound it has been empty for over a year. My grandmother was ill for several months before her death and stayed with relatives in Redruth. The garden is a wilderness and the house needs completely redecorating. As I am away at sea much of the time a task of such importance must be handled by someone I trust.'

Caseley still didn't understand why he had insisted she stay.

'I want Miss Bonython to take charge.'

She felt her eyes widen as she stared at him. He didn't mean it. He was having a joke at her expense.

Teuder frowned. 'You want *Caseley?*'

Jago nodded. 'Such a task needs someone with an eye for colour, style, and flair.'

Flinching at his irony, she gritted her teeth as a wave of fury and embarrassment broke over her.

Her father shrugged. 'I'm bound to say I've never noticed any talent in her for such things.'

'Nevertheless, I want her to do it.'

'No,' Caseley said. 'It's impossible. I have too much to do at home.'

'Get on, girl,' Teuder scoffed. 'Rosina can run the place with one hand tied behind her back. She's got Liza-Jane and Ben, and Mary Clemmow.'

'Father,' Caseley stepped forward, pleading. 'There is still so much to do here. This is only your first day back.'

'Miss Bonython,' Jago cut in. 'I do not expect

93

you to devote the whole of your time to my house. An hour or two each day to supervise however many workmen you deem it necessary to employ will be sufficient. I have no desire to interfere with your other commitments.'

'See? You're making ponds out of puddles again. I'm not saying you haven't been useful. But I can manage without you for a couple of hours a day.'

Caseley tried. 'Father, you're only just getting your strength back.'

'And wasting too much of it arguing with a stubborn young miss who should show a bit more gratitude,' he snapped.

'Gratitude? For what am I supposed to be grateful? I did not ask, nor do I want–'

'Don't try my patience too far,' Teuder warned.

'Perhaps it is merely a question of confidence,' Jago said, his voice smooth, his gaze implacable. 'Miss Bonython, I have no doubt you possess talents that would be a source of considerable surprise to those who feel they know you so well.'

Shock drained the blood from her head leaving her dizzy. She reached blindly for the chair back and gripped it. It was blackmail. Either she agreed or he would tell her father how she had run the yard well enough to escape detection by everyone except Toby.

But if she gave in now, where would it end? How many more demands would he make? What choice did she have? Another attack like this morning's could finish her father.

Now she knew why Jago Barata had wanted her here. Yet his request – demand – made no sense. He had accused her of lacking any sense of style or fashion. So *why* was he entrusting her with his house?

'Come, Miss Bonython,' he drawled. 'I have never yet seen you lost for words. Many women would consider such a request an honour.'

Caseley raised her head. Though she dared not say the words she longed to hurl at him, she made no effort to hide her contempt. He totally ignored it.

'But you must not feel overwhelmed. A simple yes will do.'

'Goddammit, Caseley. What's the matter with you?' Teuder snapped. 'I've never known you so contrary. A deal is a deal, and if Jago's agreement is dependent on you refurbishing his house then I want your word, and an end to this wilful self-ishness.'

The injustice stung and she had to swallow twice before she could utter a sound. 'As you wish.'

'That's settled then.' Jago leaned over to shake Teuder's hand. 'With your permission I shall call for your daughter this afternoon and take her to see the house.'

'Please do not trouble yourself, Captain,' Caseley said quickly. 'If you will leave the key and the address, I can manage perfectly well alone.'

He held her gaze for a moment then bowed. 'Until three, Miss Bonython.'

As his footsteps receded down the passage, Teuder rubbed a hand over his face. 'Where were we? Ah yes. Tresawle's ketch. Check the dates in the ledger, Caseley. See if we can fit him in.'

Chapter Eight

The ground and first floor sash windows of the stone-faced house were multi-paned oblongs. Those on the top floor were square. Shallow granite steps led up to an open porch with a flat roof supported by two granite columns.

Reluctantly, Caseley followed Jago up the path as the driver turned the cab in the road and bowled back towards the top of High Street.

Rosebeds on either side of the mossy flagstones were choked with weeds. Summer sun and salt-laden winter gales had flaked paint from the window frames and the heavy front door. The house looked neglected and sad.

Catching a movement, Caseley glanced sideways. In the house next door a lace curtain twitched and was still. She looked down at her feet, wondering if it belonged to anyone who knew her or her family. She had not been near this end of town for several months.

'At last,' Jago muttered as the lock finally yielded. Withdrawing the key he opened the front door. The top half of the inner door had panels of stained glass surrounding a frosted panel, which maintained privacy while admitting light when the front door was open.

'Your first job,' he said over his shoulder, 'will be to have all the locks and hinges oiled.'

Caseley barely heard him. The wide hall was

laid with terracotta tiles patterned in cream and green. Their colours were muted by dust that covered smears of long-dried mud trodden in by many feet.

The paintwork was dull and scratched. The wallpaper showed scrapes and tears and in some places had peeled away from the wall. Cobwebs hung like grey lace over the gas mantles. The glass globes were dusty and flyblown and one was cracked.

Her first impression was one of decay. Yet, against her will and in defiance of her expectations, Caseley liked the house. Now empty and neglected, once it had been filled with the laughter and chatter of a large family. Echoes remained and welcomed. It occurred to her that here she would never feel lonely.

Abruptly shutting off the thought, she was relieved that the gloom hid the betraying colour in her cheeks. She turned to see Jago watching her with an arrested expression on his face. His grey eyes gleamed like a cat's.

'It is fortunate you enjoy a challenge, Miss Bonython. You certainly have one here.' He opened a door to her left and gestured for her to enter, following close behind. 'At least I shall be spared the expense of dust covers,' he remarked as they surveyed the empty room.

His footsteps were loud on the dusty wood floor as he crossed the dim room to the window and folded back the wooden shutters. Several moths fluttered from faded curtains of crimson plush.

'I loathe that colour.' Brushing dust off his hands he returned to the hall.

97

Caseley followed him through the door opposite into another bare room. The opened shutters revealed lumps of soot from the chimney lying scattered over the blue and white glazed tiles in front of the grate.

The lace casement curtain fixed across the sash had frayed at the edges and along the bottom. Cobwebs stretched from the gas-lamps on either side of the fire to the mantelshelf. Lighter patches on the wallpaper showed where once pictures had hung, and a newspaper, yellow with age, lay in a corner.

'Why did you say that?' Caseley directed the question at Jago's broad back as they entered the large kitchen after a quick glance into another empty room that faced the back yard.

He glanced over his shoulder. 'Say what?'

'That I enjoy a challenge. You know nothing about me.'

The kitchen was large and airy with a Cornish range on one wall above which was suspended a wooden frame for drying or airing clothes. Beneath the window was a stone sink with a wooden draining board. An oblong wooden table stood in the centre. The terracotta floor tiles were covered in dust and muddy footprints.

'You're wrong, Miss Bonython. I know a lot about you.' His voice floated out from the walk-in larder. 'Before you accuse me of invading your privacy,' he closed the door and turned to face her, 'what I have learned comes from my own observations. Until we were introduced, I was not aware Teuder Bonython had a daughter.'

Why should he have known? Her father and

uncles would have had no reason to mention her. 'What about Toby? You must have asked him—'

'My only question was if your father's illness had had any effect on the yard. The rest he volunteered.'

Strangely, it did not occur to her to doubt him. She turned away. Toby hadn't intended it, but she felt betrayed. She crossed to the door that led out to the yard and washhouse. Jago followed.

'Toby Penfold thinks very highly of you. He says the men do too. Though judging by your behaviour toward me, I cannot imagine why.'

She swung round, a stinging retort ready on her lips. But seeing his mocking smile and the glint in his eyes she realised he was deliberately trying to provoke her. *Why?* If she asked him he would probably deny it. In any case, she did not care. Her chin rose.

'Do not make sport with me, sir.' As his eyes narrowed she swallowed her anger and shrugged. 'I have known those men and their families since I was a child. They have my affection and my respect.'

'And I do not?' His tone bantered, but beneath it lay something darker.

'You have given me little cause—' she broke off and took a deep breath. 'My opinions are of interest to no one but myself.' Despite her determination not to react, his goading unnerved her. Why was he doing it? What did he want from her? She walked past him back into the hall.

'Are you ready to see upstairs?' When she nodded he gestured for her to lead the way.

The carpet had been removed and the wide

staircase rang hollow beneath their tread. Caseley hesitated on the landing. Jago simply waited behind her, so she pushed open the right-hand door.

The rails and knobs on the huge brass bedstead were tarnished and dull. A few feathers were all that remained of the mattress and pillows. Hearing him come in, she focused her gaze on the floor, the planks scarred where heavy furniture had been dragged across them.

The tiny fireplace with its black-lead surround was framed by green and white porcelain tiles decorated with a flower pattern. Old newspapers had been stuffed into the chimney and grate.

'This was the room my grandparents shared all their married life,' he said, looking round. 'All their children were born in that bed. Perhaps mine will be.'

Abruptly Caseley crossed to the window.

'Are you not fond of children, Miss Bonython?' His voice followed her and she could feel his ironic gaze between her shoulder blades.

'I have no experience of them.' She gazed across the harbour towards the village of Flushing basking in the afternoon sunshine.

'But you would like children of your own, would you not?'

Beneath her enfolding cape, Caseley cupped her elbows, unsettled by his questions. 'Captain, we are barely acquainted. Such talk is not proper.'

'Not proper?' he mocked. 'Since the moment we met your attitude and behaviour towards me has been barely civil, let alone *proper*. You are in no position to invoke convention now. I merely asked–'

She whirled round, hands clenched at her sides, her face burning. 'Why are you doing this?'

His features tightened. 'Such innocence,' he mocked. 'Such wounded vulnerability.' Two strides brought him to within inches of her. She flinched from the tension he radiated, the anger he was fighting to control. His eyes glittered and she saw her own image reflected in them, pale but holding her ground.

'You give me no peace.' With a muttered oath he turned away, rubbing one hand across the back of his neck.

'Then why am I here? You don't like me. I irritate you and make you angry. So why–'

He looked at her over his shoulder. 'Your father and I have an agreement.'

'Which need not include me. You had no right to demand my involvement. Why do so when you must know dozens of women who would be only too pleased to refurbish your house for you, and remain afterwards to–' She broke off as horror washed over her.

She had never, *ever* behaved like this. Though he brought out the worst in her, her wilful, wayward tongue had handed him the ammunition with which to shoot her down.

'I beg your pardon, Captain Barata.' Seeking refuge in formality, she clasped her hands tightly. 'It is not my habit to be–'

'Rude and ill-natured?' he supplied, his eyes gleaming with amusement. 'But that is precisely why I wanted *you*, Miss Bonython. I need not lose a moment's sleep wondering how to get rid of you once the job is completed.'

Caseley caught her breath as the arrow found its target. 'You will not release me from this – this charade?'

'Agreement,' he corrected.

'Blackmail,' she flung back. 'As we are dispensing with convention, let us be completely honest. You used blackmail to get me here.'

'Yes, I did,' he said calmly, surprising her. 'Now tell me you hate the house. Tell me that the task of making it a comfortable, welcoming home neither interests nor appeals to you.'

'I–' she stopped. She moistened dry lips, willing herself to say the words. If she did, would he let her go? Unlikely. He would twist them to suit himself. And he still held the trump card: his threat to tell her father.

But those were not the reasons she remained silent. She could not say she hated the house, because she didn't. It was a happy house. With care and thought it could be made beautiful.

Now she had seen it, the challenge fired her imagination and offered a much-needed respite from the pressures she faced at home and in the office. To say she hated it would irreparably damage something she had sensed as they moved from room to room, something fragile and precious. She turned away.

'This will not be spoken of again.' It was an order. 'You are here, that is enough.'

She looked out of the window at quay punts ferrying provisions out to two barques and a brigantine moored in the middle of the river.

102

'To do it properly will cost a lot of money.'

Jago came to stand beside her. 'I expect it will.'

'Perhaps you should give me a figure, a limit.'

'Are you a spendthrift?'

She glanced at him briefly. 'No.'

'Do you intend to cheat me?'

'No!'

'Then it's unnecessary.'

'Naturally I shall keep accounts, and all the invoices will be retained for your inspection.'

'As you like.' His disinterest was plain.

'Captain Barata, you are not taking me seriously.'

He turned towards her. 'Are you concerned that I cannot afford it?'

'No, of course not.' But the warmth climbing her throat to her cheeks betrayed her.

'Forget about the money. I have enough in the bank here to cover the initial work and by the time I return from Spain I shall have the rest.'

Caseley risked a sidelong glance. He had the look of a man who had just made a far-reaching decision. But the harshness of his chiselled profile discouraged questions.

He turned to her. 'Shall we look at the remainder of the house?'

After climbing the flight of narrow stairs that led to the servants' bedrooms and the attic, they returned to the landing and entered the second front bedroom. It was a mirror image of the first, except that it was empty.

Once more Caseley was drawn to the window. A brig laden with granite was coming down-river from Penryn. Passing ships moored in the King's

Road she headed out towards Trefusis Point and the Carrick Roads, and on into Falmouth Bay. As they watched, the main staysail and flying jib were hoisted. Caseley sighed.

'I believe it is common for wives and daughters of owner-skippers to sail with them on occasion,' Jago said. 'Did you and your mother ever accompany your father?'

'We did once. But I was very young and remember little about it. Ralph, my brother, was away staying with friends, and Father took Mother and me up to Southampton.'

'You have not been to sea since?'

Caseley darted an uncertain glance at him. 'Why do you ask, Captain?'

'You gaze at those ships with such yearning. Is the sea in your blood? Or do you simply seek escape from all the problems besetting you?'

His gentleness startled her. She had grown used to being defensive, prepared for battle, trusting neither him nor her own reactions. But for the moment at least, they appeared to have a truce.

'You make me sound like a coward.' She tried to smile.

'You are many things, Caseley Bonython. But not a coward, never that.' The smile in his deep voice sent a quiver through her. 'So, answer my question.'

She looked out of the window. 'A little of both. The past months have been so ... full.' She shrugged lightly. 'I am a little weary.'

'Is there no one you can turn to? No one from whom you can seek help or comfort?'

She shook her head. 'My grandparents are

dead. My closest female relatives are Aunt Helen and Aunt Margaret. Aunt Helen is a dear, but she has a young child and does not enjoy good health. Aunt Margaret–' she looked up at him. 'Have you not met Uncle Thomas's wife?'

'Not that I recall.'

Caseley sighed. 'If you had, you would remember. Aunt Margaret has fixed ideas about everything and does not approve of me.'

'That I can understand.' Jago's tone was dry. 'What about your mother?'

Caseley looked down at her hands. 'My mother is dead.'

'When and how?'

Though taken aback by his bluntness, it did not offend her. She told him about the event that had shattered her life and of which she seldom spoke.

'My father – it was too painful for him. His first wife and son had died of diphtheria, you see. He and my mother – I remember them as very happy together. He was so proud of Ralph, my elder brother. And as the youngest and the only girl I was indulged.' She smiled at memories.

'He bought me dolls and loved to see me in pretty dresses. But Ralph was his favourite. A son to replace the one he had lost. An heir who would inherit–'

'Never mind your brother,' Jago was impatient. 'What happened?'

'An accident. A stupid, senseless accident.' Caseley wrapped her arms across her body. 'Mother had hired a pony and trap to take me out for a birthday treat. She loved to drive herself. But when we went out as a family, Father wouldn't let her. He and Ralph used to take turns while Mother and I rode in the back.

'She took me round Castle Drive. It was a beautiful spring day. The sun was shining and there was a breeze off the sea. The hedges were full of primroses and red campion. Bluebells lay like a carpet among the trees. We could see the fishing fleet out in the bay. The outer harbour was busy with ships entering and leaving Falmouth, their masts crowded with canvas. I remember seeing the steam ferry coming past St Mawes Castle.' She paused for a moment as images crowded back, still vivid.

'We had just rounded Castle Point when two fighting magpies flew out of the hedge right in front of us. The pony took fright. It reared then started to bolt. Mother wrenched on the reins. One wheel hit a fencepost and the trap turned over. We were both thrown out onto the road. The pony trod on my foot and crushed it. Luckily the coastguard was doing his round and saw what happened. He got help and they pulled me away and managed to calm the pony.

'I couldn't understand why Mother didn't come to comfort me. My foot was already swollen and hurt dreadfully. My new dress was dirty and torn and streaked with blood from all the grazes. She just lay there by the hedge, not scratched at all, just very pale. Then someone said her neck was broken.'

Caseley had not realised she was crying until Jago turned her towards him. He wiped the tears from her cheeks with gentle thumbs then cupped her face between his hands.

Her vision was blurred. As scalding tears spilled over her lashes, her breath caught in her throat, and her heart stuttered, missing a beat.

He was gazing at her with a dark intensity that made her tremble. She sensed a battle raging in him and felt herself grow hot. His rough hands so gentle on her face made her crave more. She wanted his arms around her; wanted to be held. The need, the hunger, terrified her. She gripped his wrists and drew his hands down.

'Forgive me – I am not usually so weak.'

He released her. Turning away she fumbled for her handkerchief, quickly wiped her eyes and swallowed the painful ache in her throat. 'I have not spoken – tried not to think– Telling you brought it back. I miss her.'

'There is no shame in grief,' he said quietly. 'And no one could ever call you weak.'

She looked round, pushing a loose curl back from her damp forehead. 'But–' she stopped as one dark brow rose, daring her to argue with him.

'Who took care of you?'

'Rosina, Mrs Renfree, our housekeeper. She was widowed young and has lived with our family since I was a baby. She's been wonderfully kind to both Ralph and me. As I grew up Father insisted I take responsibility for running the household. I couldn't have done it without her help. But it changed our relationship. She said that was as it should be. But–' She stopped, shook her head.

'You were lonely.'

She looked up quickly. How had he known? How had he heard what she hadn't said? She gave a tiny nod.

Holding her gaze he rested one elbow on the sash and linked his fingers. 'I am my father's only son. He has always been ambitious, for himself and for me. He has family connections in Mexico. So after he had made enough money from his business interests in Spain, he bought into silver mines there. He also breeds and sells pedigree cattle.

'I remember as a small child being placed on a pony and led around his estate in Castile. He told me that one day it would all be mine. But I did not want it. I wanted to go to sea. The day I told him was the day I grew up. I saw part of him die and knew I was responsible.

'But I also knew I had to carve out my own destiny. For a long time we both suffered. He considered me ungrateful. I was angry that he did not understand my need to be my own man, the man he had raised me to be. The family took his side.' He shrugged.

Caseley stared at him. This arrogant, demanding man was admitting loneliness? She felt a rush of empathy. 'And now?'

He moved away from the window. 'Now, there is great affection, and even greater respect. Each of us has a star to follow. We must be true to ourselves or risk the consequences.'

'My brother–'

'I know about your brother. He is older than you, yet still a child. When he finds the courage to be honest with himself then he will become a man.'

'You sound – hard.'

'Perhaps. I am not a patient man. But I demand

no more from others than from myself.'

'Not everyone is as strong as you.' She was amazed at her own temerity in speaking so openly to him.

'We are all capable of far more than we imagine.' Reaching out he caught her hand. 'You, for instance: who would have suspected such strength, such capability?'

Acutely aware of the latent strength in his warm fingers, struggling with the emotions his touch aroused, she took refuge in tartness. 'You certainly have an unusual way of paying a compliment.'

He laughed softly, his teeth very white against his dark beard. He studied her face, his gaze growing shuttered as his amusement faded and she grew hot under his scrutiny.

Releasing her hand, he turned once more to the window.

'Has your father spoken to you of his intentions?'

She struggled to adjust. His moods changed swiftly and without warning. 'I don't understand. What intentions?'

'You know he is dying.' Though the words were blunt, his tone was not unkind. She was about to deny it, to say what she so wanted to believe, that her father had many months of life ahead of him. But the awareness in Jago's eyes stopped the words before they reached her lips. She nodded, unable to speak.

'Does *he* know?'

'Yes.' She cleared her throat. 'But we have not spoken of it. He wants everything to continue as before.'

'So he has not told you what he plans to do with the yard?'

She shook her head. 'I assume he will leave it to Ralph–'

'Who does not want it,' Jago pointed out.

Caseley shrugged helplessly. 'I don't know. I don't want to think about it.'

'You must.'

'Why?' she cried. 'What is it to you anyway? Why should you care–' she stopped abruptly as dread gnawed a hollow inside her. 'Unless–'

'Unless?'

'You want the yard. You have shares in *Cygnet*. You want Will's job as senior captain. But why this?' She flung her arm wide in a gesture that encompassed the house. 'How does this fit into your plan?'

'It doesn't.'

'Then why ask me such questions? Why drag *me* into your dealings with my father?'

Tension shimmered between them as he gazed at her, slate-eyed and tight-lipped. Abruptly, he turned away. 'Why indeed?' he muttered in harsh self-mockery. 'Come, I will see you home.'

Caseley walked quickly from the room before he could touch her. Even his formal gestures of politeness, his palm cupping her elbow, a handshake, set her heart pounding and heightened her confusion. Rather than ask herself why, it was safer to avoid all contact.

'We can get a cab from the Greenbank Hotel,' he said as he locked the front door.

A middle-aged woman wearing a blue and white printed cotton day dress and a straw hat

110

stood in the tiny front garden of the house next door. She held a pair of scissors and was snipping the dead heads off some roses. Caseley guessed she had been behind the twitching curtain.

''Afternoon,' the woman said with a bright smile.

'Good afternoon,' Jago replied pleasantly. Caseley merely nodded.

'Moving in, are you?'

'Not just yet,' Jago said before Caseley could open her mouth. 'There's a great deal to be done first.'

The woman nodded. 'Been empty for a while, it has. Still, it's some lovely family home.' Her sharp eyes flicked between them. 'Plenty of room for children. I got four so I know what I'm talking about. Now they've built that there new sewer, we're having one of they proper flushing water closets. Always had a privy up the garden before. But 'tis no joke in the winter. Nor when the children are ill. All that to-ing and fro-ing is enough drive you mad. I expect you'll be having one put in?'

'I expect so,' Jago agreed, and placed a hand in the small of Caseley's back. 'Please excuse us. Nice to have met you.' He flashed a charm-filled smile and the woman simpered like a dewy-eyed girl.

Caseley walked quickly down the path. The warm pressure of Jago's hand on her waist was too possessive. She had not the sophistication to ignore it. Nor could she control the rapid pounding of her pulse.

'Why did you do that?' she hissed as they

111

reached the pavement and were out of earshot.

'Do what?' he appeared surprised but removed his hand. 'I was under the impression you wished to leave.'

'I was – am. I didn't mean that,' she retorted. 'Why did you allow that woman to think that you – that we–' she felt heat in her face and wished she hadn't said anything. 'You know what I mean.'

'Does it matter what she thinks? I feel no obligation to explain myself to her. Do you?'

'No. But–'

'Then why worry? We both know the truth. Why should we concern ourselves with the opinions of people who don't matter?'

Caseley said nothing as her thoughts whirled like windblown leaves. Maybe he was right. How could they explain without causing even more speculation? Besides, what was the truth? Certainly there was no attachment between them. Though no longer strangers, they were not friends. She irritated him. He infuriated her.

Her life and his were becoming inextricably tangled. Her father claimed there were good reasons. Jago would not explain his. And she – she didn't know what she felt.

He was silent, abstracted, as they rode back to the other end of town. Her thoughts fluttered like a cage full of birds. Yet despite the tension that vibrated between them, this afternoon had subtly altered their relationship.

The direction her life was taking seemed fraught with danger. But it was outside her control and there was no turning back.

'When do you intend to begin work on the house?' His abrupt question made her start.

'I – I hadn't thought,' she blurted in total honesty.

'I would like to move in this year.' His tone was dry. 'Hotel life has lost its appeal. May I suggest you start tomorrow?'

'I can't. I haven't had time to–'

'I will go to the bank in the morning. Aside from oil for all the hinges, you will first require a plumber and a mason. The house is already connected to the main water supply so the installation of a proper bathroom with a geyser for hot water, an overhead shower above the bath, and a new water closet should have priority, don't you agree?'

As she'd had no idea where to start, Caseley was relieved. 'Where should the bathroom go?'

'Where would you propose?'

About to tell him it was none of her business, she caught the warning glint in his eye and decided not to risk antagonising him. She closed her eyes and tried to recall the layout of the house.

'That small room behind the main bedroom on the first floor?' She turned to him. 'Then the waste pipes could go down the wall into a drain at the side of the house and join up to the new sewer.'

'I see I shall be free to devote my attention to other matters.'

The implied compliment warmed and terrified her. 'What about the tradesmen?'

He shrugged. 'You have lived in the town all your life. You should know who best ones are, and who to avoid. Your task is to organise the work and the people to do it. I will arrange the finance.'

'But – the wallpaper, curtains, furnishings – what colours...'

'I leave that to you,' he waved a dismissive hand.

'No. I cannot take that responsibility. What if you hate the things I choose?'

'Why should I?'

'Because,' her chin rose, 'because I have no taste, no sense of style.' She tried to suppress anxiety and deep lingering hurt with anger. 'You implied as much when you pressed my father into agreeing this arrangement.' She shook her head. 'None of this makes sense. You say you want only the best. So why pick me? Why–'

'Enough!' His tone made her flinch. 'I do not plan to abandon you entirely. I shall follow progress with great interest.'

'I do not doubt it. Waiting for my first mistake. What then? More taunts? More derision?'

'God give me patience,' he muttered. 'Cruel tyrant that I am, I did not wish you to feel I was watching your every move. I wanted you to have time to–' He controlled himself with an effort. But Caseley's heart sank as she saw his expression harden. 'Surely there is nothing unusual in what I ask? Do not all women consider men totally without judgement in such matters?'

'But... I am not... This is *your* house, *your* money.'

'Precisely. Mine to do with as I please.' As the hansom rocked to a halt, Jago leaned towards her, his eyes gleaming. He tilted her chin, making her burningly aware of their closeness in the confined space. 'And it would please me very much,' he said softly, 'if you would do as you have been asked, accept that I trust you, *and stop arguing.*'

Chapter Nine

Still wearing his nightshirt, his clothes over his arm, Thomas crept across to the door. Hearing the bedsprings creak he tensed.

'Thomas?' Margaret's voice was thick with sleep. The bed creaked again as she sat up. 'What time did you get in last night?'

He turned the doorknob, still clinging to hope of escape. 'Don't let me disturb you, my dear.'

'I'm awake now, so you can stay right here.'

Reluctantly, he released the handle and turned back, dropping his clothes on the ottoman at the foot of the bed.

'Well? I'm waiting.' Margaret's mouth was tightly pursed as she removed her bed cap and began to unplait her hair.

'I told you I would be late.' His attempt to placate succeeded only in sounding defensive as he pulled on his trousers before taking off his nightshirt. 'It was business.'

'At that time of night?'

'People have commitments. They aren't always available during the day.' His hands trembled as he buttoned his shirt.

'I was worried sick. You know what this town is like at night. All those lewd women. They don't even wait for darkness. Shameless, they are.'

Thomas glanced up. 'You were afraid I had been kidnapped by lewd women?' He felt a trace of wistfulness.

'There's no call to be vulgar. I heard something shocking yesterday. You should have been here so we could discuss what to do.'

The roaring in his head made Thomas sit down suddenly on the ottoman, his back to his wife. His heart was racing and perspiration beaded his forehead and upper lip. *He had been found out.*

No, he hadn't. Teuder had not done the audit yet. When he did there would be nothing to find. It had taken him until midnight but he had altered the books so the losses did not show. Now the money was back in the bank, all the figures balanced.

He sucked in a shaky breath. Everything was fine. Colenzo would not say anything. The man was a shark. But as long as the repayments arrived on time he'd keep his mouth shut.

Could Luke have let something slip? Brandy and bitterness might have loosened his tongue, made him careless.

Dare he risk continuing? But if he didn't, how would he be able to repay Colenzo? Why had Luke been talking to that arrogant half-breed, Barata?

'Thomas, you're not listening to me,' Margaret nagged. 'It's a disgrace. Lord knows what people will think of us now that Caseley has got involved with that – that person. I don't know what Teuder

116

is thinking of to allow it.'

Straightening her voluminous nightgown she stood up.

'Where *is* that girl? She knows I must have my warm water in the mornings. You have no idea what I have to put up with, Thomas. Then you stay out half the night—'

'Shut up, damn you!' His voice teetered on the edge of desperation.

'Ohhh,' Margaret collapsed onto the bed, one hand flying to her mouth. 'How could you speak to me like that? Here I am, worried out of my mind—'

'What about *me?*' Thomas turned on her. 'Don't you ever think about *anyone* but yourself? What does it matter who Caseley takes up with? You have a daughter of your own. If you must worry, then worry about her.'

'I am!' Margaret wailed. 'It's her I'm concerned for. Can't you see what might happen?'

The violence had drained away, leaving him spent and shaking. 'What are you talking about?'

'Teuder must know. In fact he must be encouraging this – liaison between Caseley and Captain Barata—'

'Who?' Thomas croaked. '*Who* did you say?'

'I wish you'd listen. Barata, Jago Barata. You must know him. He's one of Teuder's captains, master of the *Cygnet*. Thomas, what if Teuder is planning a match between them? God knows, Caseley hasn't much to recommend her. But then that man is not like us. He probably doesn't have the same tastes we do, or the same idea of beauty for that matter.' Margaret's pursed and bitter

117

mouth indicated that as far as she was concerned, Jago Barata had no taste at all. 'If Teuder sees this man as the only hope of a husband for Caseley, he might do something foolish.'

'No,' Thomas whispered. Shock and fear were paralysing his ability to think.

'Caseley is twenty-one, and lame,' Margaret went on. 'Any man prepared to wed her will seek a sizeable dowry. Ralph has no interest in the business. What's to stop Teuder leaving the yard to Caseley? If he does that and she marries Jago Barata, what will become of us then, Thomas? You, me, and Charlotte?'

'You might have it all wrong. I've met Barata. He doesn't look like a man who could be bought.' Thomas recalled cool grey eyes and lightning appraisal. He had felt his soul stripped bare and his guilt exposed. Glancing back as they left the dining room he had seen the speculative gaze following Luke and himself.

'Three times that man has been into the office to see her. Even Richard noticed and you know how blind he is. Mrs Cox in the Post Office told me that Captain Barata has acquired a house up along Greenbank. She expected me to know all about it seeing that Caseley is my niece, and he was seen entering and leaving the house accompanied by a young woman with a limp and reddish-brown hair. That's Caseley all right. So what's going on?'

'I don't know.' Thomas felt panic churn like acid inside him.

Caseley glanced up as her brother entered the dining room. He was freshly shaved, his hair neatly combed. His shirt was crisp and his coat and trousers had been brushed and pressed. Though pale, his eyes red-rimmed, he looked better than he had for days.

'Hello, Ralph,' she smiled. 'You're up early. Would you like some breakfast?'

'Just coffee.' He shuddered. 'I don't know how you can face food at this time of day.'

'I don't know how you manage without it,' she replied lightly, pouring his coffee as he sat down opposite.

'What are you doing?' He indicated her note-pad, pencil, and other pieces of paper beside her crumb-strewn plate.

'Trying to work out the best order for jobs to be done.'

'Now Father's back at work–'

'Not for the business. The list is for Captain Barata's house.'

'Ahhhh.'

She ignored the inflections in her brother's tone and continued writing.

'How is it coming along?'

'Faster than I expected. Mr Endean was due at a house in Florence Terrace but a family bereavement meant the work had to be postponed. So he was able to come right away. The inside plumbing should be finished by the end of the week. When the plaster has been made good and the other repairs completed, the decorators can begin.'

'My, my,' Ralph raised his cup in mocking salute. 'You have been busy.'

'Sometimes I feel it's running away with me,' Caseley admitted. 'I had no idea how much there was to do. Which is why getting it all in the right order is so important.'

'What does the good captain think of progress so far?'

Suppressing a pang, she riffled through the papers, pretending to search for something. Though he had promised not to watch her every move, she had expected a visit, braced herself in anticipation. But he hadn't come.

Ignoring the surprise and unease shown by the plumber and other tradesmen she consulted hadn't been easy. She had met the same reaction in shops when she enquired about materials.

The salesmen were polite but evasive, making it clear that 'the gentleman's approval must by confirmed by his visit in person before an order could be accepted.'

The second time this happened, Caseley gathered her courage, stood her ground, and asked to speak to the manager. Quaking inside, she informed him that she alone was responsible for the purchases she wished to make. The order was of considerable value, and she expected to pay at the end of the month like any other respected customer. If he was unable to meet her demands, she would take her business elsewhere.

Lavish apologies for the misunderstanding and thinly disguised curiosity had accompanied offers of assistance to locate anything else she might require. She had longed to tell someone about it, to share the experience and laugh at her own bravado. But there was only one person directly concerned, one person who would understand.

'Captain Barata has not visited yet. But I'm

sure he will be impressed. Mr Endean takes great pride in his work. He's also very quick and keeps the man and boy who work with him busy all the time.'

'Doesn't it worry you? I mean you hardly know the man. I'm talking about Barata, not Mr Endean.'

She shrugged to hide the doubts that were her constant companions. 'He and Father made the arrangement.'

'So you said. But you must admit it's rather odd. He's expecting you to do something that would cause most *wives* to hesitate. Why *you?*'

'I have no idea.' She rose and carried her cup to the sideboard. That question had kept her awake night after night. All too aware of her many defects, she could not fathom the reasoning behind Jago Barata's demand. They struck sparks off each other every time they met.

To cope with the loss of her mother, her father's absorption in the business and her brother's unhappiness, she had always striven for calm, balance. But from the instant she and Jago Barata met, she had been buffeted by violent emotions.

She loathed his arrogance and cutting irony. Yet he stirred yearnings that no self-scolding or rationalisation could banish. He could be cruelly derisive yet moments later reveal an understanding that left her breathless.

He was a man of the world in the widest sense: of dual ancestry, well educated, widely travelled and independently wealthy, leading life on his own terms. What could she ever be to him apart from briefly useful?

121

'Why me?' She raised slim shoulders. 'I don't know. Captain Barata is very busy. He needed someone to organise and oversee work on the house. It was my misfortune that I happened to be there at the time.'

Even as she spoke, innate honesty made her conscience prick. Certainly she had felt like that to begin with, but now? She gazed up at the overcast sky. The cloud, thick and low, promised rain before the day's end.

'Father approved the idea and it was agreed between them.'

'But you have no experience.'

'I know, and so I told them.' Returning to the table she leaned over to gather the papers together. 'It didn't make the slightest difference. They are very alike in their stubbornness.'

Ralph pushed back his chair and stretched out his legs, regarding his sister with a mixture of curiosity and admiration. 'Aren't you nervous? It must be costing him a bundle. What if you make a pig's ear of the whole business?'

'Thanks, Ralph.'

'You know what I mean.'

She nodded, hugging the bundle of papers to her chest. 'I admit I was terrified at first. But Mr Endean has taken me under his wing. He put me right on several matters. I've got the best mason in town in George Tallack. He'll be starting in a couple of days. He and Mr Endean have worked together many times. I think Mr Endean may have persuaded him to take this job. I know he's usually very busy. I still get butterflies in my stomach about the furnishings. Colours and textures are such a personal choice. But Captain Barata trusts me.' She shrugged, trying to ignore the combined thrill and chill that tingled through her.

'I don't know how you fit it all in. Aren't you exhausted?'

'I expected to be. But now Father seems so much better– You should have seen his face when Toby and I took him round the yard yesterday afternoon. The men gave him such a welcome. He roared at them for wasting time when they should have been working, but there were tears in his eyes. Dr Vigurs was right to let him go back.'

Seeing his shuttered expression she moved quickly on. 'Even though the house is in a far worse state now than when I first saw it, with holes in the walls and dust everywhere, it has a lovely atmosphere. It will be beautiful when it's finished.'

'Take care, Caseley,' he cautioned. 'Don't put your heart into it. It's not yours, nor ever will be.'

'I'm fully aware of my limitations. But I can't – won't – do less than my best.'

'Listen, I didn't mean–'

'I know, and it's all right.' She didn't want to hear his awkward apology, knowing that she lied. Deep in her heart she wondered what it would be like to be mistress of the house. She banished the thought. She did not need that in order to walk through the rooms, touch the furniture she had chosen, see the colours she had blended to create harmony and welcome.

Besides, being mistress of the house would require that she also be Jago Barata's wife, a thought that terrified her as much as it admittedly intrigued.

123

She flashed him a bright smile. 'So why are you up early looking so smart?'

He stood up, shooting his cuffs. 'I am off to work.'

'What? Has Uncle Richard–?'

'I'm not going to Bonython's. It's not for me, and never will be. I am waiting on Mrs Edwin Lashbrooke to make preliminary sketches for a portrait. But I need to go into town first to pick up one or two things.'

'You're going to paint *Frances?* But how – when–?'

'I wasn't commissioned directly,' Ralph admitted. 'Jason Blarney was going to do it. But he cut his hand on a broken bottle – of linseed oil,' he added as Caseley frowned. 'Anyway, Frances wanted the portrait done at once and Jason recommended me.'

'Ralph, I'm so pleased for you.' Caseley limped around the table and clasped her brother's hands. 'I know how much you want to paint. If this portrait is a success it could mean more commissions. Who knows where that might lead? You have a wonderful talent and this is a great opportunity.'

She made herself stop. She wanted to tell him not to waste it as he had wasted so many others. Not to seek solace in alcohol if he could not immediately achieve the perfection he sought. But saying such things might create doubts in his mind.

'I'll show them.' His eyes glittered. 'The doubters, the gossips, Father. I'll show them all.'

'I know you will.' Reaching up she kissed his cheek.

Grinning, he squeezed her fingers before crossing to the door. He paused, listening. 'He's on his way down.'

'Have you told him?'

Ralph shook his head.

'Why not? He would be pleased for you.'

Her brother regarded her with a bitter smile. 'Poor Caseley. You try so hard. I know you mean well but surely you've learned by now that nothing I do will ever please Father? I am doubly damned. I don't want the yard and I am not Philip.' He walked out.

She heard him say good morning, heard their father's gruff voice demanding to know where Ralph was going, and when did he intend to start accepting his responsibilities, behaving like a man. But the words lacked heart and hope. They were uttered out of habit and were answered by the sound of the front door slamming.

Jago Barata packed with an expertise born of practice. His white shirt was open at the neck, the sleeves rolled halfway up his forearms. Two canvas bags lay on the bed. Into the smaller he placed the clothes he would need while in Spain, plus toiletries. The rest of his belongings went into the larger bag.

A flurry of telegraph messages between himself and Ramon Gaudara over the past three days had established that Guadara had received Felipe's letter and reached Juan at the mine. The quicksilver was being sent to the port of Santander for him to collect. Now the blockade had been lifted, Bilbao was chaotic as all the shipping companies

125

sought desperately to clear the backlog of waiting cargoes.

Though the fighting had not reached the mine area, it had been impossible to move anything in or out.

Packing reminded him of how little he possessed. When he left his father's house and travelled to Bilbao to begin his career at sea, he had arrived there with several bags and a chest.

Sailing with Basques whose reputation as seamen was renowned throughout the world, he had learned quickly. His love of the sea in all her many moods, coupled with technical skill, a sixth sense regarding the weather, and nerves of iron, soon gained him a reputation that rivalled those of his teachers.

Realising that light was the only way to travel he had sold everything but basic necessities. He moved from ship to ship, line to line, always seeking the best, oblivious to discomfort or length of voyage, caring only for the captain's skill and what he could learn.

Having worked his way up from ordinary seaman to mate, he sat the examinations necessary before he could captain a ship in foreign waters. Two years later he had his own command, a small two-masted schooner sailing out of Bilbao, carrying oranges, lemons, salt, wine, and brandy. The ship was his home and cabin space so limited there was simply no room for personal possessions.

It was on that schooner he had first come to Falmouth. Now he owned a house here. Since his parents had moved to Mexico he had no personal ties to Spain. Here, at last, he had a home of his own and an opportunity to put down roots.

He dropped the shirt he was rolling onto the bed and flexed his shoulders, stretching his arms high and wide then running both hands through his hair. Tension lay like a yoke on the back of his neck as he looked out of the window.

Below in the busy street carts and cabs delivered goods and passengers. Two women wearing short capes and beribboned bonnets entered the grocer's opposite, where signs advertised provisions, patent medicines, pure Ceylon tea, and coffee roasted daily on the premises.

To the left was a boot and shoe shop, the wares displayed on hooked poles resembling strange trees. Next door the Supply Stores invited inspection of Devenish's Celebrated Dorset Ales in casks or bottles at popular prices, fine wines from the wood, and choice ginger wine.

Alongside was the second of George Downing's butcher's shops. Short and rotund, George stood by the window display between two pig carcasses suspended on steel hooks from an overhead rail. A blue and white striped apron covered the front of his starched white coat and a straw boater was set at a jaunty angle on his balding head. Jago's frown deepened. Why did he want a house? A house was a tie, a responsibility, and he valued freedom. He came and went as he pleased, limited only by wind and tide.

Yet had not the impersonal anonymity of hotel rooms begun to pall? After eighteen years of criss-crossing the oceans, was it not time he had somewhere of his own to come back to?

Thinking of the house brought Caseley to mind.

What infernal impulse had goaded him to insist on her help? Correct in her guess that others would have jumped at the chance, her reluctance had intrigued and irritated.

His accusation that she gave him no peace was the naked truth. Since their first meeting he had been haunted by her. Why?

She was not beautiful. Her cheekbones were too pronounced, her chin too firm, her eyes too large, and her mouth too tempting. Her hair might have the healthy shine of a polished chestnut but its springy waves and curling tendrils were untameable. She had no sophistication.

A flash of insight needled him. Enticing, amusing, worldly women had passed over the surface of his life without leaving a ripple.

Caseley Bonython touched him as none of them ever had. Straight-backed and slender, she had a presence that made her limp irrelevant. The way she held her head, the way she seemed so often poised for flight, reminded him of a gazelle.

She was defiant, quick-tempered, and impulsive. She was also intelligent, courageous, and loyal. Amusing though her anger and dislike of him had been, it had also jolted him. Not given to introspection, he found examination of his own behaviour disconcerting.

Often pursued, he was now the pursuer. He could not comprehend what drove him, for she threatened his whole way of life. Drawn to her, he deliberately kept his distance except to goad her, as if antagonising her might destroy in him the need he perceived as weakness. But his conscience wracked him and the guilt became anger directed, perversely, at her.

Picking up the rolled shirt he pushed it into his bag. He needed to get to sea again. The whisper of the night wind, the hiss of the bow cutting through the water, and the vastness of the dark sky glittering with patterns of stars would clear his head.

Though this room would be let in his absence the manager had promised to look after his spare bag until he returned. He had considered taking it up to the house and immediately dismissed the idea. Once he left possessions there he would have committed himself. He was not sure he wished to do that.

For three days he had stayed away. He had plenty to keep him busy. But too often his thoughts strayed. To Caseley. To Caseley in his house.

Anger and self-disgust burned in his gut. He should never have forced her to do it. Doubtless she would have her revenge by stuffing the place with grotesque furniture and ugly useless ornaments. The house would be desecrated with clashing colours and suffocating designs. There would be frills and fringes and lace and his money would have been wasted.

Yet the thought that, despite hating him, she would create a comfortable welcoming home was far more unsettling.

The door burst open and Louise whirled in. Slamming it shut she leaned against it, her voluptuous breasts straining against the orange material of her tight-fitting jacket.

'Why didn't you tell me?' Her eyes were bright

with accusation and excitement. The tiny hat, a confection of straw, feathers, and ribbon, tilted forward on her high-piled hair, sat slightly askew. 'Why did I have to hear it from Amy Cox?'

After a moment's utter stillness Jago continued pushing the last few items into the larger bag.

'Good morning, Louise.' His tone was cool. Brief fury swiftly contained. 'I thought it was understood that *I* would arrange our next meeting.'

'I know, Jago. But when I heard, I didn't know whether to believe it or not. I *had* to–'

'What exactly have you heard?' Drawing the cords tight to close the neck of each bag he knotted them, lifted both to the floor by the door, then scanned the room to make sure nothing had been forgotten.

'That you've bought a house up Greenbank. Is it true?'

'No,' he said evenly. 'I have not bought a house.'

'But Amy said–'

'Mrs Cox might at least make sure her information is accurate before she spreads it around the town.' Weariness tempered Jago's irony. 'The house was a bequest in my grandmother's will.'

Louisa's face lit up and she launched herself at him. 'Oh, Jago, that's handsome. I know you never liked me coming here. You was worried about people seeing us.'

'Seeing you, Louise,' he corrected. 'I am answerable to no one. But your husband is at this moment in his shop opposite the hotel entrance.'

'If he's got a customer, he wouldn't notice the

Queen herself,' Louise scoffed. 'But we won't have to worry no more now, will us? I just wish you'd told me yourself. It hurt awful hearing it from that old gossip.' Wrapping her arms around his neck she pressed close to him, moving sinuously. 'You was keeping it for a surprise.' She rained kisses onto his cheek, his bearded jaw, and finally his mouth. 'God, I've missed you,' she breathed.

He lifted his hands to break her hold. 'I have to go, Louise. I'm due at the yard. *Cygnet* sails tomorrow.'

'Be gone long, will you?' she murmured between kisses. Feeling his body's response to her provocative movements she drew her head back to give a roguish smile.

'Can't go yet, can you, my lover,' she drew the tip of her tongue along her upper lip.

His hands tightened. Images of Caseley tumbled through his mind like windblown leaves. He shuddered and ran his hands down Louise's back, pressing her hard against him. This he understood. This posed no threat.

Chapter Ten

Caseley finished the letter she was writing, addressed the envelope, then passed both across the desk for her father's approval and signature. Her thoughts strayed to the house on Greenbank.

Recalling her conversation with Ralph at breakfast she realised that in only a few days her life had taken on new purpose. But it was very different from the crushing obligation to keep the yard running smoothly. She found she was constantly thinking about colours, textiles, and furniture that would enhance the best features of each room.

The ladies' magazines Aunt Margaret had bought in a bid to 'sharpen up your fashion sense, my dear,' had been retrieved from the cupboard and pored over for their soft furnishing advertisements. She had ignored glances heavy with significance that Rosina exchanged with Liza-Jane, more concerned with working out colour balances.

'Pull yourself together, girl.' Her father shattered her reverie. 'If that's the last of the letters you may as well go.'

Caseley started. 'I'm sorry. Was there something else you wanted me to do?'

'No,' he grudged. 'It's all done for now. I suppose you'll be going up to Greenbank?' His pale gaze was shrewd and Caseley felt warmth creep into her cheeks as she stood up and placed her chair neatly against the wall.

'Not immediately.' Was he implying that she spent too much or too little time at Jago Barata's house? She wasn't about to ask.

Lifting down her short cape from the hook on the back of the door she swung it around her shoulders. 'I have some shopping to do first. Would you like me to walk you home?'

'I would not. I'm going to the yard. Sam is coming with me. I shall be better for some fresh air. It gets stuffy in here. All this damn paper. You be on your way.' He paused. 'Coming on all right, is it?'

'I think so.' She fastened the cape, put on her hat, and picked up her music case. Instead of business letters and ledgers it now contained colour charts, lists of building and plumbing materials, and invoices. 'It's difficult to tell at the moment. I'll know better when it's finished.' *Then it will be too late.*

It was one o'clock before she reached the other end of town. She had visited all the furniture repositories, comparing styles, quality, and price, making copious notes. So much was needed: a dining table and chairs, a sideboard, a sofa and armchairs, at least two small tables, a clothes press for each bedroom, a blanket chest, a dressing table, stools or chairs for the kitchen.

Then there were all the soft furnishings: curtains, rugs, cushions, bed linen, towels, tablecloths, and napkins. She had not even started on crockery, cutlery, glassware, and kitchen utensils.

She was tired and hungry, and the burden of choosing what was right for the house *and* its enigmatic owner had begun to weigh heavily. For an instant she was tempted to ignore the display in the large window of Joseph Roskruge's Drapery Emporium and simply order curtains for every room in the crimson plush he loathed. It would serve him right.

But pride triumphed over her brief dream of vengeance. Pausing to take a deep breath, she entered the shop, hearing the bell tinkle over her head as she pushed open the door.

Half an hour later she left carrying a package

containing samples of curtain material in jade velvet, maroon and ivory regency stripe, and an oyster-coloured fabric with a silken sheen and a subtle pattern of leaves.

Restored by a cup of hot chocolate and a toasted teacake at Alice Teague's refreshment house on Market Strand, she climbed the steep length of High Street. Reaching the brow of the hill she could see the river. The water looked cold and grey reflecting the heavy sky, and the wind had a keen edge.

After announcing her arrival to Mr Endean, for whom she had had a second key cut, she went back downstairs. Removing her cape she hung it over the newel post and went into the drawing room. She unwrapped the fabric samples and stood against the back wall, trying to visualise the room fully furnished.

Each day she became more concerned that the décor complemented the rooms, enhancing their proportions and emphasising the light.

The chesterfield she had seen in Prout's, with its buttoned upholstery of dark green velvet, would look equally well with the regency stripe or the oyster curtains, and perhaps two rosewood balloon-back chairs. A small rectangular sofa table could stand where she was now, and another in the corner holding a jardinière. But for the right-hand wall behind the door, which would be more suitable, the mahogany bureau or a bookcase?

She caught herself. What did it matter which she chose? Once finished she would see none of it again.

The knowledge was painful, but she had to keep it at the forefront of her mind. Doing the job to the best of her ability was one thing. But she must not become emotionally involved. She must not *care*. Jago Barata had made his reason for selecting her abundantly clear. *'I need not lose a moment sleep wondering how to get rid of you once the job is complete.'* She was simply the means by which his property would be made habitable without any involvement from him other than paying the bills.

Caseley left the empty room and walked down the passage to the kitchen. It was better that he had stayed away. The urge to ask his opinion, his preference, would have been too strong to resist.

She looked down at the three pieces of material she still held and shook her head in bewilderment. How could he show so little interest in what was, after all, *his* home? Did he really not care? Was that why, without a qualm, he could delegate such a personal matter to a virtual stranger?

But surely no mere stranger could have divined her loneliness? He had even spoken of his own. The fact that he had done so had shaken her more than the revelation itself.

He had trusted her. And for a few precious moments she had opened like a flower to the warmth of his understanding. He recognised that she felt the loss of her mother more keenly now than in her childhood.

He had spoken of her family with brutal frankness, demanding answers as if by right. For two people who had known each other barely a week

135

their arguments had had a startling intimacy.

Her father, her brother, and her two uncles were the only men she knew well, though she had seen more of Toby and Will Spargo in recent months. But nothing had prepared her for the impact and complexity of Jago Barata. She doubted anything could.

The crash of the doorknocker echoed through the house. Caseley returned to the hall and saw the plumber's lad on his way downstairs. 'It's all right, Ross. I'll answer it.'

He continued on down. 'I got to go uplong and tell Mr Tregaskis he can bring the bath and all down now. Mr Endean's ready for 'em.' He waited at the bottom of the staircase.

The outer door was opened back to the wall and through the coloured glass Caseley could see a woman silhouetted on the step. A neighbour perhaps? Bringing an offer of help or a cup of tea as a cover for curiosity? She opened the door and Ross slipped out, ducking his head politely before disappearing down the path.

The visitor was plainly startled. Caseley's gaze skimmed the high-piled hennaed curls crowned with a chic feathered hat tilted forward over one eye, a vivid orange jacket decorated with gold frogging and cut a little too tight, and an orange and black taffeta skirt with a cascade of flounces reaching to the dusty granite step.

'Good afternoon, Mrs Downing. Can I help you?'

Louise quickly retrieved her control. But the smile that stretched her painted mouth did not reach eyes as hard as sapphires and bright with suspicion. 'You're Caseley Bonython.'

Caseley gave a brief nod. In a close-knit town like Falmouth everyone knew everyone else by sight if not by name.

'Father better, is he?'

'Yes, thank you.'

'You're some long way from home. What you doing up here? Friend of the captain, are you?' Her tone was light, artless, but her gaze was as sharp as a blade.

'No,' Caseley replied after a moment's hesitation. Friendship meant the gentle warmth of long acquaintance, empathy and loving attachment. Not friction, wariness and flaring tension. 'Not exactly. I am doing a job for him.'

'What job is that?'

Caseley was taken aback by both the impertinence of the question and the inquisitorial tone in which it was asked.

'Forgive me, I don't wish to appear rude, but my reasons for being here are not your concern.'

Louise's eyebrows arched. 'Me and the captain is friends. Very *close* friends. So whatever is going on in his house certainly does concern me. Told me all about it he did, this very morning.' She nodded sharply, daring Caseley to doubt her. 'Now if you'll just move aside, I'd like to come in and look over the place. I don't think Jago would be very pleased if I was to tell him you kept me standing out here.'

Without a word Caseley stepped back and Louise swept past her into the hall. As she closed the glass door, her fingers froze on the knob as she recalled Rosina and Liza-Jane gossiping. *Foreign,*

Liza-Jane had said. *It wasn't just once that Louise Downing had been seen leaving the Royal Hotel after ten in the evening.*

Caseley closed her eyes, hearing the echo of Jago's voice. 'For some reason hotel life has lost its appeal.' The pain was so sharp, so piercing, that for a moment she couldn't breathe.

'What's going on up there?' Louise jerked her head towards the stairs at the sound of a hammer falling to the floor, male voices, and footsteps moving about.

Caseley's throat was so dry she had to cough before she could speak. 'Captain Barata is having a bathroom installed.'

Louise poked her head round the drawing room door then walked all the way in.

Had Jago sent her to the house? But why would he do that? There was nothing to see yet. Perhaps it had been her idea to come. Clearly she had not expected to see Caseley, which was odd. Surely Jago would have explained what she was doing here? He must have realised that if Louise came to the house it was likely they would meet. Perhaps he did not care. Perhaps he considered it none of her business. It was his house and he could open his door to whomever he chose. Certainly Louise was making no effort to hide their relationship.

'What's this here job you're s'posed to be doing then?' Louise demanded over her shoulder as she wandered across to the window, inspecting the chipped paintwork and peeling wallpaper with distaste.

'Overseeing repairs to the house and selecting suitable furnishings.' Had she jumped to the

138

wrong conclusion? Could Liza-Jane have meant someone else? The desperate hope shrivelled and died. Had Louise not just announced their *'very close friendship'*?

Why this stupid pain? Only for a few brief minutes had he treated her with anything other than amusement or impatience.

'A room this size will take some filling up,' Louise frowned. 'Still, I can see a nice china cabinet over by that there wall.' She tapped one gloved finger against her chin, cupping her elbow in her other hand. 'And a sofa covered in dark red brocade with a valance and chairs to match. A big round table with one of they chenille cloths with a bobble fringe round the bottom would fill up the space a bit, and a fire screen, and some ornaments on the mantelpiece. I fancy one of they glass cases with dried flowers or stuffed birds in. I could have this place looking handsome. A bit of pretty paper on the walls, something with a nice bright flower pattern, would look just right in here.' She glanced at Caseley. 'What are you smiling at?'

'I wasn't smiling,' Caseley replied truthfully. Louise's vision was so close to the revenge she had planned she should find it amusing. But she didn't. Nor could she have done it, not to this house.

'I dunno what he asked you for,' Louise sniffed. 'Got an eye for colour, I have. Everyone say so.' Her hard gaze defied argument. 'Why *did* he ask you?' Her critical gaze flickered over Caseley's simple blouse and skirt and her expression was one of open scorn.

'I have no idea, Mrs Downing.' Only bitter

stubborn pride held Caseley's voice level and stopped her snatching up her cape and running from the house. 'Captain Barata arranged it with my father.'

Ralph had warned her not to put her heart into it. She had heard his words and truly believed her commitment was only to the task. It had taken the arrival of Jago Barata's mistress to rip the blinkers off. In her secret heart she had hoped that by creating a beautiful and tranquil home for him he might see her in a different light.

Hot with shame and embarrassment she allowed herself no respite. What a *fool* she was. Clinging to the few moments' conversation they had shared upstairs, she had hoped, so wanted to believe, that it had forged the first tenuous strand of friendship. How could she have been so naïve, presumptuous, *stupid?* She was useful, nothing more.

Had he been referring to Louise when he said that once a determined woman gained access to a man's house it was difficult to dislodge her? That would explain why he had insisted on her instead. After all, she posed no threat.

It was doubtful he had ever regarded her with anything other than irritation or pity. She cringed inside, recalling how gently he had wiped away her tears. He'd have done as much for a child.

She had revealed so much, betraying her grief and uncertainty. He had crushed her defences like eggshells, making her aware of her vulnerability, attracting and terrifying her at the same time.

Despite her denials she had dared to dream foolish dreams and, like Icarus, had been scorched by flying too close to the sun. But no one would ever know. She'd had years of practice at hiding her feelings. She straightened, holding herself tall and proud.

'Show me the rest, then,' Louise commanded.

'Certainly, Mrs Downing.'

When they returned to the hall after looking into every room on the ground floor, Louise suddenly remembered another engagement and left in an excited rustle of skirts and clicking heels.

Caseley closed the glass door. She would write to Jago and tell him she would not be doing any more work on the house. His 'close friend' Mrs Downing had, during her visit, shown such interest and offered so many suggestions, he might prefer to enlist *her* services in preference to someone who had not wanted the job in the first place.

He could hardly argue with that. Given his total lack of interest, Louise Downing's choice of red brocade sofa and flower-patterned wallpaper would suit him as well as the more restrained décor she had envisaged.

Returning to the drawing room and settling herself on the bare wooden seat in the bay window, she took pen, ink, and paper from her case. She would write the letter now and leave it at the hotel on her way home.

She wrote quickly and when she had finished laid the paper aside to dry while she re-corked the ink bottle and put away her pen. After reading it through once more, satisfied that it was businesslike and revealed no emotion whatever, she folded it carefully and slid it into her case. She would buy an envelope at the stationer's next to the old Town Hall.

Louise Downing appeared not to care who knew of her relationship with Jago Barata. But he had never given any hint that he had a mistress. Perhaps he considered it none of her business. Indeed it wasn't. But she would not leave an unsealed letter in a public place for any prying eyes to read.

Did Mr Downing know? Surely he could not, for what man would accept such behaviour from his wife? Yet according to Liza-Jane, Jago was not the first lover Louise had taken. So how *could* George Downing have remained in ignorance?

Caseley felt confused and revolted. Did the sacrament of marriage mean nothing to any of them? She remembered Jago's cruel smile as he taunted her about the bed upstairs. Louise Downing's manner had been one of defiant pride and possessiveness.

That he might be the 'fancy-man' Liza-Jane had spoken of had never occurred to her. It lessened him in her eyes even as it crystallised the yearning she had felt for him. She understood Spanish, tide tables, and balance sheets, but not men, especially a man like Jago Barata.

It no longer mattered. When she left the house in a few minutes she would have severed her connection with him. Now her father was back in the office and had Sam to accompany him to and from the yard, she could take time off and stay away from places where her path and Jago's might cross.

She needed time to regain her balance, put all the upheaval behind her. She had been intimidated, bullied, and blackmailed. Yet the touch of his hand on her flushed and tear-wet cheek, his rare gentleness and insight, the sheer power of his personality, had awakened deep and powerful emotions.

She felt a frisson of fear remembering his voice, flat and cold, delivering his ultimatum. Why had he sent Louise Downing to the house? Why put her in charge of the refurbishment and not his 'close friend', who clearly believed *she* should have been asked?

Whatever his reasons, his threat to tell her father of her deception had made refusal impossible. But two could play that game. She would make public his relationship with Mrs Downing–

No, she wouldn't. In any case, the threat had no power because according to Liza-Jane it was common knowledge already.

She put on her cape, tossed the material samples onto the window seat, and picked up her case. She could not leave without saying goodbye to Mr Endean. He was visibly disappointed when she cut short his description of blue and white porcelain tiles she might like for the bathroom walls. Excusing herself, she ran downstairs, eyes stinging, biting hard on her lower lip to stop it quivering.

The first drops of rain were already falling as she hurried along the high pavement. But no matter how much distance she put between herself and the house she had only to close her eyes to recall every detail of every room.

Her hat had no brim and the slanting rain, blown by the wind, raised little puffs like smoke as it hammered onto the dusty road, darkening it and turning it to mud. It soaked into her cape and skirt and ran cold down her face, mingling with her tears. In front gardens flowers bowed their heads, and trees dripped as their leaves were washed clean.

The heavy clouds parted and the rain eased as Caseley reached the stationer's. Pausing on the step she dried her face with a wisp of lace handkerchief. She bought an envelope, slid the letter inside, and sealed and addressed it, hotly aware of the tremor in her hands and the assistant's curiosity.

By the time she reached the Royal Hotel a watery sun was shining. People had left doorways in which they had taken shelter and the street was becoming busy again.

She walked up the steps and into the noisy crowded foyer. The smell of wet clothes and tobacco smoke caught in her throat. She eased her way through to the desk. Waving to attract the attention of one of the uniformed messenger boys she handed him the envelope.

'Please see that Captain Barata receives this as soon as possible.' She dropped a coin into his other hand.

The boy touched his cap with a forefinger. 'Yes, miss.' He tucked the envelope into a long rack on the wall beside the board on which numbered hooks held keys.

Turning away, Caseley fought her way to the door. It was done. She had regained control of her life and salvaged a little dignity. There would be a price to pay. But she refused to think about that now.

Rosina met her in the hall. 'Soaked, you are,'

she scolded, taking the sodden cape and holding it at arm's length. 'Get up they stairs and change while I make you a nice cup of tea. How didn't you get a cab instead of walking all that way and getting drenched?'

'I had some errands.' Caseley removed her hat and pushed wet curls back from her forehead.

'So how's it coming on then?' Rosina's expectant smile faded. 'What is it, my bird? What's wrong?'

Caseley shook her head, fighting for control. 'I–' she cleared the thickness from her throat. 'I shan't be doing any more up there, Rosina.'

The housekeeper's jaw dropped. 'What d'you mean? Why not? I know it haven't been easy, but 'twas far better than working in that there office all day and bringing more home to work on half the night. I can't believe the captain don't want you up there no more. Not after all he done to get you there in the first place.'

Caseley started towards the stairs. 'Who knows how Captain Barata's mind works, Rosina.'

'What happened?' Rosina's face puckered in concern.

'I knew he didn't like me much,' Caseley's throat ached. 'But to send Louise Downing–' She swallowed hard then shrugged. 'It's not important.' She tried to smile. 'Father will have to be told and that won't be easy.'

'*Louise Downing* was up the captain's house? What's the woman thinking of? You *sure* he knew she was there?'

Caseley shrugged again. 'Apparently he told her about the house this morning. It's none of our business, Rosina.'

She started up the stairs. If only she could go away. But that was impossible. She could not leave her father, especially now. Nor would it make any difference. She could not out-run her thoughts.

'I'll get you that tea, my treasure,' Rosina called after her. 'Oh, afore I forget, your father's in the parlour. He said he want to see you soon as you come in.' She dropped her voice to a whisper. 'He can wait till you've changed and got something hot inside of you. White as a sheet you are. Go on now, bird.' Muttering indignantly, she hurried away to the kitchen and Caseley continued up the stairs.

Having changed her clothes for a full-sleeved bodice of pale green sprigged cotton over a plain skirt of pine worsted, her hair held back in two combs and falling loose in heavy waves down her back, she approached the parlour.

The hot tea had soothed her tender stomach and restored some colour to her cheeks. She reached for the doorknob. *She* would tell her father about the figures she had pretended were his. But not yet, not until she was certain there was no alternative. First she had to tell him she would no longer be a party to his agreement with Jago Barata.

She knocked lightly and went in. Her father was in his usual chair beside the hearth. The fire was lit and despite the heavy, dark overcrowded furniture, the glowing coals made the room feel cosy.

'You took your time,' he grumbled, resting his head in the angle between the high padded back and winged side.

146

'I got caught in the rain,' she apologised and started forward. 'Father, there's something I–'

'It will have to wait.' With the impatient gesture of one bony hand he scooped up an opened package from the scalloped-edged round table beside his chair. 'This arrived in the afternoon post.' He pulled out a folded sheet of paper and an envelope sealed with red wax imprinted with a signet.

'It was addressed to me as consul for Mexico, it's from a group of Spaniards with interests in both countries. They want the documents in the sealed envelope taken by hand to Spain and placed into the hands of Canovas del Castillo, leader of the royalists.'

Caseley was horrified. 'Father, you can't. You've been ill. You're not strong enough for such a journey. Anyway, why were the documents sent to you? Why not to the Embassy in London, or direct to Spain?'

'If you'll hold your tongue a moment, I'll tell you.'

She flushed. 'I beg your pardon.'

Teuder Bonython sucked in a breath. 'When these men heard that certain members of the royalist party were trying to safeguard their own futures by dealing in secret with the rebels, they sent similar packages, one direct to Spain, the other to the Embassy in London. Both these packages contained false information. Their suspicions proved well-founded when that information was offered for sale to the rebels. Knowing their usual routes of communication are compromised they have approached me. It is a great honour, Caseley, proof of their faith in my integrity.'

'I understand that, Father. Truly I do.' Crouching by his chair she placed her hand over his. 'But you must see it's impossible for you to go? Can you not confide in Mr Fox? He is Vice-Consul for Spain–'

'And as such is bound by oath to serve whichever government is in power. Spain is currently a republic. So how can he honour his pledge *and* handle documents that might assist the restoration of Queen Isabel's son, Alfonso, to the throne?'

'How do you know what's in the documents?'

'When Jago was describing the situation in Spain he spoke of del Castillo, though he was not complimentary.'

The mention of Jago's name sent an uncomfortable tingle along Caseley's nerves. 'Does he know about this?' She indicated the package.

'No one knows. And no one must find out. Secrecy is vital. I've told you only because I have no choice.'

'Father–'

'Will you stop fussing and listen!' His face suffused with angry colour. 'I *know* I can't go, Goddammit. I'm too weak.' His head fell back. 'Besides, if I'm to die soon I want to be here, not in a strange country torn apart by bloody civil war.'

'Oh, Father.' Her eyes filled at this acknowledgement that his time was running out.

'None of that,' he muttered. His hand rested briefly on her bent head. 'I cannot go to Spain, Caseley. So you must.'

Chapter Eleven

Her head jerked up. 'Me?'

'Yes, you.' Her father was impatient. 'There's no one else I can trust.'

'When–?' Her voice emerged as a dry croak.

'I'm trying to tell you.' Wincing, he pressed the heel of his hand against his chest.

She jumped up. 'Where are your drops?'

His eyes were closed, his forehead trenched with lines of pain. 'I want brandy.'

Catching sight of the small tray standing on a table in the corner she rushed across, and with shaking hands poured water into the glass then picked up the medicine bottle.

'No, I can't be doing with fog in my head. There are things you need to know. Pour me a brandy. Please, Caseley?'

He never *asked*. Demands, orders, instructions, she was used to those. She had never heard him plead.

He tried to smile, but it was no more than a twitch of purple-tinged lips. 'Humour an old man. I'd as soon spend what time is left to me in my right mind.'

Replacing the medicine bottle on the tray she took a small bunch of keys from her skirt pocket, went to the chiffonier, and unlocked the doors of silvered glass. The neck of the bottle clattered against the glass as she poured. Her father was facing death and sending her away.

She handed him the spirit and watched as he swallowed half of it in one gulp, his lips peeling back from his teeth as he shuddered. Replacing the bottle she re-locked the doors.

It was three years since, in an effort to curb Ralph's drinking, her father decreed that all money and alcohol in the house be kept under lock and key. It had not worked. Ralph still got drunk. Only he did it in town, on credit, pawning his belongings, mortgaging his allowance, or at the expense of his friends.

Her father sighed deeply. The harsh grooves in his face softened as he relaxed. 'You sail tomorrow morning. Officially you are going on my behalf to sign a new trading agreement with Señor Miguel Spinoza, for whom we will carry iron ore. I had Thomas work out the figures with our attorney this afternoon. The contract is perfectly legal. A telegraph message has been sent to say you're on your way.'

Caseley wrapped her arms across her body. Despite the glowing fire and the warmth in the room, she was chilled to her bones.

'But *where* am I going? And how am I to get there?' She had arrived home fighting a tangle of emotions and working up the courage to tell her father about actions she had taken on his behalf, only to have all of it brushed aside as irrelevant.

Now, with no warning or time to prepare, she was being sent to Spain on a matter of vital importance and secrecy.

'I spoke to Toby this afternoon. *Cygnet's* repairs are finished. Jago is sailing her to Santander to

150

collect a cargo. You will sail with him.'

The room went dark. With a noise like rushing water in her head, feeling as though she might shatter into a million fragments, Caseley reached blindly for the back of a chair. She collapsed onto it as her knees gave way. Her father was still talking.

'...Should take three or four days, depending on the weather. I've always said there are worse storms in the Bay of Biscay at the end of summer than in January. Still, you'll be safe enough with Jago.'

She closed her eyes. *Safe?* Only an hour ago she had planned never to see him again, to lick her wounds in private. That they were self-inflicted, the result of her own gullibility and foolishness, did not make them hurt less.

Now she had to spend at least a week on a boat with him. A week that would allow neither respite nor escape. Having received her letter he would know she was aware of his relationship with Louise Downing.

She had deliberately kept it brief. But he was astute. What if he had seen through the polite formality to the anguish beneath? She had been so naïve. How would she survive a week of barbed shafts delivered with careless skill and lethal accuracy? She couldn't. It was impossible.

'You might show some interest!' Her father's bellow made her jump and her head flew up. 'I don't expect you to understand how much it would have meant to me to go. All these years I've been consul, authenticating signatures, signing crews on and off, arranging sightseeing tours for visiting dignitaries, and acting as agent for trade contracts. All these years of routine, then this comes along.' There was hopelessness in his headshake.

'I've always been a practical man, happiest at sea or in the yard. Now I'm too old and sick to go to Spain myself.' He thumped one fist on the arm of his chair. 'And I can't trust my son to go in my place.'

For the first time Caseley began to comprehend the enormity of his disappointment. Immersed in her own problems, she had not realised how deeply her father had been hurt by Ralph's rejection of the inheritance that was more than merely a business.

The consulship was a position of trust and prestige, a public honouring of moral and financial integrity. Though not hereditary, in the case of a family business the post often passed from father to son. But there was no chance of Ralph retaining it.

Hard-pressed to cope with all her father demanded of her, plus the intolerable strain of keeping secrets from him, she had not looked beneath the surface, hearing only his complaints, orders, irascibility.

He made a weary gesture and closed his eyes. 'It's not you I'm railing at, girl. But what was the point of it all?'

Pushing herself out of the chair, Caseley knelt in front of him. He had little time left. He had seen two wives and his elder son die. Then all he had worked for, all he had built and nurtured had been tossed aside by his remaining son. She was under no illusion. She could never take the place of the sons he had regarded as his stake in the future. But she had a choice: to give the knife a final twist, or do this one last thing for him.

He would never know what it cost her. But in going to Spain she would not be haunted by the anguish of 'if only' and 'too late'. She licked paper-dry lips.

'I won't let you down, Father. The documents will be delivered as safely and secretly as if you had taken them yourself.'

Opening his eyes, he gazed at her. 'If only you had been a boy.'

Patting his knee, she rose to her feet. She was less than a son to her father and less than a woman to Jago Barata.

'What was it you wanted to tell me when you came in?'

She turned away to put his brandy glass on the table. 'Nothing important.' She offered her arm. 'Shall we go and have dinner?' Her stomach was a small hard knot and the thought of food made her feel queasy. 'I expect there are other things I should know. Who will meet me? How will I know him?'

Later, she bathed and washed her hair in the slipper bath in front of her bedroom fire, refusing to think about the lack of facilities aboard the schooner. Rosina laid skirts, blouses, and underwear on the bed.

Shrouded in a white cotton nightgown, Caseley perched on a padded footstool beside the fire, her head tilted as she brushed her hair.

Rolling each item of clothing to minimise

creasing, Rosina paused, a smile dimpling her plump cheeks. 'I'd give good money to see Louise Downing's face when she hear about this.'

Caseley glanced up. 'About what?' She swung her hair to the other side and resumed brushing.

'You and the captain sailing to Spain together. She'll be mad as fire. Still, 'tis time he come to his senses.'

'We're not sailing *together*, Rosina.' Caseley's cheeks were burning. She was too close to the flames. 'We both have business there. There's no more to it than that. He doesn't even like me.'

Rosina snorted. 'Don't you believe it, bird. I'll fetch clean towels for you to take.'

When the last item had been neatly tucked into the leather portmanteau, Rosina had gently rubbed Caseley's upper arm. 'Be all right, will you?'

She nodded. She would keep out of his way. When he was in the cabin she would go on deck. When he was on deck she would stay below.

'I'll be fine.' She crossed to the shelf to choose a book.

She hadn't expected to see him again, and wished it wasn't necessary. She had defied him. He would be angry.

Dawn had just broken when she left the house next morning. Her sleep had been restless and her eyes felt hot and gritty. But the cool air was fresh after the rain. It rippled over her face like silk, sharpening her senses.

The smell of frying bacon wafted from a nearby house on the stirring breeze.

She looked both ways before crossing the muddy road. But apart from a brewer's dray laden with casks turning into the yard of the Dock Inn, there was no traffic and few people. She closed the tall gate behind her and walked through the quiet yard towards the quay and slip, her bag bumping against her leg. Passing the sawpits and the golden dunes of sawdust, the silent sheds and the timber pool, she saw *Cygnet's* tall masts.

The jibs and topsails were loosed, the foresail set and the huge fore-and-aft mainsail partly hoisted. Gulls screamed mournfully as they wheeled overhead. The breeze sang in the rigging and made the shrouds slap against the masts.

Her hull protected from the rough stone quay by cork and rope fenders, the schooner floated on the rising tide, held only by a single rope at bow and stern. Smoke rose from the curved chimney of the cooking shack bolted to the deck behind the foremast.

Her footsteps faltered and she stopped. Where was everyone? 'Hello?' She cleared her throat and tried again. This time her voice was at least audible.

A head popped out of the cooking shack. She beckoned and the skinny boy glanced round to make sure it was him she was waving at before he crossed the deck to her, wiping his hands on a grubby cloth.

'Yes, miss?'

Caseley smiled at him. 'What's your name?'

'Laity, miss. Martin Laity.'

'I'm Miss Bonython. Will you help me aboard?'

Startled, the boy's glance jumped from her bag

155

to the companionway hatch and back to her. 'Aboard *'ere*, miss?'

'Yes.' Caseley tamped down impatience. 'If you will take my bag, I'll get over the side by myself.'

The boy glanced round again then backed away. 'I'd better git the cap'n.'

'Please take my bag first.' She hefted it onto the gunwale. Taking it reluctantly, the boy set it on the deck.

Caseley gauged the distance between the vessel and the quay. Though it wasn't far, Jago could at least have put out a ladder or a gangplank. Was he deliberately trying to make it difficult for her? He must know this was the very last place she wanted to be.

The gunwale was several inches above the quay. Gathering her skirts in one hand, Caseley placed one foot on it and held out her hand to the boy. She would not think about the gap between quay and ship, and the cold grey water slopping between the two. Flushing crimson, he grasped her fingers, steadying her as she jumped down. She winced as she jarred her damaged foot.

'What's going on?'

She stiffened at the familiar deep voice, and kept her gaze lowered as she shook out her skirt and picked up her bag, giving the boy a brief smile.

'Thank you, Martin.' She could feel her face burning as she met Jago's eyes. 'I had a little difficulty getting aboard.'

'Get back to the galley, Martin,' Jago dismissed him without a glance.

Caseley braced herself, waiting for him to mention her letter.

156

'Aye, sir.' The boy scuttled away.

His expression unreadable, Jago folded his arms, his skin brown against the rolled-up sleeves of a white shirt. A red kerchief loosely knotted around his throat emphasised the blackness of his beard.

'Now that you are on board, perhaps you will tell me why. We are due to sail shortly.'

Had he simply accepted her decision? While she longed to believe that, she couldn't because it would be totally unlike him. Not saying anything now could only mean he was saving it for later.

'Did my father not tell you?'

'I haven't seen your father.'

Though her promise made it necessary, lying to him was far harder than she expected. She moistened dry lips. 'There is a trade agreement that must be signed–'

'Then I suggest you give it to me and return home.'

Caseley stared at him. Why was he pretending not to know what she was talking about?

'I can't give it to you. If you didn't speak to my father then Toby must have told you.'

Jago frowned. 'Told me what?'

Caseley swallowed, her parched throat making an audible click. 'That you have a passenger for this trip.'

Jago nodded. 'Yes, I was told. He's already aboard. He arrived last night.'

'Who did?'

'Antonio Valdes.'

Caseley was totally confused. 'Who is Antonio Valdes?'

157

Jago's expression darkened. 'The passenger I am taking to Spain. Why are *you* here? Sam could have brought this trade agreement down. Is it money? Do you need more? The bank has my instructions. You have only to speak to Mr Buller. As for the house, this is neither the time nor the place for such discussions.'

Money? The house? He was talking as though *he had not received her letter.* The deck heaved beneath her feet. His last words brought back vivid memories of Louise Downing's visit and her own awakening to the true situation. But he was right in one respect. This was not the time to talk about his house or anyone connected with it.

She raised her chin. 'As far as I am concerned, Captain, there is nothing to discuss. Obviously there has been a misunderstanding. My father told me he left a message with Toby that you were to expect a passenger.'

'Yes. Antonio Valdes.'

'No.' Caseley was firm. 'Whoever this person is, and whatever his reasons for wanting a passage to Spain, he is *not* the passenger my father meant.'

'No? Then who–?' He broke off, his gaze darting to the heavy bag clutched in her white-knuckled hands. *'You?'* She gave a single nod. 'Why?'

'I started to tell you.'

'Ah yes. Trade contracts.' Hands on his hips he studied her but before he could speak, a man appeared behind him. He had fair hair, a narrow face, and wide-set eyes that sharpened as they saw her.

Distracted by his sudden emergence, uncomfortable beneath his intent scrutiny, she turned back to Jago, lowering her voice. 'Perhaps you had better explain the misunderstanding to Señor Valdes. No doubt he will be able to find another berth within a few days.'

As the newcomer approached, Jago swung round. 'If you will kindly go below, Señor Valdes, Martin will bring your breakfast. I will join you shortly.' Politely phrased it was nonetheless an order.

The man stopped. Slightly built, he wore a superbly cut dark coat and ochre waistcoat over grey check trousers. His linen was spotless and a garnet pin glowed in the folds of his cravat. Caseley guessed him to be a few years older than her but younger than Jago. Surprise and displeasure crossed his face.

'Forgive me, Captain. It was not my intention to intrude.' His voice was heavily accented and betrayed a pique at odds with his apology. Bowing, he returned to the companionway.

Caseley looked at Jago. 'Why didn't you tell him?'

He leaned towards her. '*I* am master of this ship,' he said softly. 'I am not obliged to explain my decisions.'

'Your point is taken, Captain.' Her heartbeat thudded so loud and fast she feared he might hear it. 'If you have decided Señor Valdes can remain aboard then so be it. But my father and I have a prior claim in ownership. I am here, not through choice, but on his instructions in a matter of some urgency. So if you will show me to my cabin, you need delay your departure no longer.'

He masked it quickly but she saw shock. 'You cannot sail with me.'

Why was he doing this? Her father had told her it was all settled. 'On the contrary, Captain, I can and I must. The error was yours, not mine. I am undertaking this voyage in my father's name because he is not well enough.' Her voice nearly faltered but she caught it in time. Anger bubbled up lending her strength. 'Were he standing here you would not attempt to force him ashore.'

'Were he here, the situation would not arise,' he retorted.

In the tense silence he rubbed one palm across his beard. 'Will you not consider another vessel?'

Feeling his rejection like a slap she took a breath then shook her head. 'That is not possible. I need to–' Recognising the audacity of his suggestion she stopped. 'Why should I? This confusion is not *my* fault.'

'So you are determined to stay?' His tone implied a warning but against what she had no idea.

'Believe me, Captain Barata, it gives me no more pleasure to be here than it gives you to see me.'

He studied her for several seconds, frowning slightly. 'Are you aware of the conditions?'

She nodded. 'My father warned me we might encounter rough weather.'

'I was not referring to the weather.'

'I do not expect all the comforts of home, Captain.'

His gaze was thoughtful. 'Once we leave, I will not turn back.'

She glanced towards the town. Once the ship sailed she would be on her own with no one to whom she could turn for advice if anything went wrong. *She had survived the past two months. She could survive this.* She thought of her father.

'I told you.' Her voice sounded thin and strained. 'I have no choice.'

'For trade agreements.' He was openly sceptical.

'They are very important.'

'They must be.'

Uncertain, she glanced at him. Their eyes locked. She wanted to look away but his steady gaze held her fast. She was acutely conscious of his physical presence, his stillness. The grey eyes were no longer cool but questioning.

The yearning she had fought so hard to deny surged over her like a breaking wave and she fought to retain her balance, barely aware of holding her breath.

Seeing his expression change, sensing his retreat behind a barrier as solid as a wall, she remembered Louise. Louise who had age-old eyes, a full-lipped mouth, and a voluptuous figure, who spoke possessively of Jago, regularly visited him at his hotel, and now laid claim to his house.

Her lashes lowered. She was grateful for the pain. Where was her pride? Could she so easily forget how cynically he had used her? She raised her head, drew herself up.

'My cabin, Captain?'

He regarded her for a moment longer, then leaned forward to take the bag from her nerveless fingers, anger flashing across his face as she flinched. Silently he gestured for her to precede him. She stopped as they reached the double doors of the companionway, now latched back.

He pushed the sliding top further open to reveal a spiral staircase with perforated brass treads and a wooden handrail that curved out of sight.

Misinterpreting her hesitation he went ahead of her and waited halfway. 'It's not as steep as it looks. You'll soon get used to it.'

She glanced over her shoulder in one last agonising instant of doubt, glimpsing the little tower atop her father's house. The breeze was like cold breath on her neck and suddenly she was afraid.

She thought of Ben helping her father wash and dress for the day while Rosina prepared breakfast and Liza-Jane worked through her morning chores. Maybe Ralph was awake and thinking about the portrait.

There was no going back. Placing one foot on the top stair, she gripped the teak rail and followed Jago down.

He pointed to a door at the bottom of the companionway. 'This is the mate's cabin. Do you know Nathan Ferris?'

Caseley shook her head. 'We've not met. I believe he lives over at Feock with his wife and children.'

Jago merely nodded and opened a door facing forward. 'This is my day room.' He stood back to let her pass.

A salt-stained and grubby canvas bag stood against an upholstered bench seat. The cabin narrowed towards the stern. Though not large, it was light and airy thanks to a large skylight that had a brass oil-lamp suspended below it.

Panelled in wood, the cabin had two shelves

edged with thin rails at the aft end. The lower one held rolled charts. The upper was crammed with books, a tin of oil, and several small tools. A barometer and a clock were set into the panelling above them.

A table between the two upholstered bench seats was hinged to fold down and provide more floor space. A small stove stood on a stone slab in front of the forward bulkhead with a coalscuttle and basket of kindling beside it.

Jago dropped her bag on the table. Pulling back the dark curtain on the far side of the stove he stepped aside.

Caseley saw the space had just enough room for a bunk and a small cupboard with a hinged lid on top, which she guessed would contain a small removable washbasin, and a single door below. A reefer jacket lay on the grey blankets and she glimpsed a canvas bag beneath the bunk.

Without a word he crossed the cabin, pushed open a sliding door on the locker above the seat, and beckoned her forward.

Aware of his mocking gaze, Caseley looked in. The sea-berth was six feet long, just over two feet wide, and contained a thin mattress, several folded grey blankets, and a pillow covered in blue and white striped ticking.

She remembered enough about the layout of a schooner to realise this was not a deliberate attempt to embarrass or frighten her off. The crew slept in the fo'c'sle; the master and mate had cabins aft. There was no extra accommodation. These vessels were built for carrying cargo, not passengers.

163

She turned to Jago. One dark brow rose but he did not speak. Nor did he smile. Was he expecting accusation? Complaint? A hasty retreat?

Caseley cleared her throat. 'If you are offering me a choice, I'll take the sleeping cabin, thank you.'

He gave a brief nod. She thought she saw fleeting approval but dismissed it as wishful thinking.

There was a tap on the door and a man poked his head into the cabin. 'Ready to warp out, skipper.' Catching sight of Caseley, his eyes rounded, darting from her to Jago.

'Thanks, Nathan.' Jago opened the door wider. 'Miss Bonython, allow me to introduce *Cygnet's* mate, Nathan Ferris.'

'How do you do, Mr Ferris.'

The mate was visibly surprised as Caseley extended her hand. She saw Jago's mouth twist and recalled their first meeting and her refusal to acknowledge their introduction.

Nathan quickly wiped his hand down the side of his trousers before taking her hand and giving it a single careful shake. 'How do, miss. I seen your father down here yesterday. Not looking too bad, is he?'

'No, he is much better,' she agreed, feeling Jago's eyes on her. What else could she say? People saw what they wanted to see. Even when they guessed the truth they would cling to the old adage about life and hope.

'Take you topside, shall I, miss? We're casting off d'rectly and–'

'That won't be necessary,' Jago broke in. 'Miss Bonython is sailing with us.'

The mate blinked. 'Ah. Right. Well. If you'll 'scuse me, miss, I'd best get on.' He touched his forehead in salute. 'Soon as we're under way I'll move my stuff down the fo'c'sle, skipper. 'Ammer can rig me 'ammock.'

Jago clapped the mate's shoulder. 'I'm much obliged, Nathan.'

The mate nodded and left.

Caseley looked at Jago in relief. But before she could speak, he shook his head.

'No. Señor Valdes has Nathan's cabin. You will remain here.' She opened her mouth to protest, but he didn't give her the chance. 'While you are aboard I am responsible for your safety.' His tone implacable, he reached for the door handle.

Caseley burned with fury and indignation. Everyone aboard would face the same dangers should the weather turn wild. So he was simply making her pay for insisting on sailing aboard *Cygnet*.

She should have known better than to expect consideration. He had made it clear from the moment they met that as far as he was concerned she deserved none. But with him in it the cabin felt very small.

Unexpectedly he turned. As her chin lifted his mouth curved in a caustic smile. 'For what it's worth,' he spoke quietly, 'our enforced proximity will be no easier for me.' He left, closing the door behind him.

Caseley pressed her palms to her hot cheeks. Never had she felt so wretchedly out of place.

Through the open skylight she could hear orders being shouted, the squeak of ropes through blocks, and the rattle of steering gear. She leaned against the doorjamb, her fingers pressed to her trembling lips as she tried to swallow the lump that threatened to choke her.

Her father was depending on her. At worst the voyages out and back would take ten days. Given good weather it might only be a week. Then she would be free of Jago Barata.

The cabin was stifling. She needed air. Quickly wiping the wetness from her cheeks, she walked out, closing the door behind her. She refused to think about the coming night and the ones to follow. Gripping the handrail she climbed the companionway and stepped out onto the deck.

Already clear of the quay, *Cygnet* was swinging round, her bow pointing towards Trefusis. She saw Jago at the wheel. He ignored her, gazing forward to where Nathan and two other men were hauling on ropes, setting the two huge fore and aft sails and sheeting home the square topsail. Even the boy Martin was involved, darting to help wherever he was needed.

The bow came into the wind then with a crack like a pistol shot, the sails filled, and the schooner surged forward.

Caseley moved to the starboard side and stood close to the mainmast rigging. *Cygnet's* raking stem cut through the choppy water like a knife as they passed the north arm of the docks and headed out towards Black Rock and the English Channel.

The sky was a pastel wash of lemon, pale green, and turquoise. Slivers of high thin cloud were edged with rose. With the breeze cool on her face and the deck moving beneath her feet like a living creature, she watched spellbound as the rising sun peeped over the headland behind the St Anthony lighthouse, unrolling a carpet of liquid gold before them.

When she looked back for one last glimpse of the town, it was already out of sight.

Chapter Twelve

Dazzled by the sunrise, Caseley watched Nathan and the two crewmen trim the sails. Hauling in and loosening ropes, winding them in figures-of-eight around two-pronged wooden pegs with speed and dexterity, they ensured that each sail drew its dull share of wind.

'Jimbo!' Nathan bawled at a stocky figure in the bows. 'Coil they jib sheets down clear for running. Likely the skipper'll gybe when she's clear o' the Point for a broad reach down past the Lizard.'

Jimbo raised a hand in acknowledgement. Where the bight of rope fell from a peg he laid it in a wide circle on the deck. He added several more turns finishing with the loose end. Quickly flipping the whole coil over, he neatly overlapped both sides of the centre into a figure-of-eight with an extra loop in the middle.

If the sail had to be loosed in a hurry, once the rope was free of the peg it would rise from the coil with no risk of knots or tangles.

As the men worked swiftly round the deck

tidying all the loose ropes, she wondered why they were lifting them off the deck and hanging them over stanchions or on the gunwale. Then Martin hauled a bucket of seawater in over the side. As he sloshed it over the deck and began scrubbing with a short-bristled broom, she realised she had not heard Jago issue one word of command.

'The captain runs, how you say, a tight ship, no?'

The soft voice so close to her ear made her jump. She turned quickly.

'Antonio Valdes,' he introduced himself and bowed his head without breaking eye contact. 'It is an unexpected pleasure to have the company of such a beautiful young lady.' His brown eyes were soft and languid, his smile admiring. 'Tell me I am not dreaming. I see this apparition before me, with hair as rich as cinnabar. Does she have a name?'

Suppressing a smile, Caseley offered her hand. 'I am no ghost, Señor Valdes. My name is Bonython. Do tell me, what is cinnabar?'

Instead of shaking her hand he raised it to his mouth. Ignoring the convention that a gentleman stopped short of actual contact, he touched his lips to her knuckles.

When Jago had done the same, his touch had stirred new and powerful emotions in her. This felt impertinent.

Firmly withdrawing her hand, she saw surprise and speculation in his gaze. She realised he would take advantage of the slightest encouragement. Yet his lavish compliments were balm to her bruised heart.

He leaned on the gunwale beside her. 'Cinnabar is the red ore from which quicksilver comes.' He paused, smiling as he studied her. 'Is there beneath those lovely tresses a silvery spirit that slips through the fingers, unwilling to be captured?'

His tone was light, bantering. Though she lacked experience in the art of flirting, Caseley recognised the skill in others. Perhaps Antonio Valdes was merely seeking to relieve a tedious voyage in a socially acceptable manner with no offence intended. But unease riffled over her skin like a cat's paw of wind on still water.

'My hair has been compared to many things, sir.' She recalled childhood taunts of *carroty, conker,* and *radish-head.* 'Though of a more mundane nature.' Before he could comment, she deliberately shifted the conversation away from herself. 'Are you involved in mining?'

'No, though there are quicksilver mines where I come from. Also coal, iron, and zinc. But I would not have you think that is all Asturias can offer.' He smiled into her eyes, his narrow face enthusiastic. 'Along the coast are small fishing settlements at the foot of sheer cliffs. Behind these, maize grows on rolling hills. We do not have frost, so dates ripen in the sun and oranges scent the air with their blossom. In the west are the mountains, wild and rugged and capped with snow.'

'You paint a vivid picture, Señor.'

'It is a vivid country, Señorita. Oviedo's cathedral has one of the finest church towers in Spain. It is the burial place of ancient Asturian kings. But most of the people live in small villages. Beside each house there is another, very tiny. This is … *horreo…*'

'A granary?' Caseley supplied.

His eyes narrowed briefly then he laughed. '*Sí,* a granary. You speak Spanish?'

'Very little.' Her response was pure instinct. There was no logical reason to deny her fluency in the language. But the warmth in his smile had not reached his eyes. Her wariness returned. 'Do go on.'

'The granaries are built on four legs to protect the maize of each household from rats and mice. The mountain ham of Asturias is famous through all Spain.' His smile faded. 'Forgive me. I think I am boring you.'

'Not at all,' Caseley said with perfect truth. 'I enjoy learning about other countries. Reading books is never as informative as listening to someone who lives there. What is so special about the ham?'

Once again something about his warm open smile disturbed her. She glimpsed hints of satisfaction and smugness that made her wonder if she had been manipulated into asking the questions. But what would be the point? Besides, she *was* interested. Why pretend otherwise?

'It has a unique flavour,' he said. 'The ham is laid in the snow high in the mountains so the sun may cure it. The cold snow stops the meat spoiling. It becomes a beautiful dark red in colour. Sliced very thin it is almost translucent. To eat it with ice-cool melon,' he bunched the tips of his fingers and kissed them, 'is a wonderful experience. Now, beautiful miss, you must tell me about yourself. Where is your home?'

'In Falmouth.' Caseley saw him look over her shoulder. As she started to turn, Jago spoke.

'A few moments of your time, Miss Bonython?' He did not even glance at Valdes. Cupping her elbow, he indicated that she should precede him aft.

Valdes straightened from the rail with languid grace and bowed to her.

'I enjoyed our conversation, Miss Bonython. Captain.' With a brief nod he made for the companionway and disappeared down the stairs.

'Well, Captain Barata?' Caseley matched his coolness. 'You have my attention. What do you want?'

'Martin needs to finish swabbing the deck. You and Señor Valdes were in the way.' He guided her towards the stern. 'You also risked getting your head knocked off.' Without waiting for a response he turned to Nathan. 'I'll take the helm. Make ready to gybe.'

'Aye, skipper.' Stating their course, the mate relinquished the wheel and hurried forward, shouting orders to Jimbo and Hammer.

Watching the smooth, sure movements of the crew as they hauled in the two booms to which the fore and aft mainsails were laced, Caseley forgot her anger.

Jago turned the wheel slowly, watching the sails to see when the wind left them. 'All right, boys,' he shouted, and spun the wheel. Nathan released ropes on the port side and the huge booms swung across. One passed right where she had been standing.

Jimbo and Hammer hauled in the starboard

171

sheets and, as the sails filled, made them fast. Heeling slightly, *Cygnet* leapt forward on her new course. The two crewmen went forward to trim the jibs and staysail and Jago checked the compass suspended just inside the day room skylight as Nathan returned.

'Keep her steady on this heading. If the wind holds we should make Ushant before sundown.'

'Only a hundred miles, skipper?' the mate grinned. 'Slowing up, are 'e?'

Caseley waited for the explosion. But to her amazement it never came.

'If you'd had my lay-over,' Jago snorted, 'you would not smile so readily.'

'Need a wife and family, you do,' Nathan advised.

Jago's laugh was brief and humourless. 'You married men want to see everyone else enslaved.'

She might as well have been invisible.

The mate's grin widened. 'Well, if 'tis a prison to have a warm bed and a woman to match waiting for me after every trip, I aren't in no hurry to break me chains.'

Jago shrugged. 'Who needs marriage for that?'

Caseley's heart was wrenched. He certainly didn't. Not when he had someone else's wife waiting for him.

'Git on.' Nathan shot him a dry look. 'If you think 'tis the same, you got a lot to learn.'

'Mind your tongue,' Jago growled, his expression severe. But as he cupped her elbow once more she saw the glint of laughter in his eyes and envied them their comradeship.

'Nathan and I have faced death together on

several occasions,' he said. 'Our lack of formality–'

'Does not indicate lack of respect. I'm aware of that.'

He nodded. 'You and your housekeeper share a similar rapport.'

He remembered.

'I will show you around the ship.'

'That is kind of you, but–'

'Kindness does not enter into it. If we are to complete this voyage quickly, the crew needs to concentrate on their tasks without concern for passengers. If you are in the wrong place at the wrong time you could endanger both them and yourself. Besides, despite your brave claim about not expecting the comforts of home, surely even you require certain amenities?'

Caseley felt a blush scald her face as he indicated an oblong wooden hut. Almost his height, it was set across the deck.

'This is the wheel shelter,' he announced, then opened a door in the side. 'This is the lamp store and paint locker.' Caseley peered in, wrinkling her nose at the strong smell of oil, varnish, and turpentine. 'There is a door on the other side into our lavatory. Though it's a basic bucket-and-chuck-it, there is a proper wooden seat. As we don't usually carry passengers there's no lock. To avoid embarrassment I suggest you tie a piece of cloth to the door handle when–' he made a small gesture leaving the sentence unfinished.

Torn between wishing she had never set foot on the boat, and gratitude that he had anticipated her needs, all she could do was try to match his

173

cool matter-of-fact manner.

He pointed to the teak rubbing boards fixed at hip and shoulder height to the front of the shelter behind Nathan.

'They give some support during the long watches. The wooden grid is to stop the helmsman losing his footing on a wet deck.'

'Does the rain make it slippery, then?' she asked, determined to be seen to be taking everything in her stride.

He threw her an oblique glance. 'Large seas breaking inboard are a greater concern.'

Caseley swallowed as her imagination instantly conjured terrifying visions.

He guided her forward. His hand under her elbow was warm. It offered strength and comfort; reminding her of the soul-baring moments they had shared in his house. Before she had opened the door to Louise Downing who had shattered every foolish dream.

Passing the companionway he knocked his knuckles against a large covered tank with a copper dipper attached to it by a line. 'Our fresh water. And this' he pointed to a cask harnessed to the tank, 'contains salt beef. Bread, fruit, and condensed milk are stored in a zinc-lined cupboard below the sea berth in my day room and apportioned daily. Vegetables are kept here in the galley shack.'

Looking in, Caseley saw Martin crouched in front of the black cooking range, shovelling coal through a hole in the flat top. Pots and pans surrounded a small stool. One pan contained a sharp knife and a huge ladle. A curved chimney

174

pipe rose from the back of the stove and belched thick smoke into the air.

As they reached the mainmast, Caseley gazed up in awe.

'One hundred feet from keel to masthead,' Jago said. 'The foremast is five feet shorter. Cargo hatches.' The large wooden covers were almost hidden beneath coils of rope, buckets, a wooden ladder and a small rowing boat mounted on a cradle.

In front of the foremast the two crewmen were sitting on the deck, binding frayed ends of rope with fine cord. Both nodded respectfully at Jago and glanced sideways at Caseley, eyes bright with curiosity.

'Hammer, Jimbo, this is Captain Bonython's daughter.'

The men scrambled to their feet, grinning at Caseley's surprise.

'You're twins,' she blurted.

'Yes, miss.' Jimbo touched his brow with a stubby callused forefinger. ''Ammer's eldest by ten minutes, but we don't fight over it. He got the beauty,' his finger strayed to a puckered scar running down his cheek. 'But I got the brains.'

'And a quick tongue,' she smiled. His grin widened.

Jago's grip tightened. 'This is the fo'c'sle, the crew's quarters.'

Caseley peered through the small, whale-backed hatch with a latched door and ring handle now hooked open to reveal a steep ladder.

'It looks very dark.'

'Since I had the skylight installed, the crew get

175

as much light and fresh air as I do.'

'You make it sound like a luxury.'

The twins had abandoned any pretence of working and were watching, open-mouthed.

'The point I was making, Miss Bonython, is that much of my work is done in my day room. All theirs is done on deck, and they eat in the mess.'

'That's right, miss,' Jimbo began, but was instantly silenced by Jago's glare.

Caseley could feel the anger radiating from him and wished she had not spoken so hastily.

The schooner's bow rose and fell, parting blue-green masses of water and tossing it aside in hissing waves of white foam that left streaks in her wake.

'We'll go below.' Jago was abrupt, hustling her aft along the canting deck and down the companionway. 'The mess is through there, next to Nathan's cabin. You'll see it later.'

She turned to face him in the small space. 'Why have you brought me down here now?'

'So that you can move your gear into the sleeping cabin while I mark the chart and write up the log.' Opening his day-room door he pushed her gently inside and closed it behind them.

'But – but you haven't moved your things out yet,' she stammered, nervous of disturbing his possessions, knowing she was an unwelcome intruder.

'We do not carry servants.' His tone was cold. 'You insisted on coming, so while on board you will pull your weight.'

'That's not what I meant.' The implied criticism stung. 'I was not trying to avoid doing anything,

176

and I certainly don't expect to be waited on. It's just – I'm not used to handling other people's belongings.'

'If *I* don't object, I see no reason why you should.' Bending over the table, he picked up a ruler and pencil and studied the chart.

Caseley glared at the broad, white-shirted back. She had never met anyone who stirred so many conflicting emotions. Compared to Jago Barata, Aunt Margaret was a novice.

'Leave my bag under the bunk,' he said without looking round. 'There's no room for it out here. Just change the pillows and blankets over. We do not run to sheets or lacy counterpanes. But as you said, you are not expecting home comforts.'

Caseley refused to be drawn. She could feel his antagonism. It seemed to come and go. But as she had no idea what provoked it or how best to react, silence seemed the safest course.

She remade both bunks, noticing with relief that though the blankets were coarse, they were clean. After pushing his bag to one end under the bunk so she could fit hers in, she straightened up. Brushing her hands down her skirt, she stood, uncertain, in the narrow doorway. Seated on one of the bench seats, Jago was apparently engrossed in the notes he was making in a leather-bound book resting on the chart.

Caseley cleared her throat. 'Unless there is anything else you wish me to do here, Captain, I thought I might help Martin in the galley. He–'

'No,' Jago looked up. 'You will not interfere with the running of this ship.'

'I have no intention of *interfering,* as you put it.

177

I simply wanted to help. Martin–'

'Is a member of my crew, and perfectly capable of carrying out his duties by himself.'

'I wasn't suggesting–'

'Can we drop the subject, Miss Bonython?'

'I cannot win. If I don't help, I'm lazy. If I try to, I'm interfering. There's no pleasing you, is there?'

'That remains to be seen.' He leaned back, turning the pencil in his fingers, his expression was enigmatic, his eyes unreadable. 'What is the present state of the house?'

The question stopped her breath. She should have known he would ask. Of course he would want some idea of what had yet to be done. A band of tension tightened round her skull. Moistening her lips she steadied herself against the sleeping cabin's door-frame.

'Mr Endean has almost finished. When I left yesterday he was about to install the bath and hand basin. The inside repairs will be complete by the end of the week. After that,' her throat closed forcing her to swallow. 'After that you may arrange for the painters to start.'

'I, Miss Bonython?' He slid from the bench and rose to his feet. 'That is *your* job.'

She looked at him. She had hoped, how desperately she had hoped, that he would behave honourably. Instead he was playing with her.

'Not any longer.'

He frowned. 'We have an agreement.'

'Had.' She folded her arms, recognised the move as defensive, and quickly unfolded them, clasping her hands instead. 'Under the circumstances you

178

cannot expect me to continue. Nor can you want it.'

'What circumstances?' His apparent puzzlement was too much.

'I told you once before, Captain. Now I'm telling you again. I will not be made sport of. You must find your amusement elsewhere.' In spite of her anger, she kept her voice low. The skylight was open and their voices would carry. Their business was private. She would not be responsible for it becoming gossip.

'You received my letter. You know full well Mrs Downing will make it impossible–'

He took a step towards her, his expression ominous. 'What letter? What has Mrs Downing to do with the house?'

'Everything!' Caseley flung at him. 'Why this pretence? Surely you are not concerned for my sensibilities? After all,' fury and bitter hurt spilled over despite her resolve to remain calm. 'I am only the hired help. Or I was,' she corrected immediately.

Jago seized her shoulders, his face thunderous. 'I don't know what you're talking about. I never received any letter.'

Caseley brought her arms up as a barrier between them. 'I took it to your hotel. One of the boys put it into the rack behind the reception desk. I saw him. You *must* have received it.'

'When did you take it there?'

'Yesterday afternoon.'

'Apart from an hour ashore to arrange an outward cargo, I have been on board *Cygnet* since yesterday morning. I did not return to the hotel

179

last night and no mail has been delivered to me here.'

'Oh.'

'Why should you imagine Mrs Downing has any connection with my house?'

'Imagine?' A harsh, painful laugh tore from Caseley's throat. 'I did not imagine her arrival on the doorstep. Nor did I imagine– She was very specific about–' She could not go on. Hot colour suffused her face and throat. She lowered her lashes to veil the anguish her pride refused to let him see.

'Louise Downing went to the house yesterday?'

'You should know. You sent her.' Caseley bit hard on the inside of her lower lip to stop it trembling.

'Is that what she told you?'

'Yes – no – but she intimated–'

'What happened? Why did you feel it necessary to write this letter I never received?' He radiated tension.

Caseley tried to pull away, but his fingers tightened, biting into her flesh. They would leave bruises.

'Tell me,' he demanded.

She could not meet his eyes. 'M – Mrs Downing announced herself as a "very close friend" of yours. She left me in no doubt that she did not approve of my presence in the house, or of me working for you. That being so, I thought it best to withdraw and allow her to take over.'

'Oh you did, did you? You've got the devil's own cheek.'

Her head jerked up. *'What?'*

'You appear to have overlooked the fact that it

is *my* house. *I* decide who will work on it. How dare you involve Louise without consulting me.'

'I didn't–' Caseley gasped.

'Had I wanted her to have anything to do with it, I would have asked her.' His eyes were fire over ice.

'But she said–'

'I don't give a damn what she said. You should not have let her in.'

'*I* should not–?' Caseley's voice rose to a squeak. 'I couldn't stop her. She was there at your invitation.'

'She wasn't.' He was grim.

'She said – she said you would be angry if I didn't let–' she stopped. It was pointless to continue. 'Anyway, she wants to do it.'

'And you don't?'

'I never did. You know that.'

'I know the *idea* did not appeal.' His tone softened slightly. 'But now you are seeing it change and come to life, are you still so set against it?'

She did not reply.

'Look at me, Caseley. Tell me.'

'I–' Her throat was parched. The lie would not come. 'That is not important.'

'It's the only thing that matters,' he said quietly.

'To you.' He did not understand at all. How could she have thought him intuitive, aware? He saw nothing, cared for nothing but his own selfish desires.

'I want you to finish it.'

'No.'

'Why not?'

She raised her eyes to his. 'I've given you my reasons.'

'Louise will not come to the house again. You have my word.'

Pride stiffened her spine. 'It's your house. You can please yourself whom you entertain, or involve–'

His breath hissed. 'You–' He yanked her towards him and her eyes flew wide as she saw his fury. 'Who in God's name do you think you are? What gives you the right to–' He stopped suddenly, eyes narrowing. The speculative gleam in their smoky depths made her tremble inside. 'Unless...'

Bracing her fists against the hard wall of his chest she pushed with all her strength.

'Caseley?' He sounded stunned.

'Let me go,' she panted, struggling violently. 'I hate you!'

A rap on the door froze them both.

'Yes?' Jago snapped.

Martin's voice came through the wood. 'Dinner, Cap'n.'

'We'll be right there.'

Seizing her chance, she pulled free. He made no effort to hold her. She was shivering yet perspiration pricked her temples and upper lip. Her heart pounded against her ribs. She rubbed her arms, the flesh tender where his grip had crushed it.

'After you,' he said solemnly, gesturing towards the door.

'I'm not hungry.' Her voice was husky and unsteady.

'I told you once, and I'm telling you again, while you are on board you are under my pro-

182

tection. You will not go hungry. Nor,' he forbade the idea even as it occurred to her, 'are you going to disrupt the routine of the ship by having your meals served in here. Now, will you walk to the mess, or must I carry you?'

She lifted her chin. 'And who will protect me from *you*, Captain?'

One dark brow rose. 'What makes you think that will be necessary?'

Wrenching the door open she stormed out of the day room, wanting to scream with frustration. How did he always manage to twist her words?

As she entered the mess, Jimbo, Hammer, and Martin scrambled awkwardly to their feet bumping against the wood table and making the spoons clatter against the enamel plates. It cost effort, but she smiled.

'Where shall I sit?'

'Beside me,' Antonio Valdes said from behind her, indicating two places on the bench opposite the twins. She sat down and he slid in beside her.

Jago took his place at the head of the table and ladled out steaming stew from a large iron pot with a ring handle and lid, serving the crew first in order of rank.

Antonio Valdes looked astonished, then annoyed, as Jago poured meat and vegetables onto his plate. He muttered something in Spanish but seemed unwilling to issue a challenge.

Caseley was served last. She murmured her thanks and the meal began.

Chapter Thirteen

There must have been conversation, but no one addressed her directly. By serving her last Jago was making it clear that despite her financial interest in the vessel, the crew's welfare took priority. Antonio Valdes took it as a personal slight. She did not. Besides, she had other things on her mind.

Barely tasting the food, she chewed and swallowed, her thoughts fluttering like a jarful of moths.

The sound of her name on Jago's lips had jolted her. Had he been anyone else she might have ignored it, or told him that such familiarity had no place between them. How could she do that? He was like no one else she had ever known.

Recalling the look on his face as comprehension broke through his scowling anger, embarrassment dewed her skin so her shift clung uncomfortably. It hadn't occurred to her that her weary remark might be construed as jealousy. Only when she saw his expression change did she realise how it must have sounded.

About to protest, she had imagined the sardonic twist to his mouth, his dark brows lifting in mocking disbelief. What exactly was her grievance: his use of her first name? Or that he recognised a truth she had denied even to herself. Anything she said would only convince him he was right. Yet in his eyes her silence served the same purpose.

Still, though he might *assume,* he could not be certain. To say nothing and keep her distance was her only hope of hiding her fear and shame. There was something pathetic and ridiculous in yearning for a man to whom marriage meant nothing, who already had a mistress, who was contemptuous of those who condemned him, and whose regard for her extended only as far as her usefulness.

A touch on her arm jerked her out of her thoughts. Antonio Valdes's fingers lingered as she turned. Hammer and Jimbo had risen from the table and were listening as Jago gave them quiet instructions. Martin was on his way out of the mess carrying the empty cauldron. The table was cluttered with dirty plates and cutlery.

'Señorita, tell me,' he coaxed softly, 'what has caused your cheeks to take their colour from winter snow instead of summer roses? If a man is responsible,' he paused, 'I will kill him for you. To mar such beauty with sadness he no longer deserves to live.'

Caseley forced a smile. 'Your gallantry does you credit, señor,' she said lightly. 'Indeed, you are correct. It is a man who occupies my thoughts. A man about whom I care deeply.'

Hammer and Jimbo had gone but Caseley was aware of Jago pausing to listen. She ignored him but could not control her stuttering heartbeat.

'And he does not return your affection.' Antonio made it a statement.

Though she held her smile steady, Caseley knew a moment's anguish. For all his lavish compliments, Antonio Valdes did not *expect* anyone to

185

love her.

As if realising he had made a slip, the Spaniard gazed into her eyes. 'What a fool he must be.' His voice was vibrant, his frown intense.

He had given her the perfect opportunity to offer a reason for her preoccupation. It meant accepting Antonio's true evaluation of her appeal rather than the extravagant compliments he poured over her like rich cream. But what did that matter? Was it not the truth?

'On the contrary, señor,' she corrected, 'my father loves me very much.'

From the corner of her eye she saw Jago's mouth twitch and with a murmured, *'Touché,'* he too left the mess.

'Your *father?'* Antonio repeated.

'He has been ill, and I worry about him. I fear that on occasion my concern outweighs my manners. If I have been a poor table companion, I trust you will forgive me.'

He seized her hand, pressing warm, moist lips against her knuckles. 'Lovely señorita, there is nothing to forgive. Such devotion must be admired. Come, let us go up on deck. There is little air down here, and though the furniture is adequate...' his shrug expressed disdain.

Caseley hesitated, unsure of committing herself. More than anything she wanted to be alone, to rest and think. She slipped out of her seat and as they reached the bottom of the stairs, glimpsed Jago in the day room seated at the table writing in the log. She would find neither peace nor privacy in his company.

'I should enjoy a spell on deck. My father

186

warned of rough weather, so we should make the most of the sunshine.'

'I sincerely hope your father was wrong.' Their feet rang on the brass as Antonio followed her up the stairs. He moved two coils of rope and a bucket further along the cargo hatch, clearing a space for them both to sit.

Caseley looked up at a brilliant blue sky scattered with puffball clouds, enjoying the warm breeze on her face. 'Are you not a good sailor, Señor Valdes?'

'Alas no.'

'Then to risk such discomfort you must be anxious to return to Spain.' She was simply making conversation, being polite while half her mind was with the man downstairs.

'I am. Are you aware of events in my country, señorita? The battles? The terrible loss of life?'

Caseley nodded. 'I have read newspaper accounts, but I doubt they describe the true extent of the people's suffering. You have my sympathy, Señor Valdes.'

'We Spaniards are renowned for many things: our wines from Jerez, the windmills of Castile, Seville oranges, the Pamplona bullfights, and even Andalusian flamenco. But it is our fierce pride and religious fervour that sets the Spanish character above all others.'

Caseley considered his statement arrogant, but courtesy would not allow her to argue. Yet though she had not observed anything remotely religious about Jago Barata, other than his occasional blasphemy when she irritated him beyond bearing, and though he was only half-Spanish, he certainly

187

possessed his full share of arrogance.

Antonio smiled, revealing small even teeth. 'I, however, have avoided such excessive rigidity of character. I am altogether more ... flexible. A trait my beloved family finds unsettling. But we do agree that it is exhausting to belong to a country which last year had four different presidents.'

'Four?' she echoed in surprise.

'Yet at this moment we do not have even one. Our last president, Castelar, was ousted in a military coup and now General Serrano is back in power.'

'At school I was taught that Spain is a monarchy.'

'Indeed it was, until six years ago when Queen Isabel abdicated.'

'I thought a king or queen reigned until they died. I cannot imagine Queen Victoria abdicating.'

'The lives of the two queens have little in common,' Antonio said. 'The forty years of Isabel's reign saw the worst scandals and excesses in Spanish history. My people have always been tolerant of small weaknesses in our royalty. But Isabel's behaviour went far beyond the forgivable. At times the court resembled a brothel. Even when the king was alive there was public doubt over who fathered certain of her children.'

Caseley turned her head away, shaken that he would repeat such scurrilous gossip to her.

'Once the junta had got rid of the queen,' he continued, oblivious to her discomfort, 'they declared that due to Isabel's appalling immorality the Bourbon family had forfeited all rights to the crown. When General Serrano was made regent everyone believed it'd be the dawn of a new era.'

His tone held cynicism Caseley did not understand. 'Wasn't it?'

'Appointing General Prim as prime minister, Serrano decided Spain would remain a monarchy, but a limited one, with the real power invested in two chambers...'

'Like our Parliament?'

Antonio nodded. 'However, this provoked a revolt among those who were disgusted with the monarchy and wanted Spain to become a republic.'

'But how could the country remain a monarchy if the royal family was no longer permitted to reign?' Caseley was astonished that a queen could behave in such a manner, and a country could be squabbled over.

'Serrano made Prim offer the throne of Spain around Europe.' Once more bitterness curled his mouth. 'But no one wanted it. Eventually he persuaded Amadeo, the second son of King Victor Emmanuel of Italy, to accept it. Amadeo might even have been a good king for my country.' Antonio shrugged.

'Might have been? But he *accepted* the crown.'

'Yes, he did. But the day Amadeo arrived in Spain, General Prim was murdered.'

As she caught her breath, Antonio spread his hands. 'Amadeo could not speak our language and no longer had a mentor to help him unravel our tangled politics. After two years he gave up the struggle and abdicated.' Antonio lifted one exquisitely tailored shoulder. 'So General Serrano is back in power for a second time. But he has lost

189

patience and now rules as a dictator. Thus my country is relieved of a freedom it could not handle.'

Caseley thought she detected a note of approval. But the impression was fleeting as his tone changed to one of frustration.

'Yet still there is no peace.'

'Why not?'

'Though there are those who support the republic, many of the Spanish people find it totally abhorrent. We are a Catholic country and the monarchists consider the present system a godless regime. But even if the clamour to restore the monarchy gained sufficient power, how are we to choose between two men who both claim to be the rightful king, and who both have armies of supporters?'

'*Two?* But how is that possible?'

Antonio took a breath. 'Over a hundred years ago, Philip V, the first Bourbon King of Spain, passed a law that said no female could succeed to the Spanish throne. Many years later this law was reversed. But the reversal was never made public until Isabel's father, King Ferdinand, announced his wife's pregnancy and declared that boy or girl, the child would be the next sovereign of Spain.'

'Yes,' Caseley nodded, 'and so she was.'

'Indeed. But under the *old* law, Ferdinand's brother, Don Carlos, would have inherited the throne. He and his supporters distrusted the new liberal ideas of Ferdinand and his queen, and were furious with what they considered sacrilegious interference with Divine Right. So the vendetta began. Now Carlos's grandson, also named Car-

190

los, claims to be the legitimate heir to the throne. Meanwhile the Royalists want Isabel's son, Alfonso, to rule.'

Hearing Alfonso's name reminded Caseley of the package, her reason for being aboard *Cygnet*. Trepidation made her tremble inside as she recalled the documents, wrapped in the disguising contract and sealed inside another envelope, hidden among her clothes.

Concerned about her father, desperately anxious to fulfil what might be his last request, and burdened with the realisation of her feelings for Jago, she had pushed the package deep into her bag and out of her mind.

In her possession was something that could have a profound effect on the future of Spain. In the hands of either faction the package would be explosive. But which side was right?

She was only a courier. As soon as she handed the package over, her job would be done and she could go home.

'I fear I have bored you,' Antonio broke into her thoughts.

'Not at all. I appreciate you taking the time to explain.'

'So now you understand it will be easier.'

Caseley wasn't sure what he meant. 'Your people must be suffering greatly during this unrest.'

He moved one shoulder in a careless gesture. 'It is the price of progress.' His gaze sharpened. 'But the instrument of change is within reach.' He smiled. 'Now let us talk of other things. You were telling me about your father.'

'Was I?' Caseley could not remember doing so.

'He sounds a most accomplished man. The name of his shipping agency is not confined to Cornwall. Juan Rodriguez speaks most highly of him.'

'You know Señor Rodriguez?' Caseley asked eagerly. 'I have corresponded with him on my father's behalf and found him charming.' The wine merchant's letters with their courteous old-world phraseology had created in Caseley's mind an image of a tall, silver-haired man of proud bearing and the impeccable manners of a grandee.

'Not personally,' Antonio admitted after a moment's hesitation. 'But his views were passed on in conversation.'

'Oh, I see.' How foolish of her to assume that simply because he was Spanish, Antonio Valdes might know people with whom her father did business.

'Managing such a thriving concern would be demanding even without the added burden of illness,' he gushed. 'Then there are his consular duties. I have heard you are of great assistance.'

Startled, Caseley caught herself. Showing concern would convince him she had something to hide. She softened her dismissive gesture with a smile. 'You flatter me, señor.'

'And you are too modest, señorita. A young woman helping her sick father in such masculine domains as shipping and politics? How could that pass unnoticed?'

Her unease increased. 'My help – such as it was – consisted of paperwork relating to cargoes. It simply released my father from routine matters during his recovery.' What was Antonio Valdes's

192

interest? Where had he obtained his information? Had he learned it from Jago?

Perhaps he had asked who she was and why she was aboard. The thought of them discussing her father or herself was unnerving. She had never pictured Jago as a gossip. In fact the idea seemed impossible. But was it? He had no reason to consider her feelings. Indeed, up to now he seemed to have made a point of not doing so.

She realised she was very much alone. As her skin tightened in a shiver she was overwhelmed with relief to see Nathan approaching. Hammer had taken over the wheel.

'Skipper says to come for tea, miss.' The mate sketched a salute. 'You an' all, sir.'

Caseley stood up at once, clinging to the hatch cover for support as she shook out her skirt. Though a command rather than an invitation, it provided escape from a conversation she suspected was more than polite interest. 'There is no hurry,' Antonio protested. 'Let us ignore this tea and take our meal at a more civilised hour.' He patted the hatch beside him.

His warm smile did not disguise his irritation and Caseley was surprised at his thoughtlessness. She remained standing, gently rotating her crippled foot to ease its stiffness.

'Señor, I understand it is the custom in Madrid to take one's evening meal at ten or even later. In English cities dinner may be served at any time between seven and nine. But in Cornwall our habits are different. On board ship tea is not simply a drink. It is the last meal of the day. I'm sure it will be possible to get a mug of cocoa later

193

in the evening when the watch changes. But a seaman's main meal is served in the middle of the day, not at the end.'

He spread his hands, palms up and lifted his shoulders. 'I must submit to this barbaric arrangement or starve?'

Caseley gave a brief nod. 'It would appear so.'

He sighed. 'Then I will come.' He stood and offered his arm.

Though reluctant to take it, she knew it would be foolhardy as well as churlish to refuse. The deck was rising and falling as the schooner cut through the darkening water, and after sitting for so long she had pins and needles in her foot. Yet she knew her instincts had been right when he rested his other hand on top of hers.

'We will talk again, beautiful señorita. We have much to discuss, you and I. Like a flower of many petals you hide yourself.' His voice was husky, his smile intimate. 'But I will pluck those petals one by one.'

Fear trickled, ice-cold, from the nape of her neck to the base of her spine. Pulling her hand free she gripped the handrail and started down the stairs. The intense stress of the past few days had made her over-sensitive. Why else would his words, spoken in such vibrantly romantic tones, sound like a threat?

As she reached the bottom of the stairs with Antonio close behind, Jago emerged from the day room. His cool grey gaze flicked over them both, but it was Caseley he addressed.

'Martin has put hot water by the stove should you wish to wash your hands.'

'Th – thank you.' Caseley stammered in surprise.

He nodded without expression and would have walked on into the mess had Antonio not put out a languid hand to stop him.

'And I, Captain?'

Jago turned his head slowly, looking at the Spaniard's fingers on his shirtsleeve. Only when Antonio had removed them did he raise his head.

'You may do as you choose, Señor Valdes. There are buckets on the cargo hatch and an ocean all around you.'

He nodded briefly and moved on.

Caseley glimpsed barely concealed rage in Antonio's shrug. Excusing herself, she entered the day room and closed the door.

Lifting the lid on top of the cupboard to reveal the basin, she picked up the bucket. It was only a third full but given the movement of the ship, she feared more would end up on the floor than in the basin. Imagining Jago's reaction to that, she set the bucket down again, fetched her soap and towel, and knelt to wash her hands.

Jago need not have agreed to Antonio making the voyage on *Cygnet*. After his initial mistake in believing the Spaniard was the passenger he'd been expecting, he could have refunded whatever Antonio had paid for the trip and referred him to Fox's or Broad's to arrange another berth.

So why had he insisted Antonio remain aboard? It wasn't for the money. Jago was a wealthy man. Given the animosity between them, what reason would be strong enough to force each into the other's presence? The matter had to be urgent.

Antonio had admitted needing a fast passage to Spain. Why? Was it connected with the unrest? Or was it that, like Jago, he had business interests that were under threat? What had he meant by saying that now she knew it would be easier?

Checking her appearance in the mirror, she tidied her hair. She was becoming far too inquisitive. This was a result of listening to Rosina and Liza-Jane gossiping.

Pierced by homesickness she pictured the kitchen: Rosina, red-cheeked from the heat of the range, bustling about getting tea, Liza-Jane holding the doors open for Ben as he brought in the coal. She thought of her father dozing by the fire. Was he all right? Would Ben remember to give him his drops at bedtime?

Fretting was pointless. There was nothing she could do. Placing the bucket between the stove and the cabin door she returned to her bag and lifted out a cloth-wrapped parcel.

When she slipped into her seat the men had already begun eating. For once she was glad Jago Barata set his own rules. Nathan pushed a plate of thickly sliced bread spread with butter towards her, interrupting what he was saying to point to a jar of jam.

''Tis raspberry, miss. Susan, my eldest, made six pound of it this year from our own bushes.'

'Thank you, Nathan.' Realising there was no serving spoon and unwilling to embarrass him she dipped into the jar with her knife.

'Tea, miss?' Jimbo held the battered iron kettle over the mug in front of her. Remembering her father's tales of tea the colour and consistency of tar, she hesitated. But longing for a hot drink overcame her doubts.

'Yes, please.' Dark brown and steaming, it wasn't as bad as she feared. Without a word, Jago placed a jug of condensed milk in front of her and her spirits rose. Lifting the bundle from her lap she set it on the table and opened the cloth.

'These were baked yesterday–'

'Saffern *and* a hevva cake,' Jimbo gasped in awe. 'I 'aven't tasted saffern cake for months. Bless your 'eart, miss.'

'I'll cut 'n,' Nathan insisted as Jimbo reached for the knife. 'Leave it to you and we'll only get half a dozen slices. By your leave, skipper?' he added quickly, glancing at Jago who nodded. His gaze met Caseley's, and his barely visible nod suffused her with warmth. Quickly she looked away. Aware that cake was a rare treat, she had brought it for the men not to win his approval.

'You won't want none, Mart.' Jimbo shook his head at the boy, who was staring round-eyed at the two cakes. One was deep yellow-gold and studded with currants and lemon peel. The other was a square slab just over an inch thick, full of dried fruit. The top was crunchy with sugar and scored in a criss-cross pattern.

'I do too want some,' the boy yelped, blushing as everyone grinned and he realised he had fallen for Jimbo's teasing yet again.

The cakes were sliced and everyone took a piece with a decorum Caseley found touching.

'Cap'n, is it all right if Nathan finish what he was saying 'bout that boat from Peru?' Martin asked.

Jago gestured to the mate. 'Carry on, Nathan.'

The mate washed down the last crumbs of his cake with tea. 'Well, knowing 'twas a long trip home and the captain's mortal remains wouldn't keep, the mate had the body stuffed with *guano–*'

'Excuse me,' Antonio broke in. 'What is this *guano?*'

'Bird shit,' Jimbo said, 'begging your pardon, miss.'

Caseley swallowed and simply nodded, hard-pressed to hide her smile. After a bewildered moment, Antonio's eyes widened and he studied the slice of saffron cake on his plate.

'They buried the coffin three foot deep in the hold,' Nathan continued. 'When the ship reached Falmouth, they dug 'n out and he looked as good as the day he died. Smelled a bit ripe, but you can't have everything. Anyhow, they took 'n over to St Ives where he come from, and buried 'n there in the churchyard like he always wanted.'

''Tis the lime,' Jimbo announced. 'Keep a body in lime for years you could.'

'Know about that, do you, boy? Got a few in your garden, have you?'

'Jimbo, tell 'em about Captain Evans,' Martin nudged the stocky seaman. 'Go on.'

Jago poured himself another cup of tea.

'Well, Hammer and me wasn't on board ourselves, but our cousin Arfie was. He swore 't was God's honest truth. See, Captain Evans was master of *Odette,* a tea-clipper out of China. He took sick with some bug out there. The cap'n I mean, not Arfie. Anyhow, he died. Cap'n's wife was with 'n and she said she wasn't going to have

198

'n buried in no heathen country. He had to be brought home. Well, you know what the heat is like out there. He wasn't going to be very sweet after three weeks at sea.' A master storyteller who relished his audience's attention, Jimbo paused.

'The cap'n had always run a dry ship. Both he and Mrs Evans was teetotal and they never allowed so much as a drop of liquor on any vessel under his command. But there was only one way missus was going to get her man home for burying all in one piece, so to speak. She had to have 'n put in a barrel filled up with alcohol.'

His grin gleeful, Martin wriggled on the bench.

'That's almost poetic,' Jago mused.

'Pickled,' Nathan guffawed. 'And the poor soul wasn't even alive to enjoy it.'

'Ah, but that isn't all,' Jimbo said quietly, his eyes dancing as everyone turned to him once more. 'Mrs Evans couldn't understand how the crew was so cheerful, specially after they was caught in a typhoon four days out. She asked the mate and he told her that though the cap'n was gone the whole crew was uplifted by his spirit. That was God's honest truth too. When *Odette* reached port and the barrel was opened, the cap'n's body was fresh as a daisy. But there wasn't a drop of alcohol left.'

After a moment's stunned silence, the small mess erupted in laughter. Shocked, Caseley couldn't suppress her giggles. Excusing herself, she returned to the cabin for her paisley shawl and, swirling it around her shoulders, went up on deck.

Hammer was at the wheel. He nodded shyly

199

then gazed resolutely forward as, embarrassed but determined, she passed him and opened the door in the side of the wheel shelter.

When she emerged, her chest hurting from holding her breath against the carbolic-laced stench, she saw Martin a few feet away. He had the heavy copper stern light on deck and was topping up the oil and trimming the wick.

She made her way forward to the companion-way. Leaning against the side, she wrapped the shawl more closely and looked westward to the setting sun. As the huge orange ball sank towards the sea, the sky changed from deep rose to pale pink and gold. The small clouds that had speckled the sky during the afternoon had melted away.

'Looks like she's set fair again tomorrow,' Nathan said, appearing at the hatch. 'If the wind hold steady, we should make port in three days.' He nodded at her and went aft to take the wheel from Hammer.

Caseley watched the sun disappear, swallowed by the ocean. Jimbo and Martin moved about on deck. The port and starboard lights in the mainmast rigging glowed ruby and emerald. At the stern an arc of white light played over their wake. No longer warmed by the sun the breeze was chilly. She shivered and, bidding Nathan goodnight, went below.

Reaching the bottom of the stairs she heard Jago's voice. Pitched too low for her to distinguish the words, there was no doubting his anger. She hesitated, unsure what to do. Then she realised the voices were coming from Nathan's cabin, now occupied by Antonio Valdes.

Quickly entering the day room she closed the door. Warmth radiated from the crackling stove and the mellow lamplight made the cabin feel cosy. The chart was rolled up and pushed to the back of the table and the leaf had been folded down.

As she tossed her shawl onto her bunk there was a single rap on the door. She opened it and stood back as Martin staggered in, a loaded coal-scuttle in one hand, a bucket half-full of steaming water in the other.

'Beg pardon, miss. I had to kick 'n 'cos I had both hands full.' He set the coalscuttle on one side of the stove, the bucket on the other, closest to the sleeping cabin.

'Thank you, Martin. How thoughtful—'

'Cap'n's orders, miss,' he blurted, blushing. ''E said you got the place to yourself til ten.'

'Oh. I see.' Recovering, she smiled at him. 'You must be busy enough without these extra duties. I'm very grateful.'

''Tisn't no trouble, miss.' As he reached the door he grinned over his shoulder. 'Handsome bit of cake that was.' He hurried out, pulling the door shut behind him.

Taking off her jacket, Caseley fetched her soap, towel, and nightgown. Starting to unbutton her bodice, she glanced up and realised that the sky-light was an illuminated window revealing most of the day room to anyone who cared to look in.

Hot with embarrassment, she carried her things back into the tiny sleeping cabin and dropped them on the bunk. She could not pull the curtain over for that would cut out all the light. Instead

201

she placed the bucket in the doorway and moved round behind it. There wasn't much room, but at least she could not be seen.

Twenty minutes later, after a strip-wash that left her feeling clean, fresh, and very tired, she pulled on her nightgown. After brushing and braiding her hair into a thick plait that fell over one shoulder, she put on her cape. Slipping her bare feet into her shoes she opened the door, starting as she came face to face with Jago.

'Where are you going?' He raked her with angry eyes.

'I – to empty this.' She hefted the bucket forward. 'Martin will need–'

'I'll see to it.' He was curt.

'Thank you.' She turned away.

'Caseley?'

She looked round. His voice held a note she had not heard before. In the lamplight his expression was forbidding and his eyes glittered.

'Yes?' Her heart thumped.

He stared at her, unspeaking. The tension emanating from him hinted at an inner battle. He shook his head. 'Nothing. Go to bed.' He turned and lifting the bucket in front of him, went swiftly up the stairs.

'Goodnight,' she murmured, and quietly closed the door.

Caseley woke with a start and for a moment could not remember where she was. Then it all flooded back. She lay, listening intently, waiting for a repeat of the sound that had woken her. But apart from the rattle of the steering gear, the creaking of the ship's timbers, and the hiss of water against the hull, there was nothing.

Pushing back the blankets she swung her feet to the floor and peeped round the half-drawn curtain into the day room. It was empty. The lamp was out and the grey light of dawn filtered through the skylight. She saw the bucket, once again half full of steaming water. It must have been the door closing that woke her.

She washed quickly and put on the same skirt and blouse she had worn the previous day. She had replaced the bucket by the stove and was in front of the mirror brushing her hair when the door opened.

She whirled round as Jago walked in, her hair flying like a red-gold banner. Their eyes met, held. She saw his hair was damp. His beard gleamed as if that too was wet. In one hand he carried a brass sextant, in the other a towel.

His shirt was open to the waistband of his trousers and she glimpsed black, curling hair on his chest. Realising suddenly that she had been staring, and hot beneath his amused gaze, she turned back to the mirror, wielding the brush with fierce strokes, sweeping through the tumbling mane until it crackled.

Jago dropped his towel on the bench seat and replaced the sextant in a lined wooden box lying on the table beside the open log. Aware of him close behind her, she lowered her arms and turned, ready to move out of his way. He reached up to stow the box in a locker.

'You slept well?' he asked without looking at her.

'Yes. I didn't expect to but—Yes I did. It must be all the fresh air.' She felt nervous, jumpy. 'And the movement. I'm hungry too.' She edged out from behind the table. 'Is breakfast ready?'

'Give the boy a chance.' His tone was mild but it brought a flush to her cheeks. 'Hold that a moment, will you?' He pushed the rolled-up chart into her arms and leaned down to raise the table leaf, slotting the supporting leg into place.

As he straightened she offered him the chart. Ignoring it, he lifted a lock of hair that had fallen forward over her shoulder, studying it as though mesmerised.

Common sense told her to step back, or knock his hand away and bundle her hair into its confining net. But she couldn't move, couldn't breathe.

He lifted his gaze and their eyes met. She swallowed. Her heart skipped a beat. Holding the chart in one hand and her brush in the other, she felt trapped, helpless. She wanted to run, but there was nowhere to hide. Still his hand moved in her hair, running it through his fingers as if testing its weight, its texture.

'Listen to me.' He spoke softly. 'Stay away from Valdes.'

The words seemed to come from far away. Then they registered, bringing her back to reality with a jarring thud.

'Why? You have refused my offer of help. You tell me I must not distract the crew. Señor Valdes provides pleasant company and conversation.'

Jago's lip curled. 'So I noticed. Nevertheless, I think it wiser that you do not spend time with him.' Gently he twisted her hair around his hand,

204

preventing her from moving. 'Do I make myself clear?'

'What is your objection?' She pushed aside her doubts about the Spaniard, whose cheerful flirtatious countenance had twice cracked to reveal an entirely different personality.

'Did you not want us out of your way?' She moved, expecting him to release her hair. Instead he tightened his grip. Shock rather than pain caused her breath to catch and tears to form. She blinked them away.

'You are not stupid, so don't play the fool,' he grated. 'Valdes is a Basque. He has a silver tongue but few scruples. If he believes you have something he wants, he will stop at nothing – and I mean *nothing* – to get it. *Now* do you understand? You are playing with fire, Caseley.'

'No,' she began, intending to tell him she knew full well that Antonio Valdes was not serious, that his flattery and conversation were only a means of passing time. But she froze as she recognised an alternative interpretation of Jago's warning. If she had something? The documents? Was that why he had explained in such detail about the political situation in Spain?

No, it could not be. No one but she and her father knew about them. The package had come direct from Mexico, the seal unbroken. Even if by some terrible misfortune Antonio Valdes was aware of their existence, he could not know they were in her possession. Her father would never have betrayed that trust and she had said nothing. Nor would she. Even Jago had no idea of the real reason she was aboard. *Or did he?*

205

His warning echoed in her head. 'You have something he wants.'

Did Jago know? If so, how had he found out? Did it mean he was in league with Valdes? She could not believe that. Their patent dislike of each other was no pretence. But nor would it matter. Jago was half-Spanish. He would care about the country of his forefathers. He would have his own beliefs about what was right for Spain.

If he and Antonio Valdes were of the same mind, and were offered the opportunity to assist their chosen leader, where would Jago's loyalties lie? With the Cornishman whose schooner he commanded? Or with the Spaniard he loathed? Yet what if that apparent loathing was indeed a ruse?

All this raced through her mind at lightning speed. No matter what either of them suspected, they had no proof, and she would not break her oath of secrecy to her father.

Not knowing whom to trust, she could trust no one. She had to pretend the documents did not exist. Future conversations with Antonio Valdes would require extreme caution. But right now she needed to convince Jago that Valdes's interest was purely personal.

'You—' Her voice cracked and she had to clear her throat. 'You are mistaken. Señor Valdes is a gentleman.' She desperately hoped he would interpret her trembling as indignation. 'He would not take advantage. Anyway,' she said recklessly as he shook his head in disgust, 'you are in no position to condemn my behaviour, or anyone else's.'

Immediately the words were spoken she wished them unsaid. His face darkened ominously and his eyes turned as cold as arctic seas. Releasing her hair, he gripped her shoulders, his fingers digging into her flesh.

The brush fell unnoticed to the deck. Her breath sobbed in her throat as he pulled her towards him and her hands flew up to fend him off. Her heart leapt in a dark tangle of fear and shocking excitement.

One hand snaked round her waist, the other grasped the nape of her neck, effectively immobilising her. One black brow rose.

'Jealous, Caseley?'

'Don't be ridiculous.' She meant it to sound scathing, a rebuff of his massive conceit. But the look in his eyes and the unyielding hardness of his body against hers were stopping her breath, sapping her will.

'Let me go,' she pleaded, her voice unsteady. She could feel her strength ebbing and a treacherous weakness stealing along her limbs. 'I – I'm sorry.'

He frowned. 'For what?'

'Anything. I should not have said... Don't, please ... don't...' Her voice faded to a strangled whisper as his head lowered to hers, blotting out the light.

'Hush,' he said against her mouth. For a moment neither moved. Then a tremor rippled through him. As Caseley's hands pushed against his chest, his lips covered hers.

Chapter Fourteen

She hadn't known what to expect: perhaps demand, even anger. But his mouth moved on hers with heart-stopping tenderness. Her eyes closed and she was falling, flying. His lips were warm, soft. Helpless against their gentle pressure hers parted.

Her heart cried out to him as her body lost its rigidity and became pliant. It fitted against his as if created for this moment, for him.

Her fingers spread, sliding through the silky black hair. Beneath the searing heat of his skin she could feel the rapid thunder of his heartbeat, and was awed.

With a groan he tore his mouth from hers, his breathing harsh, and she gave a soft inarticulate cry of loss. Gripping her upper arms he held her away, his face a taut mask. His eyes blazed with emotions she did not understand.

Releasing her without a word, he turned swiftly and strode out. She staggered against the table, hearing the clang of his quick footsteps on the stairs.

Bereft, she lifted a hand to touch her mouth. Reaction set in and she began to shake, hugging herself as she trembled. An aching void yawned in the pit of her stomach.

Shame and doubt bubbled up like marsh gas. He had a mistress. Why had he kissed her? A whim?

Punishment for her defiance? Why had she let him? Not merely allowed, but responded, welcomed. She had been waiting without knowing what for. Now she knew. But that joyous moment of recognition had been shattered into jagged shards by his rejection and abrupt departure.

A wrenching sigh sobbed in her throat. Why had he come into her life? He had stirred hopes she had deliberately suppressed, disrupted an existence she had tried to fill with meaning by caring for her father, running the house, and shouldering the responsibility of protecting him and the business.

It would have been better if she had never met him. She would have dreamed, yearned, but she wouldn't have *known*. Knowing made loss agonising.

She pressed her fingertips to the throbbing ache in her forehead. The day had only just begun. There were meals to attend and the crew to face, as well as Antonio Valdes. She *had* to pull herself together.

She ran her tongue over her lips, tasting him. She could still feel the sensation of his mouth on hers, still smell his skin. She scooped up the now-cool water to bathe her face again and erase every trace. But it was too late. Jago Barata had left his mark on her as surely as if he had used a branding iron.

She could not begin to guess at his motive. He had seemed reluctant but driven. As his lips had touched hers, his hunger and barely controlled violence had shocked her. Yet she had not been frightened, nor had she fought.

His mouth had softened like a sigh, and he had stirred an aching sweetness so exquisite her heart had stumbled. Then he had gone, leaving a gaping wound.

With unsteady fingers she twisted her hair into a thick coil on her nape and anchored it with pins. She would not think about him. She could as easily stop breathing. His presence was all around. She was living in his cabin. She had slept in his bunk. His hand had penned the flowing writing in the log. And her body still quivered from his touch

There was no escape.

Unwilling to face a truth she had no idea how to deal with, she avoided the mirror. Instead she tidied away her soap, flannel, and toothbrush, folded her nightgown, plumped the pillow, and straightened the blankets on her bunk. The tasks soothed her so that when Martin knocked she was able to open the door and greet him with a mask of calm firmly in place.

''Morning, miss. All right if I fetch the bread and milk? Breakfast'll be ready in a few minutes.'

'Thank you. I'll bring the bucket—'

'No, miss. Cap'n wouldn't like that. You leave 'n there and I'll fetch 'n d'rectly.'

Her stomach clenched into a small hard knot as she sat down opposite Hammer and Jimbo. Making an effort to smile she returned their greetings, dreading the moment when Jago would join them. Antonio came in, freshly shaved and trailing the scent of soap and cologne. Nathan followed, his expression betraying amusement and scorn. Caseley realised Jago must be at the wheel. That meant he would eat later.

Relief left her weak. For a moment she wondered if he might be avoiding her, but dismissed the notion. He had made it clear that her presence on board would not be permitted to affect the ship's routine.

So she had to hide a start of surprise when she heard Hammer ask Nathan why the skipper was on an eight to noon watch when he had already put in an extra two hours during the night.

The mate shrugged. 'He'll have his reasons. He want you to check the repair on the spare mainsail and re-stitch 'n if he's loose, all right?'

Hammer nodded, his mouth full.

'Going to strip and grease the dolly winch, he was,' Jimbo put in.

'That'll keep. Do 'n after.'

Antonio frowned at the boiled oatmeal Nathan ladled onto his plate, then turned to Caseley.

'Buenas dias, guapa señorita.'

'Good morning, Señor Valdes.'

He studied her. 'Something is wrong. What is it? You must tell me.'

Caseley looked at her plate, and carefully lifted a spoonful of oatmeal to which she had added treacle and a little milk. Surely it could not be that obvious? The others had greeted her quite normally. There had been no lingering glances or questioning frowns. He was guessing, she realised. More than that, he seemed hopeful. Pushing thoughts of Jago to the back of her mind, she closed a door on them.

'You are mistaken, Señor. Nothing is wrong. Why should you think there is?'

211

His gaze was speculative, assessing. 'Because–' he answered in Spanish, 'yesterday I was a brute. I told you sad tales of my country. These are not your problems. But to engage your interest, your sympathy, I did this cruel thing. I asked questions, wanting to learn about you and your family. My only excuse is that though Fate has brought us together, it is for so short a time. But you will be in my heart forever.' He brought his head close to hers. 'Do you believe in love at first sight, señorita? I did not,' he paused, 'until yesterday.'

Caseley looked away from his smouldering gaze, and toyed with her oatmeal, her cheeks on fire.

Nathan pushed the jug of milk towards her, his frowning gaze darting between her and the Spaniard.

She did not know what to say. For an instant she had been tempted to laugh. But he was so abject, so sincere, she felt ashamed of the impulse.

Then, like a feather brushing over her skin, came realisation. His impassioned plea had been made entirely in Spanish. Despite telling him yesterday that she spoke little of the language, she had been too taken aback to interrupt or claim that she did not understand.

She glanced up, met his gaze, and saw only admiration. Maybe she had been wrong about him. Maybe her overwrought imagination had seen intrigue and threat where none existed. His forcefulness and inquisitorial manner had unsettled her. But, as Miss Amelia had often remarked, the Latin temperament was volatile, impatient, and passionate, and thus not easy for the cool, phlegmatic English to understand.

Caseley had wondered how Miss Amelia knew. Had she reached this conclusion through her studies of Spanish art and literature? Or had she in her younger days known a man like Antonio Valdes? Had she loved and lost?

'*Madre de Dios*,' he swore under his breath. 'I am a clumsy fool. My head counsels silence but my heart must speak. And the heart is always stronger, *no es verdad?* Your pardon, señorita, I beg you.'

Caseley was thoroughly unsettled. She had not invited his attention – had she? Could she, simply through not wanting to appear discourteous, have given him the impression that she welcomed his declarations? She didn't.

Perhaps someone more experienced might laugh them off and do so without causing offence. But she didn't have that experience. No one had ever spoken of love to her. Common sense told her he didn't mean it. He was exaggerating, though she had no idea why.

Nathan cleared his throat. 'Come on, miss. You got to do better 'n that, else the skipper'll have my hide.' He indicated the plate she had hardly touched. 'Want a drop more milk do you?'

Unable to watch her himself, Jago had detailed the mate to do it and no matter what his own feelings were, Nathan would obey his captain.

'No, thank you, Mr Ferris, this is fine.' She made herself swallow a spoonful of the glutinous porridge. She knew she needed the nourishment. Nor did she want to put the mate in the position of having to report her. She sensed his

213

discomfort, and none of this was his fault.

'What is this?' Antonio demanded in a low voice. 'The captain is surely exceeding his authority. It is unforgivable. I will speak with him.'

'No.' Caseley surprised herself with her firmness. 'That is not necessary. Captain Barata is responsible for my welfare while I am aboard. He is only saying what my father would say were he here.'

Antonio leaned towards her. 'What would your father say to you sharing the captain's cabin, señorita? Is that also necessary for your welfare?'

Caseley's face flamed. 'I – I–'

'Señorita,' he interrupted with smooth concern. 'You are a lady of sensitivity, as yet unmarried. Such an unorthodox arrangement must be deeply distressing for you. When I learned you were to travel with us I offered my cabin. I was told to mind my own business. It seems the captain is a law unto himself. But what are his reasons for forcing such embarrassment upon you? No man of honour would.'

'Please excuse me, señor.' Caseley pushed her barely touched plate away and stood up.

'Can you trust him?' Antonio hissed. 'What does he want from you?'

'Miss–' Nathan began.

'It's all right, Nathan. I'm– I just need–' Shaking her head she fled.

She wanted to hide in the day room, not see or speak to anyone. She needed to think. She hadn't had time to wonder how the arrangements might appear to anyone else. The crew had made little of it. But they must be curious. Unless– Had this

214

happened before? Were they used to seeing a woman on board?

No. Instinct told her that was not so. If they showed little reaction it was because they were well-disciplined and they trusted Jago. His reasons were not their business. But clearly Antonio saw something sinister in it, and he had re-awakened all her doubts.

Jago had said it was for her protection. Against what or whom? *He* had kissed her. *He* was trying to stop her talking to Antonio. *Why?*

She hesitated at the bottom of the stairs. She did not want to see Jago. The memory of his kiss was still too vivid. Just thinking of it made her heart turn over. But she *had* to go to the wheel shelter.

Her heart quickened as she climbed the stairs. The breeze was fresh and tasted of salt. All the sails were full. She clung to the top of the gunwale as she made her way aft, the wind blowing into her face over the port quarter.

Jago stood behind the massive oak wheel, the wind billowing his shirt, his booted feet apart, balanced against the schooner's motion. His hands rested lightly on the varnished spokes and his gaze shifted from sea to sails then to the compass as he held their course, harnessing the power of wind and current to coax all possible speed from the graceful vessel.

The schooner's bow rose and she was suddenly conscious of the size of the seas around them. The deep water was inky blue and streaked with foam blown back from the wave crests. Carried forward on a rolling mass of water, *Cygnet* met a cross sea

215

with her head down. As her prow carved a path through, a cloud of spray flew skyward and Caseley gasped as some of it caught her, stippling her blouse and trickling down one side of her face and neck.

'Get below,' Jago bellowed as she gripped the rail with one hand using the other to wipe cold salt water from her stinging eyes.

She shook her head and released the rain to lurch across to the wheel shelter.

'Are you sick?' He had to shout above the din created by the wind shrieking through the sheets and shrouds and the creaking blocks.

'No,' she yelled back, her face burning as she fumbled with the latch.

With a brief nod he looked down to check the compass once more. He might have been a stranger. Yet his strong arms had held her close and his mouth had caressed hers with a sweetness she would never have suspected in him.

She almost fell into the tiny shack. Fortunately the bucket was empty except for a puddle of carbolic whose powerful smell caught in her throat. She wondered which of the crew had the unenviable task of cleaning it and sympathised, realising how much she took for granted at home.

As she swayed back to the companionway she could feel Jago's eyes on her. The temptation to look round was almost irresistible. But pride gave her the strength she needed. He had walked away without a word. Even now, though they were alone on deck, not by a word or a smile had he so much as hinted that anything had occurred between them.

Maybe as far as he was concerned it hadn't. Maybe it had slipped from his mind, an impulse acted on and dismissed. Not important enough even to be regretted. Simply forgotten.

She hurried back to the day cabin, her head down, nearly tripping in her haste to be alone as scalding tears spilled down her cheeks. Hurt, bewildered, hating herself and him, she curled up on the bunk. But the harder she tried to untangle her thoughts, the more confused she became. What to believe? Whom to trust?

At dinnertime, pride and reluctance to give Jago reason to criticise her forced her into the mess. She ate as much as she could, conscious of his rare glances, and remembered to thank Martin, who reddened and was at once teased by the rest of the crew.

Escaping back to the cabin, she brought a book from her bag and curled up in one corner at the stern end of the bench to read.

Jago came in a little later. The atmosphere changed in an instant, becoming charged with tension. Bending over the table to enter details of their course and the weather into the log he asked if she had everything she needed. She thanked him politely and said she did. Then he left. But the tension lingered on.

Towards late afternoon, Antonio Valdes knocked softly, claiming an urgent need to talk to her. She did not open the door, grateful for the barrier as she pleaded a headache. After sowing further seeds of doubt as to her safety under Jago's so-called protection, he left.

Tea followed a similar pattern. When, to settle an

argument, Jimbo wanted her opinion about the best way to cook pigs' trotters, Jago answered, deftly steering the conversation away from her. Yet instead of feeling excluded or rebuffed, she was relieved and grateful. The men took their cue from him. While giving her an occasional nod or smile to acknowledge her presence at the table, they left her alone.

Only Antonio persisted in trying to draw her out. But after his third attempt to begin a private conversation with her in Spanish earned him a cutting rebuke from Jago, he subsided into simmering silence.

As soon as she had finished eating, Caseley excused herself, left the table, and went up on deck. Hammer was at the wheel and after a nod and smile, made a point of checking the compass and looking up at the sails as she went to the wheel shelter.

When she came out the sun had set, leaving a blood-red stain on the horizon. In the twilight, stars were beginning to appear. A cold pale moon hung low in the dusky sky. With nothing but sea all around her she felt very small and insignificant. She moved down the deck, staying on the seaward side, filling her lungs with cold fresh air as she gripped the rail and gazed out across foam-tipped waves.

Thinking about home she wondered how her father was. She did not hear Jago's footsteps. But she was suddenly aware of him behind her. She could feel his presence, the warmth of his body across the inches that separated them. Tension crawled along her nerves. She shivered, craving and dreading his hand on her shoulder or cupping her elbow. But he did not touch her.

'Come below.' His deep voice was gentle, but the words were an order. There was nothing to be gained by arguing. She obeyed without looking round.

When she reached the day room, Martin had lit the stove and the cabin was warm and welcoming. Her heart quickened and a mixture of fear and anticipation rippled through her as Jago followed her in and closed the door.

Chapter Fifteen

She walked to the table and stood with her back to him, waiting.

'I have a request,' he spoke quietly.

She stiffened, mentally sifting through all the requests he might make. Only one sprang to mind. She half-turned, not meeting his eyes. 'If this concerns Antonio Valdes–'

'Valdes is the least of my concerns at the moment. I want you to write some letters.'

She swung round in surprise, watching as he opened a locker and took out a metal box. Lifting the lid he removed several sheets of paper covered in his bold scrawl. Laying the sheets on the table, he took out fresh paper, a pen, and a bottle of ink. Clearing a space on the shelf, he set the box on it out of the way.

'As you see I have already made notes. The letters are to my father's agent in Madrid, the Bilbao port authority, the British consul there, and one to Señor Esteban Cervantes who is a ship broker in Bilbao with contacts in other Spanish ports.'

'Why me?'

Jago sat down and pulled the log towards him. 'You have a neat hand and you write fluent Spanish.' He paused. 'Besides, I am very busy. You are not.'

It was no more than the truth. She slid onto the bench opposite. Picking up the scribbled notes she began to read through them, then looked across at Jago who met her startled glance with perfect calm.

She resumed reading, scanning the pages faster and faster. Then she went back and re-read to make sure she was not mistaken.

When she finished she looked up in disbelief. 'You are selling your schooner, *Cara*, and disposing of all your business interests in Spain?'

'Ah, my writing is not as poor as I feared.' He picked up his own pen and began to make entries in the log. 'I know I can leave the correct phrasing to you,' he said without looking up.

'Why?'

He reached up and tapped the barometer, making another entry on the page. 'You are practised at writing business letters for your father. The one concerning the steam pumping engine for the silver mine in Mexico was an excellent example. Write something along those lines.' His dark head was bent over the log.

'No, I meant why are you selling everything?'

He looked up then, turning the pen between his

fingers. One corner of his mouth lifted. 'Caseley, I asked you to write some letters, not question my decisions.'

The flush started at her chest and rushed up to her scalp. His rebuke was far milder than she deserved. 'I beg your pardon. I did not – that was impertinent of me.'

She drew fresh paper towards her and lifted the first sheet of notes. But she could not focus on the words. This was his private business. Yet though he would not tell her *why* he was selling all his Spanish interests, and she certainly had no right to ask, clearly he did not object to her knowing.

In asking her to write the letters it was as if he *wanted* her to know. Why? Perhaps he was simply using her to get a tedious chore done quickly while keeping her occupied and away from Antonio Valdes.

Why had he said that Valdes was the least of his concerns? He had been concerned enough to forbid *her* any contact with the Spaniard.

Some sixth sense told her Jago was watching her. Feeling a warm tide creep up her face she peeped up from under her lashes and met his ironic gaze. Quickly picking up her pen she uncorked the ink, moved the notes to one side, dipped the nib, and began to write.

For a while the only sounds were the creak of the ship, the thump and hiss of water along the hull, and the scratch of pens. Then Jago broke the silence.

'Do you know the name of the ship carrying that engine to Mexico?'

Caseley looked up, shaking her, head. 'I don't, but Uncle Richard should.'

'I called into the office the day before we sailed. Unfortunately he wasn't there.'

'Is it important?'

He shrugged. 'The cargo I'm collecting is also bound for Mexico. It would have saved time if I could have got it on the same ship.'

'Will there be room? The engine is not small and is additional to the load already booked in. What is your cargo?'

'Mercury,' Jago replied. 'Ten iron containers of quicksilver. My father needs it urgently at his mine.'

'Oh.' She nodded.

Jago watched her for a moment then started to laugh, a deep-throated sound, full of warmth. She glanced at him and her heart leapt, for the warmth was also in his eyes, along with a teasing light. 'Go on, then.'

'I don't know what you mean,' she retorted, feeling her colour rise and helpless to stop it.

'Yes, you do,' he shot back. 'You have a questioning mind, Caseley. It's one of the things I–' He broke off abruptly. He was gripping the pen so hard she tensed, expecting it to snap. Then he continued. 'You want to know what the mercury is for.' He made it a statement.

'Yes,' she admitted. 'I did wonder.'

'It's used in the refining of silver.'

'I thought silver was found in nuggets, like gold.'

Jago nodded. 'It can be, has been, in some places. Nuggets weighing hundreds of pounds have been dug up in Mexico and Canada. But most silver is a by-product of other ores such as copper, lead or zinc. Before my father moved to Mexico and left them to me, he owned refineries in Oviedo and Ciudad Real in the south of New Castile. Mercury is used in the extraction process.'

Resting her elbows on the table, Caseley supported her chin on her fists. Heat from the crackling stove and soft lamplight made the turbulence of wind and ocean outside seem far away. The conversation's shift to less personal topics had helped her relax. Though the atmosphere in the tiny cabin still held the tension that seemed inevitable when they were together, over it lay a new and gentler intimacy.

'How does it work?' she asked.

Jago studied her, a faint frown creasing his forehead. As the silence lengthened and his scrutiny continued, she became self-conscious. Why did he stare so?

'You really want to know?' His tone held both surprise and irony.

'I would not have asked otherwise. Haven't you just commented on my curious mind? But if you're too busy—'

'No, I—' Setting the pen aside, he leaned back, stretching his arms out, his strong brown hands spread flat on the table. 'You constantly surprise me, though I should know better. First the ore is finely ground,' he said before she could respond. 'Then it is mixed with water and mercury and shaken. The mercury breaks up into globules and dissolves the silver in the ore. When this amalgam is heated the mercury evaporates, condenses, and is collected for further use while the silver is left behind. Inevitably some mercury is lost during processing, so my father has regular shipments sent out to him. But the fighting has caused disruption and shipments have been delayed.'

Glancing at the clock he rose to his feet, his black curls almost touching the deck-head at the edge of the skylight. He went to the door. 'I'll send Martin with some hot water. Don't worry about finishing the letters tonight. We won't arrive in Santander until late tomorrow.' He held her gaze for a moment.

His grey eyes seemed to pierce her soul and she looked down. She carried too many secrets and their weight was becoming an intolerable burden. The door closed quietly.

Alone again, she realised how easily he had captured her attention, re-directed it, allowing her to forget for a while her doubts and fears.

Self-disgust consumed her. She had only to listen to Jago to be drawn under his spell. Had it taken only a single kiss to demolish her defences, destroy her sense of balance? She had no idea where she stood in his estimation. Was *useful* all she would ever be to him?

Antonio had declared himself in love with her. Yet his fervent whispers inspired only laughter and unease, though good manners demanded she conceal both.

When Jago had kissed her, his heart had beat against her palm as hard and fast as her own, and Antonio's warnings had crumbled to dust.

She buried her face in her hands. Jago's kiss had shown her something she had never known.

Then he had left without a word, leaving her tortured by dreams that had no future.

She was neither beautiful nor experienced in the arts of pleasing a man, and Jago Barata could have his pick of women who were both.

She pictured Tamsyn and Liza-Jane. Love had made them happy. They glowed with pride and contentment. For her, love was a double-edged sword of ecstasy and pain that would destroy her if she did not fight it.

Sitting up, she dropped her hands and looked at the notes. Her eyes burned and her head felt heavy. Smothering a yawn she gathered all the papers neatly into the tin. She still had another day in which to complete them.

She undressed, then brushed and braided her hair. Worn out by stress and the ship's plunging and rising, she climbed into the bunk, turned onto her side, and closed her eyes.

When she woke, grey light at the edge of the curtain told her dawn had broken. Sitting up and pushing the heavy plait back over her shoulder, she recalled troubling dreams and a vague memory of a quiet voice drawing her out of the nightmare that had smothered her. Her feverish body had calmed and she had slipped once more into sleep, this time deep and restful.

Hot water waited in the bucket beside the stove. After washing, she put on a clean shift and fresh bodice of cream cotton sprigged with tiny green and yellow flowers. She loosened her hair from its braid, brushed it thoroughly then twisted and coiled it into a net on her nape held in place by hand-painted slides.

She arrived in the mess as Jago was finishing his breakfast.

'Good morning.' His searching look as she sat down made her heart contract.

'Good morning,' she nodded round the table.

''Morning, miss,' Nathan, Hammer, and Martin responded then turned to Jago who was issuing the daily orders. Antonio did not smile and his narrowed gaze held bitter condemnation.

Guessing what was in his mind, Caseley was tempted to try and reassure him. The impulse swiftly passed. She owed him no explanations. She had done nothing wrong.

She ate a small dish of oatmeal and a ship's biscuit spread with treacle. After a cup of hot strong tea, she quietly excused herself and went up on deck, enjoying a sense of wellbeing she had never known before. Unwilling to examine it, she simply accepted, and was grateful.

Jimbo was at the wheel and bawled a cheery greeting. ''Morning, miss. 'Andsome day, isn't it?'

With her visits to the wheel shelter tactfully ignored by the crew, her embarrassment lessened each time.

When she emerged, Antonio was waiting near the companionway and begged her to come to his cabin. 'I have proof you are in grave danger,' he muttered urgently. 'Señorita, you are being led into a trap.'

Before she could ask him to explain, Jago appeared. Not sparing the Spaniard a glance, he took her arm in a gentle grip. 'Would you care to take a turn around the deck, Miss Bonython? Or are you ready to complete my letters?' While speaking he led her to the hatch and followed her down the stairs to the day room.

Unnerved by Antonio's hoarse warning and her inability to fight Jago's effect on her, she stopped at the door. 'Will you stop treating me like a – a prisoner?' she hissed as he leaned past to open it.

He raised one dark brow. 'I wasn't aware of doing so.'

'No, you call it protection,' she retorted, heat climbing her throat. 'I don't need it.'

'I think you do.' He was calm, implacable.

'I was only on deck a few minutes. I needed to– I wanted some fresh air.'

He nodded, guided her gently inside the cabin and closed the door. Only then did he release her arm. Without the warmth of her palm it felt cold and she rubbed it absently.

'What poison was Valdes dripping into your pretty ears this time?'

Caseley was shaken. How did he know? He could not have heard. *Pretty?* She struggled to concentrate. 'What do you mean? Why would he–?' His steady gaze stopped her. Why did she find it impossible to lie to this man?

'You have something he wants, Caseley. He will use any means he can to gain your confidence and destroy your trust in me.'

Pausing, he turned a page of the log over and back.

'The usual method for a man to get his way with an inexperienced, impressionable young woman is to tell her he had fallen helplessly in love with her. Even normally sensible and intelligent women are

227

too easily taken in.'

'You speak from experience, no doubt,' she flung at him, mortified as she recalled Antonio's declaration.

'I have never found it necessary to resort to such tactics.'

No, he wouldn't have. She turned away and limped to the table, not wanting him to see her hurt, her shame. Was it so obvious that she had never been sought after, never desired, never been in love? She closed her eyes, gripping the edge of the table. Just for an instant she had believed Antonio's declaration. Jago knew, and pitied her. She cleared her throat.

'You don't like him.' Her voice sounded thin.

'No, I don't.' There was no emotion in Jago's reply. He was simply stating a fact.

Caseley turned. 'Then why did you accept him as a passenger?'

'I owe his family a debt. They have business connections with my father. When I set up as a merchant-trader with my own schooner, they gave me cargoes.'

'But surely that was simply a business arrangement? Not a personal debt.'

Jago's chin lifted. 'To me it was a matter of honour. They had helped me. I was in a position to return the favour.'

'But how did he know you were going to Spain?'

'Valdes visited Bonython's office the day before we sailed and enquired for an urgent passage to Spain. Your Uncle Richard was out but had left word with Thomas Bonython regarding the cargo of pilchards he had arranged for me to carry to

Santander. Thomas told Valdes I was due to sail the following morning. When he arrived at the yard I assumed he was the passenger Toby had warned me to expect.'

Caseley realised he had answered all her questions without hesitation, questions she wasn't sure she had the right to ask. But would he answer this one?

'Why don't you like him?'

Jago's features hardened. 'He has no concept of honour.'

Caseley's mouth twitched in an ironic smile.

'You find that amusing?' He was sombre and she thought she had never seen him look so haughty or so Spanish.

'No. As a matter of fact he said the same of you, because of...' Her brief gesture encompassed the day room and sleeping cabin and her face grew warm.

'I see.' Neither his tone nor his expression gave anything away.

'You must have other reasons.' She wasn't sure how far she dared press, yet his explanation seemed too nebulous. Because she wasn't Spanish she might not fully appreciate their code of ethics. Even so, to her his dislike of Antonio Valdes felt personal.

'We have nothing in common,' he was brusque. 'Valdes lives on his wits and his family's generosity. It is years since I last saw him. But I have heard rumours of scandals and of his involvement with various political factions.'

Caseley's stomach tightened and it cost effort and willpower to remain perfectly still.

229

'Whether they are true I neither know nor care,' Jago went on. 'But right now he has you in his sights. Once Valdes steps ashore in Spain my debt is paid. Until then you are at risk, and I will do whatever I consider necessary to ensure your safety.' He did not smile.

Her gaze fell away and she shivered. Despite his flat tone she detected anger and impatience. Certain phrases he had used resurrected her uncertainty. It was as if he knew about the package and was giving her the opportunity to confide in him.

She clasped her arms across her body. Her heart was telling her what she wanted to hear, that she could trust him. It was a siren song, insistent and persuasive. But as she recalled the way he had treated her in Falmouth, how he had manipulated, blackmailed ... then there was Louise Downing...

'You're trying to frighten me.'

The glacial façade cracked. His eyes blazed as his hand shot out and gripped the back of her neck.

'Being frightened would be wise, Caseley,' he growled as she gasped and her hands flew up to clutch his wrist. 'We are sailing to a country torn by civil war, where friendship counts for nothing against heritage and tradition. Santander is Basque territory. I learned to sail with Basques. I worked, ate, and slept with them. They were my second family. But I am Castilian, an outsider. Now, because of the unrest, I am suspect. Think about that, Caseley. I am your only protection. But I too could be in danger.' He released her and she stumbled backwards, trembling.

He thrust his hands into his pockets, as if fighting the urge to touch her again. 'For the love of God, see sense. Let me deliver the ... contract.'

Had that tiny pause been deliberate? Was he telling her he knew whatever she was carrying was more valuable and more dangerous than any business agreement? No, he was only guessing. He couldn't be sure. Her instinct told her she could trust him. But trusting him would mean breaking her promise to her dying father.

As his gaze held hers, she wanted so much to tell him, to explain. She shook her head, the words torn from her. 'I can't.'

'So be it,' he muttered and strode out.

Chapter Sixteen

Caseley stared at the door. Doubts tore at her like talons; so did grief. Rousing herself she lifted down the tin. But as she worked on the letters her thoughts kept straying.

Tossing down her pen, she paced up and down the small cabin, rubbing her arms. Trapped, stifled, she wished she had never heard of Spain, Antonio Valdes, or Jago Barata.

She stopped, head bowed, staring at the wooden floor. She didn't mean it, not about Jago. In the short time she had known him he had caused her rage, frustration, jealousy – and unimagined happiness. He had transformed girlish dreams into a woman's desire, and kindled a spark of love that, no matter how starved of nourishment, or how low it burned, would never be extinguished.

Despite all the lacerating doubt and uncertainty, she could not regret that. Nor even if it were possible – would she want to go back to being who she was before she met him.

Once they returned to Falmouth her father could tell him the truth about her journey. Would he understand? Or would he reject her for her lack of trust? It would be too late then to change anything. In any case, he would return to his house, and the possessive arms of Louise Downing.

She tensed against knifing pain. Quickly wiping her eyes, she returned to the table.

Addressing the envelope to Ramon Gaudara, she folded the letter and slipped it into the envelope for safekeeping. Was the civil war the reason Jago was severing all his connections with Spain? That would still not explain his decision to sell his schooner.

As owner-master he could collect and deliver cargoes anywhere in the world. He was not confined to Spanish ports or waters. It did not make sense that he would sell the only vessel he owned outright.

Selling the silver refineries would bring him a large amount of money. What did he need it for? He had demanded and been given the post of senior captain with Bonython's. He would be sailing *Fair Maid* to the Azores in December at the start of the fruit season. His seamanship would ensure a fast passage and consequently a high price for his cargo. So *why?* And why *now?*

By dinnertime she had completed all the letters. After the meal, Jago returned with her to the cabin. She sat opposite him while he read each one. She, had worked hard on them and, considering how brief his notes and instructions had been, she was pleased with the result. But they were going out in his name, so it was his opinion that mattered.

When he had finished, he gave a brief nod and bent over the table to scrawl his signature at the bottom of each sheet.

Caseley wrapped her arms across her waist. She knew better than to expect gushing compliments, but could he not have managed a simple thank you? Disappointment vied with anger and her effort to mask both made her tone sharp.

'Am I to take it they are satisfactory?'

He looked round. 'Do you doubt your own ability?'

'I – no – but–'

He cut across her confusion. 'Then you must know they are exactly what I wanted.'

'Would it have cost you so much to say so?' Rising, she turned away. As tears pricked she was furious at her weakness. What was she, a child? Praise asked for had no value. She knew she had done a good job. That should have been enough.

'I'm ... sorry.' The word was uttered with difficulty as though unfamiliar to him.

Wearily she shook her head. 'It doesn't matter.' She waited for him to go. Instead he came up behind her. She could hear him breathing. *Don't touch me,* she prayed silently, her tongue paralysed by the knowledge that she wanted him to.

His hands, warm and heavy, clasped her shoulders. She caught her breath and her eyes closed. Slowly, deliberately, he turned her round.

She kept her eyes lowered.

'Caseley?'

She did not respond, terrified to meet his piercing gaze, all too aware that evasion was impossible, the truth would be there for him to read. Then what would she see in *his* eyes? Amusement? Irritation? *Pity?*

'Caseley, look at me?' he said softly.

She gave her head a tiny shake.

His hand came up and grasped her chin. Her skin burned beneath his fingers. She tried to pull away. His grip tightened.

'Look at me!' It was harsh, a command.

Her lashes lifted long enough for her to see his bearded face, his glittering eyes so frighteningly close, before tears splintered her vision.

He muttered an oath then his mouth came down on hers. He released her chin and his arms encircled her, drawing her against him.

Honed by the physical demands of handling a large schooner in all weathers, his hard-muscled body was unyielding but warm. His lips trailed fire across her cheek and down her throat, then returned to her mouth with a tenderness that spoke of iron control.

Caseley felt a strange contraction deep inside and liquid sweetness surged through her limbs. She drew in a long sobbing breath as her hands slid over his shoulders and into the thick hair curling on his neck.

Crushed against his chest, she could feel his

heart pounding, knew her own matched it. He released her mouth and as she rested her forehead on his shoulder, he laid his bearded jaw against her temple. His quick breathing feathered her ear. Her legs trembled uncontrollably. No matter what happens, she thought, I have had this moment.

'Caseley?' His voice was little more than a vibration.

'Yes?'

'Say my name.'

She opened her eyes.

He tilted her chin up with his forefinger. 'Say my name.'

'Jago.' She tested the syllables shyly, speaking them aloud for the first time. 'Jago.' She smiled.

He did not smile back. Stepping away, he slid his hands down her arms to grasp her fingers. 'Whatever happens in the next two days,' he raised her hands to his lips, kissed each one in turn, 'trust me.'

Caseley felt a dart of fear and a shudder rippled through her. Had he picked up her thoughts, or had she sensed his?

About to say more, instead he let her go. 'We should sight land in an hour. I want you to come topside. But you must stay beside me at the wheel. The wind is shifting and we'll have to change tack several times as we approach the harbour entrance.' He glanced at the barometer once more, frowning briefly. But when he looked at her, his expression softened. 'All right?'

Aware that his question had nothing to do with joining him on deck, she nodded. He left and she went into the sleeping cubicle to fetch the short

235

jacket that matched her skirt. Events were in motion over which she had no control. Yet strangely she felt calm. There had been no confiding, no explanations. Yet without a word being spoken their relationship had changed.

Leaning against the gunwale a few feet from Jago as the deck canted, Caseley was relieved to be on the higher side. With all sails full, the schooner drove through the water at speed, her fine stem cutting a path and tossing aside a foaming bow wave that bubbled and sparkled in the sunlight.

Wind and sea had changed since she was on deck earlier that morning. Busy with the letters, she had heard the grating clank of the steering chains, the squeal of ropes through blocks, and the loud rippling snap of sails refilling as the course changed. She had not registered their significance.

Now with time to look, she noticed that instead of coming from one side of the stern, the wind was blowing over the port beam. No longer a steady breeze, it was fitful and gusty.

The sea had dulled to pewter grey, and dark rolling masses of water streaked with foam surged towards them from the southwest.

Caseley glanced at Jago. Meeting her gaze he gave a small shrug. Clearly he had no idea what was brewing either. To her surprise Caseley found his honesty a comfort. A smile that pretended everything was fine would have been patronising as well as shutting her out to worry alone. Recalling his frown as he checked the barometer, she looked from sea to sky.

Though the sun still shone, it was through a fine

veil and a large ring encircled it. She knew that meant rain was on the way. The puffball clouds had become torn and ragged as they scudded across the filmy sky. A frisson of nervousness made her glad they would soon be safely in port.

The uneasiness gripping her now was different from that she had experienced earlier when Antonio Valdes came on deck. His eyes had darted from her to Jago and back. As bitter realisation thinned his lips to a tense white line, he had stumbled past her to the wheel-shelter.

She had adjusted to the increased pitching without even thinking about it. For Antonio Valdes, so sure of his invincibility, to have his advances spurned, his machinations foiled, and his *machismo* demolished by seasickness must be devastating.

Despite knowing that he would have used her for his own ends without a moment's hesitation, she still pitied him as he emerged from the lavatory, his colour a blotchy greenish-white as he wiped his mouth with a handkerchief clutched in trembling fingers.

It crossed her mind to offer help. But even before she intercepted Jago's warning glare, she abandoned the idea.

Not only had Antonio failed to sweep her off her feet, he recognised the bond between her and Jago. Though he had no idea of its significance, the fact that it existed rubbed salt into his wounded pride.

Having his seasickness exposed to their joint gaze made him a very dangerous man. Looking neither left nor right, his dignity in shreds, he staggered back to the companionway.

Jago beckoned to Caseley. 'You'll find Martin in the galley shack. Tell him to take an old bucket down to Valdes. By the look of him he won't make the stairs next time.'

The afternoon wore on. Nathan took over the wheel while Jago fetched the sextant and took sightings.

'See that double flash?' Caseley followed his pointing finger. 'That's the Caso Mayor lighthouse.'

'What's the one on this side?'

'Santa Marina Island. Our course will take us between two islands, Santa Marina and Mouro. The river curves round past Magdalena Beach and Puerto Chico up to the wharves of the main harbour.'

At teatime there was none of the leisurely pace and chatter of previous evenings. Caseley ate with Nathan, Jimbo, and Martin while Jago and Hammer remained on deck. Antonio Valdes did not appear.

Afterwards Caseley went to the cabin. Dragging her bag out she lifted it onto the bunk and felt among her clothes for the package. From now on it would be safer to keep it on her person. As her fingers closed around it she heard the door open. Her heart leapt into her throat.

'Caseley?' Jago's voice reached her through the drumming of blood in her ears. Lifting the short flared skirt of her jacket, she pushed the bulky envelope into her waistband, smoothing the material flat again.

'Yes?' Leaving the bag where it was, she emerged from the cubicle, unrolling her gabardine cape.

'What do you want that for? Are you cold?'

She shook her head. 'Not at the moment. But it may be chilly later when we go ashore.'

'Go ashore?' A frown drew his dark brows together.

'You said we would be in port this evening.'

'So we will.'

'Then I must go ashore and deliver the c – contract.'

'*Tonight?*' His gaze was shrewd, penetrating.

She nodded, swallowing to try and lubricate her dry throat. 'My father said Señor Spinoza wanted me to go to his house the moment we arrived.'

'Surely he meant during office hours? We will not be moored up much before eight. How can you be sure anyone will be there?'

She shrugged helplessly. 'I – my father said as soon as we arrive. I must follow his instructions. That is why I'm here.' Would he try to stop her? What would she do if he did?

He gazed at her for what felt like a long time. Her fingers tightened on the cape. 'Please, Jago. I have no choice.' She saw a muscle jump in his jaw then he inclined his head in a brief nod.

'All right, come up on deck. I don't want you out of my sight.'

She glanced at him but there was nothing romantic in the grim set of his mouth and narrowed eyes.

'One moment.' He caught her arm as she reached him in the doorway. 'What is the address where you are to meet this...'

'Señor Spinoza. I have it here in my pocket.' As

239

she felt for the folded scrap of paper her father had given her the evening before she left, her fingers brushed against the bulky shape of the package making it rustle. She felt heat flood her face and could not meet Jago's eyes as she passed him the address. *Please don't let him have heard.*

'What are you hiding, Caseley?' His quiet demand sent chills along her arms.

She had to tell him as much of the truth as she could without breaking her word to her father. 'I did not bring a purse or reticule with me, so I am carrying the contract in my waistband to leave my hands free for getting on and off the boat.'

His expression gave nothing away as he took the small piece of paper and Caseley folded the cape over her arm to occupy her trembling hands.

'I know this place,' he murmured. 'It's in the old town, not far from the harbour.'

She followed him up the stairs, taking up her position on the port quarter as he reclaimed the wheel. The setting sun was hidden behind a mass of grey and violet cloud and the sky had an eerie yellowish hue. Though it wasn't cold she felt gooseflesh erupt on her arms.

Ahead loomed the Spanish coast. In the fading light Caseley could just see purple mountains rising behind the smaller hills over which spread the town of Santander.

At Jago's command, Nathan and Hammer lowered the large foresail while Jimbo took in the flying jib. Next the square topsail was hauled up and the staysail dropped. *Cygnet* was now in the river. Shielded from the wind by rolling hills, the water was calmer.

240

Their progress had slowed and Martin was in the bow, checking the depth of the channel with a marked and weighted line, singing out the fathoms as the schooner made her way upriver.

'Why is he doing that?' Caseley asked.

'We're going in on an ebb tide,' Jago said, 'and the river has a lot of shifting sandbanks.'

'Wouldn't it have been safer to take on a pilot?'

'Anchor in the bay and wait until morning? Possibly. But I know this river well and I want to get home as quickly as you do.'

She stayed silent after that. Her fingers strayed to the package at her waist. She wanted to be rid of it as soon as possible. Naturally she wanted to see her father again, to watch his face as she told him she had done as he asked, and the documents had been safely delivered. But then what? What was there for her to look forward to?

Why was Jago so anxious to get back? He had his father's quicksilver to trans-ship – and there was also his house. He had only seen it once. He would want to see for himself how she had spent his money. And of course there was Louise.

Where do I stand in all that, Caseley wondered. She had refused to do any further work on the house. Jago had said Louise would not bother her any more. But he had not said he would give her up. If he did not, then the kisses that moved her so deeply, the attraction, antipathy, respect, dislike, admiration, and fury he stirred in her, had meant nothing to him. She was no more than a passing fancy.

Doubts crept in, quiet as cats, and tore at her with unsheathed claws. What did she have to

241

offer a man as well travelled, as sophisticated and knowledgeable as Jago Barata?

It was almost dark when they reached the harbour. Huddled in the warm folds of her cape, Caseley watched as Jago guided the schooner in alongside one of the quays lit by brightly burning lamps. He ordered Jimbo to make fast the stern line only. The seaman leapt ashore, apparently unsurprised.

She caught Nathan's sleeve. But he only grinned as the bow drifted out and, caught by the current, swung the schooner round to face down river once more. Jimbo trotted down the quay, ready to catch the bowline Hammer threw to him.

'Why did J – the captain do that?' she asked quietly.

'To save time,' the mate explained. 'Skipper said we might want to get away quick.'

Once *Cygnet* was securely moored, Caseley looked expectantly at Jago and started towards the midsection of the schooner, ready to disembark. His hand shot out and caught her arm before she could take a second step.

'No one leaves this vessel until the cargo has been unloaded and the quicksilver brought aboard and stowed below.' He looked over Caseley's shoulder. 'That includes you, Valdes.'

'Enough of this foolishness,' Antonio snapped. 'You cannot keep me here against my will.'

'Nor do I wish to.' Jago was perfectly calm. 'But you have been ill. You are still weak and, I believe, feverish. A few hours' rest while we unload will help you recover. Believe me, señor, I have no wish to detain you. Jimbo, escort Señor Valdes to

242

his cabin.' He walked away before the Spaniard could draw breath to argue.

'This way, sir.' Jimbo's gesture was polite, but his eyes were alert and his strong stocky body was twice the width of Antonio's slender frame.

To Caseley's surprise, instead of storming off in a rage, Antonio shrugged in apparent acceptance.

'I'm going to find the wharfinger,' Jago told Nathan. 'We'll get no help at this time of night. But the space is booked and paid for so he can't refuse to open the warehouse. Set up the winch and start unloading onto the quay.'

'Let me go with you,' Caseley pleaded softly. 'I can deliver the contract and be back on board before the men have finished unloading. Then I won't delay departure.'

Jago's glare froze her. 'Have you taken leave of your senses? You want me to let you go off into town, alone, at this time of night?' A harsh whisper, his voice vibrated with impatience. 'In the name of all that's holy, you live in a port. How could you be stupid enough to suggest such a thing?'

'Then send one of the men with me. I–'

'They are all needed here.' He bit the words off. 'When the work is completed, *I* will take you to deliver this contract. Until then, you stay right where you are.' He sprang onto the gunwale then leapt onto the quay. Striding quickly towards a row of warehouses, he disappeared into a shadowed alley between two of them.

Chapter Seventeen

Caseley leaned over the schooner's side and looked down into the black oily water. In the lamplight she saw a rainbow broken by bits of cork and frayed rope floating on the surface as water slopped between the quay and *Cygnet's* hull. She shivered.

Even with two sound feet she would be wary of jumping that gap. It wasn't very wide. But the schooner was riding two feet below the quay and the top of the gunwale was narrow, wet, and slippery. Hampered by her long skirts, it would be all too easy to slip and find herself trapped between the wooden hull and stone quay, unable to climb, up and no one able to reach her as filthy black water filled her nose and mouth, dragging her down...

'Beg pardon, miss?' Nathan said, and she looked up gratefully. 'Mind brewing up a nice cuppa tea, would you? Only Mart got to help getting the hatches off, and all.'

'No, Mr Ferris, I don't mind at all. I'd be glad to.' Had it been the mate's idea or Jago's to keep her occupied? She rubbed her hands. 'It seems colder all of a sudden.'

'Weather's changing.' He lifted his head to sniff the wind. 'That there sunset was a warning. We'll have some blow in the next day or two.' He grinned at her. 'You get that tea, and I'll see about

244

this here cargo.'

Caseley filled the kettle from the fresh water tank and set it on the stove in the galley shack after stirring up the fire. Then she went below to the day room to fetch more tea for the tin, and the condensed milk. Closing the day room door behind her she turned towards the stairs and gasped.

'Oh! You startled me.'

Standing in the doorway of his cabin, Antonio Valdes watched her. 'So,' he said softly, as he looked her up and down. 'I was too late.'

Unease battled anger and Caseley felt warmth flush her throat and cheeks. 'Please excuse me, Señor Valdes, I am busy.' She took a step towards the stairs but he blocked her path.

'Is he a good lover?' His mocking tone insinuated otherwise.

'I ... he is not my lover,' she blurted in shock, then wished she had not spoken as he raised disbelieving eyebrows. Even discussing it with Valdes, she was playing into his hands.

He shrugged. 'My apologies, señorita. Perhaps you do not like men.'

'I do not like men who insult my intelligence, señor,' she retorted. 'Nor do I like men who pretend feelings they do not have.'

'You suggest I am guilty of this?'

'Can you deny it?'

He smiled with disarming candour. 'I underestimated you, señorita. I do not encounter many women whose brains match their beauty.'

'Then perhaps you should review your choice of company. Now if you would kindly step aside, Mr Ferris is expecting me on deck.'

He did not move. 'Señorita, I beg you, listen to me. Do not risk more danger. Give me the package. I will ensure it reaches those who have the best interests of my country at heart.'

So there it was. Out in the open at last. There could be no more doubt about the true nature of his interest. Caseley frowned in puzzlement.

'Señor, I am sorry if the recent troubles have cost your family money. But I do not think one contract for the transport of iron ore will restore their fortunes. Please excuse me.'

His hand fastened around her upper arm. Fear flooded through her as rage and frustration contorted his face.

'Let go of me.' Somehow she held her voice steady though her stomach was knotting painfully. *Please somebody come.* If Valdes became violent there was little she could do to defend herself.

'You think you are so clever,' he hissed, lapsing into Spanish. 'Don't you see, you are playing right into his hands? Jago Barata is a half-breed. He does not live in Spain. His father fled to Mexico to avoid the troubles. What are the morals and loyalties of such a man? He has left the ship, no? Where is he now? You do not know. Who is he with? What are they planning?

'I have followed that package from Mexico. I care about the future of my country. The monarchy must be restored and Don Carlos must establish a new dynasty.' Saliva had gathered at the corners of his mouth, and his eyes had the feverish glitter of a fanatic. 'Spain needs his strength and his courage. Give me the package, now!'

Booted feet clanged on the stairs and Jago appeared. There was icy anger in his narrowed gaze. 'Take your hand off her.' He turned. 'The men are waiting for their tea, Caseley. See to it, will you?' he said evenly.

She glanced from one to the other then ran up the stairs. As she reached the top she heard a fist connect with flesh, a sharp cry, then a muffled thud. Her pleasure at Antonio Valdes's punishment was unladylike and deplorable. She ought to feel guilty. But she didn't.

Hurrying to the galley shack she looked over her shoulder and saw Jago emerge from the companionway, sucking his knuckles. He did not even glance in her direction but went straight to the winch, sending Hammer onto the dockside to roll the barrels to the warehouse after Martin had unloaded them from the net.

Caseley carried out mugs of tea and the last of the cake. Nathan, who had been on the winch rope with Jago, called Jimbo up from the hold and beckoned Martin and Hammer back on board. While the men talked softly, sipping and chewing, Jago took Caseley to one side.

'We won't be finished for several hours. Drink your tea, then go below and get some sleep.' He didn't give her a chance to protest. 'There's nothing you can do to help. I'll call you the instant the hatches are battened down. You have my word.' Still she hesitated, but his next words convinced her.

'I have no wish to frighten you, but it's likely we'll run into bad weather on our return trip. You'll get little rest then. Make the most of this chance.' It made sense.

'And, Caseley?' She looked up. 'Lock the door.'

A brisk tapping woke her from a fitful sleep. She had not removed any of her clothes, so it took her only moments to refasten her skirt and button her jacket. Pausing only to slip her feet into her shoes, she hurried to unlock the door.

Jago stood on the threshold. 'Ready?'

'I just need a moment.' She turned to re-enter the sleeping cubicle, limping badly, wishing there was time to wash her face and clean her teeth. Tendrils of her hair had escaped the confining net and curled on her forehead and in front of her ears.

'Put on your cape. We must go at once.'

Slinging the cape over her arm she returned to the day room, tucking her wayward hair back into the net. 'What's happened? What's wrong?' Her ankle turned again and she winced.

'Are you all right?'

She nodded quickly. 'It's just my foot. It's always stiff when I first get up. It will be fine in a moment.'

'Are you sure?'

She sensed there was more behind the question than concern for her comfort.

'Yes, truly. It's better already.' She put her weight on it, rocking back and forward as she checked that the package was secure in her waistband. 'Now, please tell me what's wrong?'

'Valdes has gone. I didn't expect– But when I sent Hammer down to check, he'd disappeared. Did you hear anything?'

Caseley shook her head. 'Does it matter?' He must have accepted that she wasn't going to betray any information concerning the documents. 'Perhaps he has returned to his family.'

'Not yet. He hasn't given up, Caseley. We don't know where he is or how many friends he may have locally. So, yes, it matters.'

She bent her head, pretending to fasten her cape, knowing her fiery blush must give her away.

'Come on.' He put his hand under her elbow. 'Let us finish this charade.' His tone was unexpectedly bitter and she dared not look at him.

She felt sick with a fear that had nothing to do with the dangers attached to delivering the package. If Jago knew what it contained – if he hated her for not trusting him – she wrenched her thoughts away. She had a job to do for her father, the most important job of her life. Focus on that. Forget everything else.

As they crossed the deck, Caseley saw that *Cygnet's* gunwale was just above the level of the quay. She noticed Martin filling an iron cooking pot with water and marvelled at the boy's stamina. He had worked alongside the men all night and was now preparing breakfast.

But where were the others? She was about to ask when Jago called her name sharply from the quay. She scrambled onto the barrel he had placed as a step. He held out his hands and she grasped them as she put her feet on the gunwale and jumped down onto the quay, automatically taking her most of her weight on her sound foot.

He kept hold of her hand and she ran to keep up with him as they quickly crossed the deserted wharves, weaving between silent sheds and warehouses.

They left the harbour area and as they turned onto a cobbled street that climbed towards a small, whitewashed church with a square tower, dawn was breaking.

Tall, flat-walled houses with oblong windows and small iron balconies bright with geraniums lined both sides of the street. But the height of the buildings filled the narrow thoroughfare with shadows. Dark doorways and alleys between the houses resembled gaping mouths.

Caseley slipped on the damp stones. Jago's grip stopped her falling. In the momentary silence as she regained her balance and flexed her foot, she heard a soft slithering on the cobbles behind her. She looked round quickly but could see nothing in the gloom. Her throat was tight and dry.

'Someone is following us,' she whispered.

He did not appear surprised, merely nodding briefly. 'It's not far now. Once we reach the church—'

Whatever words of comfort he had intended to offer remained unspoken as he glanced over his shoulder.

The sound of soft laughter from higher up the hill made them look forward again and Jago clasped her hand tighter.

'Sitting ducks.' Antonio Valdes regarded them with malicious pleasure as he and another man came slowly down the hill towards them.

A chuckle from behind them made Caseley whirl round and she clutched Jago's hand as fear bloomed inside her. Two more men were coming up the hill.

All three wore heavy dark trousers that ended

just below the knee, coarse stockings criss-crossed with leather thongs, and crude shoes. They had dark waistcoats over their shirts, loosely knotted scarves or kerchiefs at their throats, and on their heads the bright red woollen *boina* of the Carlist cause.

Jago drew Caseley towards him. 'They will try to separate us,' he warned.

Fear had robbed her of speech. She had never imagined Valdes would go to such lengths. How naïve, how foolish she had been. She could feel Jago's heartbeat against her back, slow and steady. His body was tense and one arm encircled her waist.

'Get the girl,' Valdes growled.

The men were closing in, moving forward slowly and relentlessly. Now she could see they were carrying short staves. Their eyes gleamed with savage excitement. Swarthy and unshaven, they grinned as they slapped the wooden clubs against dirty hands. She could smell their stale sweat.

'Once you've got it,' one whispered hoarsely to Valdes in heavily accented Spanish, 'what about her?'

He shrugged. 'Do as you like.'

'No,' she whispered, pressing back against Jago, raw fear turning her blood to ice water and her legs to jelly.

She felt Jago fumble at his belt and saw the flash of a blade as he held his hand low and slightly away from his body. He turned his head quickly, gauging which of the two pairs were nearer, then gave a piercing whistle. Thrusting Caseley behind him, he lunged with lightning speed at the two

251

men on the lower side.

Neither was prepared for the sudden attack. One slipped on the damp cobbles and fell backwards. As Jago caught the other a sweeping blow, the man yelled in pain, dropped his club, and clutched his arm. His shirtsleeve turned red and wet, and blood oozed between his fingers and dripped onto the cobbles.

The man who had fallen scrambled to his feet and lunged forward as Antonio darted towards Caseley.

'Take Barata,' he panted to the man beside him and seized Caseley's arm, trying to dodge the punches she was aiming at his head and shoulders. She kicked at his shins but was hampered by her skirt and petticoats. Terrified, she fought with all her strength as he tried to wrench her away from Jago.

Then she heard the sound of running feet and the sickening thud of fist on flesh. Valdes released his hold.

'Don't you fret, my 'andsome. We'll see the buggers off,' Nathan grinned and pitched into the battle.

Leaning against the wall, Caseley dragged in sobbing breaths and tried to control the trembling that racked her. The three Basques were wielding their clubs with horrific ferocity. They weren't defending themselves. They wanted to kill.

But Hammer, Jimbo, and Nathan were no easy prey. Using only fists and razor-sharp reflexes that allowed them to duck the blows, they quickly disarmed the attackers. Then they separated them.

Jago had re-sheathed his knife and as Hammer reeled back after taking a fist to his temple, Jago felled the Basque with a right cross, followed by a left hook. The man's head snapped back and he was unconscious before he hit the cobbles.

Aside from the quiet order from Antonio and the Basque's query about what to do with her, the incident had taken place in silence. Though the fighting was vicious, apart from gasped breaths, grunts as a fist landed, and the scuffle of feet on the cobbles, there was little noise.

A hand closed around her ankle and Caseley choked back a scream. Looking down, she saw Antonio Valdes sprawled at her feet. He twisted his head to peer up at her, his narrow face contorted in a smile that radiated malice.

'You stupid bitch. You think you've won? How do you intend to get back to England?' His weak laugh became a cough.

Caseley stared at him for a moment. *Cygnet.* Martin was alone on the schooner. Rage filled her. Stamping on his wrist, she wrenched her ankle free then bent and slapped his smiling face with all her strength. The force of her blow split his lip and smashed his head against the cobbles. She ran to Jago.

'The boat,' she gasped, dragging him free. 'Valdes has done something to *Cygnet.*'

Jago didn't ask questions. 'Nathan, get back to the wharf as fast as you can. Martin's in trouble.'

Seizing Caseley's arm he hurried her up the street, past the church and into an alley. Halfway along there was a heavy wooden door studded with iron nails. To one side a rope led through a

253

small hole in the stone archway surrounding the door. Jago tugged it hard.

The wait seemed interminable but was probably no more than half a minute. The door opened to reveal a short plump man with receding hair dressed in dark clothes.

'Señor Spinoza, please,' she said quickly. 'I am Caseley Bonython. My father is Teuder Bonython, the consul for Mexico. But he is unwell and could not come himself. This is Jago Barata, my father's senior captain.'

Stepping back, the man gestured for them to enter and closed the massive door. They followed him across a small courtyard then through a maze of cool passages, finally emerging into a wide hall. Opening a door on the far side, the man ushered them into a spacious, book-lined study containing a huge carved desk, a brass-topped hexagonal table and several leather armchairs.

'Señor Spinoza will be with you shortly.' He inclined his head politely and would have left had Caseley not clutched his arm.

'Please ask him to hurry. We must get back to the harbour. We were attacked on our way here and–'

Gently detaching her hand, he glanced from her to Jago then walked out.

Chapter Eighteen

As Caseley withdrew the crushed, wrinkled package from her waistband, the door opened. The man who entered was about sixty, tall and gaunt, and wore a full-length belted robe of crimson quilted silk with a white silk scarf knotted like a cravat at his throat.

Seeing the silver hair, small goatee beard, and the fine-boned aristocratic features of a grandee, Caseley was shaken. He was exactly as she had imagined Señor Rodriguez. The other man remained near the door, silent and watchful.

'Señor Spinoza?' Caseley asked the tall man.

He nodded. 'You have something for me?' His tone was polite, but Caseley noticed he had not bothered with greetings.

At her hesitation Jago muttered, 'For God's sake, Caseley, give it to him so we can get out of here.'

She glanced at him, holding the package tightly, feeling its altered thickness. Remembering her father's instructions, that she was only to hand over the documents if she was told the name of the place where the young king was, she moistened her lips.

'I believe you have visited England, sir,' she said.

He smiled slightly. 'I did, many years ago. I have a young acquaintance at Sandhurst Military

Academy. He is staying with one of the instructors whose address is One, The Terrace. Apparently it is known as Tea Caddy Row, though I have yet to discover why.'

Caseley offered the crumpled envelope and the thin man took it. But when he saw it was already open his face changed and as he raised his eyes to hers she glimpsed steel beneath the velvet courtesy.

'I beg your pardon, sir. I had to be certain.' Turning away, she withdrew the second envelope with its distinctive and unbroken seal from within her blouse. Her shaking fingers fumbled as she refastened the buttons.

'You are your father's daughter,' the thin man said.

Jago placed an impatient hand on the small of her back. 'Forgive us, sir, but we must hurry.' He propelled her towards the door.

'Please accept our sincere thanks, Miss Bony-thon. You also, Captain Barata. *Vaya con Dios.*'

As they raced back to the harbour, she was so relieved to have honoured her promise and delivered the package, she assumed Jago's silence was due to concern for Martin and the others.

Though she ran as fast as she could, her uneven gait and the slippery cobbles would have caused her to fall more than once but for his firm grip on her hand.

Her breath burned in her throat, her heart pounded, and she could not suck enough air into her lungs. Beneath the heavy cape and fitted jacket her cotton blouse and shift clung to her skin as perspiration beaded her back and trickled between

256

her breasts. Again she stumbled, and once more he pulled her upright and forced her to keep running.

People were beginning to appear and paused to stare with mingled curiosity and suspicion. But none got in their way. A swift glance at his set features convinced Caseley he would simply have knocked aside anyone who tried to stop them.

The sun had risen. But instead of the pastel shades of a mellow autumn morning, low grey clouds with flame-tipped ragged edges filled the eastern sky.

They passed the warehouses and reached the wharf. As they rounded the corner Caseley saw black smoke belching from *Cygnet's* wheel shelter. She was too breathless to speak. But Jago cursed with bitter fluency as they covered the last few yards and saw Martin, his face smeared with soot and tears, helping Hammer hurl buckets of water onto the flames.

The staysail was set. Jimbo and Nathan, their faces contorted in effort, were hauling on the mainsail halyards, but the weight of the gaff and enormous canvas sail was too much for them.

Catching sight of Jago and Caseley, Nathan yelled to Jimbo to cast off. Hopping nimbly onto the quay, Jimbo loosed the bow line. Jago swept Caseley up into his arms and threw her over the gunwale. Then, waving Jimbo back on board, he cast off the stern line himself and jumped the widening gap between quay and ship.

Lifting Caseley to her feet, he took her hands and wrapped them around the polished spokes of the wheel.

'Head her into the channel,' he pointed. 'Aim for

that buoy.' Then leaving her he hurried forward bellowing, 'All hands to the mainsail! Martin, put that bloody fire out!'

Caseley clung to the wheel. Still breathless and shaking from their headlong dash, she didn't have time to worry about the enormity of the task Jago had set her.

She glanced shoreward. Men were gathering on the quay. Was Antonio there? She couldn't see him. Nor did she recognise the men who had attacked them. Under the staysail, the schooner was drawing away from the quay. The menace in the crowd's silent watching made her throat close and she swallowed. Then smoke drifted across, obscuring the scene and she quickly looked ahead.

With Jago and Nathan on one rope, Jimbo and Hammer on the other, the four men hoisted the peak and throat halyards controlling the inner and outer edges of the sail, hauling on them evenly to send up the gaff to which the edge of the sail was laced, parallel to the boom.

The rhythmic squeal of blocks and rattle of mast hoops finally stopped. Jago passed the throat halyard under a cleat to hold it fast, while Nathan threw his full weight on the taut rope to pull the edge of the sail nearest the mast up tight. Nathan's effort enabled Jago to take in a few more inches of rope. When the throat halyard was finally secured, Hammer and Jimbo swiftly hoisted the peak, made it fast then coiled the loose ends of rope over the belaying pins. Not a word had been spoken.

Jimbo ran forward to trim the staysail and hoist the jib as Hammer and Nathan scrambled aft once more to help Martin who was working feverishly while sobbing with shock and exhaustion.

Jago eased out the mainsheet. The boom swung to starboard and the sail filled. Caseley felt new weight on the helm. Clenching her teeth so hard that they ached, she eased the wheel over. Cygnet responded. Bowsprit pointing towards the river mouth, the schooner surged forward.

Caseley could hear a low crackling, and felt the heat through the back of the wheel shelter. Thick smoke and choking fumes billowed from the open door as the man drew bucket after bucketful of water from over the side and hurled it into the paint store.

Gulls screamed overhead and further down the river brightly painted fishing boats scurried back to the protection of Puerto Chico, the little harbour.

Caseley's knuckles were white as her grip on the spokes tightened. Everyone else was making for shelter. They were heading for the open sea and the approaching storm.

They had no choice. She knew that. Had they stayed in port – it did not bear thinking about.

'I reckon we've beat the bugger,' Jimbo yelled in triumph, his sweating blackened face appearing round the wheel shelter.

The smoke was thinner, paler now it was mixed with steam, and the voracious crackling had stopped. But the fumes still caught in the throat, and were joined by the acrid stench of charred wood and burnt paint.

Jago came to the wheel. 'I'll take it now.' His tone was curt and he didn't look at her as she stepped aside.

'Hammer, see what can be salvaged,' he shouted over his shoulder. 'Chuck the rest overboard. Nathan, you and Jimbo set the lower topsail, then the foresail and secure all hatches. Martin,' he beckoned the boy forward. 'What happened?'

Caseley leaned against the shoulder board, massaging the stiffness from her fingers as she listened.

Martin's eyes were red-rimmed and bloodshot, his face and clothes smeared with oily soot. Wiping his nose on the back of his hand, he shifted from foot to foot.

'I was in the galley when they came,' his voice was hoarse, rasping from the smoke. 'Three of 'em there was. One had blood all down his arm. They had torches. I went for your gun, Cap'n. I – I thought it would scare 'em off.' He rubbed one bare grimy foot against the other.

'How else could you have defended the ship?' Jago said calmly. 'You were here alone.'

A smile lit the boy's weary face. 'Gave 'em some shock, I did. They didn't expect that.' His expression clouded. 'One was trying to burn through the bow mooring line. Another had just throwed his torch down the fo'c'sle. That's when I fired. I got 'n in the leg.' He faltered.

'Good.' Jago nodded. 'What was the third man doing?'

'Trying to smash the day room skylight. But when he seen me coming, he kicked the door of the paint store and chucked his torch in. Then he jumped back on the wharf with the others. Laughing they was – not the one I shot. He was on the ground. I didn't know what to do first what with smoke coming out of the paint store *and* the fo'c'sle. I thought of all our clothes and gear down there–' he stopped.

'Good lad. Fire is far more dangerous below deck than above.'

'But by the time I'd put 'n out the paint store was well alight. Soon as they bast– Basques,' he corrected quickly, his gaze darting to Caseley, 'seen Jimbo and Hammer come back they took off, dragging their mate with 'em. Jimbo told me to keep going with the buckets while they made ready to leave soon as you got here.'

'Where was Nathan?'

'He come just a couple of minutes later with bags of fresh bread rolls and oranges. He said we wouldn't have time for revittling, so he'd took care of it.'

Jago grasped the boy's thin shoulder. 'I'm proud of you, Martin. You showed great courage and presence of mind.' The boy shrugged and shuffled his feet, but the dirt on his face could not hide his blush of pride. 'Where did you put my gun?'

'He's over there, Cap'n, on the hatch cover.'

'Put it away, then clean yourself up and turn in for a couple of hours.'

'I'm all right, Cap'n.'

'Do as you're told, boy. I'll need you later.'

'Aye, sir.' Martin shambled forward to collect the gun, rubbing his eyes, his mouth opening in a wide yawn.

'Jago?' Caseley said. 'Shall I make tea?'

He nodded briefly, checked the sails and compass then glanced over his shoulder to see how

Hammer was doing. Looking anywhere, Caseley realised, but at her. 'While you're in the galley,' he added, 'see if the oatmeal can be salvaged.'

She hesitated, wanting to ask him what was wrong.

'Go on, then,' he snapped. 'What are you waiting for?'

Stung by his tone, she turned to the companionway, fumbling with the fastening on her cape. He was tired. They all were, but responsibility for the ship and crew rested squarely on his shoulders. Her presence had been an added burden.

But they had both achieved what they had set out to do – he had his cargo, she had delivered the package – so why was he so angry? Was he blaming her for the attack?

As she thought about it she realised he had every right. Had she not been aboard it would not have happened. *Yes, it would.* Whoever had carried those documents would have been a target. Had her father been fit enough to make the journey himself Antonio Valdes would have employed different tactics. But the objective would have been the same.

Roughly folding her cape, she wedged it behind the chocks on which the dinghy rested. She was too hot and sticky to wear it and it would be awkward in the galley. But there wasn't time to take it below and she didn't want it blown away.

The wind whined and moaned in the rigging. As another gust caught her, Caseley felt its force like a giant hand on her back and was glad to reach the shelter of the shack.

She lifted the lidded iron pot from the stove top

and put it on the zinc sheet on the floor. Then she riddled out some of the ashes, fed a few sticks and some more coal into the stove, and opened the damper to coax a flame from the glowing embers.

Taking the kettle she went out, holding tightly to anything within reach as the deck heaved under her feet. The fresh water tank was just over half full. Thank heaven Martin had reacted so quickly. Had the water been contaminated or the tank punctured, they would have had to put into one of the French ports. It might have been days before they could leave. And Jago was anxious to get home.

At the back of her mind, warning bells were ringing. Something wasn't right. But the harder she tried to fathom what it was, the more it eluded her.

Back in the galley she set the kettle within the fiddle rails to boil, then crouched and lifted the lid off the iron cooking pot. Inside a thick, black tarry substance coated the sides and bottom. That must have been the source of the smoke.

She gritted her teeth and scraped loose as much as she could then lurched across to the rail with the pot.

'What are you doing?' Jago demanded.

'It's burnt,' she shouted back and tipped the mess into the dark rolling water, momentarily dizzy as it came up towards her then fell steeply away. Turning, she crossed to the fresh-water tank, but before she could draw the dipper out, Jago shouted again.

'Have you no sense? You use seawater for a job like that.' He sounded furious.

Caseley flushed. 'I'm sorry. I didn't–'

'Think? That seems to be a habit of yours. Don't just stand there, get some food ready.'

She flinched. There was no teasing note to take the sting out of his criticism, only barbed impatience. He *meant* to hurt.

Caseley turned away, catching Nathan's eye. He winked in sympathy. But his expression turned harder and puzzled as he glanced towards the man at the wheel. He grabbed a bucket with a rope tied to the handle and swung it over the lee side, drawing it up full.

'Here you are, miss.' He set it on the deck be the galley doorway. 'You'll find a tin of sand just inside there. Use a handful or two on a cloth. Scour it out 'andsome, that will.'

'Thank you. Nathan...' she hesitated. 'Can I ask you something?'

The mate regarded her steadily. 'Depends.'

She recognised the warning. She could ask, but he might not answer. 'I've never been at sea in a storm. I know it's going to get worse, and I'm sure J– the captain knows exactly what he's doing, but...' she glanced nervously at the straining sails.

Nathan followed her gaze, and his stern expression softened. 'Think we're carrying too much canvas, do you?'

Caseley looked at the iron pot and shrugged. 'Like I said, I don't–'

'Nathan!' Jago bellowed.

The mate ignored him. 'The minute the skipper sees the wind driving her head under, we only got to release the ropes from they pins and the sails will drop. There's far more danger in being

264

close to shore in a storm. So he's making sea-room before the wind get too strong and we have to reef down.'

'Nathan, get over here!'

The mate lifted his head, his ruddy features tightening. 'Aye, *sir.*' She wasn't alone in finding Jago's hostile behaviour unusual.

The kettle boiled. Despite the sand, it was going to take time to get the pot clean, so Caseley put it aside and made the tea. Leaving it to brew, she collected her cape and went towards the companionway, clutching at the hatch cover and skylight for support.

'Given up already?' Jago snorted.

She winced and a lump formed in her throat, making it ache. Why was he doing this? She opened the hatch door and latched it back. 'I'm going to fetch the milk and some jam for the rolls.' She looked at him over her shoulder. 'Do you want yours in the mess, or would you prefer it where you are?'

His gaze held hers for a moment and in his smoky eyes she saw self-loathing and a plea. Startled, she felt her heart contract. Immediately he looked away.

'Everyone stays on deck.'

Cold and distant, his tone was totally at odds with the powerful emotions she had just glimpsed.

Retrieving the rolls, Caseley split and spread them with jam, then poured the tea. Unable to fill the mugs more than halfway without the tea slopping over the rim, she realised with growing dread that the sea was much rougher. Setting the mugs and the plate of rolls on a battered tray, she made her way carefully aft.

Working in the snug warmth of the shack, she had managed to shut everything out, clinging for comfort to the normality of domestic chores. But out on deck ink-dark seas loomed over the gunwale. Spindrift fogged the air. The wind tore at her hair and clothes as the first drops of rain splashed into her face.

She glanced up, gasping as a wall of foam-streaked water bore down on them. The stern lifted and Caseley staggered, crying out as the tray tilted and the mugs began to slide. But Nathan reached her just in time and grabbed the tray as the sea passed beneath them.

'All right, miss. I got 'n.' He grinned. She tried to smile back but her mouth wouldn't respond. Though she told herself there was no need to be frightened, that the crew were experienced sailors who regularly faced storms like this, her body wasn't listening. Her throat was dry, her skin dewed with the sweat of fear. She shivered as her heart galloped.

Nathan shouted to Hammer and Jimbo. Dressed in oilskins and sou'westers, they skittered along the canting deck, brightening at the sight of food.

'Take a mug down to the boy, shall I, skipper?' Jimbo said through a mouthful of bread and jam.

Jago nodded and, swallowing his tea in two gulps, replaced his mug on the tray Nathan held and took a roll. 'Hammer, fetch my oilskins, and Nathan's while you're down there. Where are you going?' he demanded as Caseley followed Hammer towards the companionway and Nathan took the tray back to the galley.

'For my cape,' she pointed, glancing at the darkening sky.

He shook his head. 'Go below.'

'But what about dinner?'

'Martin will see to it. That's his job.'

Something snapped. Not stopping to consider the consequences of matching his anger with her own, Caseley whirled round as large raindrops fell onto her unprotected head and soaked into her jacket.

'If you tell him to, Martin will cook dinner, tend the fires, help on deck, and work until he drops. He would die sooner than let you down. But he's totally exhausted. If you put him to work now he's quite likely to have an accident. That may not bother you, but I'm not prepared to have it on *my* conscience.'

She paused only to take a breath, her chin high. 'No passengers, you said. *I* can cook. *I'll* make dinner.' Turning her back on him she limped furiously towards the galley, clinging to the rigging as the schooner pitched and rolled.

'Miss Bonython!'

The icy rage in his voice froze her and apprehension shuddered down her spine. Yet though every nerve was stretched tight, she turned and met his gaze.

'*You* dare lecture *me* about conscience?'

'I want to help, that's all.' Head down, she dived into the galley. Sinking down onto the little stool she closed her eyes. Never in her life had she spoken to anyone like that. Nor had she ever seen such anger directed at her. She loved him and hated him, and it was tearing her apart.

267

She pressed her fingers hard against her forehead and sucked in a deep sobbing breath. Then she reached for the cooking pot and another handful of sand.

Chapter Nineteen

Cygnet drove on through steepening seas. Focused on each task, Caseley took no notice of the rain lashing the roof of the little shack or the water washing over the schooner's deck. She heard orders shouted, the thud of running feet, the rattle of blocks and mast hoops, and the clacking of the patent reefing gear as the fore and mainsails were reefed down.

Having got the pot clean, she needed fresh water to rinse it out and prepare the vegetables. But her cape was still jammed behind the dinghy, and without some form of protection she would be soaked to the skin in seconds.

Looking round the cramped galley she found a piece of old sail canvas. It was stiff and smelly but would have to do.

Holding it over her head and shoulders with one hand, she screwed up her eyes against the driving rain and stumbled out to the tank.

The wind shrieked, whipping the tops off the waves so the air was full of salt spray. The rain was so heavy and the cloud so low, it was impossible to tell where sea ended and sky began.

She struggled back to the galley, water streaming

down her face and the canvas to soak into her long skirt. She set the bucket down and immediately half of it slopped onto her shoes and ran over the floor. Rinsing the pot twice she threw the water down-wind out of the door, then lurched outside again to the salt beef barrel.

The smell of the meat made her feel sick. As she fought nausea, swallowing hard, she considered abandoning her attempt to cook a meal. The men would understand. They knew she had no experience of conditions like this. No one would think any the worse of her. They were probably amazed she had stuck at it so long.

Clinging to the barrel as the deck heaved and dropped beneath her feet, she recalled Jago's bitter taunt. 'Given up already?' That had been an hour ago. It had got much worse since then.

'Damn you,' she whispered as the rain hammered onto her back. Slamming the lid back onto the barrel, she fastened it down with fumbling fingers then, clutching the chunk of gritty fat-marbled beef, slithered back to the shack.

She made up the fire once more, deeply grateful for its crackling warmth. Hunched on the tiny stool, a chopping board on her knees, she cut up the meat, potatoes, onion, and turnip and scraped it all into the deep pot, covered it with fresh water, and jammed on the lid.

She rinsed and wiped her hands on a scrap of towel, fitted extra guard rails round the stove top to prevent the pot sliding off, then peered out of the doorway, clinging to the frame.

The seas were white and breaking. The topsails had been taken in, so had the aft gaff. The schooner was running with the reefed foresail and the staysail.

As the bow reared, two figures, oilskins slick with rain and spray, struggled to loosen the foresail halyards. The wet ropes had contracted and were wire-taut. The schooner climbed, the reefed sail filled with a deafening clap, and the staysail split.

Feet pounded forward along the deck. In the flying spray Caseley could just make out two figures releasing ropes and hauling in the tattered sail while a third unlatched the scuttle to dive below to the locker for the spare.

Salt stung her eyes and burned her face. Petrified, she could only cling to the doorframe. How long could *Cygnet* take such punishment?

A mountainous sea toppled aboard just in front of the mainmast and washed down the foredeck, swirling round the windlass in a welter of foam, reaching the knees of the men working frantically to free the torn sail.

One of the men slipped and fell, hitting his head on the windlass as he went down. Caseley's hand flew to her mouth and she choked back a scream of panic.

Working with desperate urgency to free the split sail so a replacement could be bent on, the man in front hadn't noticed. His mate lay face down in the water that streamed across the deck and out of the scuppers.

Another huge wave broke over the side, sweeping the unconscious figure against the gunwale.

Heedless of the danger, Caseley dashed forward. Icy water filled her shoes and soaked the bottom of her skirt and petticoats.

'Caseley! No!'

She heard the roar of anguish, fury and warning but kept going. Rain beat down and within seconds her hair was a wet, straggling mass. Her jacket offered little resistance to the spray-laden gale and before she reached the foredeck she was soaked to the skin. But all her thoughts were focused on the man sprawled against the gunwale.

Gasping against the force of the wind, she staggered along the deck, grabbing whatever offered a handhold, until she reached him. Crouching, she turned his head. It was Jimbo. A cut above his ear oozed blood. The swelling had spread to his temple and was already beginning to turn purple. His eyes were closed, his face pinched and white.

The tough, chirpy little man who amused them with his tales and had pitched into the vicious fight with no weapons but his callused hands, looked shrunken, vulnerable, and suddenly much older.

Nathan turned, his arms full of torn canvas. His eyes widened in horror. 'Get back! Get away! It isn't safe here,' he yelled against the howling wind.

'I can't leave him,' Caseley cried. 'He'll drown.'

Another wave crashed over the gunwale driving the breath from her body as the achingly cold water cascaded past, soaking her to the waist.

She clung desperately to the windlass with one arm and Jimbo with the other, holding his head above the foam. As it drained away through the scuppers, she clasped her hands under his shoulders and began to drag him backwards towards the companionway.

271

Hammer emerged from the fo'c'sle with the spare sail, slamming and latching the hatch behind him. His jaw dropping as he saw Caseley, he lunged forward, ready to help.

'No,' she panted. 'I can manage.'

'Come on, Hammer,' Nathan bawled. 'We're losing way. If she broaches to, skipper'll be mad as hell.'

Caseley choked on a hysterical giggle. If they turned side-on to these seas, Jago Barata wouldn't have time to be furious. He'd be drowning with the rest of them. *She wasn't ready to die. She had only just started to live.*

The schooner nose-dived once more and she had to strain to prevent Jimbo's dead weight dragging her back towards the bows. Her fingers kept slipping on the wet oilskin. Her back felt as if it was breaking and her arms were being torn from their sockets.

Cold to her bones she sobbed for breath. Black spots danced in front of her eyes and she bit her lip to stop herself screaming as she felt her fingers slip. She adjusted her grip once more. Then as *Cygnet's* head came up she managed to drag Jimbo a few feet further.

Hammer and Nathan staggered along the deck.

'Where shall us put 'n?' Hammer was asking. 'Mart's just coming up, bleddy fo'c'sle's awash.'

'My cabin,' Nathan said, rain and spray dripping off his chin. 'All right, my bird, we got 'n.' He had to prise Caseley's fingers loose.

Dimly she heard Jago shouting to Hammer to take the wheel. Painfully she straightened up, clinging to the smooth heavy frame of the skylight.

Every muscle ached and she was shaking violently.

There was movement around her, scuffling and grunts as Jimbo was manoeuvred through the hatch and down the stairs. Then a hand closed around her upper arm.

Blinded by rain and spray she raised her head, blinking to clear her vision and felt her heart wrenched as she focused. There were dark shadows beneath Jago's eyes and lines of strain she had not seen before. His lips were bloodless, his expression chilling.

Silently he guided her ahead of him down the stairs, his firm grip holding her up when she would have fallen. As they passed the mate's cabin she heard the rustle of oilskins, Jimbo moaning, and Nathan berating him for having two left feet.

They reached the day room just as Martin clattered down the stairs wearing oilskins two sizes too big for him.

'Make a pot of tea, now,' Jago ordered before the boy could speak.

'Aye, Cap'n.' The boy whirled round and raced back up again, slamming the hatch door.

'Get those wet clothes off.' Shutting the door Jago pushed her towards the sleeping cubicle. Stripping off his waterproof and sodden coat, he crouched in front of the stove, his wet shirt clinging to his broad back and muscular shoulders, and began to set a fire.

Cygnet pitched and Caseley collided with the door frame, sliding slowly down the wall. She wasn't even cold any more. She just wanted to sleep.

Jerked to her feet, she was shaken roughly.

'Open your eyes. Damn you, Caseley Bony-thon, look at me. You are going to get undressed and into dry clothes.' He shook her again. 'Do you hear me?' His fingers dug into the tender flesh below her shoulders.

She felt her face crumple and hot tears seeped through her lashes and slid down her face. 'I'm tired.'

Cursing under his breath, Jago held her up with an arm around her waist and unfastened the buttons on her jacket. Water dripped from her skirts onto the floor in a steadily widening pool. Pulling the jacket off he tossed it aside and reached for the waistband of her skirt.

Vaguely aware of what was happening, Caseley struggled weakly.

'Keep still,' Jago snapped, pushing the heavy skirt and petticoats down over her hips.

'Leave me alone.' She tried to fend him off, fighting the lethargy of cold and exhaustion that had sapped her strength.

'And let you die of lung fever? Not on my boat.'

'It's not your boat,' she mumbled.

'While I'm master she is. Now get the rest of your clothes off.' Releasing her, he reached into the cubicle, took one of the blankets from the bed, and shook it out. 'Do you hear me?'

'Yes, I hear you,' she flung back. 'But I'm— I can't—' She could feel her face burning. 'Please look the other way.'

'For God's sake,' he said through gritted teeth. 'I've seen naked women before.'

'No doubt you have. But I'm not Louise Down-ing.' The moment the words left her lips she

274

wished them unsaid. He held the blanket out to her and, as she took it, turned away.

'No, you aren't. There is no comparison.'

Stiff and cold, her fingers dug into the rough wool as she tore her gaze from the wet cotton clinging to his broad back and fumbled with the buttons of her blouse.

She had walked onto the knife and he had twisted it. He had only been using her: first his house, then the letters she had written for him here on board. Had she been a challenge?

He had blackmailed her into obedience and she had completed her own destruction by falling in love with him. He had never lied. She wasn't important enough for that. He knew she knew about Louise and had made no secret of his desire to get back to Falmouth as quickly as possible.

'Are you done?'

Blinking back scalding tears, she clenched her teeth determined not to allow a quivering chin to betray her, and hastily tore off her remaining garments. Gathering them into a bundle she tossed them onto her skirt.

'Yes,' she whispered, wrapping the blanket around her.

'Then come over here by the stove.' His voice was rough as he picked up her shoes from where she had kicked them and set them to dry. He went into the cubicle again, this time bringing her towel.

'Turn around.'

'I–'

'Your hair is dripping. It will soak the pillow.' He turned her firmly around and removed the

275

slides and net.

As the heavy coil fell loose down her back, Caseley heard his soft intake of breath, felt his fingers brush her neck and shoulders as he lifted the wet mass to wrap the towel around her head and squeeze the water out.

The crackling stove radiated heat and now she was free of her saturated clothes, the aching cold was gradually ebbing. Though scratchy against her bare skin, the rough blanket offered comfort.

He began to massage her scalp through the towel, his strong fingers soothing. The tautness at the base of her skull started to ease. Her eyes closed, then flew open again as she realised what was happening. Not only was she falling under his spell once more, his quickened breathing told her he knew it.

She whirled round, careless of the pain as she wrenched free. Her bronze-gold tresses tumbled over her shoulders and the towel fell to the floor between them. She glimpsed hunger in his eyes before shutters came down and his features hardened.

'Leave me alone.' What she had intended as an angry demand emerged a weary plea. Backing away she caught her heel in the blanket, bumped against the table, and fell onto the bench seat. Could she possibly look any more awkward and ungainly? *No comparison.* It was a blessed relief to sit down.

About to speak he clamped his mouth shut and turned away, raking a hand through the wet curls plastered to his scalp. He spun round, making her jump.

'Had I left you alone, do you really believe Antonio Valdes would have been so polite? Do you imagine he would have stopped at seduction, or even rape?' His tone was brutal.

'He would have thrown you to his thugs, watched while they had their sport, then left you to die in the gutter. You have a lot to answer for, Caseley. Your lies might have cost me the *Cygnet* and my crew.'

'I never–' she flinched and fell silent as he raised a warning finger.

'There was no contract.' His scorn was withering. 'Ricardo Spinoza has as much interest in iron ore as I have in dressmaking.'

She gaped at him. 'You *knew?*'

'From the moment you stepped on board.' His words fell like stones into a pool, the ripples spreading ever wider.

Caseley swallowed. 'How?'

Jago slid onto the seat opposite, rested his forearms on the table. As he placed one hand over the other she saw grazes and bruising on his knuckles. *He had hit Antonio and fought the Basques to protect her.*

'Your Uncle Thomas is a frightened man. My guess is he's in deep financial trouble. Not only is he scared, he's bitter. All it took was a couple of drinks, a little sympathy, and he was telling me how much he resented your father checking his every move. Especially when he found out a contract had been drawn up for a company your father admitted did not exist. A contract that was a cover for a special assignment that would make all your father's years as a consul worthwhile.'

Caseley closed her eyes. He had sworn her to secrecy, trapped her in a web of deceit. *No one* must know, he had said. But aware he had little time left, he had been unable to resist the temptation to tell Thomas, as proof he was still a man of consequence.

She opened her eyes, saw him watching her, and looked away.

'Sam mentioned the package from Mexico,' Jago went on. 'He was fascinated by the stamps and seals. My father's last letter spoke of aid from ex-patriots supporting the restoration of Alfonso to the Spanish throne. Toby warned me to expect a passenger who had urgent business in Spain.'

'Señor Valdes?'

'Having followed the package from Mexico, he called on Thomas. Smoothing your uncle's ruffled feathers with liberal doses of charm and money—' he raised one eyebrow and her protest remained unspoken. 'He extracted the information he needed. Guessing you would be carrying the package as your father was unlikely to trust anyone else, Valdes allowed me to think he was the person I had been told to expect.'

Caseley clutched the blanket tighter. All she could do was listen.

'Then you turned up with that ridiculous story. Had the contract been genuine, *I* would have dealt with it on your father's behalf. So the pieces began to fall into place.'

Bitter anger swelled inside her. What a blind fool she had been. 'You knew. All the time, you *knew.*' Suddenly she recalled incidents whose significance had escaped her at the time.

278

He had never asked her why Valdes would go to such lengths to capture a contract. He had not asked because he already knew. He had warned her off the Spaniard, but never said why. And she, unused to dissembling, had dared not call his bluff and ask, for fear of letting something slip.

He had *expected* the ambush. He had been carrying a knife, and had sent Nathan, Jimbo, and Hammer on ahead because he anticipated trouble.

He had known which was Señor Spinoza's house. Shocked and anxious after the attack, she had not noticed when he led her to a concealed side entrance instead of the front door.

Though neither of them had given any sign of knowing one another, the silver-haired Spaniard had accepted Jago's presence without question, even during her handover of the documents. Not once had Jago asked about the *second* envelope.

'You–' her entire body burned with rage and mortification. 'Why didn't you say something?'

'Why didn't you?' he countered immediately.

'My father swore me to secrecy.'

'Some secret.' His contempt had the sting of a whiplash. 'I daresay half Falmouth knew.'

Caseley's chin lifted even as her lips quivered. 'Not from me.'

'No. You kept your word to a sick old man, and nearly got yourself and the rest of us killed.' He passed a hand across his face. 'Why wouldn't you trust me?'

'Trust you?' Her voice cracked on a laugh that was half sob. Hadn't she yearned to do just that? Hadn't she ached to confide in him, draw on his strength, and share the awesome responsibility?

But she had given her word. *Oh Father, how could you?*

Yet she could not find it in her heart to blame him. He was old and ill. He had seen so many of his hopes destroyed. Even this, his last and most important task as consul, he'd been forced to delegate. Jago Barata had known all this, and had said nothing.

'What reason have you ever given me to trust you? You barged your way into my life, bullied and blackmailed me to get me to do what you wanted.' Her breath hitched. 'You made me think ... made me hope... What sort of a man are you?' She hurled the words like missiles, desperate to hurt him as he had hurt her. 'You have a mistress in Falmouth you can't wait to get back to, yet that didn't stop you forcing your attentions on me.'

Had she not been so devastated by his revelation, so hurt by his duplicity, she might have recognised the tightening of his features and swift turn of his head as the guilt and self-contempt they were. But in her misery she saw only impatience, the arrogance of a pirate who accepted no terms but his own, who had always taken what he wanted, heeding neither refusal nor rebuff.

He started to reach across the table.

'Keep away,' she warned. 'Don't touch me.'

He let his hand rest on the table. 'Or what? You'll scream? Who would hear you?'

Fear crawled along her nerves. He was right. While *Cygnet* was fighting for survival in the teeth of a storm, the crew, *his* men, had their hands full.

He lifted a handful of her damp dishevelled hair,

closing his fist on it. 'I haven't known a moment's peace since I first laid eyes on you. And for that you will pay.' Opening his fingers he let her hair spill over the grey blanket like liquid bronze. 'But not here, not now.'

Gathering the remnants of her dignity, she tilted her chin. 'Spare me your threats.' Her knuckles gleamed white as she drew the blanket close. 'I owe you *nothing*. There was a time when I thought we might be friends.'

Her throat tightened and she swallowed to clear it. 'I was wrong. Once we reach Falmouth your problem is solved, for I never want to see you again. Until then, I will keep out of your way and you will oblige us both by ignoring me. I am not your *responsibility*.'

She slid out of the seat and crossed to the cubicle.

'Do you really hate me so much?' he asked quietly.

She paused in the curtained doorway, digging her thumbnail hard into the pad of her index finger. It was a trick she had used before. Inflicting a small pain to hold off the larger one about to engulf her. She glanced over her shoulder, willing her voice steady.

'I do not hate you, Captain Barata. To hate someone they have to matter.' She walked into the cubicle and pulled the curtain across. Curled into a ball on the bunk she closed her eyes in silent, desperate agony.

Chapter Twenty

The storm passed, leaving in its wake a heavy swell and an exhausted crew.

Kept busy repairing damaged sails or splicing and whipping frayed and broken ropes, the men did not linger over meals. Instead they took every opportunity to catch up on sleep. They had all appreciated the stew. But Caseley had been unable to swallow more than a couple of mouthfuls.

On Jago's orders, Jimbo had rested for twelve hours. But he had refused to stay in bed any longer.

Caseley approached Nathan at the wheel. 'I realise this is an imposition, but would you mind if I used your cabin for the remainder of the voyage?'

After a moment's hesitation ripe with surprise and speculation the mate nodded. ''Tis all right with me, miss. But you better check with the skipper.'

Caseley went down to the day room, knocked then opened the door, and went in. Jago was seated at the table writing in the log.

'May I speak to you?'

'Yes.' He continued writing in his bold scrawl.

She cleared her throat. 'Now Jimbo has moved back to the fo'c'sle, I would like your permission to move into Nathan's cabin until we reach Falmouth. He has no objection but said I must ask you first.'

He raised his head then leaned back against the panelling, studying her with piercing intensity.

It cost her dearly to hold his gaze as she forced herself to add. 'I think you will welcome my absence and the return of your privacy.'

The silence stretched. Then he nodded. 'As you wish. When do you–'

'Now. I'll just collect my things.' Braced for a biting comment, his agreement came as a relief. Yet she was acutely aware of him watching as she removed her bag.

Wearing her spare green skirt and a pin-tucked cream shirt-blouse, she had pushed her other clothes, stiff with salt after drying in front of the stove, into her bag. Even looking at them brought back painful memories.

Nathan's cabin was not much bigger than Jago's sleeping cubicle. After stowing her bag, Caseley sat on the bunk for a few minutes. But with the only light coming in from gaps at the top and bottom of the door, she was suffocating. Putting on her salt-stained jacket she quickly buttoned it then hurried up the brass stairs to fresh air and the wide expanse of sea and sky.

The crew gave her friendly nods when their paths crossed but focused on their work, eager to get home.

Jago spoke little. When he did his tone was cool.

It was for the best, she told herself. He had shown he was not to be trusted. Wretchedly miserable, she grieved for the intimacy they had shared.

As they crossed the Bay of Biscay heading towards Falmouth she realised how hard he was driving himself. From dawn until nightfall he was either at the wheel, supervising and helping with repairs, or bent over the charts and log.

No matter what hour of the night she slipped from the mate's tiny cabin, unable to sleep, desperate for escape from her tormented thoughts, she saw light from the oil-lamp under the dayroom door.

Did he never rest? With a sudden fierce yearning for revenge she hoped not. Why should he be granted the blessed relief of oblivion when it eluded her?

Before meeting him she had been trying hard to come to terms with the limitations of her life. Yes, she had been lonely. Especially when there was no task demanding her attention, when the household slept and the new day had yet to dawn.

In those dark hours she pined for a man who might love her in spite of her limp, her boyish figure, and her coppery hair. A man she could love and respect, a man to share her thoughts with, to have children with, grown old with. Yes she had yearned, but it had been manageable.

Until *he* came, shocking her into quivering awareness, kindling wild hopes and soaring dreams, only to trample them. He had broken her heart, leaving her nothing but aching misery and the pitiful rags of her pride.

At least he had never known the depth of her feelings for him. But that was small consolation.

Midmorning on the fourth day after leaving Santander, *Cygnet* sailed into Falmouth. The sun shone in a cornflower sky, the sea sparkled like sapphires. Only a short time ago they had been fighting for their lives.

Quay punts and rowing boats criss-crossed the water ferrying goods and passengers to and from bigger ships moored to huge buoys.

Jago was at the wheel. Acutely conscious of him, she had chosen a spot well out of everyone's way. She could not have borne to stay below.

'Right, boys.' Those two laconic words were all Jago said. Yet within minutes the foresail and jib had been dropped, the square topsail hauled up, the mainsail reefed a couple of points, and the peak lowered.

She drank in the sights and smells. Nothing had changed yet everything was different. She had not wanted to make the voyage. But the events and emotions she had lived through had changed her forever. Right now her heart felt like a raw wound. But even the deepest wounds healed. Eventually.

Just before they reached the yard slipway and quays, Nathan, Hammer, and Jimbo lowered the mainsail. At Jago's nod, Martin released the stay-sail halyard. The canvas dropped into a pile on the foredeck and the schooner glided gently in alongside the wharf.

After securing the fore and aft lines, Hammer and Jimbo moved about the deck furling and lashing the sails. Martin began to unfasten the hatch cover and Nathan set up the winch.

She gazed across the yard over the sheds to the little tower on her father's house, its windows glistening in the sunlight. Home. No longer enough. But it was all she had.

She started to turn away. A shout made her glance back. Toby was hurrying towards the ship. His trousers hung in baggy folds from the belt beneath his belly, and his rolling gait made him rock from side to side. Worry furrowed his face as he beckoned urgently.

'Quick, my 'andsome. They want you uplong.'

She knew at once. 'He's not...?' She could not bring herself to say it.'

Toby shook his head. 'No. Doctor's with 'n now. Ben come over and told me and said for you to get on home the minute you come in.'

'I'll just fetch my things.' She whirled round and bumped into Jago who caught her arms to steady her.

'I've already sent Martin down.' As he spoke the boy appeared, his young face puckered in concern as he held out her bag and cape.

Shaking off Jago's hands, she seized her belongings from Martin. 'Thank you,' she managed and the boy touched a knuckle to his forehead in salute. Her world was crumbling. It was too soon. Months, the doctor had said. Why now? Why so *soon?*

'I'll come with you.' Jago was close behind her as she limped to the schooner's side where Toby waited.

'No!' she rounded on him, her voice low and intense. 'He's the sick old man who nearly cost you the *Cygnet* and the lives of your crew. Remember?'

He shook his head, abrupt and impatient. 'I spoke in the heat of the moment–'

'Stay away.' Her voice broke on a sob.

Brilliant sunshine glinted on Jago's black curls as he stood like a rock, allowing the tide of her hurt and fear to smash against him. 'If there is anything you need, anything I can do–'

'*I* can give my father everything he needs,' she broke in, not allowing him to finish. She hated the sympathy in his eyes, hated her need, the longing for his support and strength surging through her, hated *him.*

'I managed alone before. I'll manage now. Go to your *friend,* Captain Barata,' she hissed, heedless of the round-eyed stares of the crew who, sensing something was wrong, had moved towards them. 'Go and find the peace you have missed so much. You need never see me again.'

She tossed her bag and the gabardine cape onto the wharf, then stepping onto the barrel and up onto the gunwale, jumped down into Toby's arms, wincing as the hard landing jarred her foot.

'All right, are you?' Anxiety creased his lined, weathered face, and she knew he was not refer-ring solely to her concern over her father.

Not trusting herself to speak, she nodded quickly. As she snatched up her things, she heard Jago snap at the men to get back to work. There was a cargo to unload and transfer.

She hurried away from the schooner, the pain in her chest excruciating. *Jago.* She kept her gaze resolutely forward. Aware of Toby's worried glances, she hoped he would interpret the scalding tears that streaked her cheeks as fear for her father.

'See you across the road, shall I?' he offered as they reached the yard gates.

She shook her head. 'No. I'm all right, Toby. You get back. I know you have lots to do.'

'We're all thinking of 'n. And you too, my 'and-some.'

Impulsively, seeking comfort as much as giving

287

it, Caseley leaned over and kissed the bristly cheek. 'Thank you.' Her voice wobbled.

Rosina met her at the door. 'Doctor's upstairs, my bird. He said you was to wait down here and he'd be with you d'rectly. I'm going to make you a nice cuppa tea.' As she spoke she took Caseley's bag, dropped it in the hall, and steered her firmly past the stairs and into the dining room. 'Kettle's boiled and I got a tray all set. Now you stay there.'

She pulled out one of the carver chairs and gently pressed Caseley down into it. 'Don't you move, mind,' she warned, and Caseley knew the housekeeper's sharp eyes hadn't missed a thing.

Resting her elbows on the polished table, she buried her face in her hands as her thoughts flew like sparks from a burning log.

A few moments later she heard footsteps in the passage, a muffled exchange of words and the tinkle of china. Sitting up she took a deep breath and braced herself for what was to come. Dr Vigurs walked in, closely followed by Rosina.

'Good morning, Caseley. No, don't get up.' He studied her with a deepening frown and she realised he was seeing her pallor and the dark circles beneath her eyes.

'Father—'

'Is resting quietly. You will see him very soon, I promise. First I need to talk to you. And you appear to be in need of a good meal and a few minutes to compose yourself.'

'I'll go and get—' Rosina began.

'No, nothing to eat. I'm not hungry right now. Thank you, Rosina.'

Shaking her head, the housekeeper left the room.

Dr Vigurs pulled out another chair and sat down, half-facing Caseley. 'Pour the tea, my dear,' he ordered gently.

Starting, she straightened up. 'Of course. Forgive me. It's–' Her hand shook as she lifted the white china pot patterned with roses.

Removing his pince-nez, the doctor polished them carefully with a spotless white handkerchief. But she was aware of him watching her. Replacing his spectacles he helped himself to sugar, and motioned to her cup, indicating she should drink.

She took a sip then replaced the delicate china onto the saucer with a clatter, raising anguished eyes. 'Please, you must tell me – how – how long?'

'A matter of hours. He had the attack two days ago. To be honest, I did not expect him to last the night. But against all odds he hung on. He has asked for you several times.'

The lump in Caseley's throat was so painful she could hardly speak. 'He's not in pain, is he?'

The doctor shook his head. 'Not any more. He's tired, Caseley. He's ready to go. I believe he is only waiting to see you. No,' he pressed her hand as she started to get up. 'Finish your tea. You have had a shock. You need time to gather your strength.'

She nodded, lowering her head, gripping the fragile china cup with stiff fingers as she blinked back scalding tears. After a moment she looked up. 'What happened? What caused the attack? I know you said– But he was delighted to be back

289

at work, especially going to the yard. Something must have–' She broke off as the doctor glanced away, visibly uncomfortable.

'What? What is it? I have to know. Please?'

Robert Vigurs's features were sombre. 'My dear, I am so sorry to add to your troubles, but financial irregularities have been uncovered within your father's company.'

Caseley started so violently her cup fell over, spilling dregs of tea onto the lace tray-cloth. 'I don't believe it. Not *Father*. He wouldn't–'

'No, no, my dear. Forgive me. I did not make myself clear. Your father is in no way– The person responsible is Thomas Bonython. I understand the situation came to light when a money-lender demanded, with certain unpleasant threats, the return of his loan plus accrued interest.'

Caseley stopped breathing. *Jago was right.* She wanted to ask the doctor if he knew any more details, but held back. This was a family matter. She would speak to Uncle Richard later. She stood up. 'Thank you for telling me. I'll see my father now.'

Leaving Rosina to see him out, Caseley walked up the wide carpeted stairs. Her mind flashed back to a spiral of chased brass treads.

She lowered herself carefully onto the edge of the large bed. Her father's head and shoulders were propped up on snowy feather-filled pillows. His eyes were closed, his breathing shallow, and beneath the network of purple thread veins on his cheeks and nose, his complexion was ash-grey. He looked thinner. But the deep furrows of pain, the grooves of anger and disillusionment, had smoothed out. His face looked waxen.

It was then she realised that, despite the doctor's warning, she had not really expected her father to die. She had heard the words without accepting the reality.

She looked down at the man who had always been a giant, strong, forceful, and full of life, with hands like hams and a voice that could reach from one end of the yard to the other. During her absence he had withered into frailty.

Her vision blurred. Biting hard on her lower lip, she lifted his cold hand in hers.

Creased like fine tissue paper, his eyelids flickered and parted, opening slowly. As his dull gaze focused, Caseley smiled down at him.

'I can't leave you for a minute, can I?' she scolded softly.

One corner of his mouth lifted. 'Took your time, didn't you, girl?' His voice was weary and slurred, but the glow of pleasure in his eyes was nearly her undoing. She longed to lay her head on his chest, cling to him, and beg him not to leave her, not yet, not so *alone*.

She swallowed the agonising stiffness in her throat and kept her voice low to disguise the thickness of tears. 'Can I get you anything? Some water?' Her own mouth was dust dry.

His hand moved in hers and he turned his head a fraction on the pillow. 'Did it go all right?' The words rustled from his lips like autumn leaves.

She nodded. 'Señor Spinoza sends you his kindest regards. He said the new King of Spain has reason to be very grateful to you. So too will the Spanish people when Don Alfonso puts an end to the rebellion and restores peace.'

Teuder's rheumy eyes shone. 'He did? He said that?'

Caseley nodded.

Her father sucked air into his failing lungs. 'You didn't have any trouble?'

'None at all,' the lies were easy on her tongue. 'Everything was just as you said it would be.'

'And Jago, did he–?'

His name sent a tremor through her. She could not speak of him, even to her father. Fighting for composure, she gently pressed the frail hand.

'All the crew were very kind to me. Jimbo told some amazing yarns. The bad weather you warned of hit us on the way back. But *Cygnet* rode it out. She's a beautiful ship, Father.'

He nodded; too tired to press now he knew the mission had been successful. The groove between his shaggy brows deepened. 'Is it out yet? Do they know in the yard?'

'Know what?'

'About Thomas.'

'No. No one knows,' she said firmly, not knowing or caring if it was the truth.

'It mustn't get out.' Anxiety quickened his breath, making it rasp in his throat.

'It won't.' Caseley placed her hand over his, trying to soothe.

'I paid off Colenzo. But if word gets round...' He coughed weakly and she heard bubbling in his chest.

'It won't, Father. I'll take care of it.' Lifting his hand she pressed it to her cheek.

His eyelids drooped and tension drained out of him like water through a sieve. 'It's yours, girl,' he muttered. 'The yard, the business, all of it. Changed my will. Don't let it fail, Caseley.' His eyes lost focus. 'Ralph would have drunk it all away.' His voice trailed off. Then he rallied, his eyes opened and fixed on her face, urgent, pleading. 'Listen, girl, you must–' His face contorted in pain.

Smothering a cry, her heart beating wildly, she clutched his hand in both of hers. 'It's all right. Don't try to talk.' Tears splashed onto her hand. 'Rest now.'

The spasm passed. His breathing grew fainter. Then, his lips barely moving, he whispered, 'Philip?'

Caseley sat and held his hand, felt it grow cold. Eventually she laid it gently on the coverlet and rose stiffly to her feet. Her eyes burned and her throat ached. She went downstairs to the kitchen.

Rosina and Liza-Jane were preparing lunch. Ben came in from the garden as she was breaking the news. He put an arm around Liza-Jane's thin, shaking shoulders. Rosina sobbed quietly into her apron.

Caseley didn't think she would ever cry again. She was numb.

'Some sorry I am, miss.' Ben's open face was full of sympathy. 'I remember what 'twas like when my father went.'

'Thank you.' Many people would say those words in the next few days. Most would be thinking of their own losses, not hers. Few would care the way Ben, Rosina, and Liza-Jane did.

'Ben, will you go across to the yard and tell Toby? I think it's best if he tells the men. I'll let him know the date of the funeral as soon as it's arranged.'

He nodded then bent his head. 'Come on now, maid,' he murmured in Liza-Jane's ear. 'Best get moving. We want to give mister a proper send-off.'

Their closeness was too much for Caseley and she looked quickly away.

Rosina wiped red-rimmed eyes with the corner of her apron. 'We all loved 'n, though he wasn't always easy.' Her mouth quivered. 'Place won't be the same.' She sniffed then pulled herself together. 'Put the kettle on, Liza-Jane. Miss Caseley, if it's all right with you, I'd like to lay 'n out. You want it done proper, with respect.'

'Thank you, Rosina. I have to go out for a while.'

'But, Miss Caseley,' the housekeeper began, clearly startled.

'I'm going to see Dr Vigurs, then I'll call on Mr Nancholas.'

'Ben can fetch the undertaker. There's no call for you to–'

'There's something else I must do,' Caseley interrupted and went upstairs to put on a clean jacket. As she left the house the housekeeper was still protesting, visibly concerned.

The doctor was busy with a patient so Caseley left a message with the sour-faced housekeeper. 'Please ask the doctor to call when it's convenient. Tell him there's no urgency,' she added in the new calm voice that seemed to belong to someone else.

Mr Nancholas expressed his deepest sympathy in hushed tones while making washing motions with his hands. He urged her to inspect his range of coffins and suggested they decide upon the number and types of cab she would require for the cortège. Caseley shut off the flow by inviting him to call at the house later that afternoon. He was still washing and mouthing condolences as she closed the door behind her.

She went into the office and told Richard.

'Oh, my dear.' Taking both her hands in his he squeezed them. 'I am so very sorry.'

The genuine sympathy and kindness in her uncle's words and gesture caused a wrenching pang. But leaving a few minutes later she was still dry-eyed.

She reached the house in Florence Terrace, unaware of the route she had taken or the people she had passed.

'Are my aunt and uncle in?' she asked when the stocky maid opened the door.

The girl nodded and stepped back. 'In the drawing room they are. Want me to show you in? Only I got–'

'No, thank you. I know the way.'

Rose nodded, closed the front door and stomped back to the kitchen.

A door off the hall opened. 'Rose? Who–?' Margaret Bonython froze, paling so the rouge daubed on the flesh covering her cheekbones stood out in two bright patches. Shock and guilt chased across her face. 'Caseley! What – what a surprise.' Her forced smile was more a grimace.

Without waiting for an invitation, Caseley walked past her into the stuffy over-furnished room.

Thomas was huddled in a tall wing-backed chair beside the brightly burning fire. His face was the colour of clay, his eyes puffy and blood-shot. He flinched when he saw her. Her gaze went to the glass in his trembling hand and she smelled the pungent aroma of whisky.

'I suppose *he* sent you,' Thomas said. 'I can't work today. I'm not well.' His gaze slid away from hers. He did indeed look ill.

Caseley sat down, her back very straight. She folded her hands in her lap and looked from one to the other.

'I know.' She saw Thomas flinch.

'What did he want to tell you for? He had no business...' He gulped the whisky, the glass clattering against his teeth.

Margaret wrung her hands. 'It was simply an unfortunate misunderstanding. Anyway, it's all settled now.' Her mouth stretched in a travesty of a smile. Caseley remained silent. 'Thomas only borrowed the money,' she blustered. 'He was going to pay it back. If that stupid Luke Dower hadn't got himself arrested by the customs men–'

'Margaret–' Thomas croaked.

'Oh, be quiet,' his wife snapped.

'Luke Dower?' Caseley held her aunt's gaze.

'It was all his fault,' Margaret babbled. She leaned forward in an armchair upholstered in emerald green velvet, determined to convince. 'Thomas didn't know anything about the gold coins. It was supposed to be honest business. He was to be an agent, handling goods for clients abroad. Only Luke never paid Thomas when he should have. Then your dear father decided to

296

check the books.' Her mouth pursed. 'So Thomas had to borrow off Colenzo to repay what he'd borrowed from the business.'

'Are you saying that if Father had not returned to work when he did, Uncle Thomas would not have had to borrow from Colenzo?' Caseley's calm seemed to reassure her aunt.

'That's right. I knew you would understand.'

'He would simply have continued stealing from the family business?' Caseley went on as if her aunt had not spoken. 'He would have entered into further arrangements with known criminals in order to make more money for himself?'

Margaret's eyes bulged and her mouth sagged open then snapped shut like a trap. Indignation swelled her bosom.

'It was all your father's fault. How are we supposed to maintain any kind of standard on the pittance he pays? Keeping up appearances costs money. Not that *you* would understand. You don't know the first thing about style. Prices are going up all the time. We have a position to uphold–'

'So you would *steal* to maintain it?'

Margaret didn't even hear her. 'I told your father it wasn't our fault. I told him he would have to pay Colenzo off for the sake of the family name. Like I said, no one need ever know. Luke Dower won't talk. Even if he does, Thomas will swear he had no idea there was anything dishonest–'

'Margaret,' Thomas pleaded.

'Shut *up*,' she spat, her expression venomous. She turned back to Caseley. 'Everything will just go on as normal. That's in everyone's best interests, isn't it? It won't do your father any good to make a fuss, him being a consul and everything. That's what I told him anyway. Now it's all tidied up we'll say no more about it.'

Caseley stood up. 'When did you discuss this with my father?'

'When? The day before yesterday. Of course it all fell on my shoulders. *He,*' she glared at the slumped figure of her husband, 'wasn't fit for anything.' She turned a suspicious gaze on Caseley, her mouth pursing again. 'Not that it's any of your business. There's no call for you to be hanging around the office, not now your father is back. Far better that you leave business matters to those who understand them.'

'Like your husband?' Caseley suggested.

Margaret flushed an ugly brick colour. 'You mind your tongue, miss. We all know why you spend so much time in the office and down at the boatyard. Got your eyes on that Spaniard, haven't you? It's disgusting. Your father should know better.'

Caseley walked to the door. Her heart drummed against her ribs as she turned to look from her uncle's drunken misery to her aunt's malice.

'My father died this morning,' she said through stiff lips. 'The pair of you killed him.'

In the silence that followed her footsteps were loud on the hall's tiled floor. She pulled the front door closed on Thomas's groan and Margaret's shriek, and drew a deep, shuddering breath. Never had she felt so tired.

Chapter Twenty-one

It was nearly four when she got home. Messages of sympathy were beginning to arrive. Liza-Jane, her eyes pink-rimmed and swollen, had time for little but answering the door.

Rosina brought a bowl of chicken soup to Caseley in the dining room, refusing to leave until she ate it all. "'Tis nice and easy to swallow, bird.'

'I can't, Rosina. My stomach hurts.'

'It probably think your throat have been cut. You're hungry, bird. That's what's wrong. Come on now. You want to do your best for your father, you need to keep your strength up.'

Caseley lifted the spoon and sipped. For a moment she feared her stomach would rebel. But as she swallowed the hot aromatic soup, she felt the knots loosen. After several more mouthfuls, warmth slid along her veins and the dull ache at the back of her skull receded.

Rosina talked of the past, reminding Caseley of incidents long forgotten, laughing and crying over Teuder's irascibility and his kindness, so often hidden beneath noise and bluster.

'You could get 'n to do anything so long as you convinced 'n it was his idea all along. Men!' She stood up, shaking her head with a fond sad smile. 'Break your heart they do, but 'twould be a dull old world without them.'

Caseley was spared having to respond by the

sound of the front door slamming. She had seen questions in Rosina's eyes. They were too close for the housekeeper not to have recognised that aside from her father's death, she was deeply unhappy.

'You stay there, miss.' She patted Caseley's shoulder. 'I'll see what's going on.' She hurried out. Hearing her voice, sharp and scolding, Caseley tensed.

The door swung open and her brother lurched in. His clothes were creased and stained, his hair dishevelled, and he needed a shave. Under his arm he carried a large, flat, oblong object wrapped in brown paper. He had the slow blink she had come to dread and seemed to be having trouble focusing.

Caseley turned away, propping her elbows on the table as she covered her face with her hands.

'Wass' matter? Why's Rosina been crying? And skinny Liza? For God's sake, I was only away a couple of nights.'

Caseley looked at him. She felt distanced from everything and oddly calm. 'It isn't about you, Ralph. Father died this morning.'

'Oh.' He dropped the parcel onto the table then slumped into a chair, resting his head against the high wooden back. 'Sudden, wasn't it?'

Evidence of his dissipation was clear in his slack mouth, sallow complexion, and the pouches of skin beneath his muddy eyes.

'Is that all you have to say?'

'What do you expect?' he retorted angrily. 'Grief? Why should I pretend something I don't feel? We never got on, you know that.' He rubbed

300

a hand across his eyes. 'I've been staying with Jason.'

'Why, Ralph?'

'Why what?'

His vacant expression ignited a spark of anger that flared hot and bright. 'Why stay with Jason? Why not come home? Why be drunk at this time of day?'

He didn't answer and her anger died as quickly as it had flamed. How nice it would be to go to sleep and not wake up.

With unsteady hands Ralph ripped the paper off the parcel to reveal a freshly painted canvas. He pushed it towards her.

Lifting it she turned it towards the light, looking carefully at the portrait. Posed against a background of crimson drapes a pretty girl with corn-coloured hair wore a low-cut bodice that framed her white shoulders in a froth of lace. She caught her breath as she saw it: the sulky wilfulness behind the sweet smile, a restless boredom in the china blue eyes. She glanced away then looked again. But it wasn't her imagination. It was there, real and clear. She looked at her brother in awe.

'Ralph, it's brilliant. But–' She stopped, reluctant to add to his misery.

'But,' he agreed, his careless shrug not deceiving her for an instant.

'They didn't like it.' Caseley stated. How could they?

'The Tidburys said it was nothing at all like their daughter. How, when she was the prettiest girl in the entire town, had I managed to make her look so plain? The Lashbrookes, including her husband

301

Edwin, simply looked uncomfortable. They know that painting is a true likeness, but prefer to pretend it isn't.'

'And Frances?' Caseley was curious. 'What did she say?'

'She burst into tears and wanted to know why I hate her so much. I don't hate her. I hardly know her.' He shrugged. 'I painted what I saw.' His hands, long-fingered, talented and grimy, hung over the arms of the chair. 'Anyway, they refused the portrait.'

'So you went and got drunk for two days.'

Tense and furious he half-rose then fell back onto the chair, his features softening into the familiar expression of petulance and self-pity. 'How could I expect you to understand?'

Caseley laid the canvas down. 'I understand this. You have to choose. If you can see Frances Lashbrooke's character reflected in *her* face, you can see the same, good and bad, in other people. Ralph, you can commit yourself to your painting, honour your vision and talent, and accept the rejections that are bound to come. Or you can give up, live in a bottle, and be a failure who lacked the courage even to try. If you choose to paint I'll help you all I can. But I won't give you the money to drink yourself to death.'

'What money?' he sneered. 'You haven't got any. Now Father's gone, the house and the business will be mine.'

'No, they won't.' She spoke quietly.

It took a moment to register then Ralph's head jerked. 'What do you mean, they won't?' Shock had sobered him.

Caseley stood up. 'I was with Father when he died. Just before ... the end he told me he had changed his will.' She watched all colour drain from her brother's face.

'He didn't– You can't mean– You?'

'I didn't know, Ralph.' She guessed what was coming. 'Truly, I didn't. He was worried about your drinking. I think he saw everything he had worked so hard to build being frittered away.'

His face distorted, ugly with rage. 'You sneaky, manipulating bitch! It's mine. I'm the eldest. I was his only son, for God's sake. It's mine by right.'

'I'm sorry,' she whispered.

'What the hell will *you* do with the business? What do you know about running a boatyard? Or are *you* going to sell it? It's probably worth a bit. You could buy yourself a husband.'

Clasping her upper arms, holding the hurt inside, Caseley went to the window. She felt as brittle as fine glass, but tried to make allowances for Ralph's disappointment. Their father's decision was a bitter blow to him.

The sun was going down: another day almost over and her last link with childhood broken.

'I shan't sell,' she said, talking to herself as much as him, exploring possibilities. 'I learned a lot helping father during his illness. With Richard and Toby to advise–'

The door slammed and she fell silent.

The funeral took place three days later. The parish church was packed. The doors were left open so those left standing on the steps or in the road could hear.

303

Caseley had closed both office and yard for the day. Dressed in their Sunday best, their faces shaved and scrubbed shiny, hair slicked flat, every man and boy who worked at Bonython's followed a red-eyed Toby into the church.

At the graveside, with Richard and Helen on one side, Margaret, Thomas, and their daughter, Charlotte on the other, Caseley said her silent farewell. Ralph had not appeared.

As the finality of the moment hit her, she swayed. A hand gripped her arm, drawing her gently back. Her eyes burning behind the black veil, she glanced round, hoping, needing so desperately ... and looked into Richard's kind face, furrowed in concern.

Of course he had not come. Why would he? She had told him she never wanted to see him again. He had sent a note of condolence, his bold scrawl instantly recognisable. Her heart had thumped, her fingers unsteady as she opened the envelope. The wording had been formal as befitted the occasion. Yet he had signed it, 'As ever, Jago.'

What did he mean, *as ever?* What was there between them but lies, blackmail, and mistrust? Was that what he wanted her to remember? She needed no reminding.

Crushing the paper into a ball she had been about to hurl it into the fire. But she couldn't, and tossed it onto her desk instead. That night, unable to sleep, she had crept out of bed and lit the lamp. Sitting at her desk she smoothed the crumpled paper flat, and gazed at those three words for a long time.

The following day she was up early. Life had to

304

go on and responsibility for all her father's employees now rested on her shoulders. Passing the yard on her way to the office, she caught sight of *Cygnet,* easing away from the quay.

Stopping, she looked for the tall, bearded figure. Nathan was at the wheel. Hammer, Jimbo, and Martin moved swiftly about the deck, setting the smaller sails. She did not see Jago.

Recovering, she hurried on along the road. He was probably below in the day room, bent over the chart table, plotting their course. The image was so vividly, painfully real that she stumbled and almost fell.

With a hand against the high wall, she fought for mental balance. It should be getting easier, not more difficult. She should be missing him less, not more.

He was out of her life. It was a mutual decision. The problems between them were insurmountable. He had passed through her life like a shooting star. Brief, brilliant, tantalising her with a wish, a hope.

She was glad he had sailed again so soon. There would be no embarrassing encounters at the office. She would not have to face those mocking grey eyes. She would be able to work without hoping for, yet dreading, his footstep on the stairs, his cynical smile at her temerity to imagine she could succeed in a man's world. Far better he had gone.

Nodding to Sam she entered her father's office. A neat pile of letters had been stacked in the centre of the desk. She took off her bonnet and hung up her cape, now washed free of salt and neatly pressed. She looked at her mother's bureau. Then walked round behind her father's desk.

She had just sat down in his chair when the door opened and Richard entered. His round shoulders and puckered features made him appear more mole-like than ever.

'What's to be done about Thomas? He sent Charlotte down with a message that he is still unwell and Margaret is prostrate with grief.' He clicked his tongue.

Caseley sighed, turning the ivory letter-opener over in her fingers. 'I don't know. What are your thoughts?'

Clasping his lapels, Richard paced to and fro. 'We cannot ignore what he did. But as a partner he has a financial interest in the company. It would cost more than we can afford to buy him out, especially now. Not only have we lost the money he embezzled, we've also lost the amount Teuder had to draw to pay off Colenzo.' He stopped, shamefaced. 'Forgive me, my dear. I don't mean to reopen old wounds.'

She waved his apology away. 'It must be faced. Though it was a shock to learn how much was involved, and that Father had emptied his personal account to repay the debt.'

'Your father was an honourable man, Caseley.' Richard paused in his pacing to look at her. 'He knew the business could not have withstood such a drain on its working capital. Has it caused problems at home?'

She made a small, helpless gesture. 'I haven't told Ralph about Uncle Thomas. But he's threatening to contest the will anyway.'

'What about the bequests to Rosina, Liza-Jane, and Ben? Short of selling the house, there's nothing left to pay them.'

Caseley looked away, her eyes filling even as she smiled. 'They all insist they don't mind. Rosina said it was a lovely thought. But what they never had they can't miss. And none of them will be a party to anything that involves selling the house or the yard to give them a few pounds. All three are prepared to work for nothing if we can keep a roof over our heads.' Clenching her fists on the desktop, she raised her head to meet her uncle's concerned gaze. 'We *must* go on.'

For the rest of the day she immersed herself in work, making notes of matters to be discussed with Toby.

After one of her consultations with Richard over fees and cargoes, she paused in the doorway of his office, hugging a leather-bound ledger against her chest.

'On my way here this morning I saw *Cygnet* leave.' She strove to sound casual.

'Mmmmmn,' her uncle nodded, still studying a page of figures. 'She's gone up to Penryn to load granite for London.'

'Do–' she cleared her throat. 'Do you know if Captain Barata found a ship to take that quicksilver to Mexico?'

Richard glanced up. 'What? Oh, yes. Fox's had a barque due to leave the day you got back. They delayed it until the next tide to allow enough time to transfer the cargo.'

'That was good of them.'

'It was. Do you have a note of the date of

Lloyd's final inspection of *Fair Maid?*'

'Yes. It will be in the diary.'

'I'll send Sam for it.'

'Give me ten minutes.'

When Sam brought in the afternoon mail, Caseley was puzzled to find a letter addressed to her from solicitors, Knuckey & Son. She knew of them. They had an excellent reputation. But as far as she was aware they had never handled any of her father's business.

The envelope was heavy in her hand and she could feel an object at the bottom. As she slit open the envelope, tension tightened the back of her neck as possibilities raced through her mind. Was Ralph really going to contest the will? Had Thomas and Margaret taken legal advice, and now planned to cause more trouble?

Removing the thick folded paper, she tipped the envelope and a key slid out onto her palm. As she recognised it her heart leapt into her throat. Her fingers closing on the key, she read the letter. Then she read it again.

Though couched in polite terms the words amounted to an order. The following day she was required to go to the house of Captain Jago Barata on Greenbank Terrace to ascertain whether all the work ordered by her had in fact been completed. A key was enclosed.

She could not go back there. It held too many memories, too many poignant reminders of her foolishness. The wounds had only just begun to heal. And yet...

She had loved the house. Its indefinable atmosphere had captured her imagination. Choosing colour schemes, selecting wallpapers and fabrics, searching shops for furniture to complement each room had given her such pleasure.

Could it really do any harm to take one last look now all the tradesmen had finished? To see at least some of her ideas translated into reality? But what if Louise Downing had had her way? No, she wouldn't have. Jago had said as much. *Jago.*

At least she would be alone. Alone to remember, to think of what might have been, to bleed. Why should she put herself through that?

When she reached home that evening she had still not decided whether to go. As she took off her bonnet and cape in the hall, she could hear Rosina and Liza-Jane gossiping beyond the open kitchen door.

'She ditched 'n for Redvers Edyvean.'

'She never!' Liza-Jane gasped. 'He must be sixty if he's a day.'

'He also got two grocery stores in Falmouth and one in Penryn.'

Despite her tiredness and all the weight on her mind, Caseley could not help smiling at Rosina's dry retort as she rubbed stiffness from the back of her neck.

'Well, that wasn't the story *I* heard,' Liza-Jane said amid a clatter of dishes. 'My cousin Doreen do work for Mrs Bowden who live next door to that place of his up on Greenbank.'

Caseley froze, unable to breathe.

'Doreen couldn't help but hear the row. Going at it something terrible they was. He was mad as fire that she had turned up at his house uninvited, and about her going down the yard asking questions about who he'd took to Spain. He wouldn't let her in past the hallway. He said she had no business there, and she wasn't never to come back. She was screaming and yelling.

'Well, I wouldn't put my tongue to some of the things Doreen told me. But the gist of it was that she's gived him a bleddy good time and he didn't have no right to cast her off like a bleddy old shoe. He told her she wasn't in no position to complain. She'd started it, and she knew the rules. It was finished, he said, and if she had any sense she'd take the fifty pounds and keep her jealousy to herself 'cos she had most to lose and his patience was running out. Doreen said it all went quiet then. Next minute she seen Louise leaving. That was last week.'

'She certainly didn't waste much time,' Rosina commented. 'I reckon she's putting it out about she and old Edyvean. *She* always done the dumping before. Fifty pounds, eh? I'd say she done all right.'

Caseley's heart was beating hard and loud as she went upstairs to her room. Closing the door she leaned back against it. *Jago had ended his relationship with Louise.* Momentary joy evaporated as she realised it made not the slightest difference. He had left her first. He appeared to be severing all connections.

That had to be why the solicitor wanted all the loose ends neatly tied up. Was he selling the house? Would he still sail Bonython schooners? Or when *Cygnet* returned from London would he cut that last link with Falmouth and disappear to

310

a new life in some other part of the world? Selling his interests in Spain would make him a very rich man. He could go wherever he chose.

After another virtually sleepless night and a morning during which she found it increasingly difficult to focus on the piles of papers covering her father's desk, she made her decision. She would go to the house. She must, to exorcise the past.

Because she would be out of the office for the afternoon she told Richard about the letter. She expected him to comment or ask questions, but he simply nodded.

'Don't worry about coming back. It's been a difficult time for you. Take an hour or two for yourself.'

'Are you all right, Uncle Richard?'

He glanced up, but only for a moment. 'Perfectly. Why do you ask?'

'You look a little flushed. I hope you haven't picked up Aunt Helen's cold.'

'No, I'm perfectly well. If I don't catch you before you go, I'll see you in the morning.'

Lunchtime came. Too tense to go home and risk Rosina's sharp eyes, Caseley went to Clara Powell's teashop on the corner of Church Street. Unable to face eating anything she ordered a cup of hot chocolate. Its soothing warmth loosened some of the knots in her stomach.

She paid off the driver. The cab turned in the middle of the road and headed back towards the town centre.

Caseley walked up the granite steps onto the pavement that ran high above the rutted road

311

and walked along to the house. She hesitated at the open gate at the bottom of the path. A single rose bloomed in the weed-choked bed. The moss on the flagstones had been scraped off by the constant passage of feet.

The outside of the house was transformed. Within freshly painted frames, sparkling windows reflected the sunshine. The gossamer ropes and dead spiders had been swept from the porch and the steps scrubbed. So glossy was the black front door with its new porcelain knob and polished brass knocker, Caseley could see herself reflected in it. No longer shabby and neglected, the house looked proud, imposing. *Like its owner.*

She stood in the porch, fingering the key. Were it not for the letter she wouldn't be here. But now that she was, she might as well take a look.

She unlocked the front door. It opened without a sound on newly oiled hinges. Shutting it behind her she stood for a moment in front of the closed inner door. It was not too late. She need go no further. She drew a slow breath.

Chapter Twenty-two

Opening the inner door she stepped into the hall. It smelled fresh and new. She saw gleaming paint-work and new frosted glass globes with fluted tops on the gas mantles. Cream embossed paper added light and dimension to the space. The terracotta tiles glowed.

Her chest was painfully tight. As she pressed one hand to her breastbone she realised she had been holding her breath.

It was less than a month since she had followed Jago Barata into this house. Virtual strangers, captor and hostage, they had talked that day of childhood and loneliness, of destiny and courage and being true to oneself. That day she had begun to love him. What a blind, stupid *fool* she had been.

Tears gathered on her lashes and spilled down her cheeks. She clenched her fists. Why persist in this self-torture? How could she escape it? In spite of everything she loved him still. She should not have come. She could not have stayed away. Nor could she leave, not yet.

She walked slowly through rooms freshly painted and newly papered. Curtains complemented carpets on floors that had been sanded and varnished. Comfortably furnished, the rooms were not cluttered and so appeared lighter and more spacious than they really were. It was exactly as she had imagined.

Though she had walked in reluctantly, her heart had said *home*. She had seen through the neglect, and felt the house waiting. Unoccupied for too long, it needed people to bring it back to life.

Her breath hitched and she swallowed a sob. In such a short time her life had changed irrevocably. Her father was dead and she had not had time to mourn. Too many people needed her: Toby, Uncle Richard, Rosina. She hadn't seen Ralph since the day of their father's death.

She walked into the master bedroom and looked

313

at the pretty paper echoing the green and white flower-sprigged tiles surrounding the fireplace. Trailing her fingers along the gleaming foot rail of the brass bedstead, she stared at the bed's bare springs and saw white sheets, piled pillows, and her father's face contorted, then waxen as death smoothed away his pain.

She gripped the rail, her knuckles white and aching as she recalled Jago talking of his children yet unborn, mocking her blushes, angry for reasons she did not understand. She shook the rail, making the metal springs shiver and squeak as anguish tore her throat.

How was she to cope? Ralph, Aunt Margaret, Uncle Thomas, no money in the bank, the house to run, the business to manage... How could she go on? How could she not? Sinking onto the bedstead, she rested her forehead on her hands and abandoned herself to grief.

The sound of footsteps on the landing outside jolted her upright, dashing away tears with one hand while she fumbled for her handkerchief with the other.

If one of the workmen had returned for something he'd forgotten, she didn't want to be discovered weeping. They would know about her father. But they also knew about Louise Downing.

The door flew open.

'No.' She barely heard her voice through the roaring in her ears. Black spots danced across her vision and the room swayed.

Then Jago's arms were around her and her tear-wet face lay against his broad shoulder. Hearing the thunder of his heartbeat she wondered why it was so fast.

'Don't, Caseley.' His voice was hoarse. 'Please don't cry. I can't bear it.'

She felt him kiss the top of her head. Then he rested his cheek against her hair, holding her so tightly she could hardly breathe. It was a dream. She would wake up in a minute and he would be gone. But the warmth of his body, his unique scent, and the pressure of his arms were no mirage.

Easing his hold he tilted her chin. Looking into his face she saw exhaustion in the shadows under his eyes and strain in the lines that bracketed his mouth.

'Forgive me,' he whispered. Then his mouth covered hers in a kiss of such aching tenderness that fresh tears slid down her temples and into her hair. Holding her fast with one arm, he cupped her face gently with his free hand and kissed her again and again.

He was here. He did care. Everything else could wait. She put her arms around him, felt his warm breath on her cheek and heard a soft groan. At last he raised his mouth from hers.

'What are you doing here?' Caseley's voice was husky from weeping. 'I saw *Cygnet* leave.'

'Under Nathan's command.' He rested his face against hers. 'I arranged for him to pick up another crewman at Penryn.'

'Why?'

'I had business here. With you.'

Caseley loosened her hold enough to lean back and look into his eyes. 'What business? And how did you know I would–?'

'Be here? I instructed Mr Knuckey to write and send the key. I hoped you would want to see the house finished. Come, sit down.'

Allowing him to guide her to the window seat with its padded cushion that matched the curtains, Caseley sat with his arm around her shoulders. She recalled her uncle's reaction.

'Uncle Richard knew.'

Jago nodded. 'I have spent a lot of time with him this past week. Once I explained my plans he could not have been more helpful.'

She stiffened at the implied betrayal. It was happening again. Jago Barata was prying into her family's affairs behind her back. And her trusted Uncle Richard was helping him. She tried to draw away but his arm tightened.

'No, Caseley, you must listen.' She opened her mouth to protest but he silenced her with his own. She could not fight. Instead she welcomed his gentle exploration, deeply moved by delicacy in his touch, stirred by the powerful emotions she sensed he was holding back. When at last he raised his head, they were both breathless.

'I *had* to talk to Richard. I needed an honest assessment of the shipping agency and the yard's present position, financial status, and future potential.'

'Why?'

'Because I want to buy it.' He placed his fingers gently on her lips to silence the refusal her eyes signalled. His next words took her breath away.

'If I asked you to marry me *before* I bought the business, you might – you probably would – assume my proposal was simply a means to get my

316

hands on the yard. But if I already own it, that objection is void. If you refuse to sell, I will accept your decision. Instead I shall put into the business the equivalent of its market value. We will be equal partners.' A wry smile warmed his eyes. 'You would never settle for less.

'Richard will run the agency as he has always done. We will appoint a new accountant. The yard remains as it is, including the name. But Thomas goes. I will buy his share separately and give him a fair price.' Anger hardened Jago's features. 'But neither he nor that poisonous wife of his will ever set foot on Bonython property again.'

Caseley stared at him. 'Is there nothing you don't know?' Then like the sun appearing from behind a cloud she realised. 'Is this why you sold all your interests in Spain?'

He shrugged. 'What better reason could I have?'

Gently freeing herself she stood up. He rose as well, but did not follow as she walked to the window, rubbing her arms. It was too much to take in all at once.

'Caseley, please. Say you'll marry me.' He was not used to asking for anything and it showed. 'I've been out of my mind since you left *Cygnet*. I've spent most days with Toby, learning about the yard. I've nearly driven him mad.' He drove a hand through his black curls. 'Every evening I've been with Richard, going over the books. You mustn't be angry with them. I threatened them with dire consequences should they let a word slip.'

She felt a pang of sympathy for her uncle. It was not easy to stand against Jago Barata. In

317

truth, it was impossible.

'I paid the tradesmen large bonuses to ensure everything was completed quickly while maintaining the standards you had set.' He joined her at the window. 'This house needs you. You belong here. I saw it that first day. Everything you've done here,' he gestured, 'the colours, the furnishings, I didn't know the house could look and feel so – so like a home. You couldn't have done it if you hadn't cared.' He raised his hands in silent supplication.

Still, she did not answer.

'Is it Louise?' He started forward, stopping abruptly as she moved back. 'It's over. I ended it the day we got back. It never meant anything. I'm thirty-four years old and I've never been married. Of course there have been – liaisons.' He took two quick steps forward and grasped her shoulders. 'But I have never loved, until now. Until you.'

And there it was. She stood calm in his grip, unafraid despite his strength and the seething emotions he was wrestling. He loves me, she thought in wonder.

'You once said there was no comparison between Mrs Downing and me.'

He shook his head impatiently. 'There isn't.' He studied her, frowning, and she saw the moment he realised. 'Oh God. Caseley, I'm so sorry.'

'It hurt,' she admitted.

'There's no comparison because she can't hold a candle to you. No woman could. Don't you understand? I love you. I've fought it every inch of the way. I didn't believe– There had to be a catch. I've always done as I pleased. But every time we

318

were together I realised how different you are from the women I've known.'

'Defiant, argumentative, disobedient,' she smiled up at him through her tears. But this time they sprang from relief, and happiness too great to contain. He loved her. Jago loved her.

'Brave, beautiful, spirited, and loyal. I've treated you badly—'

'No—'

'Yes. But I'll spend the rest of my life making it up to you. Caseley, please be my wife. I need you. Come and live with me here.'

She laid her hand along his cheek, felt the warmth of his skin through the close beard. 'What about Rosina and Liza-Jane?'

'What about them?' He was impatient. 'They'll come too, of course. We'll need them, especially when the babies come. And Ben. That back garden is a wilderness. There's a ruined cottage under the brambles by the back wall.'

'About Ralph—' She watched his face set.

'He is not your responsibility.'

'I know,' she said softly. 'But he's my brother.'

'Then I suggest you give him half of whatever the sale of your father's house fetches. It's more than he deserves. Then he is on his own. It's the only way, Caseley. He has to grow up sometime.'

She had to ask. 'You would not allow him to live here?'

'No,' he said flatly.

She turned to the window and gazed out across the harbour, past the yard and the docks, towards the lighthouse and the open sea.

He came up behind her, slipping one arm

319

around her waist, the other across the front of her shoulders, holding her close.

She leaned back against his solid strength, safe within his protecting arms. This was what she had dreamed of, yearned for. This was home. *He* was home.

'My dearest Caseley,' he said against her ear, 'we have agreed arrangements for the business, your relatives, and the household staff–'

'There's just one more thing.' She turned her head against his shoulder to look up at him.

'God give me patience,' he muttered. 'What?'

'Will you still be taking *Fair Maid* to the Azores in December?'

He frowned. 'Yes, but–'

She smiled up at him. 'You'll be away for months. Can I go with you?'

His gaze reached into her soul as his arms tightened around her. 'There's nothing I'd like better. I'll speak to Toby in the morning.'

'What about?'

'It's a long way to the Azores, sweetheart,' he murmured, trailing his lips along her temple. 'A lot of nights at sea. If you think we'll be spending them in separate bunks, you are very much mistaken.'

Delicious heat flooded Caseley's body.

Roughly, Jago turned her around. 'Say it, Caseley,' he demanded. 'Say you'll marry me.'

'I love you,' she looked into slate-grey eyes she had seen as hard as granite, and cold as a winter sea. Now they held a warmth and gentleness that was for her alone. 'I'll be your partner, your friend, your...' she felt a blush climb her throat,

320

'your lover.'

'And wife.'

'And wife.'

'At last,' he murmured, and rested his forehead against hers. 'I know you're in mourning–'

She leaned back to meet his gaze. 'Jago, I really don't want a lot of fuss. Could we not be married by special licence?'

He reached inside his coat. 'I'd hoped you might consider it.' He held up a folded paper. 'There'll be gossip.'

She shrugged. 'I'm used to that. Then I was alone. Now I'll have you beside me.'

Dropping the licence onto the window seat he cupped her face and rested his forehead against hers. 'For always, Caseley.'

This Large Print Book for the partially sighted, who cannot read normal print, is published under the auspices of

THE ULVERSCROFT FOUNDATION